The Sidney Kimmel Comprehensive
Cancer Center at Johns Hopkins

Manual of Cancer Nursing

SECOND EDITION

The Sidney Kimmel Comprehensive Cancer Center at Johns Hopkins
Manual of Cancer Nursing

Brenda K. Shelton, MS, RN, CCRN, AOCN
Clinical Nurse Specialist
The Sidney Kimmel Comprehensive Cancer Center at Johns Hopkins
Baltimore, Maryland

Constance R. Ziegfeld, MS, RN
Clinical Nurse Specialist
The Sidney Kimmel Comprehensive Cancer Center at Johns Hopkins
Baltimore, Maryland

MiKaela M. Olsen, MS, RN, OCN
Oncology & BMT Clinical Nurse Specialist
The Sidney Kimmel Comprehensive Cancer Center at Johns Hopkins
Baltimore, Maryland

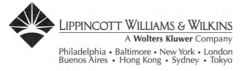

LIPPINCOTT WILLIAMS & WILKINS
A **Wolters Kluwer** Company
Philadelphia • Baltimore • New York • London
Buenos Aires • Hong Kong • Sydney • Tokyo

Acquisitions Editor: Patricia Casey
Editorial Assistant: Dana Irwin
Senior Production Editor: Tom Gibbons
Director of Nursing Production: Helen Ewan
Managing Editor / Production: Erika Kors
Art Director: Carolyn O'Brien

Design: Holly Reid McLaughlin
Cover Design: Christine Ott
Senior Manufacturing Manager: William Alberti
Indexer: Ellen Brennan
Compositor: LWW
Printer: R. R. Donnelley

9 8 7 6 5 4 3 2 1

Library of Congress Cataloging-in-Publication Data
The Sidney Kimmel Comprehensive Cancer Center at Johns Hopkins manual of cancer nursing / [edited by] Brenda K. Shelton, Constance R. Ziegfield, MiKaela M. Olsen
    p. ; cm.
    Rev. ed. of: Oncology fact finder / [edited by] Constance R. Ziegfield, Barbara G. Lubejko, Brenda K. Shelton. 1998.
    Includes bibliographical references and index.
    ISBN 0-7817-4496-2 (paper : alk. paper)
    1. Cancer--Nursing--Handbooks, manuals, etc. I. Title: Manual of cancer nursing. II. Shelton, Brenda K. (Brenda Kurtz) III. Ziegfield, Constance R. IV. Olsen, MiKaela M. V. Sidney Kimmel Comprehensive Cancer Center at Johns Hopkins. VI. Oncology fact finder.
    [DNLM: 1. Oncologic Nursing–methods–Handbooks.2
Neoplasms--complications--Handbooks. WY 49 S569 2004]
RC266.S53 2004
616.99'40231–dc22   2003065997

Care has been taken to confirm the accuracy of the information presented and to describe generally accepted practices. However, the authors, editors, and publisher are not responsible for errors or omissions or for any consequences from application of the information in this book and make no warranty, express or implied, with respect to the content of the publication.

The authors, editors, and publisher have exerted every effort to ensure that drug selection and dosage set forth in this text are in accordance with the current recommendations and practice at the time of publication. However, in view of ongoing research, changes in government regulations, and the constant flow of information relating to drug therapy and drug reactions, the reader is urged to check the package insert for each drug for any change in indications and dosage and for added warnings and precautions. This is particularly important when the recommended agent is a new or infrequently employed drug.

Some drugs and medical devices presented in this publication have Food and Drug Administration (FDA) clearance for limited use in restricted research settings. It is the responsibility of the health care provider to ascertain the FDA status of each drug or device planned for use in his or her clinical practice.
LWW.com

In recognition of our cancer patients and their families who teach us by example to value each day and take every opportunity to share your gifts with others.

Contributors

Kristen Ambrosio, BSN, RN
Clinical Nurse
The Sidney Kimmel Comprehensive Cancer Center at Johns Hopkins
Baltimore, Maryland

Janet Briel, BSN, RN, MBA
Clinical Nurse
The Sidney Kimmel Comprehensive Cancer Center at Johns Hopkins
Baltimore, Maryland

Jennifer Dunn Bucholtz, MS, RN, CRNP
Nurse Practitioner
The Sidney Kimmel Comprehensive Cancer Center at Johns Hopkins
Baltimore, Maryland

Kathy Burks, RN, BSN
Research Nurse
The Sidney Kimmel Comprehensive Cancer Center at Johns Hopkins
Baltimore, Maryland

JoAnn Coleman, MS, RN, CRNP, AOCN
Clinical Nurse Specialist/Nurse Practitioner
The Johns Hopkins Hospital
Baltimore, Maryland

Tracy T. Douglas, BSN, RN, OCN
Clinical Nurse Specialist
The Sidney Kimmel Comprehensive Cancer Center at Johns Hopkins
Baltimore, Maryland

Joanne P. Finley, RN, MS, OCN
Nurse Educator
The Sidney Kimmel Comprehensive Cancer Center at Johns Hopkins
Baltimore, Maryland

Laura Herald Hoofring, MSN, RN,CS
Clinical Specialist/Liaison Nurse
The Sidney Kimmel Comprehensive Cancer Center at Johns Hopkins
Baltimore, Maryland

Tara Kellner, RD, LD
Clinical Dietitian Specialist
The Johns Hopkins Hospital
Baltimore, Maryland

Aiko M. Kodaira, MSN, RN, OCN
Clinical Nurse Specialist
The Sidney Kimmel Comprehensive Cancer Center at Johns Hopkins
Baltimore, Maryland

Barbara G. Lubejko, RN, MS
Education Associate
Oncology Nursing Society
Formerly Nurse Educator
The Sidney Kimmel Comprehensive Cancer Center at Johns Hopkins
Baltimore, Maryland

Victoria D. Mock, DNSc, AOCN
Director of the Center for Nursing Research
Johns Hopkins University School of Nursing
Director of Nursing Research
The Sidney Kimmel Comprehensive Cancer Center at Johns Hopkins
Baltimore, Maryland

Suzanne Amato Nesbit, PHARMD, BCPS
Clinical Coordinator, Cancer Pain Service
The Sidney Kimmel Comprehensive Cancer Center at Johns Hopkins
Baltimore, Maryland

Beth L. Kozak Onners, RN,MSN
Research Nurse
The Sidney Kimmel Comprehensive Cancer Center at Johns Hopkins
Baltimore, Maryland

Michele A. Parisi, BSN, RN, RTR
Clinical Nurse
The Sidney Kimmel Comprehensive Cancer Center at Johns Hopkins
Baltimore, Maryland

Pendleton Powers, RN, BSN, OCN
Research Nurse
The Sidney Kimmel Comprehensive Cancer Center at Johns Hopkins
Baltimore, Maryland

Norrie Rabinowitz-Hirsch, BSN, RN
Clinical Nurse
The Sidney Kimmel Comprehensive Cancer Center at Johns Hopkins
Baltimore, Maryland

Carol DeClue Riley, CRNP
Nurse Practitioner
The Sidney Kimmel Comprehensive Cancer Center at Johns Hopkins
Baltimore, Maryland

Susan Sartorius-Mergenthaler, BSN, RN
Nurse Educator
The Sidney Kimmel Comprehensive Cancer Center and
   Johns Hopkins Hospital
Baltimore, Maryland

Kathy A. Shane, RN, BSN, OCN
Shift Coordinator
The Sidney Kimmel Comprehensive Cancer Center at Johns Hopkins
Baltimore, Maryland

Jane C. Shivnan, RN, MSCN
Assistant Director of Nursing
The Sidney Kimmel Comprehensive Cancer Center at Johns Hopkins
Baltimore, Maryland

Victoria J. Wah Sinibaldi, MS, RN, CS, CANP, CGNP
Nurse Practitioner
The Sidney Kimmel Comprehensive Cancer Center at Johns Hopkins
Baltimore, Maryland

Karin F. Taylor, APRN, PMH, BC
Clinical Specialist/Liaison Nurse
The Johns Hopkins Hospital
Baltimore, Maryland

Sharon D. Thompson
Research Nurse/Inpatient Clinical Coordinator
Gynecology and Obstetrics
The Johns Hopkins Hospital
Baltimore, Maryland

Nancy Tsottles, BSN, RN
Research Nurse
The Sidney Kimmel Comprehensive Cancer Center at Johns Hopkins
Baltimore, Maryland

Katherina M. Violette, BSN, RN
Clinical Nurse
The Sidney Kimmel Comprehensive Cancer Center at Johns Hopkins
Baltimore, Maryland

Jan Wemmer, MS, CRNP
Nurse Practitioner
The Sidney Kimmel Comprehensive Cancer Center at Johns Hopkins
Baltimore, Maryland

Constance R. Ziegfeld, MS, RN
Clinical Nurse Specialist
The Sidney Kimmel Comprehensive Cancer Center at Johns Hopkins
Baltimore, Maryland

Reviewers

Marianne R. Bunce, RN, MS, AOCN
Oncology Clinical Nurse Specialist
Nursing Administration
Contra Costa Regional Medical Center
Martinez, California

Cathy Churbock, RN, MSN, CCRN
Director of Education
Fayette Community Hospital
Fayetteville, Georgia

Sharon Forrester, RN, BSN, OCN
Oncology Coordinator
Saint Anthony's Health Center
Alton, Illinois

Deborah Klein, RN, MSN
Clinical Nurse IV, Radiation Oncology
Scripps Memorial Hospital
Encinitas, California

Sandra A. Mitchell, CRNP, MScN, AOCN
Lead Nurse Practitioner and Faculty Associate
School of Nursing, University of Maryland
College Park, Maryland

Carolyn Russett, RNC, BSN, OCN
Education Manager
Cape Cod Hospital
Hyannis, Massachusetts

Janet H. Van Cleave
Acute Care Nurse Practitioner
The Mount Sinai Medical Center
New York, New York

Preface

Cancer continues to be the second leading cause of death in the United States. In the past decade, there has been a major shift to ambulatory and home care for people with cancer. As costs and managed care continue to impact the delivery of cancer therapies, the community setting continues to emerge as a focal point of care. In addition, institutional reorganizations and the nursing shortage have required the work force to broaden skills and expand knowledge to meet the needs of a greater variety of patients. These factors are magnified by the increasingly complex care required for optimal outcomes of cancer treatment. As a result, nurses may care for cancer patients who participate in research protocols, experience unique side effects of treatment, or require hospitalization for more acute problems and shorter lengths of stay. This book is a reference to assist nurses in medical-surgical, primary care, and home care settings to care for persons with cancer.

The Sidney Kimmel Comprehensive Cancer Center at Johns Hopkins Manual of Cancer Nursing was written by nurses at The Sidney Kimmel Comprehensive Cancer Center at Johns Hopkins. The information reflects state-of-the-art treatment and knowledge essential to nurses caring for patients who experience a wide variety of cancer diagnoses and treatments. The purpose of this publication is to provide practical information about clinical care in a format that is quick and easy to use. The outline-structure focuses on five areas of essential information for nursing care of oncology patients.

The first section addresses cancer biology, and the second section addresses common modalities used to treat cancer. These chapters explain the basic theories and rationale for interventions and identify the unique nursing issues associated with each modality of care. Biological and alternative treatments have expanded in practice and are addressed in individual chapters.

The third section provides information about the most common cancer diagnoses and treatment. The significance and etiology of each disease or group of diseases is reviewed. Patient management is the focus of each chapter. Assessment, diagnostic parameters, treatment, nursing diagnosis and interventions, discharge planning, and patient education are outlined for each diagnosis.

The fourth section defines important aspects of patient management and focuses on frequently encountered complications of treatment and disease. This field of knowledge changes rapidly. Nurses are challenged to maintain current information about the factors that impact on quality of life and favorable patient outcomes.

The last section provides information that supports early identification of and intervention for oncologic emergencies. Structural and metabolic problems are often addressed differently in the oncology setting because of factors related to disease and treatment. It is essential that all nurses are able to identify emergent situations and act quickly and appropriately to achieve optimal patient interventions.

Our goal in writing this book is to provide nurses with a foundation of information to foster an interest and inquisitiveness in the care of individuals and families who experience a cancer diagnosis. From this beginning, we hope that colleagues will expand the body of oncology nursing research and knowledge and continue to improve the outcomes of cancer treatment.

MiKaela M. Olsen, MS, RN, OCN
Brenda K. Shelton, MS, RN, CCRN, AOCN
Constance R. Ziegfeld, MS, RN

Acknowledgments

The editors would like to acknowledge colleagues and staff of The Sidney Kimmel Comprehensive Cancer Center at Johns Hopkins and their colleagues in the Department of Surgical Nursing and the Johns Hopkins University School of Nursing. Their commitment to excellence in clinical care, research, and education makes a positive difference to individuals with cancer, their families, and the nurses who care for them.

Special thanks to Sharon Krumm, PhD, RN, Director of Nursing at The Sidney Kimmel Comprehensive Cancer Center at Johns Hopkins, who believed in and supported this project.

Contents

UNIT 3 TYPES OF CANCER

UNIT I

PATHOGENESIS

1 Carcinogenesis

Barbara G. Lubejko

I. Carcinogenesis

A. Carcinogenesis is the process by which normal cells are transformed into malignant cells.

B. Evidence indicates that an individual cancer arises from a single cell that undergoes mutations to give it a growth and survival advantage over other cells.

1. Somatic cell mutations arise from genetic damage acquired over time that is not repaired and is allowed to alter cellular functions. These are nonfamilial and may arise without a clear risk factor.
2. Germ cell mutations arise in the DNA one inherits, and they exhibit familial tendencies.

C. It takes multiple mutations of a cell's genes to create a malignancy. These mutations do not need to occur in any particular order but must affect specific types of genes for a malignancy to occur. Because multiple mutations over a period of time are required to develop most cancers, the risk of developing cancer increases as a person gets older.

D. There are three types of genes that can cause cancer when they develop mutations. These are the genes that regulate proliferation of cells.

1. Proto-oncogenes (eg, K-Ras)
   a. These genes are responsible for promoting normal cell replication. They are necessary for maintenance of many body tissues.
   b. Oncogenes are formed when proto-oncogenes are mutated. They then can overstimulate cell replication leading to continuous, uncontrolled growth and malignant transformation.
2. Tumor suppressor genes (eg, p53 gene)
   a. These genes are responsible for slowing or stopping cell replication. When tumor suppressor genes become inactivated or dysfunctional, continual and uncontrolled cellular growth with malignant transformation can occur.
   b. Inactivation of tumor suppressor genes may also impair the process of apoptosis (programmed cellular death), which is normally initiated in a cell that has irreparable genetic damage or has completed its normal number of replications. Lack of appropriate apoptosis is a precursor condition of malignancy.
3. DNA repair genes
   a. These genes repair damage in a cell's DNA before replication is allowed to occur. If the DNA repair genes become inactivated, mutations to the proto-oncogenes and tumor suppressor genes are allowed to accumulate and continue the cell's transformation to malignancy.

E. Genetic mutations can be inherited but, more frequently, are errors that occur during DNA replication or after exposure to various carcinogens.

1. Inherited mutations account for a relatively small but significant percentage of cancer cases diagnosed each year. With these syndromes, a person inherits a faulty (mutated) gene that performs a function in the control of cellular replication. This mutation can significantly increase the risk of developing certain types of cancer.

   a. Li-Fraumeni syndrome involves the inheritance of a defective p53 tumor suppressor gene. People with Li-Fraumeni syndrome have an increased risk of developing sarcomas, brain cancer, breast cancer, and leukemia.

   b. Multiple endocrine neoplasia type II (MEN II) involves the inheritance of a mutated RET (rearranged during transfection) oncogene. This leads to a greatly increased risk of developing medullary thyroid cancer.

2. Errors occur quite frequently during cellular and DNA replication, leading to translocations, additions, or deletions of genes. If these errors occur in the genes responsible for initiating cell replication (proto-oncogenes) or for stopping cell replication (tumor suppressor genes), a cell can be allowed to divide in an uncontrolled manner. If the error occurs in the DNA repair gene, the mutations will be carried forward into future generations of cells.

3. Carcinogens are substances that can cause genetic mutations and alter cellular function.

   a. Viruses can cause genetic mutations by inserting their genetic coding into the cell's DNA. Viruses have been associated with specific types of cancers.

      (1) Human papilloma virus (HPV) has been associated with cervical cancer.

      (2) Hepatitis B and C viral infections increase the risk of developing hepatocellular cancer.

      (3) Epstein-Barr virus has been associated with an increased risk of Burkitt's lymphoma.

      (4) Human T-cell lymphotrophic virus infection increases the risk of developing T-cell leukemia.

   b. Bacteria have been implicated in the development of certain cancers. *Helicobacter pylori* infections have been linked to an increased risk of gastric cancer.

   c. Tobacco use in all forms is considered to be the biggest contributing factor in the development of cancer.

      (1) Cigarette smoking has been implicated in the development of lung, head and neck, esophageal, stomach, pancreatic, kidney, and bladder cancers.

      (2) Pipes, cigars, and smokeless tobacco have been linked to lip and oral cancers.

   d. Alcohol use in excessive amounts has been tied to several types of cancer, such as oral, throat, esophageal, liver, and breast cancers. The risk is especially high in people who consume both excessive amounts of alcohol and smoke cigarettes.

   e. Environmental carcinogens include various forms of radiation, asbestos, pollution, and industrial compounds.

(1) Exposure to ultraviolet radiation from the sun has been linked to different forms of skin cancer.

(2) Exposure to ionizing radiation such as from radioactive chemicals or sources used in radiation therapy can increase the risk of cancers such as leukemia, thyroid and breast cancers.

(3) Exposure to asbestos has been implicated in the development of mesothelioma and other lung cancers.

(4) Pollutants in the air (eg, fluorocarbons) and water (eg, arsenic) at sufficient levels have been associated with higher incidence of lung, bladder, and skin cancer.

(5) Wood, leather, and metal dust created during refining procedures have been associated with nasal and sinus cancers.

f. Numerous chemicals are believed to have the potential to cause genetic mutations, thus increasing the risk of developing specific cancers. Examples include benzene (leukemia), vinyl chloride (sarcoma), arsenic (lung, skin, sarcoma), and the alkylating antineoplastic agents (leukemia, lymphoma).

g. Immune suppression and administration of immunosuppressive medications (eg, corticosteroids, cyclosporine, azathioprine) have been linked to development of hematologic malignancies (leukemia, lymphoma).

h. Hormones can play a role in the development and growth stimulation of several hormone-sensitive tumor types.

(1) Estrogen is known to play a role the development and growth of breast and endometrial cancers. The anti-estrogens tamoxifen and raloxifene have been shown to decrease the risk of developing breast cancer.

(2) Testosterone has been implicated in the development and growth of prostate cancer.

i. Diet can play a potentiating as well as protective role in the development of cancer. The role of diet in carcinogenesis is quite controversial.

(1) A high-fat diet has been linked to an increased incidence of colon, prostate, lung, and endometrial cancers.

(2) Heterocyclic amines found in certain well-cooked meats have been implicated in the development of gastric, colorectal, pancreatic, and breast cancers.

(3) Potential protective factors include fiber, fruits, vegetables, as well as calcium (colon cancer), selenium (prostate cancer), vitamins A, C, and E. Diets including a high intake of fruits and vegetables may decrease the risk of lung, oral, pharynx, esophageal, gastric, colorectal, breast, pancreatic, and bladder cancers.

(4) Exercise may also reduce the risk of developing certain malignancies, including colorectal, breast, and perhaps prostate cancers.

j. Nonsteroidal antiinflammatory agents such as aspirin may reduce the incidence of colorectal cancer by preventing the formation of adenomas.

II. Cancer-Related Terminology

A. Cancer is a group of diseases characterized by uncontrolled cellular growth and the ability to invade surrounding tissue and metastasize. Cancer can arise in most every tissue of the body. Presenting symptoms and ongoing problems experienced by the person with cancer will be related to the location of the primary tumor and metastatic activity.

B. A variety of terms are used when discussing abnormal cellular proliferation. Some of these terms apply to all tumors and some only to malignancies (Table 1–1).

III. Characteristics of Cancer Cells

A. Normal cell function and structure are closely regulated functions in the body. Cells in normal body tissues are very organized, look and act the same, and only replicate for very specific reasons (such as to replace another cell that has been damaged or become too old to perform its needed functions). Cancer cells demonstrate multiple alterations that differentiate them from cells in normal tissue.

B. Cancer Cell Appearance and Function
   1. Cancer cells are usually identifiable by their abnormal appearance. They tend to have larger nuclei and less cytoplasm outside the nucleus than normal cells.
   2. Cancer cells demonstrate a lot of variability in their overall size and shape. They are disorganized in relation to one another and may lose some of their normal distinguishing features.
   3. Cancer cells tend to be less differentiated than the normal surrounding tissue. Cells may bear no resemblance to the tissue of origin, making the parent tissue unidentifiable. Cancer cells may lose their ability to perform normal tissue functions and may gain the ability

TABLE 1-1 Tumor Growth Terminology

Terminology	Description	Comment
Hyperplasia	Excessive proliferation of normal cells	May follow exposure to an irritant and be reversible. May indicate increased risk of cancer
Dysplasia	Excessive proliferation of cells that have undergone changes in shape, size, or structure	Indicative of possible neoplastic transformation, but may be reversed with removal of irritant.
Benign	Tumors that do not invade local tissue or metastasize. Remain confined to the original site.	Problems caused by benign tumors are confined to site of tumor.
Carcinoma in situ	Excessive proliferation of cells that have remained in one location. Term may be used for severe dysplasia.	Can potentially develop the ability to locally invade and metastasize.
Malignant	Indicates the ability of a tumor to invade surrounding tissue or to metastasize.	Differentiates a cancerous tumor from a benign tumor.

to perform different functions (such as secrete hormones to amplify specific body activities).

4. Cancer cells lose the ability to recognize and adhere to cells from the same tissue. They also lose the need to stay with similar type cells, allowing them to migrate to other areas of the body.

5. Cancer cells can also lose markers and receptors on the cell surface, changing normal activities and making the abnormal cells more difficult for the immune system to recognize as abnormal.

C. Cancer Cell Growth and Metabolism

1. Cancer cells replicate regardless of the body's replacement needs. They also can replicate without being anchored to their "home base."

2. The percentage of proliferating cells in a tumor tends to be higher than for normal cells of the same tissue origin. Tumor volume doubling time is variable and reflects tumor type, vascular supply, cell loss, and hormonal influences.

3. Cancer cells divide in a random, disorganized fashion creating cells with genetic damage and alterations in structure and function.

4. Malignant cells become immortal. They are no longer susceptible to programmed cell death (apoptosis), a function that limits the number of divisions a particular cell undergoes. This function also prevents cells with genetic damage from replicating further.

5. Most cancer cells are able to survive with less oxygen than normal cells, allowing them to proliferate even with deficits of nutrients.

6. Cancer cell growth may depend on specific hormones (eg, estrogen-dependent breast cancer cells), growth factors (eg, epidermal growth factor [EGF]), or enzymes (eg, cyclins or cyclin kinases).

D. Tumors are named for the tissue from which they originate (Table 1–2). Malignant tumors derive their names from their location, behavior, tissue, and degree of similarity to healthy cells (differentiation).

IV. Metastasis is the ability of cancer cells to migrate from the primary tumor and establish colonies at different locations in the body. Although not all tumors metastasize, more than half of people with solid tumors will have metastatic spread upon diagnosis.

A. Because metastatic growth is commonly the cause of death in cancer patients, early intervention is extremely important. A combination of

TABLE 1-2 Malignant Tumor Classifications

Terminology	Source	Examples
Carcinoma	Epithelial tissue (adeno or squamous)	Adenocarcinoma (lung), breast cancer, colorectal cancer
Sarcoma	Connective tissue	Osteosarcoma (bone), liposarcoma (fatty tissue), rhabdomyosarcoma (skeletal muscle)
Leukemia	Hematopoietic cells	Acute lymphocytic leukemia, chronic myelocytic leukemia
Lymphoma	Lymphatic tissue	Hodgkin's disease, non-Hodgkin's lymphoma

early detection before a tumor has attained the ability to metastasize and adjuvant therapies to eliminate any early metastases has been shown to increase survival for many tumor types.

B. A tumor can metastasize by several mechanisms.

1. Local extension: As tumor cells lose their need to remain with similar cells, they may migrate to structures and tissues in immediate proximity to the tumor. For example, ovarian cancer is known for invading local organs such as fallopian tubes, bladder, and bowel as well as seeding throughout the peritoneum.

2. Lymphatic spread: If tumor cells infiltrate the local lymphatic vessels, they can travel to surrounding lymph nodes and create metastatic sites. Examples of malignancies known for their tendency to spread by way of the lymphatic system are breast cancer and Hodgkin's disease.

3. Hematogenous spread: If the tumor cells invade local blood vessels, they can travel to numerous sites in the body, often at some distance. Bloodstream metastasis is common in lung cancer.

4. When staging a particular tumor, the type and degree of spread are used to define the extent of the cancer. This might include:

   a. Local involvement by direct extension into surrounding tissue

   b. Regional spread through lymphatic system or seeding into local cavities such as the peritoneum

   c. Distant spread, usually through the vascular system

C. The process of lymphatic and hematogenous metastasis follows a series of specific steps. Only very aggressive cells are able to perform all these steps and escape detection and destruction during the process.

1. Angiogenesis: For a tumor to grow beyond a relatively small size, it must create its own blood supply (angiogenesis). To do this, the tumor must be able to secrete factors that stimulate blood vessel growth. These same factors may also encourage tumor cell motility.

2. Basement membrane invasion: To enter the lymphatic or blood vessels, the tumor cells must secrete enzymes that erode the vessel's basement membrane creating an opening that the cell can pass through.

3. Migration: Once in the lymphatic or blood vessel, cells are usually trapped in the first vascular bed they encounter. Here they must attach to the vessel wall and prepare to move out of the vessel.

4. Extravasation: Tumor cells again produce enzymes that erode the capillary wall and allow the cell to enter the adjacent organ or tissue. Here the metastatic cell must attach to the extracellular support matrix and replicate to create a new colony.

5. Metastatic growth: The new tumor implant grows and is nourished by the same mechanism as the primary tumor.

D. Individual tumor types tend to metastasize by a specific mechanism of spread to a particular set of organs (see individual chapters for dissemination patterns for specific tumor types). The most common sites for metastatic spread are:

1. Lung

2. Liver

3. Bone

4. Brain
5. Lymph nodes
E. Metastatic tumor cells can differ from primary tumor cells.
   1. For cells to metastasize, they must have the ability to produce the enzymes and growth factors necessary to complete the process. Only a subset of cells in a given tumor will have all the necessary capabilities to metastasize.
   2. Only a small number of cells that escape from the primary tumor are able to avoid immune detection and survive travel through the bloodstream or lymphatic system. These cells then choose a target organ and establish a colony of metastatic cells. These metastatic cells tend to be more aggressive and able to survive in the hostile environments.
   3. Metastases develop in organs where the environment contains the biochemical factors conducive to metastatic tumor growth. Future treatment of metastatic cancer may need to include techniques that interfere not only with tumor growth but also the microenvironment that supports this growth (Fidler, 2002).

REFERENCES

Collins, F. S., & Trent, J. M. (2001). Cancer genetics. In E. Braunwald et al. (Eds.), *Harrison's principles of internal medicine* (pp. 503–509). New York: McGraw-Hill.

Fidler, I. J. (2002). The organ microenvironment and cancer metastasis. *Differentiation, 70*, 498–505.

Hawkins, R. (2001). Mastering the intricate maze of metastasis. *Oncology Nursing Forum, 28*, 959–965.

Loescher, L. J. (2000). Biology of cancer. In C. H. Yarbro et al. (Eds.), *Cancer nursing: Principles and practice* (5th ed.). Sudbury, MA: Jones & Bartlett.

Loescher, L. J., & Whitesell, L. (2003). The biology of cancer. In A. S. Tranin, A. Masny & J. Jenkins (Eds.), *Genetics in oncology practice: Cancer risk assessment* (pp. 23–56). Pittsburgh, PA: Oncology Nursing Society.

National Cancer Institute. (2000). *Understanding cancer* [script]. (Publication No. 194.) Bethesda, MD: Author.

2 Genetics

Jennifer Dunn Bucholtz

I. Genetic Overview
  A. Basic Genetics
1. Information discovered in the past 20 years has advanced all aspects of cancer care including prevention, screening, diagnosis, and treatment.
2. Genetic information helps to identify and test people at risk for hereditary cancers and to offer individualized screening and prevention strategies.
3. Cancer genetic data also help diagnose and identify certain malignancies and can be used to tailor treatments based on a person's genetic profile and the tumor's genetic changes.
4. Gene therapies are now emerging to treat certain cancers.
5. Nurses need to be familiar with cancer genetics information to best help people and families throughout the cancer care continuum (Jenkins, 2002). Oncology nurses, in particular, can be instrumental in helping people and families incorporate data regarding the rapidly evolving field of cancer genetics into all areas of clinical practice (Tranin, Masny & Jenkins, 2002).
6. An understanding of basic genetics is helpful in understanding cancer genetics, inherited cancer syndromes, and targeted cancer diagnostics and therapies (National Cancer Institute, 2002: *Cancer genetics overview*).
  B. Genetic Structure
1. All genetic information is stored in the nucleus of our cells.
2. Inside the nucleus are chromosomes made of DNA proteins.
3. A genome is the complete set of DNA sequences in a species.
4. The human genome has 23 pairs of chromosomes.
5. Chromosomes contain thousands of genes, the smallest functional unit of genetic information.
6. Genes determine how a person's body will grow and function.
7. Genes come in pairs. One copy is inherited from each parent.
8. A gene can have different forms in its DNA sequence. These variant forms are called *alleles.*
9. Everyone inherits two alleles for each gene—one copy of each chromosome from each parent.
10. Not all mutated alleles or genes lead to cancer.
11. The probability that a given mutated gene will cause disease is referred to as *penetrance.*
12. Alleles can be *dominant or recessive, or x-linked.*
13. If one parent carries a dominant allele (eg, mutation in BRCA1 or BRCA2), there is a 50/50 chance of each offspring inheriting the diseased allele. This is referred to as *autosomal dominant inheritance.*

C. Genetic Mutations
1. A *mutation* is a change in the usual DNA sequence of a particular gene. Mutations can be harmful, beneficial, or neutral. The term *mutation* is commonly used to refer to changes in the DNA that affect its protein structure.
2. All cancers arise from mutations in genes that can be inherited (germline mutations) or develop over a person's lifetime from exposure to carcinogens or other mutagens (acquired or somatic mutations).
3. Inherited mutations are referred to as *germline mutations* because they are present in the ova and sperm from the parents and passed to every cell in the offspring. Because all cells contain the inherited mutation, the chance of developing cancers at earlier ages, as well as multiple cancers, is increased.
4. The majority of cancers are thought to be noninherited, somatic cancers and occur in older years of life. Somatic mutations arise in DNA of individual cells.
5. When a somatic mutation alters a gene in a normal cell, copies of the mutation will be present only in the descendants of that particular cell.
6. DNA mutations can alter protein function, resulting in a complete absence, underexpression, or overexpression of the protein.
7. Benign changes in DNA that do not alter protein function are referred to as *polymorphisms* and are used to track possible inherited disease patterns.
8. Dominant inherited mutations of the genes are found on autosomes, not sex hormones; therefore, both males and females can transmit the mutation. These mutations usually do not skip generations.
9. With autosomal recessive genes, one copy of the mutated allele must come from each parent. In general, one in four offspring will inherit the associated disease if both parents carry the mutated allele.
10. Autosomal recessive mutations may skip generations but are also transmitted equally by men and women.
11. Recessive X-linked mutations are carried on the X chromosome. Men are more likely to inherit a disease stemming from an X-linked mutation, because only one mutated allele is needed. Women are more likely to be mutation carriers.
12. Genetic testing can involve looking at a person's DNA, which is obtained most often from his or her blood and occasionally from other body fluids or tissue. Examining key proteins that can signal abnormal genes is also a form of genetic testing (eg, Her2 neu testing).

II. Cancer Genetics
A. In general, all cancer is triggered by genetic changes.
B. Most cancers stem from random mutations caused by somatic mutations over a person's lifetime.
C. It is estimated that only 5% to 10% of all cancers are caused by known inherited germline mutations.
D. Genes associated with cancer have been placed into three classes: *oncogenes, tumor suppressor genes*, or *DNA-repair genes* (see Chapter 1).
E. *Microsatellite instability* refers to an effect on a cell's inability to repair DNA mismatches. Microsatellites are repetitive sequences of DNA located on the genome. Microsatellite instability can be found in a high percentage of certain hereditary cancers (eg, this is found in about

90% of hereditary nonpolyposis colorectal cancer [HNPCC] related cancer versus 15% of sporadic colorectal cancer).

F. Normal cells turn into cancer cells by a multistep process with specific genetic events. The best example of a known multistep progression is the colon cancer carcinogenesis model developed by Fearon and Vogelstein (1990). Other cancers are believed to have similar multistep progression in genetic changes.

G. All cancers originate from a single cell. When one cell acquires enough mutations to become cancerous, it can form a tumor.

H. In the future, it is likely that additional molecular discoveries will find other cancer genetic changes and causes and will isolate additional mutations.

I. Certain families may appear to have a higher incidence of cancers that are not inherited but result from a complex interaction between multiple genes and the shared environment. These are referred to as *family clusters of cancer*.

III. Hereditary Cancer Syndromes

A. General Overview

1. Represent 5% to 10% of known cancers in adults and children (American Society of Clinical Oncology, 1999).
2. Estimated that 1 in 300 people have mutations that predispose them to cancers of the breast, colon, uterus, and ovary.
3. People who inherit genetic mutations associated with certain cancers have a high risk of developing these cancers, and at early ages.

B. Assessing for Familial Cancers

1. Because hereditary cancers represent only a small number of all cancer cases, it is important to be able to recognize people and their family members who are at high risk for inherited cancers.
2. Common features seen in families with a hereditary cancer predisposition are listed in Box 2–1.
3. Families do not need to have all of these common features to have a genetic mutation.
4. Table 2–1 lists known family cancer syndromes and the associated types of cancers.
5. Examples of features seen in specific cancer syndromes are listed in Boxes 2–2, 2–3, and 2–4.

▼ **BOX 2-1** | **Common Features Seen in Families With Hereditary Cancer**

- Cancer diagnosis in two or more close family members on same side of family
- Diagnosis of cancers occurred at earlier ages than normally seen with particular cancers
- Bilateral or multiple rare cancers
- Multiple primary tumors
- Evidence of autosomal dominant inheritance
- Tumors in family consistent with specific cancer syndrome (eg, breast and ovary in BRCA; colon, uterine in HNPCC)

TABLE 2–1 Family Cancer Syndrome, Identified Mutation, and Associated Cancers

Family Cancer Syndrome (Mutated Gene)	Type of Cancers
Adenomatous polyposis (FAP) *(APC, Attenuated APC)*	Colon/rectum, liver, hepatoblastoma, small bowel, intestine, stomach, thyroid, medulloblastoma
Ataxia-telangectasia (ATM)	Breast, pancreas, stomach, uterine, leukemias, glioma, non-Hodgkin's lymphoma, medulloblastoma, basal cell, ACA
Basal cell-nevus (PTC)	Ovarian, fibrosarcoma, medulloblastoma, basal cell
Bloom syndrome (BLM)	Breast, colon/rectum, esophagus, cervix, larynx, tongue, leukemias, non-Hodgkin's lymphomas, lung cancer, basal cell, squamous cell
Breast/ovarian (BRCA1)	Breast, ovarian, colon/rectum/prostate
Breast/ovarian (BRCA2)	Breast, ovarian, colon/rectum, prostate, pancreas, ACA
Carcinoid, familial	Carcinoid
Carney's syndrome	Adrenal, cortical, pituitary, thyroid, testicle, schwannoma
Chordoma	Chordoma
Colon (hereditary nonpolyposis cancer) (HNPCC) *(MLH1, MSH2, MSH6, PMS1, PMS2)*	Colon/rectum, biliary, liver, hepatocellular, pancreas, colorectal ACA, stomach, bladder, kidney, renal clear cell, renal transitional, ureter, uterine, ovaries, glioma, sebaceous gland
Cowden syndrome *(PTEN)*	Breast, small bowel, thyroid
Esophagus with tylosis	Esophagus
Fanconi's anemia *(FACC, FACA)*	Liver, hepatocellular, cervix, leukemias, glioma, medulloblastoma, squamous cell
Gastric cancer, familial	Esophagus, stomach, tongue
Hodgkin's disease	Hodgkin's disease
Li-Fraumeni syndrome *(TP53)*	Breast, pancreas, ACA, adrenal cortical, prostate, testicle, germ cell, ovarian, larynx, leukemias, lung, glioma, non-Hodgkin's lymphomas, osteosarcoma, rhabdomyosarcoma, soft tissue sarcoma
Melanoma *(CDKN2A, BDRF)*	Melanoma, pancreas, glioma, ACA
Multiple endocrine neoplasia 1 (MEN 1)	Adrenal cortical, apudoma, carcinoid, pancreas, islet cell, parathyroid, pheochromocytoma, pituitary, schwannoma
Multiple endocrine neoplasia 2 (MEN 2) *(RET)*	Paraganglioma, parathyroid, pheochromocytoma, pituitary, thyroid, medullary
Neurofibromatosis 1	Acoustic neuroma, glioma, meningioma, schwannoma, neuroblastoma, carcinoid, Wilms' tumor, leukemias, paraganglioma, pheochromocytoma, rhabdomyosarcoma
Neurofibromatosis 2	Acoustic neuroma, glioma, meningioma, schwannoma

(continued)

■ TABLE 2-1   Family Cancer Syndrome, Identified Mutation, and
Associated Cancers (Continued)

Family Cancer Syndrome (Mutated Gene)	Type of Cancers
Osteochondromatosis	Chondrosarcomas, osteosarcoma
Pancreatic cancer, familial	Pancreas, adenocarcinoma (ACA)
Paraganglioma, familial	Paraganglioma, pheochromocytoma
Peutz-Jeghers syndrome	Breast, colon/rectum, pancreas, ACA, small bowel, stomach, testicle, cervix, ovarian
Prostate cancer, familial	Prostate
Renal cancer, familial	Renal clear cell, kidney, renal papillary
Retinoblastoma (RB1)	Retinoblastoma, leukemias, non-Hodgkin's lymphomas, chondrosarcomas, fibrosarcoma, osteosarcoma, soft tissue sarcoma, pinealblastoma, melanoma
Rothmund-Thomson syndrome	Osteosarcoma, squamous cell
Testicular carcinoma, familial	Testicle, germ cell
Tuberous sclerosis	Paraganglioma, thyroid, kidney, renal clear cell, glioma
Von Hippel-Lindau disease (VHL)	Pancreas, ACA, stomach, apudoma, carcinoid, pancreas, islet cell, paraganglioma, kidney, renal clear cell
Werner's syndrome	Breast, liver, hepatocellular, thyroid, leukemias, osteosarcoma, rhabdomyosarcoma, neuroblastoma
Wilms' tumor (WT1 and others)	Wilms' tumor, liver, hepatocellular, adrenal cortical, germ cell, rhabdomyosarcoma, neuroblastoma
Xeroderma pigmentosum (XPB, XPD, XPA)	Breast, stomach, tongue, leukemias, lung, glioma, basal cell, melanoma, squamous cell

▼ BOX 2-2   Specific Implications for BRCA1/BRCA2 Mutation Carriers

Risk of Cancer
- ~ 50% to 85% risk of breast cancer by age 70, but increased risk of breast cancer before age 50
- ~ 15% to 45% risk of ovarian cancer
- Increased risk of multiple cancers
- Increased risk of male breast cancer especially with BRCA2

Risk Reduction Options
- Increased surveillance (yearly bilateral mammogram starting at an age 10 years younger than age of family member's cancer diagnosis)
- Chemoprevention with tamoxifen (Fisher, 1998; Gail, 1999). (Breast cancer associated with BRCA1 less likely to express estrogen receptors; BRCA2 more likely to express estrogen receptors)
- Prophylactic bilateral mastectomy (Eisen, 2000)

▼ **BOX 2-3** | **Specific Implications for HNPCC Mutation Carriers**

Risk of Cancer
- ~ 90% risk of colon cancer
- Greater risk for second cancers after first is diagnosed
- 42% to 60% risk of endometrial cancer
- 12% risk of endometrial cancer

Clinical Features
- 60% to 80% of HNPCC-associated cancers arise proximal to the splenic flexure
- Despite HNPCC colorectal cancer pathology as high grade, it has a better prognosis than sporadic tumors
- Most HNPCC is associated with mutations in MSH2 or MLH1 genes. Microsatellite instability is seen in a high percentage of DNA associated with HNPCC

Risk Reduction
- Increased surveillance
  Colonoscopy every 1 to 3 years starting at ages 20 to 25 or 10 years before earliest age of family member diagnosed with colon cancer
  Annual transvaginal ultrasound/endometrial aspirates in women starting at age 25
- Prophylactic surgery
  Colectomy
  Total abdominal hysterectomy/bilateral salpingo-oophorectomy in women mutation carriers after completion of childbearing
- Chemoprevention
  No proven chemoprevention drugs for HNPCC but many drugs in clinical trials

HNPCC: Hereditary non-polyposis colorectal cancer

6. Important tools to identify familial cancer predisposition include:
   a. A thorough, three-generation family history pedigree of all maternal and paternal family members (Figure 2–1). Having the person complete a structured family history questionnaire is helpful in obtaining a complete family history.
      (1) Pedigree should include any cancer diagnosis, age at diagnosis, whether cancer was primary or metastatic site, and, if person is deceased, cause of death.
      (2) Pedigree should include ethnic background of maternal and paternal relatives because some genetic predisposition cancers have a higher prevalence in specific populations (eg, BRCA1/2 in Ashkenazi Jewish population).
      (3) Pedigree should include precursor lesions in any family members, such as adenomatous colon polyps, dysplastic moles, or atypical breast biopsies.

▼ BOX 2-4 | **Specific Implications for FAP and Attenuated FAP Carriers**

Risk of Cancer
- 87% risk of colon cancer by age 45
  100% risk for FAP carriers
  80%+ risk for attenuated FAP (AFAP)

Clinical Features
- Hundreds to thousands of colon polyps seen in FAP in the colon and rectum. Twenty to 100 cumulative polyps seen in AFAP
- Colorectal polyps begin to appear at an average age of 16 with a range of ages 8 to 24 years
- Genetic testing for APC gene recommended at ages 10 to 12
- FAP affects 1 in 5,000 people

Risk Reduction
- Increased surveillance (AFAP)
  Colonoscopy every 1 to 2 years starting in late teens
- Prophylactic colectomy after adenomatous polyps seen on colonoscopy
- Increased surveillance (FAP)
  Sigmoidoscopy starting ages 10 to 12
- Prophylactic subtotal colectomy after polyps seen

FAP: Familial adenomatous polyposis

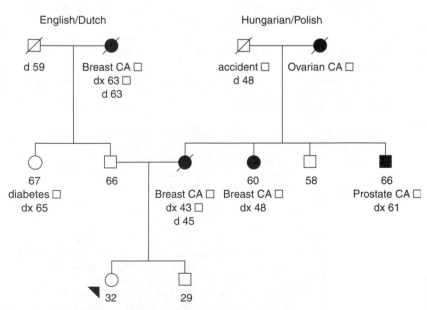

Figure 2–1. Three generation family pedigree.

(4) Pedigree should include the presence of bilateral cancer diagnoses in organs such as the breast or kidney.

(5) Pedigree should list known benign diseases or unusual physical traits of family members (eg, thyroid problems and hamartomas are found in families with Cowden's syndrome).

  b. Verification of medical records of family members with cancer/benign diagnoses if family history is not well-known or incomplete (eg, a diagnosis of cancer of the uterus may have been cancer of the ovary in a family with a predisposition for BRCA1 or BRCA2).

  c. Use family history to decide which risk assessment tool may be appropriate for the particular family. Several tools exist to help estimate a person's probability for carrying a cancer predisposition mutation (Table 2–2).

  d. Refer person with a family history suggesting hereditary cancer syndrome to an expert in genetic counseling. Experts include

TABLE 2–2 Risk Assessment Tools Used for Identifying People Potentially at High Risk for Hereditary Cancers

Hereditary Cancer	Tool	Reference
Breast (BRCA1/2)	**Claus** Estimates breast cancer risk solely on family history of breast cancer	Claus et al., 1994
	Couch Predicts probability of finding BRCA1/2 mutation	Couch et al., 1997
	BRCAPRO Predicts individual breast cancer risk based on probability that family carries BRCA1/2 mutation	Berry et al., 2002
	Myriad Genetics Predicts probability of individual carrying BRCA1/2 mutation based on personal and family history	www.BRCAAnalysis.com
	Note: All above models contained in Cancer Gene Program are available free to health professionals with signed contract at www3.utsouthwestern.edu/cancergene.	
Colorectal HNPCC	**Amsterdam Criteria I & II** Criteria of individual and family history used to recommend genetic testing	American Medical Association, 2001
	Bethesda Criteria Criteria of individual and family history used to recommend genetic testing	American Medical Association, 2001
	Myriad Genetics	www.Colaris.com

genetic counselors, physicians and nurses trained in cancer genetics, and cancer risk assessment programs (Bernhardt et al., 2000; Calzone & Biesecker, 2002).

   e. Assess person's and family members' *perception* of cancer risk. A person's subjective cancer risk may differ from a statistics-based estimated risk, but the perceived risk may be the determining factor in pursuing genetic testing.

7. Genetic counseling and cancer predisposition testing (National Cancer Institute, 2002: *Elements of cancer genetics risk and counseling*).

   a. Genetic counseling should take place before any genetic testing.

   b. Genetic counseling establishes probability of inherited cancer syndromes, perceived cancer risk, pros and cons of genetic testing, how to interpret genetic test results, and current clinical management options in risk reduction of associated cancers. Counselors need to be aware of data or lack of data regarding risk reduction measures.

   c. Genetic testing is preferably offered only when the family history pedigree suggests an inherited familial cancer syndrome for which a specific mutation has been found and can be measured.

   d. If a family history suggests a cancer predisposition, testing is best done in a family member who has a specific cancer in question.

   e. If a mutation is found, other family members can then be tested for the specific mutation identified. If no mutation is found in an affected family member, there is less convincing reason to test unaffected members.

   f. Performing a genetic test first on an unaffected family member is uninformative because a negative test does not rule out whether there is a genetic mutation in the family or in the person tested.

   g. Genetic tests are generally done on blood samples, but can be done on stored tissue samples and other body fluids.

   h. The actual genetic test is done only at a few specialized laboratories and involves sophisticated testing methods, which can be costly.

   i. The exact genetic mutation(s) to be tested for should be recommended by a genetic counselor or specialist, because some hereditary cancers may be caused by different cancer genes (eg, colon cancer may be stem from mutations in HNPCC or FAP).

   j. Molecular testing information is rapidly changing, and the ordering of genetic testing is best determined by those in the specialty area.

   k. Genetic testing requires informed consent with several components

      (1) Discussion and understanding of the people's perceptions

      (2) Assessment of motivation and goals of genetic testing

      (3) Discussion of how family history may affect cancer susceptibility

      (4) Determination of the person's cancer risk

      (5) Discussion of the potential benefits, risks, and limitations of testing, including psychological, social, economic, and family ramifications of testing

         (a) Potential benefits:

            Certainty about presence or absence of mutation with true-positive or true-negative result

            Knowledge regarding mutation risk to offspring

Help with decision regarding risk reduction options
Opportunity to inform other family members

(b) Potential risks:

Uncertainty regarding cancer risk with uncertain result

Psychological distress

Increased worry about cancer risk

Guilt regarding transmission of genetic risk to children

"Survivor guilt" in family members who test negative in known mutation family

Potential insurance, employment discrimination (Hall & Rich, 2000). Documented cases of discrimination rare, versus perceived risk

False sense of reassurance for cancer risk if test negative because may not appreciate background risk

Costs of testing and prevention options altered relationships with family members

Non-paternity issues may surface

(6) Discussion of costs and specifics about the testing process

(7) Clarification of possible testing outcomes:

  (a) Positive—a specific identified mutation is present

  (b) True positive—a person has a specific mutation present that is known to exist in a family

  (c) Negative—a specific mutation is absent

  (d) True negative—a specific mutation is not present in a person who has a known mutation in the family

  (e) Indeterminate—a change in the gene has been found, but the significance of this change is unknown regarding its role in cancer development.

(8) Discussion of medical options for people tested or not tested

(9) Discussion of alternatives to genetic testing

(10) Discussion of plan options for surveillance/risk reduction after testing or without testing

(11) Obtaining verbal and written informed consent if testing desired

(12) Scheduling of follow-up discussion after testing results received (face-to-face follow-up visit advised versus notification of results by telephone).

(13) Sharing a patient's perspective on risks/benefits and psychological impact of genetic testing can be helpful (Prouser, 2000).

8. Genetic testing in children

  a. Recommended only when family history suggests risk for high probability of associated cancer occurring in childhood years (eg, retinoblastoma).

  b. Similar to adults, test should be done only when there are effective interventions to reduce risk and the mutation test can be interpreted.

IV. Genetics in Cancer Screening

  A. As more information is learned about the specific genetic events that lead normal cells to develop into cancer cells, screening these genetic events

will be able to identify genetic markers that can find precancerous growths. (Calzone & Biesecker, 2002; Oncology Nursing Society, 2002).
  B. Genetic markers can be used to predict initiation of cancer (eg, gastric cancer genes found in dysplastic gastric polyps).
  C. Screening for genetic mutations in body fluids or secretions that might have been in contact with malignant tissues.
   Examples:
     1. p53 mutations and K-ras in stool specimens, showing a high sensitivity for predicting colorectal tumors
     2. Mutated p53 genes in urine of people with bladder cancer
     3. Mutated p53 genes and K-ras in sputum of lung cancer patients

V. Genetics in Cancer Diagnosis
  A. Evaluation of chromosome changes associated with specific cancers (eg, testing for Philadelphia chromosome in chronic myelogenous leukemia).
  B. Evaluation of genetic features of cancer cells to help determine cancer treatment response (eg, evaluation of DNA ploidy of cancer cells in neuroblastoma).
  C. Evaluation of genetic technology to predict cancer prognosis and likelihood of recurrence (eg, development of gene microarrays or "chips," which place a person's DNA on a small glass chip that then can be tested for the presence of specific mutations. This technology may help determine which people will best benefit from current cancer treatments).

VI. Genetics in Cancer Treatment
  A. Genetic information can help tailor cancer treatments and monitor for cancer progression (eg, testing for the overexpression of the oncogene HER2/neu in breast cancer patients. With overexpression, patients can be treated with herceptin, leading to a potentially improved prognosis).
  B. Gene Therapy
     1. Definition: Altering of genetic material to treat or prevent disease.
     2. Gene therapy in cancer is experimental but is being studied in clinical trials.
     3. Because genes cannot be directly inserted into a person's cell, vectors, such as retroviruses, are used for delivery.
     4. Genes can also be inserted directly into tumors.

VII. Cancer Genetic Resources: Information on cancer genetics is rapidly evolving and changing. Useful resources for nurses to stay informed and updated in cancer genetics are essential.
  A. Website Resources
     1. National Cancer Institute www.cancer.gov
        PDQ: Cancer Genetics
        Elements of Cancer Risk Assessment and Counseling
        Prevention (see individual cancers)
     2. Directory listing healthcare professionals trained in genetic counseling www.cancernet.nci.nih.gov/genesrch.shtml
     3. GeneTests (online directory of clinics/laboratories performing genetic tests for specific mutations www.genetests.org
     4. Online Mendelian Inheritance in Man (OMIM)
        Information on specific genetic disease information
        www3.ncbi.nim.nih.gov/Omim

5. National Coalition for Health Professional Education in Genetics (NCHPEG) www.nchpeg.org
B. Organizations
   1. Oncology Nursing Society www.ons.org
   2. National Society of Genetic Counselors www.nsgc.org
   3. American Society of Human Genetics www.faseb.org/genetics/ashg
   4. American Society of Clinical Oncology www.asco.org

REFERENCES

American Medical Association. (2001). *Identifying and managing risk for hereditary non-polyposis colorectal cancer and endometrial cancer.* Chicago: Author.

American Society of Clinical Oncology. (1999). *Cancer genetics & cancer predisposition testing.* Alexandria, VA: Author.

Bernhardt, B. A., Geller, G., Doksum, T., et al. (2000). Evaluation of nurses and genetic counselors as providers of education about breast cancer susceptibility testing. *Oncology Nursing Forum, 27,* 33–39.

Berry, D. A., Iverson, E. S., Gudbjartsson, D. F., et al. (2002). BRCAPRO validation, sensitivity of genetic testing of BRCA1/2, and prevalence of other breast cancer susceptibility genes. *Journal of Clinical Oncology, 20,* 2701–2708.

Calzone, K. A., & Biesecker, B. B. (2002). Genetic testing for cancer predisposition. *Cancer Nursing, 25*(1), 15–25.

Claus, E. B., Risch, N., & Thompson, W. D. (1994). Autosomal dominant inheritance of early onset breast cancer. *Cancer, 73,* 643–651.

Couch, F. J., DeShano, M. L., Blackwood, M. A., et al. (1997). BRCA1 mutations in women attending clinics that evaluate the risk of breast cancer. *New England Journal of Medicine, 336,* 1409–1415.

Eisen, A., Rebbeck, T. R., Wood, W. C., et al. (2000). Prophylactic surgery in women with a hereditary predisposition to breast and ovarian cancer. *Journal of Clinical Oncology, 18,* 1980–1995.

Fearon, E. R., & Vogelstein, B. A. (1990). A genetic model for colorectal tumorigenesis. *Cell, 61,* 759–767.

Fisher, B., Constantino, J. P., Wickerham, D. L., et al. (1998). Tamoxifen for prevention of breast cancer: Report of the National Surgical Adjuvant Breast and Bowel P-1 Project. *Journal of the National Cancer Institute, 90,* 1371–1388.

Gail, M. H., Constantino, J. P., Bryant, J., et al. (1999). Weighing the risks and benefits of tamoxifen treatment for preventing breast cancer. *Journal of the National Cancer Institute, 91,* 1829–1846.

Hall, M. A., & Rich, S. S. (2000). Laws restricting health insurers' use of genetic information: Impact on genetic discrimination. *American Journal of Human Genetics, 66,* 293–307.

Jenkins, J. (2002). Genetics competency: New directions for nursing. *Advanced Practice in Acute and Critical Care, 13*(4), 486–491.

National Cancer Institute. (2002, December 18). PDQ Statements: *Cancer genetics overview; Elements of cancer genetics risk and counseling; Genetics of breast and ovarian cancer; Genetics of colorectal cancer; Genetics of melanoma.* Bethesda, MD: Author.

Oncology Nursing Society. (2002). *Genetics and cancer care.* Project Leader: Dale Lea Halsey. Pittsburgh, PA: Oncology Nursing Society.

Prouser, N. (2000). Case report: Genetic susceptibility testing for breast and ovarian cancer: A patient's perspective. *Journal of Genetic Counseling, 9*(2), 153–159.

Tranin, A. S., Masny, A., & Jenkins, J. (2002). *Genetics in oncology practice.* Pittsburgh, PA: Oncology Nursing Society.

3 Epidemiology

Kathleen Burks

I. Epidemiologic Process

A. Goals: The goals of epidemiologic studies are to discover the causes of disease, detect and quantify risk factors, increase understanding of carcinogenesis, and evaluate preventive measures and treatment modalities.

B. Methods
   1. Observational studies
      a. *Descriptive studies* are designed to describe patterns of disease-related data in populations over time to identify clues to etiology. Data from descriptive studies are often used to develop public health priorities such as screening and prevention activities.
      b. *Analytic studies* are designed to test hypotheses about relationships between cause and outcome. There are three types of analytic studies.
         (1) *Cohort studies* are usually prospective, requiring observation of a disease-free population for a long period of time to see who develops disease (eg, the Framingham Heart Study).
         (2) *Case-control studies* examine data collected from people already diagnosed with a disease (cases) as well as data from similar people without disease (controls). Data collected include questionnaires, medical histories, and biologic specimens.
         (3) *Molecular and genetic* epidemiologic studies include elements of both cohort and case-control studies to develop understanding of the role of genetic variation and mutation in cancer development.
   2. Intervention studies use data obtained from observation and analytic studies to test means of disrupting the process of cancer development. Studies usually involve dietary, chemopreventive, screening, or lifestyle interventions.

II. Cancer Epidemiology

A. Epidemiology is the scientific study of factors influencing the frequency and distribution of disease in human populations. Cancer epidemiology is the study of these factors in relation to malignancies.

B. Epidemiologic studies are conducted to monitor the occurrence and outcomes of cancer in populations. These studies enable identification of trends in cancer occurrence and complications, as well as target areas and populations most in need of cancer screening, education, and treatment programs.

C. Descriptive epidemiologic studies deal with vital statistics, whereas analytic epidemiologic studies are concerned with causes of disease. A variety of terms are used in epidemiologic studies.

1. *Incidence rate* is the number of new cases in a given population during a specified time period. It measures the probability of developing a disease and compares rates of disease development between populations.
2. *Prevalence rate* measures existing disease in a population during a specified period of time. It reflects the burden of disease on a population and is used in the planning and distribution of health care services.
3. *Mortality rate* measures the number of deaths from a disease in a population during a specified time period.
4. *Survival* measures the number of people with cancer who are alive 5 years after diagnosis. (*Note:* This is not the same as cure rate, which measures disease-free intervals of 5 or more years.)
5. *Morbidity* is the state or condition of having a disease. This is often used to describe complications or consequences of having a disease.
6. *Host* is a person who is susceptible to disease. Many different host characteristics are studied in epidemiology, including age, sex, race/ethnicity, genetic predisposition, and preexisting disease.
7. *Environment* includes factors to which the host is exposed. Characteristics studied include place (which may be the home, workplace, city, town, region, or country), nutrition, occupation, and personal habits.

III. Cancer Statistics: A variety of cancer statistics are reported annually for the United States. These statistics include the number of new cases of cancer (incidence), the number of deaths due to cancer (mortality), and information about how long individuals survive after a diagnosis of cancer (survival).

  A. Incidence: The American Cancer Society estimates that there will be 1.3 million new cases of cancer diagnosed in 2003 (Fig. 3–1). This includes cancers of all types except carcinoma in situ (except for urinary bladder), and basal and squamous cell skin cancers.

  B. Mortality: Twenty-three percent of all deaths in the United States are due to cancer. This translates to about 1,500 deaths per day (Table 3–1).
   1. Cancer is second only to heart disease as the leading cause of death. However, when deaths are categorized by age and sex, cancer ranks first as the cause of death among females age 40 to 79 and among males 60 to 79.
   2. Lung cancer is the leading cause of cancer mortality among men and women of all ethnic groups, followed by breast, prostate, and colorectal cancers.
   3. Overall, the cancer mortality rate has been decreasing slightly since 1994.

  C. Survival: Cancer survival rates are increasing.
   1. Over the past 60 years, the percentage of people surviving for 5 years after cancer diagnosis has improved from less than 20% to about 40%.
   2. This figure represents the "observed" survival rate for cancer patients. When adjusted for average life expectancy (reflecting deaths due to other causes), a "relative" 5-year survival rate of about 62% is seen for all cancers combined.
   3. Increased survival rates most likely reflect improvements in patient management, promotion and acceptance of early detection methods, and the availability and use of medical care.

Estimated New Cases

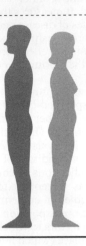

Male	Female
Prostate (33%)	Breast (32%)
Lung and Bronchus (14%)	Lung and Bronchus (12%)
Colon and Rectum (11%)	Colon and Rectum (11%)
Urinary Bladder (6%)	Uterine Corpus (6%)
Melanoma of the Skin (4%)	Ovary (4%)
Non-Hodgkin Lymphoma (4%)	Non-Hodgkin Lymphoma (4%)
Kidney (3%)	Melanoma of the Skin (3%)
Oral Cavity (3%)	Thyroid (3%)
Leukemia (3%)	Pancreas (2%)
Pancreas (2%)	Urinary Bladder (2%)
All Other Sites (17%)	All Other Sites (20%)

Estimated Deaths

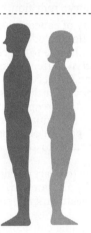

Male	Female
Lung and Bronchus (31%)	Lung and Bronchus (25%)
Prostate (10%)	Breast (15%)
Colon and Rectum (10%)	Colon and Rectum (11%)
Pancreas (5%)	Pancreas (6%)
Non-Hodgkin Lymphoma (4%)	Ovary (5%)
Leukemia (4%)	Non-Hodgkin Lymphoma (4%)
Esophagus (4%)	Leukemia (4%)
Liver (3%)	Uterine Corpus (3%)
Urinary Bladder (3%)	Brain (2%)
Kidney (3%)	Multiple Myeloma (2%)
All Other Sites (22%)	All Other Sites (23%)

* excludes basal and squamous cell skin cancers and in situ carcinomas except urinary bladder.
Note: percentages may not total 100 percent due to rounding.

Figure 3–1. Ten leading cancer types for the estimated new cancer cases and deaths, by sex, US, 2003. (Jemal, A., et al. [2003]. Cancer statistics, 2003. *CA: Cancer Journal for Clinicians, 53,*5–26.)

D. Several factors impact the patterns of cancer incidence, mortality, and survival. Chief among these are age, gender, and race or ethnicity.
   1. Age: Cancer incidence increases with advancing age. Cancer among children is relatively rare.
   2. Gender: Overall incidence of cancer is higher among males than females, with approximately 1 in 2 males and 1 in 3 females diagnosed in their lifetime. Rates are age-adjusted (ie, incidence for

females from birth to age 39 is 1 in 52, and for males 1 in 69). Incidence rates increased among females from 1987 to 1999 by about 0.3%, probably due to increased rates of lung cancer. Incidence rates among males remained relatively stable between 1995 and 1999. Cancer death rates declined in males by 1.5% per year and in females by about 0.6% per year between 1992 and 1999.

a. Males: Prostate cancer is the most frequently occurring cancer, comprising 33% of cancers in men and affecting 1 in 6 males by age 85. Lung and colorectal cancers have the second and third highest incidence. The highest mortality from cancer is from lung cancer, followed by prostate and colorectal cancers.

b. Females: Breast cancer will occur in approximately 1 out of 8 women by age 85. It is the most frequently occurring cancer among women, accounting for 32% of all cancers diagnosed. The next most common malignancies are lung and colorectal cancers. Deaths from lung cancer have surpassed those from breast cancer.

3. Race/Ethnicity: Cancer incidence and mortality vary widely among racial and ethnic groups. Racial and ethnic groups are divided into five general categories: African American, Asian/Pacific Islander, Hispanic, Native American, and white. The US Census Bureau estimates that, by the year 2050, Hispanics will comprise about 25% of the US population. African Americans, Asian/Pacific Islanders, and Native Americans combined will make up another 25%. Although targeted data collection has been lacking, some trends can be pinpointed.

a. African Americans: For the most common cancer sites, African Americans have significantly higher rates of incidence and mortality than any of the other racial and ethnic groups. Exceptions to this are breast cancer incidence and lung cancer mortality.

(1) Specifically, African Americans have the highest incidence and mortality rates for cancers of the prostate, esophagus, larynx, pancreas, and multiple myeloma. Incidence of prostate cancer among African-American males is the highest in the world.

(2) The rate of new cancers in African Americans exceeds that of white Americans by about 10%, of Hispanics and Asian/Pacific Islanders by 50% to 60%, and of Native Americans by 100%.

(3) Mortality from all cancers is 30% higher than in whites, and more than twice as high as among Hispanics, Asian/Pacific Islanders, and Native Americans.

(4) The largest decrease in mortality rates between 1995 and 1999 occurred among African-American males. However, survival continues to be lower in the African-American population as compared to whites.

(5) Later diagnosis of cancers, differences in the quality of health care, and comorbid conditions probably contribute to poorer survival.

b. Asian/Pacific Islanders: This group has the lowest rates of prostate cancer incidence. However, there is a very high rate of liver cancer, particularly among Southeast Asians, which is linked to high rates of infection with hepatitis B. Gastric cancer incidence and mortality are high among Japanese, Korean, and Vietnamese populations.

Table 3-1 Trends in 5-Year Relative Survival Rates* (%) by Race and Year of Diagnosis, US, 1974 to 1998

	Relative 5-Year Survival Rate (%)								
	White			African American			All Races		
CANCER TYPE	1974 to 1976	1983 to 1985	1992 to 1998	1974 to 1976	1983 to 1985	1992 to 1998	1974 to 1976	1983 to 1985	1992 to 1998
All Cancers	51	54	64†	39	40	53†	50	52	62†
Brain	22	26	32†	27	32	40†	22	27	32†
Breast (female)	75	79	88†	63	63	73†	75	78	86†
Uterine cervix	70	71	72†	64	60	60	69	69	71†
Colon	51	58	63†	46	49	53†	50	58	62†
Uterine corpus	89	85	86†	61	54	61	88	83	84†
Esophagus	5	9	15†	4	6	8†	5	8	13†
Hodgkin's disease	72	79	85†	69	77	77†	71	79	84†
Kidney	52	56	62†	49	55	60†	52	56	62†
Larynx	66	69	66†	60	55	54	66	67	64
Leukemia	35	42	47†	31	34	38	34	41	46†
Liver	4	6	7†	1	4	4†	4	6	7†

Lung and bronchus	13	14	15†	11	11	12†	12	14	15†
Melanoma of the skin	80	85	89†	67‡	74§	66‡	80	85	89†
Multiple myeloma	24	27	30†	28	31	33	24	28	30†
Non-Hodgkin's lymphoma	48	54	56†	49	45	46	47	54	55†
Oral cavity	55	55	59†	36	35	35	53	53	56†
Ovary	37	40	53†	41	42	53†	37	41	53†
Pancreas	3	3	4†	3	5	4	3	3	4†
Prostate	68	76	98†	58	64	93†	67	75	97†
Rectum	49	56	62†	42	44	53†	49	55	62†
Stomach	15	16	21†	17	19	20	15	17	22†
Testis	79	91	96†	76‡	88‡	85	79	91	95†
Thyroid	92	93	96†	88	92	93	92	93	96†
Urinary bladder	74	78	82†	48	60	65†	73	78	82†

*Survival rates are adjusted for normal life expectancy, and are based on cases diagnosed from 1992 to 1998, followed through 1999.

†The difference in rates between 1974 to 1976 and 1992 to 1998 is statistically significant (p < 0.05).

‡The standard error of the survival rate is between 5 and 10 percentage points.

§The standard error of the survival rate is greater than 10 percentage points.

Division of Cancer Control and Population Sciences, National Cancer Institute, 2002. Surveillance, Epidemiology, and End Results program, 1973 to 1999.

    c. Hispanics: This is a widely diverse group, composed of Mexicans, Puerto Ricans, and Central and South Americans. Rates of cancer diagnosis tend to rank in the middle of all groups. Higher rates of gall bladder, biliary tract, and stomach cancers have been noted, as well as cancer of the uterine cervix in women.

    d. Native Americans (includes American Eskimos): High rates of colorectal cancer have been noted in American Eskimos, but, overall, Native Americans have the lowest incidence of cancer, and cancer is the third leading cause of death, after accidents and heart disease. Incidence rates are high for renal cancers in men and for ovarian cancer in women.

IV. Sources of Cancer Statistics

    A. Cancer Prevention Studies (CPS) I and II: These prospective studies have been conducted by the American Cancer Society since 1959. CPS I established the link between smoking and death. The goal of CPS II is to explore the relationship between various lifestyle and environmental factors and the development of cancer.

    B. SEER (Surveillance, Epidemiology, and End Results): This project was established in 1973 by the National Cancer Institute as an ongoing study of cancer incidence and survival in the United States. It is the major source for incidence, mortality, and survival statistics.

    C. National Cancer Database: This program was created in 1989 by the American Cancer Society and the American College of Surgeons. It combines regional data into one national database addressing cancer diagnosis, treatment, and survival.

V. Implications for Patient Care

    A. Epidemiologic data are used to identify at-risk populations and individuals, and to test focused education and intervention efforts related to cancer prevention and early detection.

    B. Epidemiologic data are also used when estimating a person's risk of cancer occurrence and recurrence. Counseling can then be tailored to address methods to reduce identified risks, such as smoking cessation or increasing the frequency of screening examinations.

REFERENCES

Cartmel, B., & Reid, M. (1997). Cancer control and epidemiology. In S. Groenwald, M. H. Frogg, M. Goodman, & C. H. Yarbro (Eds.), *Cancer nursing principles and practice* (4th ed., pp. 50–74). Boston: Jones & Bartlett.

Cole, P., & Rodu, B. (2001). Descriptive epidemiology: Cancer statistics. In V.T. DeVita, Jr., S. Hellman, & S. A. Rosenberg (Eds.), *Cancer: Principles and practice of oncology* (6th ed.) [limited on-line access]. Philadelphia: Lippincott Williams & Wilkins. Available: lwwoncology.com.

Division of Cancer Control and Population Sciences, National Cancer Institute. (2002). Surveillance, Epidemiology, and End Results Program, 1973 to 1999.

Groenwald, S. L., Frogge, M. H., Goodman, M., & Yarbro, C. H. (Eds.). (1998). *Comprehensive cancer nursing review*. Sudbury, MA: Jones & Bartlett.

Jemal, A., Murray, T., Samuels, A., Ghafoor, A., Ward, E., & Thun, M. J. (2003). Cancer statistics, 2003. *CA: Cancer Journal* [On-line], *53*, 5–26. Available: Hostname: acs.org. Directory: http://caonline.amcancersoc.org/cgi/content/full/53/1/5.

Tucker, M. A. (2001). Epidemiologic methods. In V. T. DeVita, Jr., S. Hellman, & S. A. Rosenberg (Eds.), *Cancer: Principles and practice of oncology* (6th ed.) [limited on-line access]. Philadelphia: Lippincott Williams & Wilkins. Available: lwwoncology.com.

UNIT II

CANCER TREATMENT

CHAPTER

4 Biological Therapies

Brenda K. Shelton

I. History
   A. In 1895, Hericourt and Richet were first to document antitumor immune therapy in humans, defining the immune surveillance theory of cancer development.
   B. Primary barrier to development of biological therapy as a cancer treatment modality was ability to generate large quantities of immune substances, resolved by development of recombinant DNA technology in the 1970s.

II. Definitions/Overview
   A. Immune activity is the essential homeostatic mechanism protecting a person against potential pathogens and foreign tissues.
   B. Biological therapy is defined as use of naturally occurring immune substances to affect the body's immune responses. Includes activities such as:
      1. Immune stimulation
      2. Immune augmentation
      3. Immune suppression

III. Rationale for Use
   A. Proposed Physiologic Activity
      1. The discovery of individual tumor-surface antigens (tumor-specific antigens) and tumor-associated antigens has supported the belief that most human cancers have antigens capable of eliciting an immune response.
      2. Cells may spontaneously transform to malignancy or mutate after exposure to carcinogens.
      3. Once malignant transformation has occurred, the immunologic surveillance system recognizes the neoplastic cell as foreign by the presence of antigens on the surface of the tumor cells.
      4. Under normal circumstances, the immune surveillance system destroys the malignant cell in the preclinical stage; however, an impaired immune system will permit malignant cells to proliferate to clinical disease.
   B. Evidence Supporting Immunosurveillance Theory
      1. Higher incidence rates of cancer in children, elderly, people with immunodeficiency diseases, and in organ transplantation patients.
      2. Reports of spontaneous tumor regression.
      3. It has also been shown that tumors heavily infiltrated by lymphocytes may have a better prognosis than those that do not demonstrate this characteristic (Reiger, 2001).

C. Antitumor biological agents have been developed based on different proposed mechanisms of altering the host-tumor response so tumor cells are immunologically destroyed.

IV. Biology of Therapy

A. Basic Goals of Anticancer Biotherapy
1. To stimulate direct and indirect immunocompetence
2. To create tumor-specific immunity
3. To induce tumor regression when used adjunctively with other cancer treatments

B. Indications for Biological Therapy
1. Known tumor-associated antigen that can be targeted for destruction (eg, her-2-neu receptor in breast cancer patients).
2. Tumors with high lymphocytic infiltration.
3. Limited disease thought to be more responsive to immunologic manipulation.
4. Tumors for which spontaneous remissions have been reported (eg, malignant melanoma, renal cell carcinoma).
5. Existing or anticipated bone marrow suppression is the clear single indication for restorative biological therapy.
6. Prevention of rejection in organ transplant recipients and suppression of autoimmune disease mechanisms are indications for immunosuppressive immune modulators or monoclonals that target the T lymphocytes.

C. Principles to Determine Patient Eligibility
1. Tumor size: Large tumors are thought to depress the immune system, and less likely to demonstrate an antitumor response with biological therapy because of the slow immunologic destruction induced by these agents.
2. Tumor type: Patients who derive the most benefit from biological therapy have disease that has not progressed beyond stage II and who are not severely immunosuppressed.
3. Immunocompetence: Patients able to generate positive skin test reactions demonstrating active immune responses may have better antitumor response rates. Quantitative assessment of immune function is made by peripheral blood counts, immunoglobulin assays, and bone marrow aspiration.

D. Biological Therapy Administration
1. Treatment scheduling: Treatment should be timed carefully with other anticancer therapies, so the immune system can recover from the effects of these other modalities. Certain chemotherapeutic agents demonstrate synergistic antitumor activity with biotherapeutic agents (eg, 5-fluorouracil and levamisole).
2. Dosage
   a. Biotherapy is not dosed according to maximal tolerated dose (MTD).
   b. Biological therapy may exert its optimal biological effect at a dose much lower than the MTD.
   c. Optimal biological dose (OBD)—the dose which, with a minimum of side effects, produces the optimal desired clinical responses.
3. Evaluation of efficacy

    a. Traditional measures of antineoplastic therapy measure tumor size as the primary assessment of successful therapy.
    b. Biotherapeutic trials must incorporate measures of biological effects on the immune system, and immunologic assays.
    c. Stabilization of disease may be a more accurate objective than reduction of tumor because the objective of biological therapy is immune activation.

V. Classification of Biological Agents: There is no defined classification system of biological agents because many have multiple immunologic antitumor activities. The general categories and their nursing implications are listed in Table 4–1.

    A. Antitumor biotherapy uses active and passive mechanisms to enhance the nonspecific and specific host-tumor immune responses through the use of attenuated live bacteria or their products or through immuno-chemical agents. Antitumor biotherapy is further subdivided into cytokines, vaccines, and monoclonal antibodies.

    1. Cytokines are cell-killer substances modeled after normal human lymphocyte secretions that are administered to enhance normal immune defense mechanisms. Human growth factors (eg, erythro-poietin, granulocyte colony stimulating factor, granulocyte-macrophage colony stimulating factor, and platelet colony stimulating factor) are termed *cytokines* in some texts, but they do not have antitumor properties and are, therefore, described as restorative biotherapy here.
        a. Interferons—alfa, beta, gamma
        b. Interleukins—interlcukin-2
        c. Other—-tumor necrosis factors (still investigational)

    2. Antitumor vaccines are antibodies specifically engineered to destroy particular tumor antigens, theoretically making them tumor-specific, long-lived, and nontoxic. A major problem in vaccine therapy is the identification and purification of relevant antigens to be used in preparing vaccines.
        a. Vaccines may be made from animal or human models.
        b. Types of cancer vaccines determined by the transport mechanism of the vaccine: recombinant bacteria, protein peptides, nucleic acids, recombinant viruses, transduced cells, modified tumor cells (Kinzler & Brown, 2001).
        c. Immunoadjuvants involve the use of transports that primarily activate existing host immune activities rather than replace defective gene sequences (eg, bacteria, interleukin-12, granulocyte-macrophage colony stimulating factor). This category includes the single vaccine product currently licensed as an anti-cancer therapy (bacillus Calmette-Guérin [BCG]).
        d. Dendritic cells are potent antigen-presenting cells that are essential for recognition and destruction of tumor cells. Removal and cytokine activation of human dendritic cells followed by reinfusion is thought to produce effects similar to other immunoadjuvant therapies (Kinzler & Brown, 2001).

    3. Monoclonal antibodies are antibodies derived from the fusion of an antibody-producing cell, such as a B lymphocyte, and another cell.

(Text continues on page 40)

TABLE 4-1 Biotherapy Agents*

Biologic Classification and Agents	Adverse Effects	Special Nursing Implications

Antitumor biotherapy: vaccine
• Bacillus Calmette-Guérin
	• Flulike syndrome within 12–24 hours after dose; subsides within 48 hours
	  • Injection site irritation, wheal reaction
	  • Dysuria, urinary urgency or frequency if administered via the bladder
		• Protect from light.
		• Do not use alcohol to prepare skin because it can kill organisms.
		• Avoid concomitant administration of isoniazid because it may inhibit BCG multiplication.
		• Teach patient self-injection technique if applicable.
		• Reconstituted, most agents stable up to 1 month in refrigerator.
		• Prevent flu symptoms with prophylactic acetaminophen or nonsteroidal antiinflammatory agents.
		• Pretreat injection site with ice or massage to reduce injection site irritation.

Antitumor biotherapy: cytokines
• Interferon-alfa
• Interferon-beta
• Interferon-gamma
• Interleukin-2 (IL-2)
	• Flulike syndrome: fever, chills, myalgias, arthralgias, headache
	• Gastrointestinal distress: anorexia, nausea, vomiting, diarrhea
	• Elevated liver enzymes
	• Weight loss
	• Primarily IL-2
	  – Capillary leak syndrome (edema, vascular volume depletion, hypotension)
	  – Oliguria and renal insufficiency
	  – Dysrhythmias
	  – Flushing, erythema, rash, pruritus
	  – Thrombocytopenia
	  – Cognitive dysfunction: difficulty concentrating, emotional lability, confusion, hallucinations
		• IL-2
		  – Perform baseline cardiac and pulmonary function tests before therapy.
		  – Give cautiously in neurologic diseases (eg, seizure disorder), brain metastases.
		  – Be aware of wide variation in dose range, schedule, and mode of administration, affecting variability of adverse effects.
		  – Adding albumin to aldesleukin injectable is also thought to reduce injection site irritation.
		  – Use a large variety of symptom management strategies (eg, guided imagery) and concomitant medications (eg, diuretics, antipyretics, antiemetics) to abrogate adverse effects and continue therapy.
		• Adverse effects are completely reversed with cessation of therapy.

	Side effects	Nursing considerations
Cytomodulatory biologic therapy; monoclonal antibodies for diagnosis • Satumomab pendetide (OncoScint CR/OV) • Carpromab pendetide (ProstaScint)	• Fever, chills • Hypersensitivity (rare)	• Detection of ovarian or colorectal cancer (OncoScint), or prostate cancer (ProstaScint) • Premedicate with acetaminophen for flulike symptoms • Have emergency equipment available for rare circumstance of anaphylaxis.
Antitumor biologic therapy; monoclonal antibodies • Alemtuzumab (Campath) • Gemtuzumab (Mylotarg) [combined with antitumor antibiotic] • Rituximab (Rituxan) • Trastuzumab (Herceptin)	• Infusion-related chills or fever, hypotension • Hypersensitivity reaction (pruritus, rash, dyspnea, wheezing) • Nausea, vomiting • Pain at disease sites • Fatigue • Elevated liver enzymes • Bone marrow suppression—neutropenia, thrombocytopenia	• Administer as IV infusion only. • Stable for 24 hours after reconstitution if remains unrefrigerated. • Premedication with acetaminophen and diphenhydramine is recommended. • Vital signs q 15 min 3 1 hr, then q 30 min during infusion. • Have emergency equipment readily available during infusion in case severe hypersensitivity occurs. • Trastuzumab has been associated with acute onset of cardiomyopathy and congestive heart failure, especially when administered with anthracyclines or cyclophosphamide

(Continued)

TABLE 4-1 Biotherapy Agents* (Continued)

Biologic Classification and Agents	Adverse Effects	Special Nursing Implications
Cytomodulatory biologic therapy; radio-labeled monoclonal antibodies • Tositumomab + Iodine[131] (Bexxar) • 90Y ibritumomab tiuxetan (Zevalin) • Nofetumomab + technetium (Verluma)	• Acute hypersensitivity reactions—fever, chills, hypotension, bronchospasm • Bone marrow suppression—neutropenia, thrombocytopenia • Asthenia (Zevalin only)	• Must be administered by radiation therapy professionals • Observe the patient continuously for the first 15 minutes. • Monitor vital signs every 15 minutes for at least an hour. • Have emergency equipment available for rare circumstance of anaphylaxis. • Monitor for infection or bleeding.
Cytomodulatory biologic therapy; T-lymphocyte/TNF suppressing monoclonal antibodies • Adalimumab (Humira) • Daclizumab (Zenapax) • Infliximab (Remicade) [anti-TNF antibody] • Muromonab-CD3 (Orthoclone OKT3) • Natalizumab (Antegren) • Omalizumab (Volair) [allergen antibodies]	• Infection	• Implement infection prevention precautions. • Discontinue other antirejection drugs to reduce the risk of infection.
Cytomodulatory biologic therapy; fusion proteins • Denileukin difitox (Ontak) [diphtheria toxin and interleukin-2]	• Acute hypersensitivity reactions—fever, chills, hypotension, bronchospasm • Capillary leak syndrome (edema, vascular volume depletion, hypotension) • Hypoalbuminemia about 1 week after administration	• Observe the patient continuously for the first 15 minutes. • Monitor vital signs every 15 minutes for at least an hour. • Have emergency equipment available for rare circumstance of anaphylaxis.

| **Cytomodulatory biologic therapy; polypeptide antibiotics**
• Cyclosporine
• Tacrolimus | • Hypertension
• Mental status changes
• Decreased seizure threshold.
• Nausea, vomiting
• Renal dysfunction | • Plan for monitoring blood pressure, weight, and presence of edema.
• Avoid other drugs with neurotoxicity.
• Monitor blood levels as ordered.
• Monitor BUN and creatinine during therapy, and report elevations in laboratory values that may necessitate dose reduction.
• Reduce dose slowly while observing for signs and symptoms of organ rejection.
• Monitor BP frequently.
• Administer oral cyclosporine with chocolate milk to mask taste and maximize absorption. |
| **Restorative biologic therapy; hematopoietic growth factors**
• Erythropoietin
• Granulocyte colony stimulating factor (G-CSF)
• Oprelvekin (interleukin-11)
• Granulocyte-macrophage colony stimulating factor (GM-CSF) | • RBC growth factors: headache, hypertension, increased clotting tendency
• WBC growth factors: fever, chills, bone pain, leukocytosis
• Platelet growth factor: atrial arrhythmias
  Blurred vision, dyspnea
  Fluid retention (eg, edema, increased effusions)
• All: injection site erythema or irritation | • Indications for usage are lineage specific.
• Erythropoietin:
  – Monitor reticulocyte count for drug effectiveness, and reduce dose for dramatic increases in RBC count.
  – Monitor and replenish iron or transferrin for greater efficacy of treatment.
  – Monitor BP for hypertension.
  – Monitor for thromboses or risk factors for clotting
• WBC growth factors:
  – Administer 24 hours after conclusion of antineoplastic therapy.
  – Use acetaminophen or nonsteroidal antiinflammatory agents prophylactically to reduce risk or severity of flu symptoms. |

(continued)

TABLE 4–1 Biotherapy Agents* *(Continued)*

Biologic Classification and Agents	Adverse Effects	Special Nursing Implications
Restorative biologic therapy; hematopoietic growth factors		• Platelet growth factors: – Administer 6–24 hours after conclusion of antineoplastic therapy and continue after the nadir of the platelet count. – Monitor platelet count daily during therapy • All: – Pretreat with ice or massage injection site to reduce irritation.
Cytomodulatory biologic therapy; retinoids • Bexarotene (Targretin) • Alitretinoin (Panretin, 9-*cis*-retinoic acid) • Tretinoin (Vesanoid, All-*trans*-retinoic acid, ATRA) • Tretinoin liposomal	• Erythema, skin irritation with topical administration • Vitamin A toxicity—headache, fever, dry skin and mucous membranes, pruritus, bone pain, nausea and vomiting, visual disturbances • Systemic administration of ATRA produces "ATRA syndrome"—fever, dyspnea, weight gain, pulmonary infiltrates, effusions, hypotension • Systemic administration may cause: – Temporary (rarely permanent) hearing loss – Alopecia – Agitation, emotional disturbances, forgetfulness, paresthesias – Increased cholesterol or triglycerides	• Assess baseline skin integrity before applying topical agents. • Use gloves to administer any of these agents topically. • Check for hypersensitivity to any previous retinoids (eg, acne treatments, vitamin A supplements) • When giving systemic retinoids, check hepatic enzymes. • Observe for "ATRA syndrome" and treat symptomatically while discontinuing the drug.

Cytomodulatory biologic therapy; anti-angiogenesis factors
• Thalidomide (Thalomid)

- Flulike syndrome—fever, headache, arthralgias, myalgias
- Neuropathy
- Constipation

- Monitor complete blood count for drug toxicity
- Monitor for skin reactions and treat rashes symptomatically.
- Provide patient education about risk to the fetus if this drug is consumed while pregnant.

Cytomodulatory biologic therapy; miscellaneous
• Levamisole

- Flulike syndrome—fever, headache, arthralgias, myalgias
- Fatigue
- Gastrointestinal distress: stomatitis, altered taste sensations, nausea, vomiting, abdominal pain, diarrhea
- Bone marrow suppression: neutropenia, thrombocytopenia
- Dizziness

- Always give exactly on time to enhance synergistic properties with 5-fluorouracil.
- Concomitant alcohol consumption can cause disulfiram reactions.
- Inhibits cholinergic activity.
- Monitor phenytoin levels; may be higher while receiving levamisole.

---

*Specific clinical indications for each agent are included in disease-specific chapters, and this table describes an overview of the general clinical features of each category of agents.

a. Diagnostic monoclonal antibodies detect the presence of tumor cell surface antigens and provide nuclear highlighting to detect occult disease when attached to a nuclear imaging agent (eg, satumomab pendetide, carpromab pendetide).
b. Antitumor monoclonal antibodies directed against tumor surface antigens (eg, rixtuximab, trastuzumab).
c. Chemoimmunoconjugates involve the use of a targeted monoclonal antibody with an attached active chemotherapeutic agent (eg, gemtuzumab combines a monoclonal with the antitumor antibiotic, calicheamicin).
d. Radioimmunoconjugates combine a radioactive agent with a directed monoclonal antibody to aid direct application of radiation therapy (eg, tositumomab + iodine[131], ^{90}Y ibritumomab tinxetan, nofetumomab + technetium).
e. Immunosuppressive monoclonal antibodies that target T lymphocytes, or tumor necrosis factor (eg, muromonab OKT3, infliximab).
f. Monoclonal antibodies may also be classified according to their source, and the less pure human sources place patients at risk for immunologic reactions related to human antimurine antibodies (HAMA).
  (1) Murine—mouse antibodies modified and used to attach to human antigens
  (2) Chimeric—fusion of both a murine and a human component of the antibody
  (3) Humanized—antibody produced from a human antibody protein
B. Adoptive biotherapy is based on the assumption that there are tumor-associated antigens that can elicit an antitumor response when stimulated.
  1. Immunologically active cells that originate from the patient, other humans, or an animal donor are infused into the host.
  2. In autologous adoptive biotherapy, the tumor is harvested from the patient, and the lymphocytes within the tumor are cloned and nurtured, then reinfused. Use of the patient's own genetically altered tumor cells is termed *tumor-infiltrating lymphocytes* (TIL).
  3. Passive adoptive biological therapy incubates donor lymphocytes with tumor cells from the patient or with a cytokine such as interleukin-2 to sensitize the lymphocytes, then those lymphocytes are reinfused into the patient.
C. Restorative biotherapy increases the patient's immunologic competence by increasing the number of mature, functioning hematopoietic cells.
  1. Substances that enhance the production rate, differentiation, maturation, and functional ability of hematopoietic cells are called *immunologic stimulants* or *hematopoietic growth factors*.
  2. Subclassified as lineage restricted (acting on one cell type) or multilineage (affecting more than one cell type).
D. Cytomodulatory biotherapy exerts immunoproliferative or immunomodulatory functions through the recognition of tumor-associated antigens and histocompatibility (HLA) antigens on the surface of

tumor cells. This type of biological therapy is less well defined and includes agents that enhance antitumor activity, as well as target T lymphocytes for immunosuppressive activity.

1. Polypeptide antibiotics that cause reduced T-lymphocyte antigen recognition or response (eg, cyclosporine, tacrolimus).
2. Retinoids cause changes in the metabolic pathways of tumor nutrition and replication that cause apoptosis of the tumor cells.
3. Antiangiogenesis factors act by targeting the receptor sites for self-vascularization of tumor cells that are essential for tumor-cell growth and metastasis. Some receptor sites that have been identified as essential for tumor vascularization include epidermal growth factor receptor (EGFR), vascular endothelial growth factor (VEGF), angiostatin, and matrix-metalloproteinases.
4. Miscellaneous

E. Human gene therapy involves the biological technique of inserting a functioning gene into the patient's cells to reverse a defective gene or add functions to an existing cell. Gene therapy is delivered by in vivo technique (directly to the targeted cell in the body) and ex vivo technique (cell removal from the body and cell return by way of replacement genes in a retroviral vector).

VI. **Nursing Issues:** Nursing care of patients receiving biological therapy focus on educating the patient, family members, and staff members and on therapy-specific assessments.

A. Treatment Plans
1. Educate the patient on the option of a biotherapy-containing treatment regimen. Know the patient's cancer diagnosis, disease sites, goals of therapy, concomitant diseases, and information about the agents to be administered.
2. Explain the administration plan and purpose for the scheduling.
   a. Many new biotherapy regimens use biotherapy agents as adjuncts to chemotherapy, radiotherapy, or after bone marrow transplantation, to augment the host-tumor response.
   b. The biotherapy agent selected, dose, schedule, and concomitant therapies will predict the nursing plan of care.
   c. Most biological therapy plans do not permit systemic administration of corticosteroids because it is proposed to interfere with the desired proinflammatory effects of the agent.
3. Evaluate the patient's and family's cognitive, psychological, and emotional status throughout the therapy.
   a. Often, these immune therapies do not demonstrate disease regression until months after administration.
   b. The patient may also experience neurologic variations that affect the understanding of therapy and the ability to cope with its adverse effects.

B. Administration
1. Follow universal precautions during administration of biotherapy agents because they are not classified as biohazards. Many institutions, however, have elected to uniformize antineoplastic precautions and advise more conservative measures.
2. Administer biotherapeutic agents by way of intradermal, scarification, multiple puncture, intravenous, intravesical, intraabdominal,

intrapleural, or intralesional routes. (Nurses do not usually independently administer these agents intralesionally or intrapleurally.)

3. Prepare the solution and injection site according to the appropriate standard.

   a. Some biotherapeutic agents contain live organisms or biologically active substances that must be protected from extreme heat and cold and severe agitation.

   b. Use only the diluent provided when preparing biotherapeutic solutions for injection. Other diluent solutions may be incompatible with the agent or render it nonviable. Sterile water and normal saline with preservatives both contain small amounts of alcohol, which can kill the organisms in the BCG vaccine or inactivate cytokines.

   c. Alcohol skin preparation before injection may also be contraindicated because its presence on the skin surface can kill BCG vaccine organisms and inactivate some cytokines. Acetone is effective for skin preparation.

4. Test the skin for delayed hypersensitivity as a precursor to some biological therapies.

   a. Prepare and administer the agents and assess the resultant skin reactions.

   b. Carefully and accurately describe the local reactions, including measurements, diagrams, and photographs.

C. Adverse Effects

1. Reassure the patient that adverse effects of biotherapy are acute and totally reversible after discontinuation of therapy. The effects are not likely to be life-threatening and usually can be abrogated with therapy modification.

2. Observe and plan for a broad range of adverse effects to effectively implement early intervention for these complications. Variability in adverse effects or their severity can be related to patient variables (eg, immune competence, disease location) rather than drug or dosage.

3. See Table 4–2 for a summary of the most common adverse effects of biotherapy and the nursing interventions for these complications. The two most commonly experienced adverse effects are fatigue and flulike syndrome.

   a. Fatigue: Almost all patients receiving biotherapy will suffer from fatigue that may significantly alter quality of life (see Chapter 25).

   b. Flulike syndrome: Most patients will experience flulike symptoms, including chills, fever, headache, rhinitis, arthralgias, and myalgias. Assess fever patterns and associated symptoms to aid in differentiating between biologic therapy toxicity and infectious complications.

   c. Other adverse effects: Skin reactions, edema, emotional distress, anorexia, and diarrhea are other common effects of biotherapy. See chapters in Unit IV for detailed information on assessment and management of these complications.

   d. Severe hypersensitivity reaction (anaphylaxis): This is the most common reason for discontinuation of therapy, but it rarely occurs.

(Text continues on page 48)

TABLE 4–2 Management of Common Adverse Effects of Biotherapy

Symptom/Sign	Assessment	Interventions
Hypersensitivity reaction	• Monitor patient carefully in the first 5–60 minutes of first administration of a biologic agent. • Check frequent vital signs during this time period. • Observe respiratory rate and rhythm during this time period. • Check breath sounds for stridor or wheezing. • Check skin for flushing, swelling, or pruritus.	• Have emergency equipment readily available during administration of biologic agents. • When administration is intravenous, slowly titrate the infusion or administer a test dose as advised by the specific manufacturer's instructions for each agent. • Premedicate patients with acetaminophen, histamine blockers, or corticosteroids as advised by the manufacturer's instructions for each agent.
Headache	• Intensity or character (throbbing or dull ache) of pain • Timing (continual or exacerbated with exertion) • Headache location (usually frontal) • Associated visual disturbances • Associated nausea or vomiting • Exacerbating factors (eg, light, position change) • Alleviating factors (eg, eating, temporal massage)	• Administer mild analgesic medications (eg, acetaminophen). • Document patient responses to pain relief measures. • Apply cool compresses to head. • Darken room. • Avoid loud and high-pitched noises, constant noise. • Encourage rest, sleep, and quiet activities. • Avoid asking patient to make decisions or concentrate (eg, to learn a skill) during symptoms. • Implement nonpharmacologic interventions (eg, massage, acupressure, aromatherapy)
Dizziness/vertigo	• Position when it occurs • Accompanying tinnitus, visual disturbances • Other associated symptoms (eg, nausea, headache, dyspnea)	• Provide safe environment. • Assist when patient is out of bed. • Encourage use of stable furniture or walking implements if available. • Have "smelling salts" or other potent odorous substance available when patient gets out of bed. • Perform orthostatic checks at least daily during therapy or when suspicious symptoms occur. *(continued)*

TABLE 4–2 Management of Common Adverse Effects of Biotherapy (Continued)

Symptom/Sign	Assessment	Interventions
Visual disturbances	• Presence of blurred vision, diplopia, photophobia	• Patch eye if only one eye affected. • Provide safe environment. • Assist with activities of daily living as needed (eg, cutting food, putting spill-proof lids on drinks).
Mental status changes	• Emotional lability (dysphoria, euphoria) • Decreased ability to concentrate • Decreased reasoning or calculating ability lost early, before orientation • Appropriateness of behavior or responses to questions • Disorientation to person, place, time • Motor difficulties accompanying altered mental status	• Encourage rest. • Reorient as needed. • Provide a safe environment. • Check reasoning ability, calculation ability, and personality consistency on a periodic basis. • Include family members in identifying atypical behaviors that may indicate neurotoxicity. • Avoid mind-altering or sedating medications when possible. • Include written instructions of follow-up for all patient teaching performed when the patient could experience neurotoxicity.
Arthralgias (joint discomfort)	• At rest or with weight bearing • Accompanying swelling • Crepitus palpable over joint	• Administer analgesics as ordered. • Offer heat application to areas of joint pain. • Document patient responses to pain relief measures.
Myalgias	• Quality (cramping, spasmodic, or dull) • Location • Exacerbating factors • Alleviating factors	• Inability to stand without lower back or leg pain • Offer heat application to areas of muscle tension. • Make necessary referrals for the use of massage, relaxation techniques, etc. • Encourage rest periods to coincide with peak of symptoms.
Skin changes: erythema, rash, increased skin temperature	• Skin dry or moist • Rash characteristics (color, raised or flat, pruritus, distribution)	• Administer diphenhydramine as needed for pruritus. • Use lipid-based, nonscented creams to keep skin moist. • Keep nails clipped low or covered to avoid scratching induced skin abrasions.

Fever	• Temperature greater than 100.5°F (38.5°C) • Temperature increase greater than 1°C from baseline	• Measure and document temperature at least twice per shift, daily during ambulatory therapy, check every hour when febrile. • Monitor and document hydration status daily: intake and output; assess skin and mucous membranes; monitor for tachycardia, tachypnea, orthostasis, hypotension; check urine specific gravity against intake and output if dehydration is suspected. • Initiate patient education for managing body temperature; document teaching and patient's understanding of at least one management strategy. • Administer antipyretics as ordered. • Provide tepid sponge bath, etc., if unresponsive to antipyretic medications. • Provide cool, comfortable environment. • Remove heat sources such as blankets, unnecessary electrical equipment, etc. • Use indirect fans. • Encourage increased fluid intake during fever. • Assess temporal relationship to biologic medication administration, and determine if fever may be infection related; perform cultures if infection is suspected or possible. • Monitor for CNS changes with prolonged or very high fever.
Chills/rigors	• Sensation of cold/chills	• Keep chilled patient warm. • Provide emotional support during chills. • Medicate with meperidine or benzodiazepine to break a severe rigor.

(continued)

TABLE 4–2 Management of Common Adverse Effects of Biotherapy (Continued)

Symptom/Sign	Assessment	Interventions
Anorexia	• Vocalization of lack of desire to eat • Decreased oral intake • Taste alterations	• Offer small, frequent feedings. • Encourage eating foods the patient likes. • Avoid strong-smelling or strong-flavored foods.
Nausea/vomiting	• Presence, frequency, and perceived distress related to sensations of nausea, retching, and vomiting • Hyperactive upper-quadrant bowel sounds	• Offer small, frequent feedings. • Use antiemetic agents as needed. • Encourage nonpharmacologic management of symptoms (guided imagery, relaxation). • Remove plastic lids from food trays before entering the room. • Avoid potent odors (perfumes). • Encourage cold foods that may be less nausea inducing, have less odor.
Fatigue	• Apathy • Sensation of inability to feel rested • Lack of motivation • Easily tired • Decreased concentration	• Identify time periods when fatigue is at its worst (often 4–8 hours after biotherapy dose). • Give biotherapeutic agent on a schedule to anticipate the fatigue peaking during normal sleep period. • Identify specific variables causing worsening fatigue (eg, heat, argumentative situation, headache); avoid variables when possible. • Identify individualized strategies to reduce incidence or severity of fatigue. • Monitor laboratory values that may contribute to or worsen fatigue symptoms (eg, anemia, hypokalemia). • Encourage frequent rest periods alternating with mild exercise, which may increase energy level. • Assess coping strategies, tendencies for depression, or feelings of hopelessness that may be exacerbated by fatigue. • Discuss need for therapy break if fatigue is severe and unremitting.

Fluid retention	• Increased weight	• Weigh daily, report greater than 2 kg gain.
	• Dependent edema	• Assess for edema in dependent areas.
	• Dyspnea	• Evaluate intake and output every shift during hospitalization, or through a patient log during ambulatory therapy.
	• Dysrhythmias	
	• Oliguria	• Monitor urine output; fluid retention may cause decreased urine output.
		• Monitor breath sounds, respiratory rate, and respiratory effort for symptoms of interstitial fluid.
		• Monitor central venous pressure (CVP) levels in hospitalized patients; CVP may be elevated if fluid volume is high, but often fluid extravasates into interstitial spaces and CVP is low.
		• Periodically assess electrolyte values for hemodilution and low values that are common with fluid retention.
Hypotension	• BP less than 90 systolic	• Monitor BP frequently, especially if orthostatic symptoms are present.
	• BP more than 40 mmHg below baseline systolic	• Investigate origins, onset, timing, and precipitating factors associated with nausea to ascertain whether may be indicative of vascular volume depletion.
	• Dizziness	
	• Nausea	
	• Blurred vision, stars in vision	
	• Oliguria	• Monitor tissue perfusion during hypotension (eg, mental status, urine output, bowel sounds) to determine need for intervention.
	• Altered mental status	• Administer crystalloid or colloid fluid changes as ordered.
	• Decreased bowel sounds	• Administer vasopressors or inotropic agents as ordered; be aware, these agents will precipitate severe tachycardia if the patient is actually volume depleted.
	• Cool, clammy, dusky or cyanotic skin, especially of extremities	

Patient outcomes/goals:
• Patient notifies health care providers when reportable symptoms occur.
• Patient uses preventive strategies for common adverse effects.
• Patient identifies helpful strategies to abrogate symptoms and implements them independently.

D. Financial Considerations: Confirm insurance coverage for home or outpatient therapy because reimbursement for biotherapy is inconsistent and may depend on the disease, dose, or setting in which dose is administered.

VII. Summary: Biotherapy is the fourth cancer treatment modality with its growth paralleling our development of DNA technology and manipulation of immune system activities. Administration of biotherapeutic agents involves the integration of a multidisciplinary team of which the nurse is coordinator. Nursing knowledge and understanding of the science and art of administering biological therapy and nursing experience in caring for patients receiving these agents will contribute to the realization of the therapy's future applications.

REFERENCES

Armstrong, A. C., Eaton, D., & Ewing, J. C. (2002). Cellular vaccine therapy for cancer. *Expert Review Vaccine*, 1(3), 303–316.

Bedell, C. (2003). Pegfilgrastim for chemotherapy-induced neutropenia. *Clinical Journal of Oncology Nursing*, 7(1), 55–57.

Brown, K. A., Esper, P., Kelleher, L. O., Brace O'Neill, J. E., Polovich, M., & White, J. M. (Eds.). (2001). *Chemotherapy and biotherapy guidelines and recommendations for practice.* Pittsburgh, PA: Oncology Nursing Society.

Bruner, R. J., & Farag, S. S. (2003). Monoclonal antibodies for the prevention and treatment of graft-versus-host disease. *Seminars in Oncology*, 30(4), 509–519.

Buchsel, P. C., Forgey, A., Grape, F. B., & Hamann, S. S. (2002). Granulocyte macrophage colony-stimulating factor: Current practice and novel approaches. *Clinical Journal of Oncology Nursing*, 6(4), 198–204.

Buchsel, P. C., Murphy, B. J., & Newton, S. A. (2002). Epoetin alfa: Current and future indications and nursing implications. *Clinical Journal of Oncology Nursing*, 6(5), 261–266.

Bush, S. (2002). Monoclonal antibodies conjugated with radioisotopes for the treatment of non-Hodgkin's lymphoma. *Seminars in Oncology Nursing*, 18(1 Suppl. 1), 16–21.

Camacho, L. H. (2003). Clinical applications of retinoids in cancer medicine. *Journal of Biological Regulators and Homeostatic Agents*, 17(1), 98–114.

Cersosimo, R. J. (2003). Monoclonal antibodies in the treatment of cancer, Part 1. *American Journal of Health Systems Pharmacy*, 60(15), 1531–1548.

_____. (2003). Monoclonal antibodies in the treatment of cancer, Part 2. *American Journal of Health Systems Pharmacy*, 60(16), 1631–1641.

Cheng, J. D., Rieger, P. T., von Mehren, M., Adams, G. P., & Weiner, L. M. (2000). Recent advances in immunotherapy and monoclonal antibody treatment of cancer. *Seminars in Oncology Nursing,* 16(4 Suppl. 1), 2–12.

Coleman, C. (1998). Overview of biotherapy and nursing considerations. *Journal of Intravenous Nursing*, 21(6), 367–373.

Cuaron, L., & Thompson, J. (2001). The interferons. In P. T. Reiger (Ed.), *Biotherapy. A comprehensive overview* (2nd ed., pp. 123–194). Sudbury, MA: Jones & Bartlett.

Cumisky, S. (2000). BCG immunotherapy for carcinoma of the urinary bladder. *Nursing Standards*, 14(37), 45–47.

Dereure, O. (2003). Skin reactions related to treatment with anticytokines, membrane receptor inhibitors and monoclonal antibodies. *Expert Opinions in Drug Safety*, 2(5), 467–473.

Drevs, J., Laus, C., Mendinger, M., Schmidt-Gersbach, C., & Unger, C. (2002). Antiangiogenesis: Current clinical data and future perspectives. *Onkologie*, 25(6), 520–527.

Estes, J. M. (2002). Handling and disposal of monoclonal antibodies. *Clinical Journal of Oncology Nursing*, 6(5), 290–291.

Frankel, C. (2000). Nursing management considerations with trastuzumab (Herceptin). *Seminars in Oncology Nursing*, 16(4 Suppl.1), 23–28.

Fumagalli, L. A., Vinke, J., Hoff, W., Ypma, E., Brivio, F., & Nespoli, A. (2003). Lympho-cyte counts independently predict overall survival in advanced cancer patients: A biomarker for IL-2 immunotherapy. *Journal of Immunotherapy*, 26(5), 394–402.

Gale, D., & Sorokin, P. (2001). The interleukins. In P. T. Reiger (Ed.), *Biotherapy. A Comprehensive Overview* (2nd ed., pp. 195–244). Sudbury, MA: Jones & Bartlett.

Gemmill, R., & Idell, C. S. (2003). Biological advances for new treatment approaches. *Seminars in Oncology Nursing*, 19(3), 162–168.

Hendrix, C. S., de Leon, C., & Dillman, R. O. (2002). Radioimmunotherapy for non-Hodgkin's lymphoma with yttrium 90 ibritumomab tiuxetan. *Clinical Journal in Oncology Nursing*, 6(3), 144–148.

Kahan, B. D., Kirken, R. A., & Stepkowski, S. M. (2003). New approaches to transplant immunosuppression. *Transplant Proceedings*, 35(5), 1621–1623.

Kennedy, R. C., & Shearer, M. H. (2003). A role for antibodies in tumor immunity. *International Review of Immunology*, 22(2), 141–172.

Kinzler, D., & Brown, C. K. (2001). Cancer vaccines. In P. T. Reiger (Ed.), *Biotherapy. A comprehensive overview* (2nd ed., pp. 357–382). Sudbury, MA: Jones & Bartlett.

Lazar, G. A., Marshall, S. A., Plecs, J. J., Mayo, S. L., & Desjarlais, J. R. (2003). Design-ing proteins for therapeutic applications. *Current Opinions in Structural Biology*, 13(4), 513–518.

Lewis, J. D., Reilly, B. D., & Bright, R. K. (2003). Tumor-associated antigens: From dis-covery to immunity. *International Review of Immunology*, 22(2), 81–112.

Malek, S. N., & Flinn, I. W. (2003). Incorporating monoclonal antibodies in blood and marrow transplantation. *Seminars in Oncology*, 30(4), 520–530.

Mitchell, M. S. (2003). Combinations of anticancer drugs and immunotherapy. *Cancer Immunology and Immunotherapy*, Aug 26 [Epub ahead of print].

Poole, P., & Greer, E. (2000). Immunosuppression in transplantation. A new millennium in care. *Critical Care Nursing Clinics of North America*, 12(3), 315–321.

Reiger, P. T. (2001). Biotherapy: An overview. In P. T. Reiger (Ed.), *Biotherapy. A compre-hensive overview* (2nd ed., pp. 3–37). Sudbury, MA: Jones & Bartlett.

_____. (2001). Optimizing the dose and schedule of biological agents. In P. T. Reiger (Ed.), *Biotherapy. A comprehensive overview* (2nd ed., pp. 85–122). Sudbury, MA: Jones & Bartlett.

Reiger, P. T., & Khuri, F. R. (2001). The retinoids. In P. T. Reiger (Ed.), *Biotherapy. A comprehensive overview* (2nd ed., pp. 407–430). Sudbury, MA: Jones & Bartlett.

Riley, M. B. (2003). Ibritumomab tiuxetan. *Clinical Journal of Oncology Nursing*, 7(1), 110–112.

Schmidt, K. V., & Wood, B. A. (2003). Trends in cancer therapy: Role of monoclonal antibodies. *Seminars in Oncology Nursing*, 19(3), 169–179.

Seeley, K., & DeMeyer, E. (2002). Nursing care of patients receiving Campath™. *Clini-cal Journal of Oncology Nursing*, 6(3), 138–143.

Shelton, B. K. (2001). Hematological and immune disorders. In M. L. Sole, M. L. Lam-born & J. C. Hartshorn (Eds.), *Introduction to critical care nursing* (3rd ed., pp. 405–458). Philadelphia: W. B. Saunders.

Shelton, B. K. (2004). Flu-like syndrome. In C. H. Yarbro, M. H. Frogge, & M. Good-man (Eds.), *Cancer symptom management*, (3rd ed.). Sudbury, MA: Jones & Bartlett.

Shelton, B. K., Ashenbrenner, D., & Shane, K. (2002). Biological therapy. In D. Ashen-brenner (Ed.), *Pharmacologic therapy* (pp. 583–610). Philadelphia: Lippincott Williams & Wilkins.

Waldmann H. (2003). The new immunosuppression. *Current Opinions in Chemistry and Biology*, 7(4), 476–480.

Wujcik, D. (2001). Hematopoietic growth factors. In P. T. Reiger (Ed.), *Biotherapy. A comprehensive overview* (2nd ed., pp. 245–282). Sudbury, MA: Jones & Bartlett.

5 Blood and Marrow Transplantation

Jane C. Shivnan

I. History

A. Beginnings of Blood and Marrow Transplantation (BMT): The earliest recorded attempt to use bone marrow therapeutically was in 1891, when bone marrow was administered by mouth to patients suffering from anemia and leukemia. It wasn't until the explosion of the first atomic bomb in New Mexico in 1945, however, that a concerted effort was made to understand the principles of bone marrow replacement. Work in the 1950s and 1960s helped define appropriate preparative regimens and methods of bone marrow collection and administration. The 1970s saw a focus on the application of human leukocyte antigen (HLA) typing to BMT, and the use of immunosuppressive medications to prevent and control a serious BMT complication, graft-versus-host disease (GVHD).

B. Expansion of Transplantation Technology: The clinical availability of cyclosporine-A in 1983, enhanced HLA-typing methods, improved antibiotics and antiviral medications, availability of specialized blood products for transfusional support, and other supportive treatments made the 1980s a decade in which the application of this technology grew exponentially. Further refinement of GVHD prophylaxis and treatment, as well as the use of growth factors and other biologic response modifiers, supported the increased use of bone marrow for the treatment of malignancies and disorders of the immune system. The 1990s brought a significant advance with the application of pheresis technology to the collection of peripheral blood stem cells (PBSCs). This allowed transplantation to proceed without the risks of a bone marrow harvest, and often with a more rapid engraftment of hematopoietic cells. Additional advances included the extension of transplantation technology to unrelated and HLA-mismatched donors, and the increased banking and use of a rich source of hematopoietic stem cells, umbilical cord blood (UCB).

C. Future of BMT: Current research in transplantation includes investigation of the "mini" (nonmyeloablative) allogeneic BMT, designed to create a chimeric bone marrow with both host and donor cells. Donor lymphocyte infusions (DLI) and tumor vaccines in conjunction with BMT are also under investigation. These techniques have in common a focus on the graft-versus-tumor immune system response that helps prevent relapse after allogeneic BMT. Improving preparative regimens to increase relapse-free survival and minimize toxicity continues to be a focus for BMT research. In the allogeneic BMT setting, manipulation of T-lymphocyte subpopulations in the graft and continued study of immunosuppressive regimens seek to decrease the risk of GVHD.

Changes in supportive therapies provide hope for prophylaxis and treatment of infectious complications and organ toxicities. The body of nursing research investigating short- and long-term quality of life for BMT recipients and caregivers, symptom management, and the use of alternative modalities such as massage therapy and acupressure is growing rapidly. These changes in BMT modalities and supportive care promise a future of safe, cost-effective, readily available immune system treatments for many cancers and inherited or acquired nonmalignant disorders.

II. Definition

A. Blood and marrow transplantation is a complete or partial replacement of hematopoietic stem cells after an immunosuppressive and myeloablative preparative regimen (generally a timed sequence of high-dose chemotherapy with or without radiation therapy and immunosuppressives). It is a potentially curative treatment for a wide variety of malignant and nonmalignant disorders.

B. The source of hematopoietic stem cells and type of transplant selected are based on a number of factors, including diagnosis, the patient's general state of health, and the availability of an HLA-matched familial related or unrelated bone marrow donor. Table 5–1 summarizes the advantages and disadvantages of the major types (autologous, syngeneic, and allogeneic) of transplantation.

III. Rationale for Use

A. The dose-limiting toxicity for many chemotherapeutic agents and for total body irradiation is bone marrow destruction, and the resulting life-threatening aplasia. By providing a source for new bone marrow cells, BMT facilitates the use of higher, potentially more curative doses of chemotherapy and radiation therapy in malignancies such as neuroblastoma.

TABLE 5–1 Types of Stem Cell Transplantation

Type of Transplantation	Advantages	Disadvantages
Autologous: bone marrow, PBSCs or UCB obtained from self	Readily available. Lower morbidity and mortality.	Generally higher risk of relapse. May have prolonged engraftment with bone marrow and UCB.
Syngeneic: bone marrow or PBSCs obtained from identical twin	Lower morbidity and mortality than allogeneic.	Few such donors exist. Higher relapse rate than allogeneic due to the lack of graft-versus-tumor effect.
Allogeneic: bone marrow, PBSCs or UCB obtained from related or unrelated donor with HLA-identical (or near identical) phenotype	Related bone marrow has lowest risk of relapse. Mini-BMT requires less intense preparative regimen and has low morbidity and mortality.	Highest morbidity and mortality, especially with unrelated. Acute and chronic GVHD remain significant risks.

B. BMT can also be used to treat primary disorders of the bone marrow. BMT allows the replacement of diseased bone marrow with healthy cells in diseases such as aplastic anemia, thalassemia, myelofibrosis, and leukemia.

C. The observed graft-versus-tumor effect of transplanted allogeneic hematopoietic stem cells enhances the immune system's ability to control residual malignant disease and prevent relapse.

D. The usefulness of BMT as an intensive treatment modality is demonstrated by the variety of diseases treated: hematologic malignancies, solid tumors, genetic disorders, immune deficiencies, and autoimmune disorders (Table 5–2).

IV. Biology of Therapy

A. It had long been surmised that a pluripotent hematopoietic stem cell exists, capable of repopulating bone marrow and producing all of the differentiated cells made by that organ. Advances in the identification of cells through immunoassays have shown that cells carrying CD34 antigens on their cell surfaces may be pluripotent hematopoietic stem cells. These cells are found in bone marrow, UCB, and, in small numbers, circulating in the peripheral bloodstream.

B. Destruction of the bone marrow may be done deliberately to treat a primary disorder of the bone marrow or may occur as a side effect of therapy aimed at destroying tumor cells. An infusion of stem cells from a source such as bone marrow, UCB, or peripheral blood allows repopulation of bone marrow and production of red blood cells, white blood cells, and platelets. Measurable numbers of differentiated cells usually reach the peripheral bloodstream within 1 to 4 weeks of infusion.

TABLE 5–2   Diseases Treated by BMT and PBSCT

Autologous	Allogeneic
Malignant	*Malignant*
Leukemias: AML, ALL	Leukemias: AML, ALL, CML
Lymphomas	Lymphomas
Hodgkin's disease	Hodgkin's disease
Multiple myeloma	Multiple myeloma
Ovarian cancer	Myelodysplastic syndrome
Testicular cancer	*Nonmalignant*
Sarcomas	Aplastic anemia
Neuroblastoma	Thalassemia
	Fanconi's anemia
	Wiskott-Aldrich syndrome
	Severe combined immunodeficiency (SCIDS)
	Lipid storage diseases
	Mucopolysaccharidoses
	Sickle cell disease

V. Process of BMT

A. Pretransplantation Evaluation and Consultation: Before beginning the actual process of BMT, it is important to make sure that the patient is able to withstand the rigors of BMT and that the patient understands and is willing to undergo this potentially life-threatening treatment.

  1. Eligibility criteria: All patients undergoing BMT must meet specific eligibility criteria that help predict their ability to withstand this intensive treatment modality. Criteria will vary among institutions as well as for different diseases and treatment protocols, but generally include measures of organ function, disease status, and health (Table 5–3). Before starting the BMT, staff at the transplantation center collect and review patient data to ensure that the patient meets the clinical eligibility criteria for transplantation.

  2. Insurance verification: Due to the high costs associated with this intensive treatment, verification of insurance coverage or adequate financial resources is also obtained. Frequently, the patient and family must find additional funding sources within their community to finance the cost of BMT. Although direct costs such as hospitalization, outpatient treatment, pharmacy charges, and blood products are often covered by insurance, indirect costs such as housing, travel, child care, living expenses away from home, loss of income of the patient and primary caregiver, and loss of income are generally borne by the patient and family.

  3. Informed consent: The complexity and potential morbidity of the procedure must be explained to the patient as part of an informed consent process. A variety of teaching methods (videos, printed materials, discussion) are helpful in providing the patient with sufficient knowledge about the procedure, as well as its risks and potential benefits. The nurse plays an important role in reinforcing information and supporting the patient and family during this decision-making process.

B. Preparation for transplantation

  1. Intravenous (IV) access is needed throughout the transplantation process for blood sampling, medication administration, parenteral

---

▨ TABLE 5–3 Example of Eligibility Criteria for Transplant

Age	Generally ≤ 55 years for allogeneic, 70 for mini-BMT*
	Generally ≤ 70 years for autologous, syngeneic
Availability of stem cells	HLA-identical match or harvestable marrow or PBSCs
Disease status	In remission or with limited tumor burden
Organ function	Cardiac function: no cardiac disease, left ventricular function ≥ 45%
	Pulmonary function: no pulmonary disease, normal function
	Renal function: both kidneys healthy, creatinine ≤ 2.0 mg/dL
	Hepatic function: no liver disease, bilirubin ≤ 2.0 mg/dL
Other risk factors	No active infections (eg, HIV, aspergillosis)
	No other serious medical or psychiatric illnesses

*Organ function, disease status, and risk factor criteria are also relaxed for mini-BMTs.

nutrition, and blood product administration. For patients undergoing PBSC transplantation, large-bore IV access is required for apheresis. Long-term indwelling catheters (eg, Hickman or Groshong), frequently with two or three lumens, are usually inserted before transplantation to support the need for IV access. The nurse should review the procedure for insertion and care of the catheter with the patient. Nosocomial bloodstream infections are a serious risk to BMT patients, and meticulous catheter care based on research findings and national guidelines is essential. Long-term indwelling catheters are usually inserted in an operating room or fluoroscopy procedure room under local anesthesia or IV conscious sedation.

2. Bone marrow harvest is an operative procedure most often done under epidural or spinal anesthesia in adults (general anesthesia in children). During the procedure, large-bore needles are inserted through the skin and underlying tissues into the iliac crest of the patient (autologous) or donor (allogeneic). Bone marrow is aspirated into large syringes, and the needles are manipulated into different areas of the bone to maximize marrow removal. The volume removed is based on the size of the recipient and the estimated cell count of the marrow. It is filtered in the operating room to remove tissue particles and is then heparinized. Autologous marrow is usually cryopreserved using dimethyl sulfoxide (DMSO). Bone marrow donors often experience pain after the procedure and may also experience complications such as bleeding, orthostasis, loss of mobility, and infection. Full recovery from the harvest can be expected within a few weeks.

3. Only small amounts of stem cells are located in the peripheral blood, and stem calls must be encouraged to enter the peripheral blood. PBSC harvest begins with a step known as "priming" or "mobilizing" stem cells. The donor is generally given a combination of a chemotherapeutic drug (eg, cyclophosphamide) and a growth factor in a timed, sequential fashion. This stimulates existing marrow to produce and release stem cells into the peripheral blood. When the number of circulating PBSCs is deemed sufficient by analyzing serial white blood counts and differentials, the donor undergoes apheresis. During this procedure, IV access by way of a large-bore central catheter allows blood to flow through a pheresis machine, which separates out the fraction of blood most likely to contain PBSCs and returns the remainder of the cells and plasma to the patient. The PBSCs are then treated and stored in a manner similar to autologous marrow.

4. UCB is a rich source of hematopoietic stem cells and may be collected at birth for allogeneic use or for potential future autologous use. Numerous UCB banks have been created, but the standardization and accreditation of UCB banks are still in early stages. Limiting factors for more widespread use of unrelated UCB transplantation have included the low volume of stem cells present in UCB and delayed engraftment. Approximately 700 unrelated donor and 150 sibling donor UCB transplants have been performed to date (National Marrow Donor Program, 2003). Techniques to enhance

engraftment through ex vivo expansion of stem cell populations and improvements in collection techniques are under investigation.

5. The purpose of the preparative regimen of high-dose chemotherapy with or without radiation therapy is to destroy existing marrow and tumor cells elsewhere in the body; to make space for new marrow to grow, particularly in conditions such as myelofibrosis; and to provide immunosuppression, particularly in allogeneic BMT. The choice of preparative regimen is based on the disease and type of transplantation. Most preparative regimens last from several days to a week or more and may be given in an inpatient or outpatient setting depending on the method of delivery, the expected side effects, and the institution.

C. Infusion of Stem Cells: On the day of transplantation, the bone marrow or stem cells are infused into the bloodstream using methods similar to the transfusion of blood products. The volume of the stem cell product and the method of infusion vary depending on the source of stem cells and the need for additional manipulation of the product. The largest available lumen of a central line is generally used for administration. The possibility of serious side effects exists, including anaphylaxis. Emergency medications and equipment should be immediately available, and staff should receive adequate training in the administration of these stem cell products.

1. Autologous bone marrow is thawed before administration by immersion in a warm water bath. The 100-mL to 500-mL product may be administered in syringes by slow IV push or in small infusion bags. Immediate side effects are generally related to the amount of DMSO in the product and may include flushing, nausea, chest tightness, and bradycardia, and dysgeusia caused by the DMSO.

2. PBSCs and UCB are administered in a similar fashion to autologous bone marrow. Unmanipulated PBSCs may have a higher volume and, therefore, may contain higher concentration of DMSO. The infusion will generally take longer, with rest periods provided for the recipient (if necessary), and side effects are usually more frequently observed.

3. Allogeneic bone marrow is usually administered in one or two large infusion bags. Unmanipulated ABO-compatible bone marrow is similar to whole blood in appearance, and its volume of 500 mL to 2 L is usually administered over 2 to 4 hours. Bone marrow may be manipulated to remove red blood cells if the donor and recipient are ABO-incompatible or to remove selected lymphocytes to reduce the risk of GVHD. These smaller volumes of 200 mL to 600 mL are also administered over 2 to 4 hours. Side effects of allogeneic bone marrow infusions may be due to allergic reactions (fever, chills, pruritus), volume overload (edema, hypertension, tachycardia), or, rarely, intravascular hemolysis (anaphylaxis, hemoglobinuria). PBSC transplantation is also being used in allogeneic recipients. The donor goes through "mobilization" with growth factor only in preparation for pheresis of the PBSCs. PBSCs in healthy donors can often be collected through large-bore needles in the antecubital veins.

D. Recovery of Immune Function: Adequate production of white blood cells (ie, absolute neutrophil count ≥500/mm³) generally takes 10 days to several weeks, depending on the source and quantity of stem cells. Full recovery of immune function and of all bone marrow function may take several months. Generally, white blood cell production recovers first, followed by platelet and red blood cell production. Much of the person's immune memory is also lost, making patients vulnerable to both reactivation of viral infections, such as herpes simplex and cytomegalovirus, and new infections with pathogens such as varicella (chickenpox) or polio. Six months to a year after transplantation, patients are generally revaccinated against most "childhood" diseases.

VI. Nursing Issues

A. Administration: The specialized nature of BMT nursing and the intensity of the treatment provided to patients support the need for a designated setting and staff. In addition to the nursing care required, patients undergoing transplantation and their families may need significant psychological support during this difficult process.

1. Inpatient services: Beds are ideally grouped in a separate transplantation unit or as part of a hematology or oncology unit. Medical, nursing, social work, nutrition, and other discipline staff should be trained in the processes of BMT and the unique needs of BMT patients and families. There should be 24-hour access to ancillary services, such as pharmacy, laboratory, radiology, and blood bank services. Provision should be made for critical care, either through training the staff to provide critical care on the unit or training intensive care unit (ICU) staff in the basics of BMT. Survival of BMT patients who require critical care continues to improve with advances in supportive therapy. The nurse-to-patient ratio varies nationally depending on factors such as the type of transplantation and the provision of critical care but is usually not more than 1:3 on average. Specific educational needs for staff are outlined in Box 5-1.

▼ **BOX 5-1** | **Educational Needs of Transplantation Staff**

Chemotherapy and radiation therapy: administration, side effects, safe handling

Vascular access devices: care of devices, dressings, troubleshooting

Understanding BMT: immune system, types of transplantation, sources of stem cells, apheresis, DLI

BMT critical care: sepsis, congestive heart failure, superior vena cava syndrome, pneumonia, bronchiolitis obliterans, hepatic failure, renal failure, GI bleeding

Complications of transplantation: nausea and vomiting, pain, fatigue, infection, bleeding, organ toxicities, GVHD, long-term complications

Supportive measures: medications, infection prevention, assessment skills, blood product support, nutritional support

Psychosocial support of the patient and family: anxiety, depression, delirium, grief, guilt, survivorship

2. Ambulatory services: BMT outpatient services may be provided in a specialized setting or by a trained staff within an oncology outpatient department or practice. Most BMT patients require a period of close observation after discharge for complications related to transplantation (eg, GVHD, cytomegalovirus pneumonia) before they are referred back to their primary care physicians or oncologists. BMT care is shifting rapidly to the outpatient setting, with innovative programmatic changes designed to reduce the number of inpatient days required and the total cost of transplantation. Changes in transplantation methods, such as the use of PBSCs and mini-BMTs, have accelerated this trend.

B. Patient and Family Education: The patient undergoing BMT and the patient's family and friends have significant educational needs throughout the BMT process (Table 5–4). Shifting care to outpatient settings places an even greater burden on the patient and family, increasing the importance of adequate, thorough, and well-designed educational programs.

1. The nurse has an important role in teaching the patient and family self-care skills. To fully participate in care, patients need to understand the process of transplantation and to have access to information about their care and treatment.
2. The nurse may need to learn methods for teaching pediatric patients, patients who do not speak English, and patients and families with specific cultural, psychological, or religious needs.

C. Psychological and Social Support: Throughout the transplantation process, numerous stressors affect the patient and family.

1. The nurse must be skilled in assessing the psychological status of the patient and supporting the patient and family throughout the process.
2. Frequently, problems arise that require assessment and intervention from a specialized social worker, psychological liaison nurse, psychologist, or psychiatrist. For example, a patient or family member may experience anxiety or depression or may have problems with substance abuse, noncompliance, or suicidal ideation.

D. Complementary and Alternative Treatment Modalities: BMT patients may be helped by the judicious use of nonpharmacologic methods to decrease symptoms of pain, fatigue, anxiety, and depression.

1. The nurse should obtain a complete history of vitamin and herbal supplement use, as well as over-the-counter medication use. Many of these agents may be dangerous during BMT, potentiating bleeding or exposing the immunocompromised patient to microbial contamination of unregulated products.
2. Massage therapy has been shown to have beneficial effects on fatigue, nausea, distress, and anxiety in BMT patients. Acupressure and acupuncture studies have had mixed outcomes, with some studies showing no added benefit and some showing positive effects on nausea and vomiting. Music therapy, relaxation therapy, distraction, and exercise have also been found to have potential benefits for BMT patients.

E. Adverse Effects: There are numerous common acute complications of BMT that require prompt and expert nursing assessment, management, and evaluation (Table 5–5, and also see Chapters 6, 8, and 22). In

TABLE 5-4 Examples of Educational Needs of BMT Patients and Families

Pretransplant	Preparative Regimen	Stem Cell Infusion	Recovery	Discharge and Long-term Care
Process of BMT	Side effects of chemotherapy and total body irradiation	Process of stem cell infusion	Temperature-taking, reporting symptoms	Managing fatigue, resuming normal activities
Care of long-term indwelling IV catheter	Maintaining good nutrition	Possible side effects, management	Self-care activities and infection prevention	Preventing infection
Stem cell collection: process, side effects	Managing nausea and vomiting		Possible problems: infections, GVHD, VOD, mucositis	Long-term risks: relapse, sterility, chronic GVHD

TABLE 5-5 Common Complications of Transplantation

Complications of chemotherapy	Nausea and vomiting
	Diarrhea
	Hemorrhagic cystitis
	Seizures
	Alopecia
	Mucositis
	Fatigue
Complications of total body irradiation	Fever
	Parotitis
	Nausea and vomiting
	Diarrhea
	Alopecia
	Mucositis
	Fatigue
	Cataracts
Complications of bone marrow suppression	Bacterial and fungal infections
	Viral reactivation or infections
	Bleeding
	Anemia

addition to these side effects of chemotherapy, total body irradiation, and bone marrow suppression, there are some potentially life-threatening complications of BMT rarely seen in other clinical settings.

1. Veno-occlusive disease (VOD) of the liver is a side effect of high doses of certain chemotherapeutic agents, such as busulfan, and total body irradiation. It occurs in approximately 20% of patients. The disease is generally diagnosed based on the clinical symptoms of painful hepatomegaly, bilirubinemia, and weight gain, which is usually not responsive to diuretics. With VOD, the liver is characterized by fibrosis and particulate matter that blocks the venules. This can lead to hepatomegaly and eventual destruction of hepatocytes. As many as half of patients who develop VOD will die from progressive hepatic encephalopathy and coagulopathies. Efforts at prevention include dose modification of busulfan, liver-shielding during irradiation, and low-dose heparin administration. Treatments include systemic anticoagulation with heparin and tissue plasminogen activator (t-PA) or the more promising antithrombotic and thrombolytic, defibrotide. Bleeding complications have limited the use of these agents. Nursing interventions include the following:
   a. Monitor intake and output, weight gain, abdominal girth, pain intensity and location, respiratory rate and pattern, and mental status.
   b. Administer medications such as diuretics and analgesics as ordered, oxygen therapy, and blood products.
   c. Protect from injury due to aspiration, bleeding, falls, or delirium.
   d. Ensure adequate nutritional intake through use of supplements, if appropriate, or parenteral nutrition.
   e. Provide support and information to patient and family.

2. Acute GVHD is an immunologic complication of allogeneic BMT due to activity of donor-derived lymphocytes against the recipient's cells and organs (Table 5–6). Acute GVHD usually occurs within the first 3 months after allogeneic BMT and often begins as engraftment occurs. Even with fully HLA-matched transplants, acute GVHD occurs in 40% to 60% of allogeneic BMT recipients. Its incidence is higher in transplantations that are not fully HLA matched and in unrelated donor transplantations and allogeneic PBSC transplantations. Its incidence is lower in UCB transplantations and in transplantation of bone marrow that has been manipulated to remove selected groups of lymphocytes thought to be involved in GVHD; however, the risk of graft failure and relapse may be higher in these types of transplantation. Acute GVHD is life-threatening, and its treatment with immunosuppressive medications places the patient at increased risk of infections such as aspergillosis and viral pneumonias. Nursing interventions include the following:

a. Monitor for presence of skin rash, particularly on the palms, soles, ears, and trunk. Assess for increased erythema, blistering of skin, and itching.

b. Monitor for increased volume of diarrhea, abdominal pain and cramping, increased nausea and vomiting, and elevated liver function tests.

c. Administer immunosuppressant medications as ordered and monitor for signs and symptoms of infections.

d. Protect against skin breakdown and injury.

3. Chronic GVHD occurs in about 20% of long-term survivors of allogeneic BMT. It appears to be an autoimmune disorder, with features often similar to scleroderma. Patients with chronic GVHD are at increased risk for infections such as bacterial pneumonia and sepsis. Chronic GVHD can seriously limit functional ability and quality of life. Nursing interventions include the following:

a. Monitor for presence of skin dryness or rash, skin thickening or discoloration, white plaques within mouth, and dry eyes.

b. Administer immunosuppressant medications as ordered and teach patient and family about medications and signs and symptoms of infections (patient is frequently treated as outpatient).

c. Refer patient to physical therapy and encourage use of exercise program to maintain flexibility and range of motion.

d. Provide patient with items such as artificial tears and saliva as needed.

e. Ensure patient has adequate nutritional intake and refer to dietitian as needed.

f. Encourage patient and family to use support groups and other sources of psychological support.

F. Long-Term Complications of BMT: In addition to chronic GVHD, there are other long-term complications of BMT that may impact survival and the quality of life experienced after transplantation (Box 5–2). Nursing plays an important role in the early detection of these complications, as well as in helping the patient and family to manage their sequelae.

TABLE 5–6   Graft-Versus-Host Disease (GVHD)

	Target Organs	Possible Symptoms	Prophylaxis	Treatment
Acute GVHD	Skin Liver GI tract	Erythema, pruritus, pain, follicular rash, blistering, desquamation, bilirubinemia, elevated liver enzymes, profuse diarrhea, GI mucosa damage	Methotrexate Cyclosporine-A Tacrolimus Steroids Manipulating bone marrow to remove lymphocytes	Increased doses of immuno-suppressive therapy Mycophenolate Antithymocyte globulin (ATG) Monoclonal antibodies
Chronic GVHD	Skin Eyes Mouth Salivary glands GI tract Muscles Liver Vagina	Skin dryness, changes in pigmentation, thickening skin, inability to sweat, dry eyes, xerostomia, difficulty swallowing, anorexia, muscle weakness, polymyositis, fasciitis, contractures, cirrhosis, vaginal dryness and thickening	As for acute GVHD	Steroids Cyclosporine-A Thalidomide Psoralen and ultraviolet light treatments (PUVA) Extracorporeal photochemotherapy

▼ **BOX 5-2** | **Long-Term Complications**

Neurologic
Changes in attention span, memory, or ability to learn; peripheral neuropathy; leukoencephalopathy; CNS relapse

Endocrine
Hypothyroidism; decreased fertility or sterility; ovarian failure and early menopause; growth retardation

Ophthalmic
Cataracts; changes in visual acuity; sicca (dry eye) syndrome

Cardiopulmonary
Cardiomyopathy; congestive heart failure; pericarditis; pulmonary fibrosis; bronchiolitis obliterans; interstitial pneumonitis

Renal
Renal insufficiency, often a nephrotic syndrome; hemolytic uremia syndrome; hemorrhagic cystitis

Musculoskeletal
Aseptic necrosis

Other
Graft failure or dysfunction; relapse; secondary malignancy

REFERENCES

Ahles, T. A., et al. (1999). Massage therapy for patients undergoing autologous bone marrow transplantation. *Journal of Pain and Symptom Management, 18*(3), 157–163.

Buchsel, P. C., & Whedon, M. B. (Eds.). (1995). *Bone marrow transplantation: Administrative and clinical strategies.* Boston: Jones & Bartlett.

Lewis, I. D. (2002). Clinical and experimental uses of umbilical cord blood. *Internal Medicine Journal, 32*(12), 601–609.

National Marrow Donor Program. (2003). See *www.nmdp.org.*

Richardson, P. G., et al. (1998).Treatment of severe veno-occlusive disease with defibrotide: Compassionate use results in response without significant toxicity in a high-risk population. *Blood, 92*(3), 737–744.

Santos, G. (1983). History of bone marrow transplantation. *Clinical Haematology, 12,* 611–639.

Scott, P. H., et al. (2002). Survival following mechanical ventilation of recipients of bone marrow transplants and peripheral blood stem cell transplants. *Anaesthesiology and Intensive Care, 30*(3), 289–294.

Shivnan, J., Shelton, B. K., & Onners, B. K. (1996). Bone marrow transplantation: Issues for critical care nurses. *AACN Clinical Issues, 7*(1), 95–108.

Tarzian, A. J., et al. (1999). Autologous bone marrow transplantation: The patient's perspective of information needs. *Cancer Nursing, 22*(2), 103–110.

Whedon, M. B., & Wujcik, D. (Eds.). (1997). *Blood and marrow stem cell transplantation: Principles, practice, and nursing insights* (2nd ed.). Boston: Jones & Bartlett.

6 Chemotherapy

MiKaela Olsen

I. Definition: Chemotherapy is the use of various chemical agents that interfere with the replication and other normal functions of cancer cells, resulting in cell death. The modern use of chemotherapy began in the 1940s with the discovery that mustard gas causes myelosuppression in those exposed to it. Further investigation with the derivative nitrogen mustard revealed a significant antitumor effect. The continued development of chemotherapeutic agents has led to dramatic improvement in survival for people with various tumor types, including childhood leukemia, Hodgkin's and non-Hodgkin's lymphomas, and testicular cancer. As new agents are discovered, the list of chemotherapy agents continues to grow and new classifications of chemotherapy agents are being identified.

II. Rationale for Use

  A. Because malignant cells tend to divide more rapidly than normal tissue cells, chemotherapy should have a greater effect on the malignant cells.

  B. Chemotherapy provides a systemic approach to the treatment of cancer. Systemic treatment is necessary for cancers that are disseminated by nature, such as leukemias, or cancers that have metastasized.

  C. The goals of chemotherapy are cure, control, or palliation.

   1. Cure: Some malignancies may be cured with the use of chemotherapy alone or in conjunction with other treatment modalities. Adjuvant therapy is the use of chemotherapy in conjunction with a primary treatment in an attempt to eliminate any undetectable metastatic spread and to increase the chance of cure.

   2. Control: When a cure is not a realistic goal, chemotherapy may be used to control the disease. The aim is to extend the length and improve the quality of life by preventing development of new problems and symptoms.

   3. Palliation: When neither cure nor control of the malignancy is possible, chemotherapy may be used to reduce the tumor burden and related symptoms and possibly improve the quality of life.

III. Biology of Therapy

  A. Cell Cycle Phase: Cells undergoing replication move through several phases. These phases occur in both normal and malignant cells (Fig. 6–1). Cells are most sensitive to chemotherapeutic agents while they are actively dividing. Some chemotherapy drugs work only during specific phases of the cell division cycle (cell cycle specific), whereas others work throughout the process (cell cycle nonspecific).

  B. Tumor Sensitivity to Chemotherapy: Tumors with a large number of dividing cells are more sensitive to chemotherapy drugs than tumors with more cells in the resting phase. Tumors can also develop resistance to

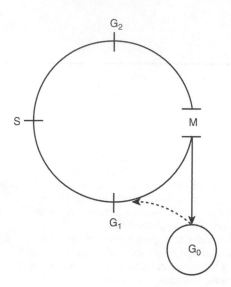

G_1 Protein and RNA synthesis
S DNA replication
G_2 Protein and RNA synthesis
M Mitosis
G_0 Resting

Figure 6–1. Phases of the cell cycle. (Porth, C. M. [1994]. *Pathophysiology: Concepts of altered health states* [4th ed.]. Philadelphia: J. B. Lippincott.)

chemotherapy drugs over time. Treatment approaches that can decrease the development of resistance include administering dose-intensive regimens (higher doses over a shorter period of time), alternating drugs with each treatment course, and shortening the intervals between treatments.

C. Combination Therapy: Although single agents are sometimes used in the treatment of cancer, combination drug therapy is increasingly becoming the norm. By combining agents, more malignant cells should be caught in a sensitive phase, resulting in a larger tumor cell kill. Several principles underlie the selection of agents for combination therapies.

1. Each drug must show efficacy in the specific tumor type.
2. The drugs chosen should have a synergistic effect or potentiate each other.
3. The drugs should have different mechanisms of action and, therefore, affect the cell in different manners.
4. The drugs should have different side effects, or similar side effects that occur at different times.

D. Repeat Dosing: Seldom will all cells in a tumor be affected by a single course of chemotherapy. Most chemotherapy regimens involve several cycles (courses) of chemotherapy repeated at specific intervals. With each repeated dose of chemotherapy, more of the cancer cells are killed, with the goal of eliminating the majority of the tumor to allow the patient's immune system to destroy any remaining cancer cells.

IV. Types of Chemotherapy Drugs: Chemotherapy drugs are classified according to how they interfere with cell division and maintenance. Table 6–1 lists commonly used chemotherapy classifications with indications and side effects.

A. Alkylating agents act by cross-linking strands of DNA, thus preventing transcription of RNA and replication of DNA. These agents can affect cells during various phases of cell division and are, therefore, cell cycle nonspecific.

B. Antimetabolites act during the S phase, interfering with DNA and RNA synthesis. These agents are considered cell cycle specific.

C. Antitumor antibiotics interfere with DNA synthesis by binding with the DNA at various points and preventing RNA synthesis. These agents may also alter the cell membrane and inhibit certain enzymes. They are cell cycle nonspecific.

D. Nitrosureas interfere with DNA synthesis and can damage the DNA helix. These agents are cell cycle specific.

E. Vinca alkaloids act in G1, G$_2$, and M phases. They block production of DNA and prevent cell division. Vinca alkaloids are cell cycle specific.

F. Taxanes prevent depolymerization of microtubules. Paclitaxel acts in the G$_2$ and M phases, whereas docetaxel acts primarily in the S phase. Taxanes are considered cell cycle specific.

G. Camptothecins act in the S phase and are known as topoisomerase I inhibitors. When topoisomerase I is inhibited, DNA damage occurs. Camptothecins are cell cycle specific.

H. Epipodophyllotoxins interfere with topoisomerase II, causing damage in the G$_2$ and S phases. They are cell cycle specific.

I. Miscellaneous agents work in a variety of ways. Asparaginase agents and procarbazine both work by inhibiting protein synthesis. These are considered cell cycle specific agents.

J. Tyrosine kinase inhibitors decrease proliferation of tumor cells and induce apoptosis.

K. Proteosome inhibitors induce apoptosis in tumor cells by blocking proteosome.

L. Hormones and hormone antagonists interfere with cellular function and growth in sensitive tissues. Corticosteroids can suppress the production of abnormal lymphocytes. Antiandrogens and antiestrogens can be administered to interfere with the replication of tumors that proliferate in the presence of these hormones, such as certain prostate and breast cancers.

V. Nursing Issues

A. Administration: Chemotherapy can be administered by several different routes depending on the drug being administered, as well as on the tumor type and location.

  1. The intravenous (IV) route allows administration of chemotherapy directly into the blood, allowing more precise control of dose and decreasing absorption issues. It is the most commonly used method.

  a. The peripheral route allows access to the blood without more invasive procedures. The peripheral route is best suited to patients undergoing short-term therapy who have healthy peripheral veins.

  b. The central route can be accessed by using a variety of central venous access devices. The choice of catheter depends on such issues as length of anticipated use, frequency with which the device will be accessed, ability of the patient and caregiver to care

(Text continues on page 70)

TABLE 6-1 Commonly Used Chemotherapy Classifications With Indications and Side Effects

Chemotherapy Agent and Classification	Adverse Effects	Special Nursing Implications
Alkylating Agents Busulfan (Myleran) Carboplatin (Paraplatin) Cisplatin (CDDP, Platinol) Melphalan (Alkeran) Cyclophosphamide (Cytoxan) Dacarbazine (DTIC) Ifosfamide (Ifex) Mechlorethamine hydrochloride (Nitrogen mustard) Thiotepa (Thioplex) Chlorambucil (Leukeran) Eloxatin (Oxaliplatin)	Myelosuppression, fatigue, nausea, vomiting, mucositis, liver and renal toxicities, second malignancies, peripheral neuropathy, suppressed sperm production and ovarian function	Seizures can occur with high doses of busulfan; administer anticonvulsant. Ototoxicity can occur with cisplatin and carboplatin. Cisplatin causes electrolyte wasting; replace and monitor electrolytes as needed. Amifostine may be used as a renal protectant with cisplatin. Myelosuppression can be delayed with melphalan (4–6 weeks in length). Melphalan and dacarbazine are irritants. Dilute drugs during administration. Hemorrhagic cystitis occurs with ifosfamide and cytoxan. Prehydration and mesna are used for prevention. Nitrogen mustard is a vesicant and irritant; administer through a side port of a free-flowing IV and flush with ≥125 mL of normal saline at the completion. Eloxatin is associated with pharyngolaryngeal dysesthesia seen in 1% to 2% of patients, characterized by subjective sensations of dysphagia or dyspnea, without any laryngospasm or bronchospasm. Thiotepa can cause severe skin toxicity in high doses.
Antimetabolites Cladribine (Leustatin) Cytarabine (cytosine arabinoside, araC, Cytosar-U) Cytarabine liposomal (DepoCyt) Floxuridine (FUDR) Fluorouracil (5-fluorouracil, 5-FU)	Myelosuppression, fatigue, nausea, vomiting, mucositis, liver and renal toxicities, rash, photosensitivity, palmar plantar erythrodyskesthesia, diarrhea, fever, interstitial pneumonitis, alopecia, hyperpigmentation of skin and veins.	Cytarabine in high doses given as a bolus infusion can cause cerebellar toxicity. Monitor patients for the inability to do rapid alternating hand movements, unsteady gait, nystagmus, slurred speech. Hold cytarabine and notify physician immediately for these symptoms. Cytarabine in high doses given in a continuous infusion causes pulmonary toxicity. Monitor fluid status and lungs closely. Cytarabine in high doses causes chemical conjunctivitis. Administer steroid eye drops as ordered. Fluorouracil is often given concurrently with leucovorin.

Methotrexate (MTX, Amethopterin Folex)
Mercaptopurine (6-MP, Purinethol)
Thioguanine (6-thioguanine, 6-TG)
Fludarabine (Fludara)
Capecitabine (Xeloda)
Gemcitabine (Gemzar)
Deoxycoformycin (Pentostatin, Nipent)
Hydroxyurea (Hydrea, Mylocel)

Warn patients to avoid sun exposure while on these medications.
High doses of methotrexate must be administered with aggressive hydration, sodium bicarbonate to alkalanize the urine, and leucovorin, which is started 24 hours after methotrexate as a rescue agent.
Pentostatin is used investigationally for graft-versus-host disease.

Antitumor Antibiotics

Bleomycin (Blenoxane)
Dactinomycin (Actinomycin D, Cosmegen)
Daunorubicin (daunomycin, Cerubidine)
Doxorubin (Adriamycin, Rubex)
Doxorubicin HCl (liposome) (Doxil)
Idarubicin (Idamycin)
Mitomycin (Mutamycin)
Mitoxantrone (Novantrone)
Plicamycin (Mithramycin, Mithracin)

Myelosuppression, fatigue, nausea, vomiting, mucositis, cardiotoxicity, liver and renal toxicities, alopecia, suppressed sperm production and ovarian function

All antitumor antibiotics are vesicants except bleomycin, Doxil, and mitoxantrone.
Administer vesicants through a side port of a free-flowing IV.
Follow institutional guidelines for bleomycin administration if test dose is required. Fever and chills frequently occur after bleomycin administration. Acetominophen can be used in the first 24 hours.
Dactinomycin is ordered in micrograms. Use caution with administration.
Red discoloration of urine can occur 1–2 days after treatment with dactinomycin, doxorubicin, and daunorubicin.
Blue/green discoloration of urine or sclera can occur 1–2 days after treatment with mitoxantrone.
Cumulative lifetime doses:
Bleomycin = 400 units
Idarubicin = 150 mg/m^2
Mitoxantrone = 140 mg/m^2
Doxorubicin = 550 mg/m^2*
*If patient has history of chest radiation, then decrease to 450 mg/m^2.

(continued)

TABLE 6–1 Commonly Used Chemotherapy Classifications With Indications and Side Effects *(Continued)*

Chemotherapy Agent and Classification	Adverse Effects	Special Nursing Implications
Nitrosureas Carmustine (BCNU) Lomustine (CCNU) Streptozocin (Zanosar)	Myelosuppression, fatigue, nausea, vomiting, mucositis, liver and renal toxicities, pulmonary toxicity, alopecia, suppressed sperm production and ovarian function	Nitrosureas are associated with a delayed nadir of approximately 4–6 weeks. Do not administer more frequently than every 4–6 weeks. Nitrosureas cross the blood-brain barrier. Carmustine is an irritant. Flush with ≥150 mL normal saline after administration.
Vinca Alkaloids Vinblastine (Velban) Vincristine (Oncovin, Vincasar, Vincrex) Vinorelbine (Navelbine)	Myelosuppression (mild with vincristine), fatigue, nausea, vomiting, mucositis, liver toxicity, peripheral neuropathy, constipation, alopecia, paralytic ileus, trigeminal nerve toxicity	All vinca alkaloids are vesicants. Administer through a side port of a free-flowing IV. If extravasation occurs, apply warm compresses per institutional guidelines. Maximum single dose of vincristine is 2 mg.
Taxanes Paclitaxel (Taxol) Docetaxel (Taxotere)	Myelosuppression, fatigue, hypersensitivity reactions, mild nausea, vomiting, myalgias, flulike symptoms, peripheral neuropathy, alopecia, cardiac toxicities, fluid retention with docetaxel	Paclitaxel premeds—steroid, h2 blocker, and antihistamine Docetaxel premeds—steroids (for prevention of fluid retention) Non-PVC tubing required for infusion of both paclitaxel and docetaxel 0.2-micron in-line filter required for paclitaxel administration
Camptothecins Topotecan (Hycamtin) Irinotecan (Camptosar, CPT-11)	Myelosuppression, fatigue, nausea, vomiting, alopecia, diarrhea	Irinotecan is associated with early (acute, during administration, or within 24 hours) and late diarrhea. Early-onset diarrhea is treated with atropine, and late-onset diarrhea is treated with Imodium. Patient teaching regarding the onset, associated signs and symptoms, and management of diarrhea is essential.

Epipodophyllotoxins

Etoposide (VP-16, Etopophos, VePesid)
Teniposide (VM-26, Vumon)

Myelosuppression, fatigue, nausea, vomiting, alopecia, hypotension, hypersensitivity reactions.

Rapid administration of these drugs results in hypotension. High doses precipitate in IV tubing and need to be diluted according to manufacturer guidelines.

Miscellaneous Agents

Asparaginase (Elspar)
Pegasparaginase (Oncaspar)
Procarbazine (Matulane)
Arsenic trioxide (Trisenox)

Myelosuppression, fatigue, nausea, vomiting, alopecia, hypersensitivity reactions, liver toxicity. ECG changes and APL differentiation syndrome with Trisenox administration.

An intradermal test dose of asparaginase may be used based on institutional guidelines.

Hyperglycemia, pancreatitis, and alterations in coagulation factors are potential toxicities that can occur with asparaginase and pegasparaginase. Monitor closely.

Polyethylene glycol (PEG) attached to the asparaginase decreases the immunogenicity and increases the half-life.

Procarbazine should not be taken with foods high in tyramine (eg, aged cheeses, avocados, bananas, beer, caffeinated beverages, chocolate, sausages, liver, over-ripe fruit, red wine, smoked or pickled fish, yeast, and yogurt).

Tyrosine Kinase Inhibitors

Gefitinib (Iressa)

Diarrhea, nausea, vomiting, rash, liver toxicity, lung toxicity, corneal erosions

Oral chemotherapy drug

Interstitial lung disease occurs in approximately 1% of patients on Iressa and can be fatal.

Imatinib mesylate (Gleevec)

Nausea, vomiting, fluid retention, neutropenia, hepatotoxicity

Check drug compatibilities carefully. Instruct patient to take with food.

Proteasome Inhibitors

Bortezomib (Velcade)

Myelosuppression, nausea, vomiting, diarrhea, anorexia, constipation, peripheral neuropathy, fever, edema, asthenia

Indicated for multiple myeloma and under investigation in other malignancies

for the device, type of treatment to be given, patient factors that may contraindicate an invasive procedure, and patient preference.

(1) Tunneled catheters may be indicated for long-term therapies that require frequent accessing of blood vessels for phlebotomy or treatment administration. They are typically flexible catheters inserted into the subclavian vein and threaded into the superior vena cava, then tunneled under the skin to a separate exit site to decrease the risk of infection and make the catheter more secure.

(2) Subcutaneous implanted ports (centrally or peripherally placed) may also be indicated for long-term therapies. These catheters consist of a soft, flexible catheter attached to a metal or plastic port with a noncoring rubber center. The centrally placed catheters are typically inserted into the subclavian vein, threaded into the superior vena cava, and connected to a port that is placed in the subcutaneous tissue. The peripherally placed catheters are inserted through the brachial veins of the arms, threaded into the superior vena cava, and connected to a port located near the antecubital fossa. The port is accessed through the skin using a noncoring needle.

(3) Peripherally inserted central catheters (PICCs) may be indicated for more short-term treatments (weeks to months). They are inserted into the brachial veins on the anterior surface of the forearm and threaded into the superior vena cava vein. They are less expensive than the other central venous access devices, but their small diameter can sometimes be limiting. (See Chapter 32.)

2. The oral route can increase ease of administration, allow for more chronic dosing of chemotherapy, and provide a route of administration for agents that cannot be given intravenously.

3. The intramuscular and subcutaneous routes can ease administration and decrease side effects for agents that are not too irritating for use by these routes.

4. The intracavitary route can be used to administer the chemotherapy into body cavities where there is tumor seeding or spread. This route is used most commonly to access the abdominal cavity or pleural space and bladder.

5. The intrathecal route is used to administer chemotherapy into the cerebral spinal fluid for patients with tumors involving the central nervous system. Intrathecal chemotherapy is administered by performing a lumbar puncture or by placing a subcutaneous intraventricular reservoir (eg, Ommaya).

6. The intraarterial route may allow delivery of higher concentrations of chemotherapy directly to the tumor, resulting in decreased systemic side effects.

B. Dose Determination

1. Chemotherapy dosing is frequently based on the patient's body surface area (BSA), ideal weight, or actual weight.

2. The BSA is a calculation derived from a patient's height and weight (Fig. 6–2). Use of the BSA allows for individualization of chemotherapy dosing with consideration of each patient's size.

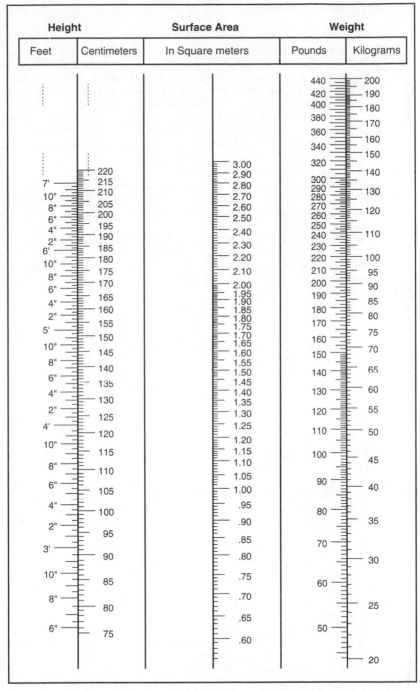

Figure 6–2. Nomogram for estimating body surface area of older children and adults. (Courtesy of Abbott Laboratories.)

C. Safe Chemotherapy Administration

1. The nurse who administers chemotherapy does the last safety check. It is important to verify that the dose was accurately calculated before drug administration. All calculations should be verified using independently obtained data (eg, height, weight, laboratory values). A second nurse should verify all calculations in order to validate that the chemotherapy doses prescribed are correct before administration.
2. Laboratory values that are pertinent to the chemotherapy agents being administered should be checked. Any abnormal laboratory values that would preclude administration of the chemotherapy should be reported to the physician.
3. If chemotherapy drugs have maximum cumulative lifetime doses associated with their administration, then the provider administering the chemotherapy should ensure that these doses have not been met or exceeded.
4. Patients and caregivers should be included in the chemotherapy administration process as another safety check. Patient education regarding the drugs, doses, side effects, toxicities, and reportable problems should be thoroughly reviewed.

D. Hazardous Drug Handling

1. Antineoplastic agents are classified as hazardous drugs. A hazardous drug is an agent that poses a significant risk to health care workers who come in contact with contaminated materials because of a potential to cause teratogenic, mutagenic, carcinogenic, or reproductive toxicity, as well as other serious organ damage.
   a. A *teratogen* can cause the development of abnormal structures in an embryo during susceptible portions of development.
   b. A *mutagen* can cause genetic mutation.
   c. A *carcinogen* can increase the risk of development of cancer.
   d. A *reproductive toxin* can potentially interfere with the normal outcomes of pregnancy.
2. Exposure to hazardous drugs can occur during preparation, transportation, administration, disposal of administration equipment, or disposal of body excreta from patients who have received hazardous drugs. Excreta and other body fluids may contain significant amounts of chemotherapy and active metabolites. Follow special handling procedures during chemotherapy administration and for 48 hours after.
3. Because it is difficult to determine safe levels of exposure to hazardous drugs, follow safety procedures when handling contaminated materials, as defined by the institutional standards.
4. There are three major routes for accidental absorption of hazardous drugs. The recommended procedures below should reduce the risk of absorption.
   a. Avoid inhalation of aerosolized particles.
      (1) Hazardous drugs should be mixed or otherwise manipulated (eg, crushed) in a biologic safety cabinet (BSC).
      (2) IV administration sets should be primed in a BSC to avoid aerosolization exposure, or the tubing should be primed with a nondrug solution before mixing the chemotherapy in the attached bag.

(3) Disruption of the IV administration set should be minimized, and connections should be wrapped with sterile gauze before disconnecting tubing from side injection ports, stopcocks, or extension tubing.
  b. Avoid contact with skin and mucous membranes.
    (1) Gloves used should be powder-free. Nitrile, polyurethane, and neoprene gloves are often used. Double gloving is recommended for hazardous drug preparation depending on the glove thickness. Protective gowns should be worn during hazardous drug preparation and administration. Gowns should be disposable, impermeable, and lint-free. Gloves, gowns, and a face shield should also be used when dealing with body fluids or excreta in patients who have received chemotherapy within 48 hours.
    (2) Gloves should be changed after completion of a task involving hazardous drugs or body excreta and whenever the gloves become torn, punctured, or contaminated. Hands should be washed before and after working with hazardous materials and whenever gloves are changed.
    (3) The work area should be limited, and a plastic-backed absorbent pad should be used to contain any accidental spillage.
    (4) Goggles or a facial splash guard should be worn during drug handling or disposal if there is a risk of splashing.
    (5) Institutional procedures should be followed quickly and efficiently in the event of spillage or contamination.
  c. Avoid accidental ingestion of hazardous drugs.
    (1) Hazardous-drug work and storage areas should be separated from places where people eat and drink.
    (2) Hands should be washed before and after working with hazardous drugs or contaminated body fluids.
    (3) Hand-to-mouth or hand-to-eye contact should be avoided while working with hazardous drugs or contaminated body fluids.
5. In the event of an accidental spill or exposure of the health care worker to the chemotherapy or to contaminated body excreta, refer to the institutional guidelines for decontamination, reporting, and evaluation.
D. Patient and Family Education
  1. Before beginning treatment with chemotherapy, give the patient information about the many aspects of treatment and care. The specific information will depend on the type of cancer, actual drugs and dosages administered, and the patient's abilities to perform self-care procedures. Consider the patient's abilities, including any impairment in vision or hearing, cultural or language barriers, age, and level of education.
  2. Discuss specific content areas with the patient and caregivers, addressing:
    a. Rationale for the chemotherapy treatment.
    b. Information about the specific drugs the patient is to receive, including how, when, and where they will be given.

  c. Expected side effects and potential management strategies.
  d. Other care needs, such as management of central venous access devices.
  e. Available resources, such as the local American Cancer Society chapter, the Cancer Information Service (1–800-CANCER), or other local support groups.

E. Adverse Effects: Chemotherapy damages cancerous and normal cells that have a high turnover rate, which adversely affects healthy cells and causes multiple systemic side effects.

 1. Infection, bleeding, and anemia: The process of blood cell production and maturation is continuous, making the white blood cells, platelets, and red blood cells vulnerable to damage from chemotherapy drugs. This can lead to decreased volumes of these blood cells, increasing the risks of infection, bleeding, and anemia (see Chapter 22).

 2. Fatigue: The most common and most distressing side effect reported by cancer patients receiving chemotherapy is fatigue. Fatigue requires a multidimensional approach due to the numerous contributing causes (see Chapter 25).

 3. Nausea and vomiting: The length and severity of nausea and vomiting depend on the agents being used, as well as on the dosing schedule being employed. Nausea and vomiting can lead to psychological distress, dehydration, and nutritional deficits and may interfere with treatment if severe (see Chapter 27).

 4. Mucositis: The incidence and severity of mucositis in patients receiving chemotherapy also vary depending on the agent and doses (see Chapter 29).

 5. Impaired tissue integrity: Vesicant drugs have the potential to cause blistering or tissue necrosis if they leak into the tissue surrounding a blood vessel or venous access device. Extravasation with resultant tissue damage can happen with peripheral or central administration of vesicant drugs.

  a. Assess the IV site for signs and symptoms of possible extravasation before and frequently during the administration of the vesicant agent. Use dressing materials that allow visualization of the site (eg, transparent dressings) throughout the infusion. To detect signs and symptoms of extravasation, observe for:
   (1) Loss of or sluggish blood return.
   (2) Erythema.
   (3) Swelling or blanching at the IV site.
   (4) Discomfort (pain, stinging, or burning) at or above the IV site.
   (5) Slowed or stopped IV flow.
  b. Teach the patient the signs and symptoms of vesicant extravasation and expected sequelae. Instruct the patient to report these symptoms or any change in how the IV site feels during and after vesicant administration.
  c. Peripheral administration of vesicant drugs should be done by IV push through a side port of a free-flowing IV.
  d. Continuous or piggyback infusions of vesicant drugs should be given by way of a central venous access device. Positive blood

return should be obtained before beginning any vesicant infusion through a central line. Ongoing blood return checks for continuous infusions of vesicants should be obtained per institutional guidelines.

   e. If extravasation is suspected:

     (1) Stop the infusion.

     (2) Disconnect the IV tubing from the IV device; attach a syringe to the IV device and try to aspirate any drug from the device or tissue.

     (3) Administer appropriate antidotes per institutional policy.

     (4) Remove the IV administration device.

     (5) Apply warm or cold compresses to the extravasation site as indicated by institutional policy for the specific agent. Generally, ice packs are used, except with the vinca alkaloids (vinblastine, vincristine, vinorelbine) for which warm compresses are usually recommended.

   f. After an extravasation, perform a site assessment at 24 hours, 1 week, 2 weeks, and as indicated by appearance and discomfort at the extravasation site. More frequent or extended assessments and notification of the physician should be performed if the patient experiences:

     (1) Burning.

     (2) Erythema.

     (3) Inflammation.

     (4) Pain.

     (5) Ulceration.

     (6) Tissue necrosis.

   g. Initiate consultation with a plastic surgeon for persistent redness, swelling, or pain, or development of ulceration or necrosis.

   h. Teach the patient and caregivers the importance of follow-up assessments and interventions after a suspected extravasation.

6. Ineffective breathing patterns: Allergic or hypersensitivity reactions can range in severity from mild (eg, facial flushing, urticaria, itching) to potentially life-threatening anaphylactic reactions (eg, bronchospasm, hypotension, anxiety). Hypersensitivity reactions most commonly occur during IV administration of an antineoplastic agent, usually within the initial 15 minutes of the first infusion of an agent. However, delayed reactions and reactions with later cycles can also occur.

   a. Review the patient's allergy history, especially drug allergies.

   b. Administer test dose of agent if indicated per institutional guidelines.

   c. Monitor the patient for signs and symptoms of hypersensitivity reactions, especially during the first 15 minutes of administration of a drug known to cause these reactions.

   d. If the patient develops signs of an anaphylactic reaction (bronchospasm, lightheadedness):

     (1) *Stop* the infusion and maintain IV access.

     (2) Stay with the patient and have someone call for help.

     (3) Obtain vital signs, oxygen saturation, electrocardiogram, and other data as appropriate to further evaluate the patient's symptoms.

(4) Place the patient in an upright position (as tolerated) and maintain a patent airway. Administer oxygen if needed.

(5) Administer emergency medications per protocol or physician's orders. Commonly used medications include diphenhydramine, epinephrine, steroids, and bronchodilators.

(6) Continue to monitor the patient's vital signs frequently until resolution of symptoms.

(7) Provide emotional support to the patient and family.

7. Alopecia: A variety of chemotherapy agents can cause hair loss. Hair loss can range from patchy loss or thinning to complete loss of scalp hair. Patients can also lose body hair, including their eyelashes, eyebrows, and axillary and pubic hair. Hair loss tends to be more severe with multidrug and high-dose chemotherapy treatment. Hair loss is usually gradual with each dose of chemotherapy, but can be rapid and abrupt as with paclitaxel administration. The hair will usually grow back at the normal rate of hair growth after completion of the treatment with chemotherapy.

   a. Assess the patient's perception of hair loss before and after the hair loss has occurred. Encourage the patient to express his or her fears and distress related to the change in appearance.

   b. Discuss with the patient the hair loss potential of the treatment regimen. Assure the patient that hair will usually grow back gradually after the treatment is completed.

   c. Discuss available resources with the patient and family, such as wig specialists; vendors of turbans, wigs, and hats; and programs to assist in their adjustment to hair loss (eg, "Look Good, Feel Good" program).

   d. Refer the patient to a mental health professional to assist in adjustment to body image change, as indicated.

8. Hemorrhagic cystitis: Certain chemotherapy agents, such as cyclophosphamide and ifosfamide, can cause hemorrhagic cystitis through a direct irritating effect on the mucosal cells of the bladder. The patient can experience dysuria, frequency and burning on urination, and may report darkening of the urine or clots or both. If severe enough, the patient may require aggressive treatment to prevent clots from obstructing the urethra.

   a. Teach the patient to monitor for and report any signs or symptoms of bladder irritation or bleeding.

   b. Instruct the patient to increase fluid intake and to void frequently. Patients receiving high-dose chemotherapy may require vigorous IV hydration. Recommend that the patient take the oral form of the drug in the morning to allow elimination of the drug before bedtime.

   c. Administer uroprotective agents (eg, mesna) and hydration as ordered to decrease the risk of hemorrhagic cystitis.

9. Renal toxicity: Patients receiving chemotherapy may be at risk for renal toxicity from the direct or indirect toxic effects of the chemotherapy. Certain chemotherapy agents (eg, cisplatin, methotrexate) can damage the renal structures. Rapid tumor lysis with release of uric acid and hypovolemia can contribute.

a. Encourage adequate fluid intake or provide aggressive hydration for patients receiving renal toxic agents. Volume expanders, such as 3% saline and mannitol, may be used as well.

b. Assess the patient's intake and output to assess hydration status and urine output, while monitoring for fluid overload.

c. When a rapid tumor kill is anticipated, follow the instructions outlined in Chapter 40.

d. For patients receiving high-dose methotrexate, perform urine alkalinization ($\geq$pH 7) to decrease renal toxic effects.

10. Impaired reproductive function: Amenorrhea, ovarian dysfunction, and impaired sperm production can occur with chemotherapy treatment. This is usually transient and more severe with intensive dose therapy and certain drugs, such as alkylating agents. The risk of infertility is also related to the patient's gender and age. Women over 30 are less likely to regain ovarian function. Chemotherapy may also cause mutations in genetic materials and malformations in developing fetuses.

a. Obtain a brief sexual history, including the importance of reproductive function to the patient.

b. Advise male patients about sperm banking options and, if available, female patients about ovum banking before initiation of chemotherapy treatments.

c. Advise patients to avoid pregnancy in themselves and their partners during treatment. Provide information about contraceptive options.

d. Advise the patient of long-term side effects and the potential for return of reproductive functioning.

REFERENCES

Baquiran, D. C., & Gallagher, J. (2003). *Lippincott's cancer chemotherapy handbook* (2nd ed.). Philadelphia: Lippincott Williams & Wilkins.

Elliott, P. J., Zollner, T. M., & Boehncke, W. H. (2003). Proteasome inhibition: A new anti-inflammatory strategy. *Journal of Molecular Medicine, 81*(4), 235–245.

Fischer, D. S., Knopf, M. T., & Durivage, H. J. (2003). *The cancer chemotherapy handbook.* St. Louis, MO: Mosby.

_____. (2000). *Cancer nursing: Principles and practice* (5th ed.). Boston: Jones & Bartlett.

Gross, J., & Johnson, B. L. (1998). *Handbook of oncology nursing* (3rd ed.). Boston: Jones & Bartlett.

Oncology Nursing Society. (2003). *Safe handling of hazardous drugs.* Pittsburgh, PA: Oncology Nursing Press.

_____. (2001). *ONS chemotherapy and biotherapy guidelines and recommendations for practice.* Pittsburgh, PA: Oncology Nursing Press.

PDR nurses handbook. (2003). Montvale, NJ: Medical Economics.

Yarbro, C. H. (Ed.). (2003). *Cancer symptom management* (5th ed.). Boston: Jones & Bartlett.

7 Complementary, Alternative, and Unproven Therapies

Joanne Finley
Susan Sartorius-Mergenthaler

I. History: Complementary, alternative, and unproven therapies have been around for thousands of years, particularly in Chinese medicine. However, these therapies seem "new" because of the public's recent, renewed interest. The public was the force behind the federal government's decision to establish a National Center for Complementary and Alternative Medicine (NCCAM) in 1999, previously called the Office of Alternative Medicine from 1991 to 1999. Complementary and Alternative Medicine (CAM) is a diverse group of therapies not considered to be part of mainstream medicine, due to questions about efficacy and safety.

II. Definitions
   A. Conventional Medicine: Accepted practice with a scientific basis.
   B. Complementary Therapies: Used with conventional medicine.
   C. Alternative Therapies: Used instead of conventional medicine.
   D. Integrative Therapies: Combination of conventional medicine and complementary therapies.
   E. Unproven Therapies: Therapies under investigation or with little or no scientific basis.

III. Rationale for Use
   A. Incidence: The incidence of CAM use ranges from 30% to 80%, and it is on the rise. CAM users are typically female, educated, younger, and of a higher socioeconomic level. The therapies most commonly used are spirituality, vitamins/minerals/herbs, support groups, relaxation, imagery, and exercise. Most users also continue conventional therapy (Jordan & Delunas, 2001; Richardson, Sander, Palmer, Greisinger & Singletary., 2000; Sparber et al., 2000).
   B. Goals: The overall goal of CAM is to create a healing environment for one's own internal healing to occur. The specific goals of CAM include:
      1. Prevention of illness.
      2. Promotion of wellness.
      3. Prevention or reduction of side effects of treatment.
      4. Improvement of immune system function.
      5. Active participation in treatment.
      6. Improvement in quality of life.

IV. Biology of Therapy Based on NCCAM Classification System (NCCAM, 2002). Tables 7–1 through 7–5 describe the risks, benefits, and scientific evidence for the various types of CAM therapies.

(text continues on page 96)

TABLE 7–1 Alternative Medical Systems

Intervention	Description	Potential Risk/Cancer Benefit
Ayurveda *Knowledge of Life*	An ancient integrated medical system from India. Uses multiple modalities to maintain spiritual, physical, and mental harmony. The combination of modalities used varies depending on the diagnosis of the patient. Diagnosis is based on critical observation, history, and physical assessment, and how the individual is connected to the cosmic universe. The treatment plan is complex and takes into account the whole person, such as diet, relationships, lifestyle, seasons, and color. Modalities include massage, yoga, guided imagery, blood letting, intestinal cleansing, dietary modifications, and herbal remedies.	*Risks:* Some aspects are harmful. Consult a health care provider before using any form. *Benefits:* No scientific evidence. Some research has been done on its use for prevention and treatment of some cancers. No conclusions can be made at this time.
Homeopathy	The use of minute amounts of plant extracts, minerals, or chemicals that are diluted in water or alcohol. Believed to aid many health problems. Solutions are carefully mixed and diluted based on individual symptoms.	*Risks:* Considered safe because of the small amounts of product. *Benefits:* No scientific evidence.
Holistic medicine	Belief system based on philosophy that the disease plus other aspects of the person should be treated as a whole to achieve a high level of wellness. Practitioners take into account the spiritual, emotional, physical, and mental attitudes of the individual. Various forms of complementary therapies are included so the individual may gain a sense of control over the disease.	*Risks:* Consult practitioner related to domain of treatment (yoga, massage, acupuncture) or for dietary changes and supplements. *Benefits:* No scientific evidence. Some aspects are recognized as complementary support during cancer treatment.
Native American healing	Basic belief that disease is caused by spiritual problems. The goal of healing is to restore an individual to a state of wholeness. To achieve spiritual balance and harmony, several techniques and rituals are used: herbal medicine, religion, shamanism, and ceremonial practices. Proponents believe that disease can be cured by these approaches.	*Risks:* Consult physician about dietary changes and purification rituals. *Benefits:* No scientific evidence. The supportive community and interventions may improve quality of life. Prayer may reduce stress.

TABLE 7-2 Mind–Body Interventions

Intervention	Description	Potential Risk/Cancer Benefit
Aromatherapy	Use of fragrant essential oils inhaled by way of humidifiers or during application of massage. Believed to enhance quality of life, help with coping, and produce feelings of well-being.	*Risks:* Poisonous. Do not take oils internally. *Benefit:* No scientific evidence. May reduce anxiety, tension, pain.
Art therapy	Use of art to encourage release of emotional conflicts and express unconscious concerns/conflicts.	*Risk:* Should be monitored by therapist. Uncomfortable feelings could occur. *Benefit:* No scientific evidence. May reduce anxiety.
Breathwork	General term used to describe various forms of deep breathing exercises.	*Risk:* Unknown. *Benefit:* No scientific evidence. May aid in relaxation and the reduction of stress.
Crystals	Used to restore energy flow, promote healing, balancing. Thought to have reenergizing effects on body's energy fields.	*Risk:* Considered safe. *Benefit:* No scientific evidence. May aid in relaxation and the reduction of stress.
Dance therapy	Use of movement to increase mobility, improve self-awareness, reduce muscle tension.	*Risk:* May have restricted movement; involves use of the joints, muscles. *Benefit:* No scientific evidence. May improve self-concept, reduce stress, pain, body tension.
Faith healing	A strong belief in a supreme being or place that has the ability to cure disease. May involve prayer; laying on of hands; visit to a church, shrine, or another kind of healing monument.	*Risk:* No curative effect, which may lead to feelings of guilt, failure, hopelessness. *Benefit:* No scientific evidence. May produce placebo effect, which may evoke peacefulness.
Feng Shui *"wind and water"*	Chinese philosophy that placing objects, furniture, rooms in a particular arrangement will promote the flow of vital energy, *qi,* thereby promoting healing.	*Risk:* Unknown. *Benefit:* No scientific evidence.

Therapy	Description	Risk/Benefit
Humor therapy	Use of laughter to promote relief from physical illness and emotional complexities.	*Risk:* Considered safe. *Benefit:* No scientific evidence. May enhance quality of life, reduce stress, anxiety.
Hypnosis	Relaxation technique used to guide a person into a trancelike state. Person enters a state of restful alertness and becomes open to suggestion.	*Risk:* Considered safe under the care of a trained hypnotherapist. *Benefit:* No scientific evidence. Approved by National Institutes of Health for treatment of chronic pain. May aid in the reduction of blood pressure, anxiety, fear. May control nausea/vomiting.
Imagery	A "mind-over-matter" methodology in which a person will concentrate on a specific problem and visualize positive outcomes to be achieved. Methods include: guided imagery, Simonton method.	*Risk:* Considered safe under the care of a trained health professional. *Benefit:* No scientific evidence. May decrease pain, nausea/vomiting, depression, stress, and may enhance immune system.
Labyrinth walking	Meditative walking along a continuous pathway that has a directed beginning and end. During the walk, a person may pray, let the mind wander, reflect on a specific problem.	*Risk:* Considered safe. *Benefit:* No scientific evidence. May reduce stress, promote relaxation, enhance spirituality.
Meditation	Relaxation technique achieved by closing the eyes or chanting a sound and concentrating on a pleasant theme to create a sense of well-being and separating self from the outside world. A self-directed or guided method for relaxing the mind and calming the body. Methods include: tai chi, aikido, Zen Buddhism.	*Risk:* Complications are rare. A person may become disoriented or experience uncomfortable feelings. *Benefit:* No scientific evidence. Approved by National Institutes of Health for the treatment of chronic pain and insomnia. May improve quality of life.
Music therapy	Use of music to soothe and promote healing.	*Risk:* Considered safe. *Benefit:* No scientific evidence. Clinical trials have shown a reduction in nausea, pain, anxiety, blood pressure, depression, insomnia. May promote social interaction, enhance quality of life.

(continued)

TABLE 7-2   Mind-Body Interventions *(Continued)*

Intervention	Description	Potential Risk/Cancer Benefit
Psychotherapy	Widely supported mind-body approach in which a person discusses the emotional difficulties of an illness. Methods include: behavior modification, cognitive therapy, group therapy, psychodynamic therapy, client-centered therapy.	*Risk:* Considered safe. May experience uncomfortable feeling. Person should be under the care of a trained therapist. *Benefit:* Research has shown a decrease in depression and anxiety, and quality of life improvement. May benefit coping skills and overall enjoyment of life, or aid in communication with health care workers.
Spirituality and prayer	Method of communicating to a higher power to decrease the negative effects of illness. Can be self-directed, done in groups or by individuals for a "sick" person in any place or at any time. Often takes place in religious facilities.	*Risk:* Considered safe. *Benefit:* Research has demonstrated quality-of-life benefits. May psychologically reduce stress and anxiety, and strengthen will.
Support groups	Education-based and behavioral supportive group to share feelings and experiences related to illness. By sharing these experiences, the person will develop a better understanding of the illness, receive emotional support, reduce stress, and form positive coping skills.	*Risk:* Considered safe. May provoke uncomfortable feelings. Caution when using online chat rooms because of the lack of information regarding confidentiality issues and verification of training/qualifications. *Benefit:* A clinical trial has shown benefits in the reduction of anxiety, fear, fatigue, and confusion. May increase treatment compliance, and enhance quality of life.

Therapy	Description	Risk/Benefit
Tai-chi	Chinese form of martial arts. Believed to balance the life force, *qi*. Form of relaxation using deep breathing methods and physical movements to prevent illness and improve health and extend life. Considered self-healing.	*Risk:* Moderately safe, but a physician should be consulted before undergoing a program because it is considered a form of exercise. *Benefit:* Research has demonstrated benefits in stress reduction; decreased blood pressure; reduction of heart disease; improvement in posture, flexibility, balance, muscle mass. Recommended for older adults to improve well-being.
Yoga	Hindu philosophy used to create a union of mind, body, spirit. Believed to cultivate the life force, *prana*. Thought to be consulted before undergoing a program because lead to a state of relaxation, peace, harmony, and happiness. Form of exercise that requires exact postures and breathing techniques.	*Risk:* Moderately safe, but a physician should some yoga positions may be physically difficult to achieve. *Benefit:* National Institutes of Health suggest benefits may provide cancer symptom relief. Research has shown control of blood pressure, respiration, heart rate, body temperature.

TABLE 7-3   Biology-Based Therapies

Intervention	Description	Potential Risk/Cancer Benefit
Chlorella	Freshwater alga containing high levels of chlorophyll. Used extensively in Japan. Believed to have cleansing effect on the body by ridding the body of toxins. Contains antioxidants. Stimulates the production of macrophages. May be taken in many forms: liquid extracts, powder, and tablet.	*Risks:* Considered safe. No adverse effect data available in humans. *Benefits:* No scientific evidence. Animal and laboratory research testing the extract suggests possible anticancer properties.
Copper	Controversial trace element found in foods. May aid the immune system and rid toxins from the body. Controversial beliefs regarding its cancer protectant and cancer-promoting effects. Available as a natural element in vegetables and fruits and as a vitamin supplement.	*Risks:* Vitamin supplements are considered safe. Do not take if diabetic (may affect glucose levels) or with Wilson's disease. *Benefits:* No scientific evidence. Laboratory studies suggest it may contain antioxidants.
Ellagic acid	Compound believed to prevent carcinogens from binding to DNA by causing apoptosis. Found naturally in fruits and nuts but especially strawberries, raspberries, and pomegranates. Available as a liquid, capsule, or powder.	*Risks:* No information available. *Benefits:* Currently under investigation. Animal studies have shown that it may inhibit tumor growth in some cancers.
Essiac tea (slippery elm bark, Turkish rhubarb, burdock root, sheep sorrel, blessed thistle, red clover, watercress, and kelp)	Mixture of eight herbs that, when infused together, is used as a tea. Strengthens the immune system, promotes cell repair, and shrinks tumors.	*Risks:* Considered safe. When taken with food, may cause diarrhea, nausea, vomiting, and headache. *Benefits:* No scientific evidence. Many testimonials. Laboratory research suggests that some of the herbs in the tea may have anticancer activity.

Therapy	Description	Risks/Benefits
Evening primrose	North American fragrant flowering plant that blooms at night. Oil is extracted from the seeds containing essential fatty acids, gamma linolenic acid and omega-3 fatty acid, that are believed to have anticancer properties. Available for administration as a tea, capsules, and gelcaps.	*Risks:* No side effects identified. Gamma linolenic acid may lower the seizure threshold. *Benefits:* No scientific evidence. Laboratory tests in animal tumors suggest that it may slow cancer growth in breast and skin cancer cells.
Flaxseed	The seed and oil from the flaxseed plant are thought to have anticancer properties. The oil is high in omega-3 fatty acids and alpha linolenic acid. Flaxseed contains lignans, a compound that functions as an antioxidant and has antiestrogen effects. Flaxseed oil is available in gel capsules and as a liquid. Flaxseed is also found in meal, flour, breads, cereals.	*Risks:* Needs to be refrigerated. Must not be used by people with inflammatory disease. Immature pod is poisonous. *Benefits:* No scientific evidence. Currently being studied in animals. One study suggests that flaxseed and low-fat diet may decrease testosterone levels and slow tumor growth in men with prostate cancer.
Folic acid	Naturally occurring B-complex compound found in many foods. It promotes development of blood cells and aids in metabolism of DNA. Available as an oral vitamin supplement and in fruit, vegetables, liver, and grains.	*Risks:* Considered safe. In high levels, may interfere with methotrexate. *Benefits:* Low levels of folic acid linked to cancer. Thought to be related to decreased immune surveillance or DNA structure changes due to low levels.
Garlic	Allyl sulfur is one of several compounds from the lily family to have anticancer and enhanced immune surveillance activities. Available in natural plant form (eaten cooked or raw) extracts, powders, capsules, and oils.	*Risks:* Large quantities may cause GI distress. Has anticoagulant properties. *Benefits:* No scientific evidence. Studies suggest it may lower the risk for some type of cancers or reduce tumor growth.
Ginger	Root of this native Asian plant is often used in herbal remedies for nausea, vomiting, and motion sickness. Available as root (fresh/dried), capsules, tablets, and tea.	*Risks:* May interfere with blood clotting, and enhance bleeding risk. *Benefits:* No scientific evidence. Believed to relieve therapy-induced nausea and vomiting.

(continued)

TABLE 7-3 Biology-Based Therapies *(Continued)*

Intervention	Description	Potential Risk/Cancer Benefit
Ginkgo	Leaf from the ginkgo tree native to Asia that may promote cancer growth. Available in multiple oral forms.	*Risks:* Considered safe. May enhance bleeding risk. *Benefits:* No scientific evidence of anticancer or cancer-causing effects.
Ginseng	The root of an Asian Perennial plant that may have cancer-protective effects. Available in multiple oral forms.	*Risks:* May interact with anticoagulants or anti-depressants. May cause high blood pressure, insomnia, headaches, vaginal bleeding, swollen breasts, and, some believe, recurrence of breast cancer. *Benefits:* No scientific evidence. Research has demonstrated potential anticancer effects.
Goldenseal	Native to the United States, the root is used for many conditions. Available for administration in multiple oral forms, douches, eyedrops, eardrops, and powder forms.	*Risks:* Multiple serious adverse effects: depression, tachycardia, diarrhea, nervousness, respiratory problems, death. Long-term use may lead to hallucinations and vitamin D deficiency. Consult physician before taking. *Benefits:* No scientific evidence. May activate the immune system. Has been studied for cardiac-stimulating properties and anticoagulant potential.
Green tea	Comes from the leaves of the native shrub plant from Asia called *Camellia sineses.* A popular tea used for many conditions including the prevention of cancer. Contains an element called epigallocatechin-3-gallate, which may inhibit the blood supply to tumor cells (antiangio-genesis properties). Usually found in tea form, but may also be administered as an extract.	*Benefits:* Mixed results from laboratory/animal studies. Some studies do show potential cancer-protecting benefit.

Inositol hexaphosphate (IP6)	Chemical found in foods that are high in fiber. Believed to inhibit or slow growth in some cancers and have antioxidant properties. Called the "natural cancer fighter." Available in many food sources and in pill form.	*Risks:* Believed to be safe. *Benefits:* Studies have shown potential reduction of lung cancers and possibly a relationship between cancer and high cholesterol.
Kampo	Popular Japanese medicine containing 210 different herbs. Formula is often individualized to each patient based on visual and auditory interpretations of the concept *sho.* Proponents claim that Kampo enhances macrophages and boosts natural killer cells.	*Risks:* Very little is known about safety. *Benefits:* No scientific evidence.
Kombucha tea	Tea made from a mushroom culture and sugar. Proponents believe that it detoxifies and promotes tissue-restoring balance to the body. Proponents also encourage the removal of all chemicals from the diet while taking the tea.	*Risks:* FDA warning to consumers that it may cause acidosis and death. Do not use if immuno-compromised. *Benefits:* No scientific evidence.
Lycopene	Natural compound found in tomatoes, watermelon, papaya, and other fruits. Believed to protect enzymes, cellular lipids, DNA, and have antioxidant properties. Available as a natural resource and capsule form.	*Risks:* None found. *Benefits:* Believed to reduce cancer growth in many cancers. Research has been focused on prostate cancer.
Macrobiotic diet	Dietary way of life based on elements of Buddhism and belief that food is sacred. A process of eating/chewing food until it is liquid. A precise way of preparing and cooking the food in a peaceful setting. Diet consists of organic whole grains, cooked vegetables, and cereals.	*Risks:* May cause vitamin and other nutritional deficiencies. Deaths have been reported. *Benefits:* No scientific evidence.

(continued)

TABLE 7-3   Biology-Based Therapies *(Continued)*

Intervention	Description	Potential Risk/Cancer Benefit
Maitake mushroom	D-Fraction, a polysaccharide, is an extract found in the Maitake mushroom that may slow tumor growth and boost the immune system. It is an edible mushroom and available in capsule, pill, tablet, and liquid forms.	*Risks:* Considered safe. *Benefits:* No scientific evidence. Studies in mice using injectable extract have shown some evidence of tumor inhibition.
Marijuana	Leaves and buds of *Cannabis sativa* grow in warm tropical regions. Delta-9-tetrahydro-cannabinol (THC) is one of 66 active biologic ingredients found in marijuana that is believed to help manage symptoms of patients who have cancer, AIDS, and glaucoma. THC is available as a pill or suppository by prescription. The raw plant may be smoked or eaten and is illegal in the United States.	*Risks:* Side effects of THC are similar to the natural plant leaves when smoked or eaten. May cause tachycardia, low blood pressure, memory loss, increased anxiety, or altered time perception. May decrease immune function. The plant material does contain carcinogens, which may increase risk of oral cancers and respiratory disease. *Benefits:* Prescription THC has been studied in patients with chemotherapy-induced nausea and vomiting. THC is used to reduce anxiety, stimulate appetite, and may have sedative effects. More studies need to be done to evaluate the effectiveness as compared to standard medications.
Modified citrus pectin (MCP)	Carbohydrate found in many fruits. Believed to slow the growth of prostate and melanoma cancers. May enhance "killer T cell" abilities. Available as a natural product, powder, and capsules.	*Risks:* Side effects are rare. Considered safe. *Benefits:* Animal research has demonstrated reduction of lung metastasis in prostate and melanoma cancers.
Noni plant	Juice from the fruit of the Noni plant, a large evergreen tree native to the Pacific Islands, is used as an herbal remedy for many conditions and is available in many forms.	*Risks:* No information available. *Benefits:* Hawaiian researchers found that mice treated with Noni juice had a longer survival time.

Omega-3 fatty acids	Nutrient source found in oils from cold water fish, flaxseed, and bears. Believed to stop the spread of some hormone-based cancers. Available as oil supplements and in diet.	*Risks:* Do not take with anticoagulants. May increase anemia in women while menstruating or may cause abdominal bloating. *Benefits:* No scientific evidence. Preliminary studies are inconclusive.
PC-SPES (PC-prostate cancer; SPES-Latin for hope)	Combination of eight herbs: chrysanthemum, licorice, saw palmetto, Rabdosia, skull cap, ginseng, isatis, and *Ganoderma lucidum.* Collectively, they contain plant chemicals and trace minerals such as copper, zinc, and calcium. PC-SPES shows promise in slowing tumor growth in prostate cancer. Proponents believe it may also stimulate the immune system. Available in oral form, but the drug is not regulated and the formula may vary.	*Risks:* Side effects are similar to estrogenlike compounds. May increase risk of thromboembolism. *Benefits:* Clinical trials have been established to study the effectiveness in men with prostate cancer who have not responded to hormonal treatment. In 2002, the drug was recalled due to contamination. Future studies are planned.
Peppermint	Widely known and cultivated plant. Oil is extracted from the flowers and leaves and used for GI and respiratory disorders. May be administered in capsule, inhaled, tea, and oil forms.	*Risks:* Considered safe. May be a skin irritant. *Benefits:* No scientific evidence. May be useful in patients with chemotherapy-induced nausea and vomiting.
Pokeweed	Berries and root of this native North American shrub are used to treat many conditions. Proponents believe it has anticancer and antiviral properties. Available as an extract, powder, and tincture.	*Risks:* Pokeweed is poisonous. Do not take with antidepressants or oral contraceptives. *Benefits:* Animal research suggests that it may have anticancer effects and may stimulate the immune system.
Saw palmetto	Berries of this palm tree are promoted as a treatment for several prostate conditions. Available in oral forms.	*Risks:* Side effects may include nausea, vomiting, headache, dizziness, and insomnia. Safety of long-term use is not known. May interfere with PSA levels. *Benefits:* May improve symptoms associated with benign prostate hyperplasia (BPH), but not established for use with prostate cancer.

(continued)

TABLE 7-3 Biology-Based Therapies *(Continued)*

Intervention	Description	Potential Risk/Cancer Benefit
Shitake mushroom	Compound lentinan is found in this native Asian fungus. Believed to have antitumor effects. Available as an edible mushroom or in extract form.	*Risks:* Considered safe. Allergic reactions have been noted. *Benefits:* Early studies have proven lentinan has antiviral properties and may also be effective against stomach and colorectal cancers.
Soybean	Isoflavones, also called phytoestrogen, are found in this high-protein Asian plant. Believed to be effective against many cancers. Available in many dietary sources: tofu, soybean extract or powder, protein bars, milk, and other dairy products.	*Risks:* Considered safe. Women taking hormonal supplements should refrain from large amounts of soy products. May cause GI distress. *Benefits:* It is uncertain how the isoflavone affects estrogen-receptor growth in breast cancers, although thought to have protective properties for breast and prostate cancers.
Turmeric	Root of this native plant of India and Asia is used as a spice in foods. The active ingredient curcumin is used for antiinflammatory conditions. Proponents believe it has antioxidant properties, which may slow growth of cancers. Available as a powder, tablet, and ointment.	*Risks:* Considered safe when used as a spice. Do not take with anticoagulants, nonsteroidals, or immunosuppressants. *Benefits:* No scientific evidence. Research in the laboratory and animals has been focused on antioxidant properties.
Venus flytrap	Native plant of the southeastern United States that has the unique ability to eat and trap insects. Carnivora is extracted from the plant and is felt to have anticancer effects and to stimulate the immune system. It is commercially available in liquid form and may be taken either by mouth, inhaled, or injected. Another extract from the plant is plumbagin.	*Risks:* No toxic effects reported. May cause nausea and vomiting when injected. *Benefits:* No scientific evidence. Both carnivora and plumbagin have inconclusive laboratory evidence.

Phytochemicals (Ascorbic acid, beta-carotene, flavonoids, carotenoids, sulfides, vitamins A, C, E)	Group of over 4,000 compounds found in fruits, beans, grains, and vegetables that have antioxidant and hormonelike properties. Promoted as a preventive and treatment for various health conditions. Believed to block carcinogens from their target organ. Available as a food source and in numerous oral supplemental forms.	*Risks:* Do not take with benzodiazepines. May be toxic in large doses. *Benefits:* Most studies have been focused on diets high in this classification of food derivative. Research suggests that, by eating foods high in phytochemicals, the risk of some cancers can be reduced. Studies indicate that the collective whole might have more benefit than select supplements.
Vitamin B complex	Dietary essential nutrient needed to maintain adequate enzyme activity in the body. Available as a food source and as oral supplement.	*Risks:* Considered safe. High doses may be toxic. Folic acid may interfere with methotrexate. *Benefits:* Research is focused on the relationship of vitamin B and the prevention of some cancers. It may lower the risk of colorectal cancer.
Zinc	Dietary mineral that the body needs to build DNA, and to regulate the immune system and cell metabolism. Believed to protect against some cancers. Available in the diet, as a spray and oral supplement.	Risks: High-level exposure to zinc is a prostate cancer risk. Benefits: Research has shown that patients with head and neck cancers, melanoma, and some forms of leukemia have low serum zinc levels.

TABLE 7–4 Manipulative and Body-Based Methods

Intervention	Description	Potential Risk/Cancer Benefit
Acupuncture	Traditional form of Chinese medicine to maintain internal balance and energy flow. Small needles are placed at specific points (acupoints) under the surface of the skin representative of different positions along the meridians. Meridians are channels of vital energy *qi* or life force.	*Risk*: Considered safe when administered by a trained professional. If administered incorrectly, could result in bleeding, convulsions, infection, fainting, nerve damage. *Benefit*: No scientific evidence.
Bodywork Movement therapy Rolfing Alexander technique Feldenkrais method Trager approach Shiatsu massage See: Massage	Use of hand, finger, elbow, and knee manipulation on the skin, soft tissue, and muscle. Techniques may vary as to the location and depth of touch.	*Risk*: Do not manipulate or massage area of bone metastasis due to risk of fractures, or directly on tumors. Use cautiously in patients with anemia, neutropenia, and thrombocytopenia. Consult physician and qualified therapist. *Benefit*: No scientific evidence. May reduce pain and stress, relieve symptoms, promote circulation and relaxation, and enhance quality of life.
Cancer salves Black salve Escharotics Botanical salve Curaderm	Application of a salve to a tumor or tumor area for healing.	*Risk*: May cause burning, severe scarring. *Benefit*: No scientific evidence.
Castor oil	Application of the oil to various parts of the body for healing.	*Risk*: Do not eat castor beans or seeds. Poisonous and may cause death. *Benefit*: No scientific evidence.
Chiropractic	Manipulation of the spine to correct any blockages that may exist between the nerves and bone. Belief is that the body has the ability to heal itself.	*Risk*: Consult physician and seek qualified chiropractors. Do not manipulate bone metastasis. May cause injury, paralysis. *Benefit*: No scientific evidence. Reduces lower back pain, encourages relaxation and stress relief.

Therapy	Description	Risk/Benefit
Colon therapy	Method of detoxifying the body by way of various types of enemas (eg, coffee enemas to clean the colon and kill cancer cells) and enable natural healing. Administration is by a colonic hygienist. A plastic tube is inserted into the rectum and continues into the colon, then a pump delivers 20 gallons of fluid into the colon. The hygienist massages the abdomen to aid in waste removal. Another tube then carries the waste and water out of the body. The process may take 60 minutes.	Risk: Machines used to deliver the water for the colon therapy are illegal. May cause electrolyte imbalance, perforation of the intestinal wall, infection, and death. Benefit: No scientific evidence.
Craniosacral therapy	Gentle massage and manipulation of the skull, spinal cord, and pelvis. Technique may correct any blockages in the cerebral spinal fluid and associated body areas, thus returning the body to a healthy state.	Risk: Seek qualified therapist. Benefit: No scientific evidence. May reduce headaches, stress, and tension, and enhance relaxation.
Heat therapy	Application of heat to a specific site, region, or whole body. The supporting theory is that heat increases the blood flow, thereby making the cancer cells more susceptible to treatment.	Risk: May cause internal bleeding. Use only by qualified physician. Benefit: Clinical trials have substantiated the use of heat therapy for the enhancement of radiation therapy and chemotherapy in some cancers. Whole body heat therapy is under investigation.
Hydrotherapy	Use of water in the forms of ice, liquid, or steam to promote healing. Water therapy can be given internally by way of enemas or applied externally.	Risk: Bacterial infection, tissue damage, and local pain. Benefit: No scientific evidence. Acceptable form of physical rehabilitation, relaxation, relief of minor aches/pains.
Hyperbaric oxygen therapy (HBOT)	Breathing in pure pressurized oxygen at 1.5 to 3 times normal atmospheric pressure. Proponents claim this treatment cures cancer and kills microorganisms.	Risk: Myopia, headaches, fatigue, sinus damage, lung damage, oxygen toxicity. Benefit: No scientific evidence to support use in cancer treatment. May aid in the healing of soft tissue due to radiation therapy.

(continued)

TABLE 7-4 Manipulative and Body-Based Methods (Continued)

Intervention	Description	Potential Risk/Cancer Benefit
Light therapy	Patients sit in front of a light box for a specific amount of time with exposure to UVA, UVB, UVC light. It is believed that UV light therapy neutralizes toxins in the bloodstream and kills infectious organisms.	*Risk:* Is considered safe. May increase aging of the skin and risk of skin cancer. *Benefit:* No scientific evidence as curative therapy. Is used as a treatment for cutaneous T-cell lymphoma and in clinical trials for GVHD. UV light is considered a conventional treatment for seasonal affective disorder.
Magnetic therapy	Use of wafer-thin magnets, placed on the body in various areas for varying amounts of time. The negative magnetic field changes the body from an acidic environment to alkaline, stimulates metabolism, increases blood flow, improves emotional well-being, and relieves pain.	*Risk:* Considered safe. *Benefit:* No scientific evidence.
Massage	Noninvasive manipulation of the body involving kneading and rubbing the skin, soft tissue, and muscles.	*Risk:* Consult a physician. Consider treatment by a trained professional. Do not massage bone metastasis or massage directly on tumor sites. Use cautiously in patients with bone marrow suppression. *Benefit:* Recognized as a complementary therapy for stress reduction, relaxation, pain relief, increased mobility, insomnia, improved circulation.
Transcutaneous electrical nerve stimulation (TENS)	Small, electric generator with electrodes used for the reduction of pain. Electrodes are placed on the skin near the area of pain. Waves of current pass through the electrodes and stimulate the muscles into relaxation, thus decreasing the pain	*Risk:* Considered safe. Should be placed by a trained therapist. May cause burning of skin. Not to be used in patients with heart problems. *Benefit:* Approved method of treatment for certain types of pain. Appears to benefit patients with acute, mild pain as opposed to chronic pain. Studies are limited in cancer-related pain.

TABLE 7-5   Energy Therapies

Intervention	Description	Potential Risk/Cancer Benefit
Polarity	Based on the electromagnetic energy field theory. Practitioners believe the body maintains both negative and positive flows of energy. Any disruption in the smooth flow of energy will cause an imbalance in the body's state of health. A trained therapist uses various hand motions on the body to clear and balance the energy flow.	*Risk:* Considered safe under the care of a reflexologist. *Benefit:* No scientific evidence. May be used as a relaxation technique. May help in pain reduction.
Reflexology	Hands-on approach to manipulate the body's energy fields. Energy flow is redirected, and the energy path becomes unblocked and realigns, thereby influencing spiritual and physical health. for quality of life and stress reduction. May aid in pain reduction.	
Reiki Universal life energy	Hands-on approach to manipulate the body's energy fields. Energy flow is redirected, and the energy path becomes unblocked and realigns, thereby influencing spiritual and physical health.	*Risk:* Considered safe under the care of a Reiki practitioner. *Benefit:* No scientific evidence. Useful as a complementary method for quality of life and stress reduction. May aid in pain reduction.
Therapeutic touch (TT)	It is believed that the flow of energy can become blocked and lead toward distress or illness. The TT practitioner uses hands to redirect and transfer a positive energy flow, thereby removing blockages and restoring balance to the body. The practitioner will move his or her hands around the body in a systematic format. The hands never actually touch the body but stay 2 to 5 inches from the body during the session.	*Risk:* Considered safe under the care of a Therapeutic Touch practitioner. *Benefit:* No scientific evidence. May improve quality of life and reduce anxiety.

(*text continues from page 78*)

- **A.** Alternative Medical Systems: Complete systems of theory and practice (Table 7–1)
  Examples: homeopathy and ayurveda
- **B.** Mind-Body Interventions: Use mind to affect body function (Table 7–2).
  Examples: meditation and music therapy
- **C.** Biology-Based Therapies: Use natural substances (Table 7–3).
  Examples: herbs, foods, and vitamins
- **D.** Manipulative and Body-Based Methods: Manipulate and/or move body parts (Table 7–4).
  Examples: chiropractic and massage therapy
- **E.** Energy Therapies: Use energy and/or magnetic fields (Table 7–5).
  Examples: reiki and therapeutic touch

V. Nursing Issues: Multiple nursing issues must be addressed when caring for patients using or considering CAM therapies. These include assessment, education, supportive care, and integration of therapies into practice.

- **A.** Assessment
  1. One of the most important tasks of the nurse is to elicit information from the patient and family.
  2. Open, accepting, and respectful communication is key.
  3. Some questions to ask are:
     a. What therapies are being used by the patient?
     b. What has the patient used in the past?
     c. What do the patient and family know about the therapies, their effectiveness and safety?
     d. How did the patient and family select the CAM practitioner?
  4. Barriers to patient disclosure
- **B.** Lack of health care provider interest
  1. Negative reaction of the health care provider
  2. Lack of health care provider knowledge
  3. Fear of legal liability on the part of the provider
  4. A thorough assessment of the patient's CAM use and knowledge is necessary to provide comprehensive care.
  5. Assess the patient's potential benefit from CAM therapies.
- **C.** What are the patient's personal strengths and weaknesses?
  1. Could the patient benefit from CAM therapies?
  2. Does the patient want information on CAM therapies?
  3. CAM therapies should be considered in any nursing plan of care.
- **D.** Education and Support
  1. An important nursing role is to ensure that patients and families have the information they want and/or need about CAM.
  2. Accurate information enables patients to make informed choices about practitioners and therapies.
  3. A multitude of instructional methods are available, such as books, pamphlets, videotapes, and audiotapes.
  4. Internet-based materials have the advantage of being current and accessible. Patients must be taught, however, to evaluate websites.
  5. Table 7–6 contains a list of CAM resources. Many of these organizations are devoted to CAM research and education.

TABLE 7-6 CAM Resources

Name of Organization	CAM Offerings	Website	Phone Number
National Center for Complementary and Alternative Medicine (NIH)	CAM research, training, and information for professionals and public	nccam.nih.gov	1-888-644-6226
Office of Cancer Complementary and Alternative Medicine (NCI)	Cancer-specific CAM research and information	occam.nci.nih.gov	1-800-4cancer
CAM on PubMed	CAM search tool with abstracts and references	www.ncbi.nlm.nih.gov/PubMed	
Food and Drug Administration	CAM safety issues	www.fda.gov	1-888-463-6332
White House Commission on Complementary and Alternative Medicine	Recommendations for public policy related to CAM	www.whccamp.hhs.gov/es.html	
Center for Mind-Body Medicine	CAM information, conferences, training, and therapies	www.cmbm.org	1-202-966-7338
American Cancer Society	CAM information	www.cancer.org	1-800-acs-2345
National Cancer Institute	CAM information and clinical trials information	cancer.gov	1-800-4cancer
Duke Comprehensive Cancer Center	"A Cancer Patient's Guide to Complementary and Alternative Medicine"	cancer.duke.edu/PatEd	

C. Integration of Care

    1. Nurses who look at the patient and family holistically will enhance their practice through integration of CAM therapies into standard nursing care or facilitation of the patient's environment to allow for use of CAM therapies.

        a. Massage and support groups are examples of activities that may be incorporated into the plan of care for the patient.

        b. Nurses may also pray with patients and teach guided imagery, relaxation, and breathing, within the scope of nursing practice.

        c. A referral should be made for therapies that require a trained practitioner, such as acupuncture and reiki, if that is what the patient desires. Questions to ask a CAM practitioner are outlined in Box 7–1.

    2. Goals of CAM therapies for patients

        a. Access the person's internal healing system. Many patients turn to CAM for an increased sense of control and empowerment. Families, too, may be empowered if they are taught CAM methods such as massage.

        b. CAM therapies allow nurses and families to spend quality time with the patient. The relationship with the patient becomes a partnership.

D. Barriers: CAM is not considered part of mainstream medicine because of several barriers (Table 7–7). Despite these barriers, CAM therapies are being sought out and used by the public with increasing frequency. It is the nurse's responsibility to assist consumers in their search for quality care by providing them with information and support.

▼ **BOX 7-1**   **Questions to Ask a CAM Practitioner**

1. What benefits can I expect from this therapy?
2. What risks are associated with this therapy?
3. Do the benefits outweigh the risks for my disease or condition?
4. What side effects can be expected?
5. Will the therapy interfere with any of my daily activities?
6. How long will I need to undergo treatment? How often will my progress or plan of treatment be assessed?
7. Will I need to buy any equipment or supplies?
8. Do you have scientific articles or references about using the treatment for my condition?
9. Could the therapy interact with conventional treatments?
10. Are there any conditions for which this treatment should not be used?

National Center for Complementary and Alternative Medicine. (2002, August). *Selecting a complementary and alternative medicine (CAM) practitioner. Bethesda, MD: Author.* NCCAM Publication No. D168 (p. 4).

TABLE 7-7 Barriers to CAM

Barrier	Issues
Lack of research	• More research is needed to substantiate CAM methods so they may be viewed as conventional medicine
Safety	• Natural products do not have same oversight as prescription drugs • Adverse effects are reported on a voluntary basis • Potency varies • Products may be contaminated • Fallacy that "natural" is safe
Reimbursement	• Insurance does not cover many therapies • Need more research to prove effectiveness
Attitudes of health care provider	• May deter open communication
Access to CAM practitioners	• May not refer to CAM providers • May not be available in all geographic locations • May lack credentialing and qualifications • May lack system of referrals

REFERENCES

American Cancer Society. (2002). *Complementary and alternative cancer methods handbook*. Atlanta: American Cancer Society Health Content Products.

Clark, C. C. (2000*). Integrating complementary health procedures into practice*. New York: Springer.

Decker, G. (Ed.). (1999). *An introduction to complementary and alternative therapies*. Pittsburgh: Oncology Nursing Press.

Eisenberg, D. M., Davis, R. B., Ettner, S. L., Appel, S., Wilkey, S., VanRompay, M., & Kessler, R. C. (1998). Trends in alternative medicine use in the United States, 1990–1997. Result of a follow-up national survey. *Journal of the American Medical Association, 280,* 1569–1575.

Jordan, M. L., & Delunas, L. R. (2001). Quality of life and patterns of nontraditional therapy use by patients with cancer. *Oncology Nursing Forum, 28,* 1107–1113.

National Center for Complementary and Alternative Medicine. (2002, May). What is complementary and alternative medicine? NCCAM Pub. No. D156. Available: http://nccam.nih.gov/health/whatiscam/.

Richardson, M. A., Sander, T., Palmer, J. L., Greisinger, A., & Singletary, S. E. (2000). Complementary/alternative medicine use in a comprehensive cancer center and the implications for oncology. *Journal of Clinical Oncology, 18,* 2505–2514.

Sparber, A., Bauer, L., Curt, G., Eisenberg, D., Levin, T., Parks, S., Steinberg, S. M., & Wootton, J. (2000). Use of complementary medicine by adult patients participating in cancer clinical trials. *Oncology Nursing Forum, 27,* 623–630.

CHAPTER

8 Radiation Therapy

Jennifer Dunn Bucholtz
Michele A. Parisi

I. History: In the late 1890s, x-rays and gamma rays were discovered by Roentgen and Curie. By the early 1900s, ionizing radiation was being used to treat a variety of neoplasms. Since that time, the ability to precisely aim radiation at tumors, minimize radiation delivery to normal tissues, and manage the side effects of treatment has greatly improved.

II. Definition: Radiation is the movement of energy through a space or medium. It causes damage or changes to the cells. Radiation therapy is a major cancer treatment that can be used alone or in combination with other therapies to cure, control, or palliate disease. It is estimated that over 50% of all people with cancer will receive radiation therapy during treatment for their disease. Radiation therapy is also used occasionally to treat benign tumors.

III. Rationale for Use: When radiation is well planned and executed, cancer cells are killed or left unable to reproduce while the surrounding healthy cells are minimally affected and can repair radiation damage.

IV. Biology of Therapy: Ionizing radiation includes x-rays and gamma rays, which are energy sources in wave formation, and particle radiation (electrons, beta, or protons). Each form causes damage or changes to cells that are penetrated, and DNA is directly or indirectly damaged.

    A. Cell Cycle Phase: Cells are more sensitive to radiation during the late G_2 and early M phases.

    B. Degree of Oxygenation: Well-oxygenated tumor cells are more sensitive to radiation than hypoxic cells.

    C. Tumor Size: Small tumors are more responsive than large tumors.

    D. Cell Ability to Repair Damage: When treated appropriately, tumor cells are not able to repair radiation damage as well as surrounding normal cells.

    E. Dose and Fraction Size of Radiation: Normal cells are able to repair radiation injury between fractionated doses better than tumor cells.

    F. Types of Radiation: The radiation source may be external or internal. Beam characteristics vary with the source of radiation and allow maximum treatment of different tumor types (Table 8–1).

V. Types of Radiation Therapy

    A. External beam radiation is an external source of radiation in the form of x-rays, gamma rays, protons, or electrons. The source is emitted from equipment that delivers radiation to the depth appropriate for each tumor. Treatment may be administered one or more

TABLE 8-1   Radiation Source, Delivery Mode, and Characteristics

Source	Equipment	Beam Characteristics
X-ray	Kilovoltage (40–150 V)	Superficial, scatters at skin barrier
	Orthovoltage (150–1000 kV)	Deep, with good skin penetration and bone absorption
	Linear accelerator (4–20 MeV)	X-rays
	Betatron (18–40 MeV)	High-energy photons
Gamma rays	Cesium-137 (600 kV)	Large source size
	Cobalt-60 (1.25–2.00 MeV)	Skin sparing, deep penetration
Photons	Linear accelerator (4–20 MeV)	Deep penetration with precession
Electrons	Betatron (10–30 MeV)	High velocity, deep penetration
	Linear accelerator (6–30 MeV)	Maximum skin dose

Adapted from Hilderly, L. J. & Hassey-Dow, K (1996). Radiation oncology. In R. McCorkle et al. (Eds.) *Cancer nursing: A comprehensive textbook* (2nd ed., pp. 331–358). Philadelphia: W. B. Saunders.

times a day. The number of treatments is determined by the size and location of the tumor and the total dose required (see Table 8-1).

B. Internal radiation is placed in or near the tumor. The source may be a sealed isotope, placed in the body, or the systemic administration of an unsealed radionuclide, given orally, intravenously, or into a body cavity.

C. Methods of Administration

  1. Intraoperative treatment exposes the localized tumor or tumor bed to electrons or orthovoltage during the surgical procedure.

  2. Hyperthermia raises the body temperature and increases perfusion of the radioactive substance at the tumor site for a defined period of time.

  3. Radioimmunotherapy allows selective delivery of radionuclide isotopes within the tumor.

  4. Radiosensitizers are chemical agents given to increase sensitivity to radiation.

  5. Radioprotectors are chemical agents that decrease the effects of radiation on normal tissue.

  6. Hyperfractionation uses smaller, more frequent doses of radiation to impact on cancer cells as they divide and grow.

  7. Total body irradiation cleanses the body of any tumor cells before the infusion of healthy bone marrow.

  8. Stereotactic radiosurgery is the precise delivery of radiation to a brain tumor with sparing of surrounding normal tissue. To achieve precision, special procedures for localization of the tumor are necessary. These tools include the stereotactic frame, the computed tomography (CT) and magnetic resonance imaging (MRI) scanner, a computerized system for calculating the radiation dose, and a precise system for delivering the radiation to the tumor.

9. The gamma knife is a radiosurgery device that enables treatment of deep intracranial lesions without the risks of open-skull surgery. The "blades" of the gamma knife are beams of gamma radiation programmed to bombard the lesion when they intersect, and to spare surrounding tissue.

10. Three-dimensional (3D) CT simulation aids in planning. The modern CT simulator is capable of interactive 3D volumetric treatment planning, which provides a digitally reconstructed radiograph (DRR). The technique provides imagery of a beam's eye view of the treatment field anatomy and contoured areas of interest, and is a more accurate beam delivery planning device.

11. Intensity modulated radiation therapy (IMRT) is an advanced form of external beam irradiation. It can yield dose distributions that conform closely to the 3D shape of the target volume (desired treatment area), while minimizing the dose to normal structures by allowing the beam intensity to vary across fields. This provides the opportunity to deliver a higher dose to the diseased area, while sparing normal tissue. This is one of the most important technical advances in radiation therapy.

VI. Nursing Issues
A. Role of the Nurse
1. Provide appropriate education to the patient and family (see VI.C below).
2. Monitor and assess the patient's and family's response to treatment.
3. Ensure that radiation protection measures are followed.

B. Adverse Effects
1. Assess for anticipated side effects and appropriate interventions. Immediate or acute side effects occur during treatment. Long-term side effects may occur from months to years after treatment is completed (Table 8–2).
2. Side effects of radiation are specific to the treatment site.

C. Patient and Family Education
1. Address both expected and emergency situations related to radiation therapy. Many patients are treated in ambulatory settings, and validation of learning is essential to ensure optimal patient outcomes.
2. Explain the onset of side effects to the patient and family. Teach the patient and family ways to anticipate and manage or avoid common side effects of radiation therapy (see Table 8–2).
3. Teach general principles of radiation therapy, such as the source of the radiation and how it works, and explain the treatment schedule (see Table 8–1).
4. Teach emergency procedures by giving instructions on when, why, where, what, and whom to call in the event of an emergency. For example, signs and symptoms of infection or significant bleeding is an emergency situation that requires immediate action.
5. Emphasize radiation safety precautions for patients with an internal radiation source (Table 8–3).

TABLE 8-2 Management of Frequent Side Effects of Radiation Treatment

Symptom	Interventions	Comments
Fatigue (I)	Alter activities of daily living to provide for rest. Participate in mild to moderate exercise as tolerated.	Due to increased metabolic rate. Begins about 3 weeks into treatment and lasts up to 1 month after treatment.
Skin reactions (I)	Skin care: avoid sun, temperature extremes, and other trauma or irritation. Keep skin clean and dry, but avoid OTC lotions, soaps, and topical treatment unless advised by the physician.	Changes should be reported to and evaluated by the nurse or physician. Skin reactions are graded: 0 = no change 1 = mild erythema 2 = severe, red erythema and tenderness and moist desquamation 3 = edema and confluent, moist desquamation 4 = ulceration, hemorrhage, or necrosis
Mucositis (I)	Increase oral hygiene care. Use nonirritating rinses. Assess and medicate for pain with topical and systemic drugs (see Chapter 29).	Diet may need to be altered temporarily. Soft, cool, or room temperature foods are often preferred. Dental care and preventive treatment before beginning radiation are important.
Xerostomia (I)	Increase hydration and assess for changes on a regular schedule. Increase routine mouth care. Use saliva substitutes for long-term problems.	Hard candy and gum may be helpful if mucositis is not a problem.
Dysgeusia (I)	Meals should be altered to accommodate for taste changes. High-protein foods are usually the most objectionable.	Taste changes may resolve or persist after treatment is completed.

(continued)

TABLE 8-2 Management of Frequent Side Effects of Radiation Treatment *(Continued)*

Symptom	Interventions	Comments
Altered functions related to head and neck radiation: dental caries, hypothyroidism, cataracts (L)	Pretreatment dental consult. Ensure appropriate protection during treatment. Assess for side effects after treatment.	Side effects are often late in occurrence.
Respiratory compromise: radiation pneumonitis, pulmonary fibrosis, and cardiac problems (L)	Teach about signs and symptoms and risk of occurrence. Assess on each follow-up visit.	Encourage patients to report these signs to the physician or nurse promptly.
Gastrointestinal side effects: nausea/vomiting, anorexia (I)	Provide high-calorie, high-protein diet in small frequent feedings, as tolerated. Use medications, as ordered, to control side effects.	Refer to dietitian if efforts are not effective.
Bone marrow suppression (I)	Monitor blood counts and administer blood or growth factors as ordered. Treatment break may be required if WBC < 2,000 or platelets < 100,000.	Be sure patients know the signs and symptoms and how to protect themselves from infection and injury.
Sexual dysfunction: infertility, vaginal stenosis, erectile dysfunction (I & L)	Ensure that shielding is appropriate. Teach about sperm and ovum banking. Women may need vaginal lubrication and dilatation.	Refer for appropriate counseling for continued dysfunction or infertility.
Secondary malignancies (L)	Teach cancer warning signals and prevention and detection guidelines.	Risks are higher in children.

I = Immediate; L = Long-Term

TABLE 8-3   Radiation Safety

Principles/Practice	Intervention
Principles of radiation safety are time, distance, and shielding.	Minimize exposure of staff and visitors by limiting the time spent with patients who have an active source of radiation.
	Keep as much distance as possible between you and the radiation source.
	As much as possible, use lead shields to protect from exposure to the source.
Sealed radioactive gamma source: cesium-137, iridium-192, radium-226	Provide private room with precaution signs.
	Place shields and equipment to dispose of a dislodged source in the room.
	Limit staff exposure by teaching self-care measures, assigning pregnant staff to other patients, monitoring exposure using film badge or dosimeter, and observing restricted visiting policy.
	Notify radiation therapy and radiation safety immediately if source is dislodged.
Unsealed source (eg, iodine-131)	Provide private room with precaution signs.
	Cover mattress, pillow, and bathroom floor to prevent and limit contamination.
	Keep all patient linens, personal items, and disposable meal trays in the room until surveyed for radioactive activity.
	Shield as required.
	Limit contacts (see sealed radioactive source, above).
	Use gloves to avoid exposure if body fluids are handled.
	Double flush toilet.
	Restrict visitors per policy.
	Notify radiation safety immediately if body fluids are spilled or contacted.
	Survey room after discharge to ensure appropriate levels of exposure are not exceeded for the next patient.
Protect staff from unnecessary exposure	Do not assign pregnant nurses.
	Provide film badges and monitor exposure.
	Rotate staff to limit exposure.
	Teach and review principles of radiation safety annually and at the time of any policy change.

REFERENCES

Brimer, D. W., Buchholtz, J. D., Iwamoto, R., & Strohl, R. (Eds.). (1998). *Manual for radiation oncology nursing practice and education.* Pittsburgh, PA: Oncology Nursing Society.

Catlin-Huith, C., Hass, J., & Pollack, V. (Eds.). (2002). *Radiation therapy patient care record: A tool for documenting nursing care.* Pittsburgh, PA: Oncology Nursing Society.

Dow, K. H., Bucholtz, J. D., Iwamoto, R., et al. (Eds.). (1997). *Nursing care in radiation oncology* (2nd ed.). Philadelphia: W. B. Saunders.

Hilderly, L. J. (1997). Radiotherapy. In S. Groenwald et al. (Eds.), *Cancer nursing: Principles and practice* (3rd ed., pp. 247–282). Boston: Jones & Bartlett.

Hilderly, L. J., & Hassey-Dow, K. (1996). Radiation oncology. In R. McCorkle et al. (Eds.), *Cancer nursing: A comprehensive textbook* (2nd ed., pp. 331–358). Philadelphia: W. B. Saunders.

Hirth, A., Pedersen, P. H., Baardsen, R., et al. (2003). Gamma-knife radiosurgery in pediatric cerebral and skull base tumors. *Medical and Pediatric Oncology, 40*(2), 99–103.

Intensity Modulated Radiation Therapy Collaborative Working Group. (2001). Intensity-modulated radiotherapy: Current status and issues of interest. *International Journal of Radiation Oncology, Biology, and Physics, 15*, 51(4), 880–914.

Stephenson. J. A., & Wiley, A. L., Jr. (1995). Current techniques in three-dimensional CT simulation and radiation treatment planning. *Oncology, 9*(11), 1225–1232,1235–1240.

Verhey, L. J. (1999). Comparison of three-dimensional conformal radiation therapy and intensity-modulated radiation therapy systems. *Seminars in Radiation Oncology, 9*(1), 78–98.

Xiao Y., Galvin, J., Hossain, M., & Valicenti, R. (2000). An optimized forward-planning technique for intensity modulated radiation therapy. *Medical Physics, 27*(9), 2093–2099.

9 Surgical Therapy

JoAnn Coleman

I. History: Surgery is the oldest treatment for cancer and, until recently, the only cure for patients with cancer. The excision of a tumor recorded on an Egyptian papyrus dating from 1600 BC may be the earliest use of surgery for cancer. More modern approaches to cancer surgery were described in 1809 when a 22-lb ovarian tumor was successfully excised. In the 1890s, Dr. William S. Halsted, a Johns Hopkins surgeon, developed the radical mastectomy procedure, which became the first surgery commonly used for cancer. Over the last several decades of the 20th century, advances in surgical technique and a better understanding of the patterns of spread of individual cancers have dramatically changed the surgical treatment of cancer. Modern anesthetic techniques, increased knowledge of antibiotic therapy, and blood component administration have greatly increased the safety of major oncologic surgery and allowed surgeons to perform successful resections for an increased number of patients.

  A. Surgical therapy is now used in combination with other forms of treatment. Multimodality therapy has led to more conservative, less radical procedures for some cancers as is seen in the options for the treatment of breast cancer. There is also a trend toward an increased use of more aggressive major operations for other cancers. Complex resections of the pancreas and liver can now be performed with less risk because of increased technology and skill.

  B. New technologies may allow for less extensive surgery, with the potential for minimal pain, less use of blood component replacement, decreased hospital stay, and a more rapid recovery. Minimally invasive surgical procedures using laparoscopy, robot-assisted laparoscopy, and video-assisted thoracoscopy are examples of the new techniques that have evolved.

II. Definition: Surgical therapy remains the primary method of treatment of most solid malignancies. In some cases, it is the only chance for cure. It is estimated that more than 90% of patients with cancer have some type of surgical procedure for diagnosis, treatment, or management of the disease and complications.

III. Rationale for Use: A major goal of surgical therapy is to resect the entire tumor and to maximize preservation of body function and appearance, if at all possible. Curative resections involve the removal of tumor along with a margin of normal tissue and regional lymph nodes. This type of resection offers the best chance of cure and provides histologic information for prognosis.

IV. Biology of Therapy

  A. Growth Rate: Slow-growing tumors generally lend themselves best to surgical treatment because the tumor is more likely to be confined to a local area. Smaller tumors are also less likely to have spread, and surgical removal is more likely to be curative.

B. Invasiveness: Any cancer cell remaining after surgery constitutes a risk of recurrence or metastasis. A surgical procedure performed for curative intent of cancer would include resection of the entire tumor mass along with a margin of normal tissue to decrease the risk of leaving residual cancer cells. Cancers with extensive invasion into adjacent structures, such as another organ, or invasion into major blood vessels or nerves could preclude a curative surgical resection.

C. Metastatic Potential: Knowledge of the metastatic patterns of individual tumors is crucial in planning the most effective therapy. Tumors that are slow to metastasize are the most amenable to surgery, whereas those that present with advanced disease are less often curable with surgical therapy alone.

D. Tumor Location: The location of the tumor in relation to other structures is a key factor in determining if it can be surgically removed. Superficial and encapsulated tumors are easier to remove than those embedded in inaccessible or delicate areas. The following questions help determine the potential effectiveness of surgical intervention:
1. Does the tumor involve major vessels or structures that cannot be resected?
2. Has the tumor spread to multiple sites?
3. Is it possible to remove the entire tumor along with a margin of normal tissue?

E. Physical Status: The patient's physical condition may influence the selection of surgery for the treatment of cancer. Careful preoperative assessment involves the evaluation of significant factors that may potentially increase the risk of surgical morbidity and mortality. Deficits should be corrected before surgery whenever possible. Nutritional status often needs corrective measures. A thorough systems assessment and a determination of the presence and severity of other medical conditions factor into the decision to have surgery.
1. The presence and severity of comorbid conditions increase with age. The elderly patient should be treated as aggressively as possible but may need additional preoperative support to be adequately prepared for surgery. Elderly patients are especially at risk for morbidity and mortality if the surgery must be performed as an emergency (eg, emergency surgery to relieve an acute malignant bowel obstruction).
2. A proposed operation may produce physiologic alterations that may be beyond a person's capabilities. The rehabilitation potential of every patient needs to be evaluated, particularly if the intended surgery will significantly alter normal physiologic function.

F. Quality of Life: Quality-of-life issues must be addressed for potential surgical candidates. Research has shown that some radical surgical procedures are not warranted either because they do not improve the end result or because they interfere unduly with the person's functional or physiologic well-being. The patient's unique needs and desires must be considered in the treatment selection process. A particular surgical procedure may be technically feasible, but it may not be the best alternative in terms of quality of life.

V. Roles of Surgery

A. Diagnosis: A tissue diagnosis is important in the planning of subsequent treatment for specific cancers. The major role of surgery in the diagnosis of cancer is the acquisition of tissue for histologic diagnosis. Various techniques are used to obtain tissue for suspected malignancy.

  1. *Aspiration biopsy* is the removal of cells and tissue fragments by aspiration through a needle that has been guided into the suspect tissue. The material is cytologically analyzed to provide a tentative diagnosis of the presence of malignant cells. Although this is a recognized method of examining cells, major surgical resections may not be performed solely on the basis of the evidence provided by an aspiration biopsy because there is an error rate substantially higher than that of standard histologic diagnostic tests.

  2. *Needle biopsy* is performed by obtaining a core of tissue through a specially designed needle placed into the suspect tissue.

  3. *Incisional biopsy* is the removal of a small portion or wedge of tissue from a larger tumor mass. This type of biopsy is usually performed for larger tumors that will require major surgery for removal.

  4. *Excisional biopsy* is the removal of the entire suspected tumor with little or no margin of surrounding normal tissue for diagnostic purposes. This is the most common surgical diagnostic procedure and is used for easily accessible tumors. For nonpalpable lesions, such as mammographic abnormalities of the breast, an excisional biopsy may be performed with the assistance of needle localization. Needle localization involves the placement of a radiopaque wire or needle into or near a nonpalpable radiographic abnormality to mark the site.

  5. *Exfoliative (surface) biopsy* is the direct smear or scrape and examination of these shed cells as found in a Pap smear or brushings or washings from a bronchoscopy.

  6. *Invasive procedures* may allow access to areas that are normally inaccessible. Upper endoscopy, colonoscopy, and laparoscopy are examples of procedures that provide access to areas for one or more types of biopsies.

B. Staging: Staging involves the pathologic examination of tissue to determine the size of the primary tumor, presence of positive lymph nodes, and extent of metastases. Surgical staging is most often performed for tumors otherwise inaccessible, or for those difficult to evaluate by any other means. Extensive surgical staging may be necessary before any major surgical procedure for cure. It provides a systematic approach to the diagnosis and treatment of malignancies.

  1. *Laparotomy:* Exploratory operations may be performed to diagnose and stage cancers with intraperitoneal involvement (eg, laparotomy done to stage lymphoma). Second-look procedures may be performed after chemotherapy to evaluate ovarian cancer.

  2. *Laparoscopy:* Laparoscopic surgery employs a laparoscope and video equipment to visualize internal structures with minimally invasive techniques. The laparoscope is placed into the peritoneum through a small incision. This is the main instrument for looking into the abdomen. Laparoscopic procedures may be used for diagnosis, staging, and treatment of a variety of tumors involving the abdominal cavity, including esophageal cancer, gastric cancer, liver tumors, pancreatic cancer, adrenal tumors, and lymphoma. Biopsies or minimally invasive surgical procedures can be performed through additional small incisions using specially designed instruments. Laparoscopy is useful in evaluating metastatic spread of tumor before laparotomy. It is useful in determining the resectability of gastric cancer, pancreatic cancer, and hepatic tumors and may prevent laparotomy in cases of unresectable disease. Curative resections using laparoscopic techniques are being used in early lesions or for specific reasons.

3. *Robot-assisted laparoscopy:* Advances in technology have enhanced the use of robotics in surgery. Surgeons can perform complex surgeries by guiding and manipulating instruments by way of a computer and robotic arms. This minimally invasive laparoscopic technique is also used to prevent pain, decrease the amount of blood component administered, decrease length of hospital stay, and promote a more rapid recovery.

4. *Sentinel node biopsy* is used to stage a tumor such as melanoma. It is performed when the nodes appear clinically negative. An isotope is injected near a lesion or the site where the lesion was removed. A scan is performed to detect the spread of the isotope. A gamma probe is then used to locate the lymph node that picks up the most isotope, thus documenting the nodal drainage pattern for the area. If the tumor spreads, it will spread to the sentinel node first. This node is then excised. A full lymph node dissection is not performed unless the sentinel node contains cancer cells. This procedure is used in a number of cancer diagnoses and treatments.

5. *Placement of radio-opaque clips* during biopsy, staging and palliative procedures is important to mark areas of known tumor and as a guide to subsequent delivery of radiation therapy in the areas.

C. Treatment: Goals of treatment may include complete excision of malignant disease, control of cancer cell growth, or relief of symptoms associated with the cancer. The magnitude of surgical resection may be modified in the treatment of many cancers by the use of adjuvant therapies. Integrating surgery with other treatment modalities requires a careful consideration of all effective treatment options. The use of effective adjuvant treatment modalities has led to a decrease in the magnitude/extent of surgery in some instances.

1. Curative surgery or definitive surgical treatment for primary cancer involves the complete removal of the malignant tumor, primary lymph nodes, contiguous structures involved, and structures at high risk for tumor spread, along with a margin of normal tissue. The treatment of many solid tumors falls into this category. Usually, a metastatic evaluation for tumor spread will precede a surgical resection for cure. This is also important for staging. The goal of surgery is important in justifying the consequences. If function cannot be preserved, the potential for cure must be great. Resection of a primary solid tumor as the principal form of treatment includes lung cancer, colon cancer, breast cancer, and prostate cancer.

2. Salvage surgery is performed after the patient fails the first line of therapy and experiences recurrence as metastatic cancer from the primary cancer (eg, liver resection for metastatic colon cancer or neck dissection for a nodal metastasis from head and neck cancer).

3. Adjuvant surgery is aimed at removal of tissues to decrease the risk of cancer incidence, progression, or recurrence. It is also performed to reduce the size of a tumor as the extensive local spread of cancer may preclude the removal of all gross disease. This is referred to as *cytoreductive surgery*. Cytoreductive surgery is of benefit only when other treatments are available and may be effective in controlling residual disease that is unresectable.

4. Palliative surgery is performed to promote patient comfort and quality of life without curing the disease. The goal of palliative surgeries is to relieve symptoms of obstruction, pressure, and pain. Palliative surgery may relieve mechanical problems such as intestinal obstruction, or may be used for the removal of masses that are causing severe pain or disfigurement.

   a. Interventional procedures for palliation of obstruction. The use of stents to maintain patency of a lumen has greatly aided in the control of symptoms and quality of life for patients with cancer. Stents may be made of synthetic material or metal. They can be placed either endoscopically by a gastroenterology endoscopist or percutaneously by an interventional radiologist. Stents may be placed endoscopically to relieve esophageal, duodenal, biliary, or colonic obstruction. Stents can also be placed percutaneously for biliary obstruction by interventional radiologists.

   b. Palliative surgeries are also used to create diversions of normal function due to the presence of tumor. Placement of nephrostomy tubes or creation of a colostomy or ileal conduit are examples of surgery for this purpose.

5. Other surgical modalities used for ablation of tumor cells in the treatment of cancer

   a. Cryosurgery uses liquid nitrogen to selectively freeze cancerous tissue, resulting in cell death. This modality is used mainly to treat gynecologic cancers and skin cancers.

   b. Lasers may be used in certain procedures. Laser is an acronym for *light amplification by stimulated emission of radiation*. This treatment modality may be associated with less bleeding and scarring.

      (1) In laser procedures, a laser is attached to a contact tip or scalpel to provide a focused form of energy to incise within a precise location and depth of tissue (eg, a laser cone of the cervix and the use of a laser during endoscopy to open obstructed lumens, particularly the esophagus).

      (2) Photodynamic therapy also uses lasers. This treatment modality involves an intravenous injection of a light-sensitizing agent that is absorbed by cancer cells, followed by exposure to laser light 24 to 48 hours later. This causes cell death. It is used for a possible cure for early stages of some skin and bladder cancers and for palliation of advanced lung, esophageal, and pelvic cancers. The patient will have

photosensitivity for several weeks after injection and should avoid exposure to sunlight during this time.

   c. Fulguration (electrodesiccation) is the eradication of cancer cells by the application of an electric current. Although rarely used, it has some application in the treatment of rectal masses and some skin lesions.

D. Treatment of Complications: Surgery is performed to treat complications of other cancer therapies, oncologic emergencies, and disease sequelae (see Unit V).

E. Prevention/Prophylaxis: Surgery is also performed to prevent cancer in high-risk individuals. Removal of precancerous lesions prevents the subsequent development of cancer.

   1. Patients with familial polyposis and those with ulcerative colitis have a propensity to develop colorectal cancer. Surgery to remove the entire colon and rectum, called a total proctocolectomy, will prevent cancer from developing.

   2. A prophylactic mastectomy may be indicated for individuals at high risk for breast cancer.

   3. Cryptorchidism places males at risk for the development of testicular cancer, thus orchidectomy may be indicated.

F. Reconstruction/Rehabilitation: Extensive surgical resections that cause disfigurement are sometimes necessary to obtain adequate tissue margins. Reconstruction techniques may be performed at the time of initial resection or at a later date/time. Reconstruction operations aim to improve structure, function, and appearance, and to repair or reduce anatomical defects from cancer surgery or therapy. Examples include breast reconstruction, facial reconstruction for head and neck cancers, and skin grafting.

G. Insertion of Devices for Other Treatment Modalities (eg, placement of vascular access devices, ommaya reservoirs, hepatic arterial infusion pumps, gastrostomy or jejunostomy tubes, and brachytherapy catheters).

VI. Nursing Issues: The surgical oncology patient requires nursing care similar to that required for any other surgical patient. However, the surgical oncology nurse must be aware of unique problems and complications related to treatment modalities for cancer and the disease process. The effect of cancer and previous cancer therapies increases the risk for postsurgical complications.

A. Diagnosis

   1. Explain the purpose of the diagnostic procedure and how it will be performed.

   2. Provide specific information regarding any preparation as with a special bowel or skin preparation.

   3. Provide additional information depending on the type of biopsy and where it will be performed (eg, in the doctor's office, the operating room, or another area such as the endoscopy suite or radiology).

   4. Offer emotional support to allay patient fears while awaiting definitive diagnosis.

   5. Inform the patient how long it will take to get the results of the biopsy. This depends on where it is performed and type of tumor cells being reviewed.

B. Treatment

1. During patient assessment, perform a thorough nursing history and baseline assessment, focusing on factors that may increase the incidence of postoperative complications. These factors include preexisting cardiac, pulmonary, renal, central nervous system, mobility, and gastrointestinal problems; any prior surgeries; bleeding tendencies; lifestyle factors such as smoking, alcohol, and drug use; and any prior cancer therapy, including the date of the last treatment.

2. Teach the patient about the planned procedure by explaining the operation, what to anticipate after surgery, potential complications, and expected outcomes. These may all vary depending on each procedure. It is beneficial to have another person with the patient to hear the instructions and education provided. This "other ear" can validate what was taught by the nurse as well as ask questions perhaps not considered by the patient.

   a. Use both written and verbal reinforcement to aid retention because perioperative anxiety impairs learning. Provide written materials, anatomical diagrams, and pictures of what the operation will involve. Explanations of special surgical techniques, such as laparoscopy, may also be useful. Referral to an appropriate Internet website may also be helpful for patient education.

   b. Explain the reason for the surgery and incorporate the use of a clinical or critical pathway/care map to educate the patient and family about the typical daily progress for the particular procedure.

   c. Prepare the patient by explaining any bowel preparation (if indicated), positioning during surgery, location of incision, placement of any tubes and/or wound drains, intravenous lines or any other special attachments.

   d. Explain what will be expected of the patient postoperatively regarding deep breathing exercises, activity, diet advancements, and self-care to optimize recovery.

3. Assess current pain management in terms of both needs and deficits.

   a. Find out if the patient is currently on any pain medications and, if so, which ones and at what dose because this will have an impact on postoperative doses.

   b. Address the patient's fears of postoperative pain and explain pain management strategies, such as patient-controlled analgesia, in order to reduce patient anxiety.

4. Facilitate discharge planning by assessing needs and available resources preoperatively.

   a. Evaluate function in terms of abilities and deficits.

   b. Evaluate support systems, community resources, and special needs preoperatively to facilitate planning for needed services. Preoperative planning for discharge needs is important as hospital stays are minimized and the access to resources may be limited. Coordination and mobilization of resources improve efficiency.

   c. Assist with discharge planning, and consult a social worker as dictated by the needs and anxieties of the patient. It is important to address the patient's fears, concerns, and perceptions about the situation, and to refer the patient to resources, such as support groups or individual counseling as appropriate.

5. Offer emotional support throughout the perioperative course as the patient comes to understand the disease, surgical procedure, and anticipated outcomes. Often, patients only hear the words *cancer* and *surgery* and forget all of the preoperative instructions. A supportive nurse-patient relationship promotes an atmosphere in which the patient is encouraged to voice fears and anxieties.

C. Postoperative
   1. As with any postoperative patient, monitor and assess the patient, prevent complications, and promote the return to normal functioning. Note that the patient's immediate needs are primarily physical.
   2. Be aware of the effects of combined modality therapies or recent anti-neoplastic treatments. The interactive and compounding effects of chemotherapy, radiation therapy, and immunotherapy produce difficult problems and place the patient at higher risk for postoperative complications.
   3. Manage pain in the surgical patient. Physical comfort is the primary focus, and both intravenous and epidural patient-controlled analgesia pumps are commonly used. Surgical oncology patients may have greater needs for postoperative analgesia, particularly if the surgical procedure is for advanced disease or if patients were previously receiving analgesics. Many oncology patients are not narcotically naïve and may have sources of chronic pain in addition to acute surgical pain. Performing a thorough pain assessment and appropriate management of pain often requires the expertise of an astute surgical oncology nurse (see Chapter 30).

D. Role of the Surgical Oncology Nurse Dealing With Adverse Effects
   1. Pulmonary problems: A postoperative temperature elevation in the first 48 hours is almost always secondary to atelectasis, not infection. Instruct the patient in appropriate pulmonary toilet, including the use of an incentive spirometer, turning, coughing, and deep breathing exercises. Encourage early ambulation to promote lung expansion and mobilization of secretions.
   2. Wound complications: Cancer patients are particularly prone to infection and bleeding. Postoperative wound healing may be impaired by nutritional status, age, dehiscence, infection, and tissue and bone necrosis after radiation therapy. Head and neck cancer patients who have had preoperative radiation therapy are at increased risk for carotid artery rupture and poor wound healing. Certain chemotherapeutic agents, including methotrexate, bleomycin, doxorubicin, and 5-fluorouracil (5FU), have been shown to modify wound healing at specific times in the postoperative period. Immunosuppression places the patient at a higher risk for wound infections. Latent cytomegalovirus may be activated by the stress of surgery. For more information on wound healing, staging, and care products, see Tables 9–1 and 9–2 and Box 9–1.
      a. Assess wounds for any signs or symptoms of infection, seroma, or hematoma.
      b. Check drains for patency and for color, consistency, and amount of drainage.

TABLE 9-1   Phases of Wound Healing

Phase	Care Focus
Inflammatory Phase • Begins with tissue trauma, ends with clean wound • Initial goals: Prevent hemorrhage, bacterial invasion beyond the wound, extension of injury • Long-term goals: Prevent bacterial invasion, eliminate nonviable tissue, support healing	• Aggressive cleaning • Maintain moisture • Disinfect as necessary • Regular reassessment
Fibroblastic Phase • Begins with clean tissue base; ends with closed wound • Goal: Begin granulation and closure of the wound	• More gentle cleansing to allow granulation • Maintain moisture for fibroblasts to be effective • Bleeding during dressing changes indicates granulation tissue is damaged
Maturation Phase • Begins with wound closure; ends after scar remodeling • Goal: Develop scar with strong tensile strength	• Continue pressure relief strategies • Maintain adequate nutrition for healing • Protect the scar tissue from injury

Hawkins-Bradley, B. (2003). Effective management of chronic wounds: Practical approaches to wound healing. Nashville, TN: Cross Country University.

    c. Monitor for other signs of bleeding, such as tachycardia, hypotension, and decreased urine output.

  3. Deep vein thrombosis/pulmonary embolism: Coagulopathies and bleeding tendencies are not uncommon in the oncology patient. Hypercoagulability and thrombosis are associated with abnormal clotting factors found in some cancer patients, placing them at increased risk for the development of deep vein thrombosis and pulmonary embolism. Certain surgical procedures, such as abdominal or pelvic surgery, also predispose the patient to deep vein thrombosis.

    a. Provide the patient with support hose and sequential compression devices on the legs to promote venous return and prevent pooling of blood.

    b. Use low-dose heparin therapy to reduce complications of venous stasis in certain patients.

    c. Encourage early mobilization and ambulation to decrease the risk of deep vein thrombosis and pulmonary embolism.

  4. Malnutrition: Nutritional depletion places the patient at risk for poor wound healing, infection, pneumonia, and increased morbidity. Surgical procedures, such as gastrectomy, place the patient at higher risk for problems of dumping syndrome, malabsorption, and changes in eating patterns.

TABLE 9–2 Wound Care Products, Level I*

Product	Characteristics	Advantages	Disadvantages	Use
Transparent films	Clear film with adhesive, allows gas exchange, and maintains a barrier to water and bacteria	Semiocclusive protection, conforms to body surface, wound is visible, facilitates autolytic débridement, less costly than some dressings	Adhesive may damage fragile skin, nonabsorbent, does not fill in dead space	Dry, shallow wounds, softens eschar, protects from friction
Hydrocolloid dressings	Occlusive, absorbs 3 to 5 times its weight in fluid, usually in a gel or paste, and may be used as a depth filler	Absorbency, protects from contamination, conforms to body surface, promotes autolysis, less frequent dressing changes	Not for use with infected wounds, high moisture environment, may dislodge with movement, adhesive may damage skin, unpleasant odor or residue on skin/wound	Shallow wounds with moderate exudates, promotes autolytic débridement, soothes painful wounds
Calcium alginates	Nonadhesive, nonocclusive, sheets or rope that facilitates autolytic débridement in moist wounds	Very absorbent, may use with infection, fills dead space, nonadhesive, extended time between dressing changes, does not disrupt wound base	Requires secondary dressing, more costly if changed frequently	Fills in depth under hydrocolloids or films, good débridement of slough after eschar is removed
Hydrogels	Sheets, gauze, or tube forms; is water-based with polymers or glycerin to add moisture, facilitates granulation and autolytic débridement	Soothes painful wounds, absorbent, conforms to body, does not disrupt wound base, may be occlusive or nonocclusive	May dry after 24 hours, may cause maceration of surrounding skin, costly, requires secondary dressing, limited absorption	Painful wounds, partial thickness wounds, surgical wounds, dry eschar or dry clean wounds, wounds with fragile surrounding skin

116

Foams	Polyurethane foams with absorbent layers and repellent outer cover, may have activated charcoal for odor	Available with or without adhesive, nonocclusive, does not disrupt wound base or cause pain on removal, absorbs exudates, helps control odor	May dry wounds, costly	Wounds with heavy exudates, skin tears, wounds with macerated edges, malodorous wounds or tumors
Exudate absorbers	Secondary dressings usually containing polymer beads, nonocclusive	Can combine with other products to decrease need for dressing changes, promotes autolytic or mechanical débridement, can be used on infected wounds, conforms to body surface, range of costs	Requires secondary dressing, may adhere to wound base and disrupt granulation	Heavy exudation, use to mechanically débride, extend dressing time with hydro-colloids and films
Moisture barriers (ointments, wipes, sprays)	Nonocclusive with zinc, petroleum, or dimethicone base	Protect peri-wound skin from friction, moisture, and adhesives, available, low cost, can be combined with other products	May prevent dressing from adhering and rub off	Prevention of skin breakdown from incontinence, protection of peri-wound skin

*Level I products are commonly available and often reimbursable, and should be used in initial interventions.

Hawkins-Bradley, B. (2003). *Effective management of chronic wounds: Practical approaches to wound healing.* Nashville, TN: Cross Country University.

▼ **BOX 9-1** | **Wound Staging**

Partial thickness wounds may be stage I or II and have the following characteristics:

Shallow, moist, painful, pink-red color, involves epidermis and dermis
Stage I: Intact skin with nonblanchable erythema
Stage II: Dermal wound or roofed blister; does not granulate to heal

Full-thickness wounds may be stage III or IV and have the following characteristics:

Shallow or deep (< or > 0.5cm, respectively), extend to subcutaneous layer or deeper, may be necrotic or infected
Stage III: Extends to subcutaneous layer, may be shallow or deep, heals by granulation, may have undermining or tunnels
Stage IV: Extends to muscle or bone, osteomyelitis may occur

5. Bladder and bowel dysfunction: Urinary retention can be a problem postoperatively. Patients who have epidural catheters for pain management are more prone to develop problems with urinary retention. Various changes in bowel patterns may also occur, depending on the type of surgical procedure.
   a. Discontinue Foley catheters as soon as possible based on the type of surgery performed. Surgery on the rectum or in the pelvis may require the catheter to remain in place longer.
   b. Monitor bowel function as appropriate for the surgery performed.
   c. Postpone diet advancement until bowel sounds are present and flatus has been passed.
   d. Monitor the patient for development of an ileus in the postoperative period.
6. Immobility: In addition to early ambulation, certain surgical procedures may require specific postoperative activity. For example, patients who have had a mastectomy should be instructed regarding arm exercises to promote the return to normal range of motion. Physical therapy may be necessary to assist the patient in returning to functional abilities. Mobility restrictions may also be indicated for certain reconstructive procedures. In addition, occupational therapists may be consulted to help patients resume activities of daily living.
E. Patient Education: Patients and families commonly want to know if all the cancer was removed and how the surgery will affect their lives. Reinforce what the surgeon has told the patient, as well as any preoperative instructions. Much repetition is usually needed because patient anxiety may have been elevated before surgery and retention of information may be poor. Discharge planning starts before the operation, mainly at the time of decision for surgical intervention. Teach the patient about the disease, the surgical procedure, and how it will impact lifestyle, activities of daily living, employment, and relation-

ships. Patients and families may need to learn how to care for wounds, drains, and equipment along with learning to deal with alterations in functioning. Review information regarding future treatment plans. When the patient and family know what to expect, they can often modify life in the home to facilitate long-term rehabilitation.

F. Emotional Support: Discuss with the patient expectations regarding the surgery and its perceived impact on lifestyle and relationships. Provide opportunities for the patient to discuss concerns and the meaning attached to the loss of a body part or function or both. Postoperatively, the surgeon will inform the patient and family of the surgical findings and what the operation accomplished. Provision of an appropriate environment for this discussion is essential. For many patients, it is after surgery that they come to the realization they have cancer.

G. Effects of Other Therapy: The interactive and compounding effects of chemotherapy, radiation therapy, and immunotherapy may produce problems and side effects for the postoperative patient. Postoperative wound healing may be compromised by effects of radiation therapy; immunosuppression places the patient at a higher risk for wound infections; and chemotherapeutic agents have specific organ toxicities that place the surgical oncology patient at increased risk for pulmonary, renal, respiratory, and cardiac complications.

VII. Follow-up: Follow-up after surgery depends on several factors, including the type of operation, the stage of the cancer, and the patient's general medical condition. If appropriate, referrals are made to medical oncology and radiation oncology for further therapy. Generally, the risk for recurrence lessens over time. Follow-up visits may be fairly frequent for the first few months to years after diagnosis and then become less frequent.

REFERENCES

Aiken, S. W. (2003). Principles of surgery for the cancer patient. *Clinical Techniques in Small Animal Practice, 18*(2), 75–81.

Ashammakhi, N., Suuronen, R., Tiainen, J., Tormala, P., & Waris, T. (2003). Spotlight on naturally absorbable osteofixation devices. *Craniofacial Surgery, 14*(2), 247–259.

Bland, K. I. (Ed). (2002). *The practice of general surgery.* Philadelphia: W. B. Saunders.

Cameron, J. L. (Ed.). (2001). *Current surgical therapy* (7th ed.). St Louis, MO: Mosby.

Chand, B., Felsher, J., & Ponsky, J. (2003). Future trends in flexible endoscopy. *Seminars in Laparoscopic Surgery, 10*(1), 49–54.

Dunn, G. P. (2002). Surgical palliation in advanced disease: Recent developments. *Current Oncology Reports, 4*(3), 233–241.

Hawkins-Bradley, B. (2003). *Effective management of chronic wounds: Practical appoaches to wound healing.* Nashville, TN: Cross Country University.

Kirsner, K. M. (2003). Cancer: New therapies and new approaches to recurring problems. *AANA Journal, 71*(1), 55–62.

Krouse, H. J. (1998). Innovations in office-based surgery. *ORL-Head and Neck Nursing, 16*(3), 20–26.

Pandit, S. K. (1999). Ambulatory anesthesia and surgery in America: A historical background and recent innovations. *Journal of Perianesthesia Nursing, 14*(5), 270–274.

Winer, W. K. (1999). Laparoscopic procedures: Innovations and complications. *Today's Surgical Nurse, 21*(1), 15–19, quiz 33–34.

TYPES OF CANCER

10 Breast Cancer

Carol D. Riley

I. Definition

A. Incidence: Excluding skin cancers, breast cancer is the most common cancer in women, accounting for 32% of all cancers in the United States. In 2003, there will be an estimated 211,000 new breast cancers diagnosed. It is second only to lung cancer as the leading cause of death in women. In the United States, a woman has a 1 in 8 risk of developing breast cancer during her lifetime, with an increasing risk in each decade of life after age 40. Worldwide, breast cancer is the leading cause of cancer death among women. The overall incidence of breast cancer in Japan is approximately one fifth that of the United States. In Western Europe, 1 in 15 will develop breast cancer in their lifetime. An increase in the incidence of early breast cancer is attributed to screening and detection.

B. Epidemiology: The incidence of breast cancer is highest in developed countries. Within the United States, breast cancer is most common in Caucasian women, followed by African-American women. Asians and Hispanics are at lower risk, and American Indian women are least likely to have breast cancer.

C. Morbidity and Mortality: Although the overall incidence of breast cancer has increased, the mortality rate from breast cancer has undergone a gradual decline. This decline in mortality is likely due to numerous factors, including earlier stage at diagnosis, advances in local therapy, and advances in systemic treatment of breast cancer.

II. Etiology

A. Risk Factors: The cause of breast cancer in humans is not known, but some factors will put a woman at a higher risk than average.

1. Gender: Breast cancer occurs almost 100 times more frequently in women than in men.

2. Age: The risk of breast cancer increases with age.

3. Demographic/social factors: More commonly a disease of the upper socioeconomic classes.

4. Family history: The risk of breast cancer doubles if there is a history of breast cancer in a first-degree relative. BRCA1 and BRCA2 mutations account for only 5% to 6% of all breast cancers. Mutations of the p53 tumor-suppressor gene may contribute to 1% of breast cancers in women less than 40 years of age. Having a BRCA1 mutation gives a woman up to an 85% risk of developing breast cancer. In addition, it increases a woman's risk of developing ovarian cancer. Having a BRCA2 mutation predisposes men to breast cancer (see Chapter 2).

5. Personal history of breast cancer, atypical hyperplasia, ductal or lobular cancer in situ increases a woman's risk of developing primary breast cancer or a second breast cancer.
6. Reproductive factors: Nulliparity or having first full-term pregnancy after age 30 increases a women's risk of developing breast cancer, particularly in the months after delivery.
7. Menstrual factors: Menarche before the age of 12 or onset of menopause after age 55.
8. Oral contraceptives: A recent study by Marchbanks and associates (2002) shows no association between past or present use of oral contraceptives and breast cancer risk.
9. Estrogen/progestin replacement therapy: On May 31, 2002, after a mean follow-up of 5.2 years, the Women's Health Initiative trial, which was looking at estrogen and progestin in postmenopausal women, stopped the trial because of patient safety. Among others, the risk of breast cancer risk was increased by 26%. The absolute risk was 38 versus 30 per 10,000. This trial, however, does not address the risk of estrogen alone on the incidence of breast cancer (Rossouw et al., 2002).
10. Dietary factors: Research does not support an association between breast cancer and dietary fat intake. The use of alcohol has also been studied, and there seems to be an association between breast cancer risk and alcohol. The American Cancer Society recommends that women consume no more than one alcoholic beverage per day.
11. Exposure to radiation: There is an association between radiation exposure and breast cancer risk. The risk is inversely correlated with age, and it is very low if the exposure occurred after the age of 40. Most epidemiologic evidence is derived for women who received mantle radiation for Hodgkin's disease at a young age.

III. **Patient Management**
   A. Risk Reduction: There is no prevention for breast cancer, but there are ways to reduce one's risk. The Gail model (Gail et al., 1999) is often used to identify the potential risk of breast cancer and evaluate eligibility for chemoprevention.
      1. Chemoprevention. The largest breast cancer prevention trial, NSABP-P1, showed a decrease in the development of breast cancer by almost 50% in women in the tamoxifen treatment arm as compared with those receiving placebo (Fisher, 1998). Women at a high risk for breast cancer should be considered for tamoxifen prevention.
      2. A newer medication, raloxifene, has shown promise in preliminary studies as a preventive agent for breast cancer. Raloxifene is approved to treat and prevent osteoporosis. The NSABP-P2 trial, the Study of Tamoxifen Against Raloxifene (STAR), will evaluate the efficacy of raloxifene in preventing breast cancer in high-risk women and will compare its efficacy with that of tamoxifen. Side effects such as menopausal symptoms, endometrial cancer, thromboembolic events, and benefits regarding serum lipids and incidence of osteoporotic bone fractures will be carefully assessed.
   B. Assessment: Screening and Early Detection: The goal of screening is to detect cancers at the earliest stage possible, because the extent of disease at diagnosis is correlated with survival.

1. Screening: The American Cancer Society recommends the following:
   a. Breast self-examination (BSE) should be practiced monthly by women, beginning in adolescence.
   b. A skilled health care professional should provide annual clinical breast examination (CBE). The CBE should be conducted close to and preferably before the scheduled mammogram.
   c. Annual mammography beginning at age 40.
2. Signs/symptoms
   a. Breast cancer is found more frequently on the left side in the upper outer quadrant of the breast. The mass may be tender or painless.
   b. Features suggestive of a malignant mass include:
      (1) Hard, painless mass that may be fixed to the chest wall.
      (2) Nipple discharge that is unilateral and serosanguineous results from a local lesion. Palpating each quadrant with one finger and observing when the discharge occurs from the duct can identify the involved quadrant.
      (3) Skin dimpling and retraction. Dimpling may look like the surface of a golf ball, and retraction alters the contour of the breast. Recent onset of nipple inversion may also result from tumor growth.
      (4) Redness, heat, tenderness, and edema are characteristic signs of inflammatory breast cancer that result from dermal involvement.
      (5) Skin ulceration is often present with locally advanced carcinoma.
      (6) Nipple changes may be moist, eczematous, dry, or psoriatic in Paget's disease of the nipple.
      (7) Peau d'orange skin changes appear as thickened skin with prominent pores. It is the result of obstructed lymphatic drainage.
      (8) Palpable lymph nodes are frequently an indication of metastasis. They are most commonly palpable in the axilla, but supraclavicular, infraclavicular, inframammary, or cervical lymph nodes may also be enlarged.
C. Diagnosis
   1. Radiology
      a. Mammography
         (1) Mammography is useful in screening asymptomatic women, evaluating palpable masses, and monitoring women who are at high risk for breast cancer. This small dose of radiation is best able to penetrate the tissue of women who are postmenopausal, over 50 years of age, and have less dense breast tissue.
         (2) All patients with any clinically worrisome breast mass should undergo mammography, and all palpable breast masses that cannot be definitely ruled benign should be biopsied.
         (3) Dense tissue, scar tissue, or breast implants can impede visualization.
         (4) Mammography findings suggestive of malignancy include an irregular or spiculated mass, clustered calcifications, solid

nodule with ill-defined borders, architectural distortion, or a focal density.

b. Ultrasound, although not approved for screening, is useful in diagnosing a breast mass in young women with dense tissue. It is often used as an adjunct to mammography and is helpful in differentiating solid masses from cysts.

c. Magnetic resonance imaging (MRI) is investigational for screening. It is more expensive but improves the sensitivity and specificity of mammography. It differentiates between solid and liquid tumors of small size. It may be the best method of visualization for women with silicone implants.

d. Positron emission tomography (PET) is being studied and is not proven for screening. It is adjunctive to mammography in patients with dense breasts. It may also be useful in patients with axillary or internal mammary lymph nodes.

2. Biopsy: Tissue is necessary to make a diagnosis of breast cancer.

a. Fine-needle aspiration (FNA) is used most often to differentiate between solid and cystic masses. It is inexpensive, causes little discomfort, and can be performed in an outpatient or office setting. It cannot, however, distinguish between invasive cancers and a ductal carcinoma in situ (DCIS)

b. Core-needle biopsy can be done with or without the assistance of ultrasound. It is appropriate for both palpable and nonpalpable breast masses and will yield enough tissue to adequately evaluate the tissue for immunohistochemistry (ie, hormone receptors [HR] and HER2/neu status). It is highly accurate and can be performed in an office or outpatient setting.

c. Stereotactic biopsy is useful in sampling small, nonpalpable lesions, but shares the same limitations as FNA.

d. Open biopsy may be required for some lesions to determine a definitive diagnosis. This is done in the operating room, is more expensive, and requires a longer period of recovery. The biopsy may be incisional, sampling only part of the tumor, or excisional, removing the total tumor.

D. Treatment

1. Staging: The American Joint Committee on Cancer (AJCC, 2002) recently developed a new staging system to take into account number of lymph nodes and micrometastasis (Table 10–1). This new system also reclassifies internal mammary nodes and infraclavicular nodes (Table 10–2).

2. Treatment plan: The treatment of breast cancer varies according to type, stage, and hormone sensitivity. The three modalities of treatment include surgery, radiation, and systemic drug therapy.

a. Surgery—Two major types of surgery are used: mastectomy and breast-conserving therapy, with or without lymph node dissection and/or sentinel node biopsy. The goal of surgery is to remove the existing tumor as well as to determine staging and prognostic information. Surgery is used primarily with early-stage breast cancer when the goal of therapy is cure. It is also used for palliation in the metastatic setting when there is a large breast mass that is ulcerating and painful.

TABLE 10-1 Definition of TNM

Primary Tumor (T)

Tis	Carcinoma in situ
Tx	Primary tumor cannot be assessed
T0	No evidence of primary tumor
T1	Tumor size less than 2 cm (including microinvasion, 0.1 cm or less)
T2	Tumor size 2 to 5 cm
T3	Tumor size greater than 5 cm
T4	Extension to the chest wall, not including the pectoralis muscle
	Edema or ulceration of the skin
	Inflammatory carcinoma

Regional Lymph Nodes (N)
Pathologic—Based on axillary lymph node dissection with or without sentinel nodes

pNx	Regional lymph nodes cannot be assessed
pN0	No regional lymph node metastasis
pN1	Metastasis in one to three axillary and internal mammary nodes (including micrometastasis, 0.2 cm to 2.0 cm)
PN2	Metastasis in four to nine axillary lymph nodes, or in clinically apparent internal mammary nodes in the absence of axillary metastasis; metastasis in four to nine axillary lymph nodes with at least one measuring greater than 2.0 cm
PN3	Metastasis in 10 or more axillary lymph nodes, or in infraclavicular lymph nodes, or in internal mammary lymph nodes in the presence of one or more axillary nodes

Distant Metastasis (M)

Mx	Distant metastasis cannot be assessed
M0	No distant metastasis
M1	Distant metastasis

(1) Breast-conserving therapy (lumpectomy) is a limited removal of the tumor and a margin of normal tissue while leaving much of the breast intact. Radiation therapy is required to complete local treatment. Lumpectomy may be a choice for women without multifocal disease who have adequate tissue for good cosmesis.

(2) Mastectomy is the removal of the entire breast. This is most often performed in women who have large tumors or multifocal disease or who are not otherwise candidates for breast-conserving therapy. This is also performed based on patient preference. Immediate or delayed reconstruction is an option for these patients.

(3) Exploration of the axillary nodes is necessary in patients with invasive breast cancers. Node dissection determines staging

TABLE 10–2 Stage Grouping

Stage 0	Tis	N0	M0
Stage 1	T1	N0	M0
Stage IIA	T0	N2	M0
	T1	N1	M0
	T2	N0	M0
Stage IIB	T2	N1	M0
	T3	N0	M0
Stage IIIA	T0	N2	M0
	T1	N2	M0
	T2	N2	M0
	T3	N1	M0
	T3	N2	M0
Stage IIIB	T4	N0	M0
	T4	N1	M0
	T4	N2	M0
Stage IV	Any	Any	M1
	T	N	

and guides physicians in treatment recommendations. In the past, a full axillary node dissection was performed; more recently, however, the sentinel node biopsy is being studied as an alternative. The sentinel lymph node is the first node to receive drainage from the breast and more likely to contain metastatic cancer cells. It is identified through visualization of blue dye injected at the tumor site and intraoperative gamma probe detection. If the sentinel node is identified, patients may avoid a full axillary dissection if the sentinel node is free of cancer cells. Sentinel node biopsy is not the standard of care. There is a learning curve associated with this technique, and there is a 9% to 15% false-negative rate. Ongoing studies are evaluating the use of sentinel lymph node dissection alone as adequate and reliable for staging.

b. Radiation therapy

(1) Adjuvant radiation therapy completes breast-conserving therapy. Fisher and associates (2002) recently reported a 20-year follow-up of patients treated with mastectomy alone versus patients treated with lumpectomy and radiotherapy. This trial concludes that there is no survival difference in early-stage disease in these two groups. This important trial paved the way for women to receive breast conservation.

(2) Postmastectomy radiotherapy in the adjuvant setting has a role that is still controversial. Two large trials (Overgaard, 1999; Ragaz, 1997) demonstrate a decrease in locoregional recurrence in patients with stage II or III breast cancer receiving postoperative radiation and improved overall survival. The American Society of Clinical Oncologists recommends postmastectomy radiotherapy for patients with large tumors (T3), or those with four or more positive lymph

nodes. The role of postmastectomy radiotherapy in patients with one to three positive lymph nodes is under debate but should be considered and discussed with patients. There are clinical trials ongoing that will answer this question of postmastectomy radiotherapy in patients with one to three positive nodes.

(3) Radiation in the metastatic setting is used primarily for pain control in patients with bony metastasis or those with skin metastasis.

c. Systemic chemotherapy

   (1) Adjuvant therapy: The decision to treat with systemic adjuvant therapy is based on prognostic factors. The two most important prognostic indicators are tumor size and number of lymph nodes involved. The goal of therapy is to prevent or stop the growth of micrometastatic cancer cells and reduce the risk of recurrent disease.

     (a) Chemotherapy has been shown to improve the long-term, relapse-free, and overall survival in both premenopausal and postmenopausal women up to age 70 years regardless of nodal status. The National Comprehensive Cancer Center Network (NCCN) guidelines are under review and revision because of the new staging system; however, current guidelines recommend that women with a tumor size greater than 1 cm or those with node-positive disease be considered for chemotherapy.

     (b) Many proven chemotherapy options are available (Table 10–3).

     (c) Results of a large intergroup trial (Cancer and Leukemia Group B Trial [CALGB] 9741) showed a survival advantage without additional toxicities in administering standard chemotherapy regimens, such as AC (see Table 10–3), in more frequent intervals, known as "dose dense" therapy. These are early but promising results (Citron et al., 2003).

     (d) The use of high-dose chemotherapy followed by bone marrow transplantation or peripheral blood stem cell (PBSC) transplantation has not been shown to work better than standard chemotherapy in the treatment of breast cancer.

     (e) Complications of chemotherapy

       (i) Side effects of chemotherapy are usually not life threatening, vary in degree, and usually follow a predictable course. According to the ECOG grading system, side effects are measured on a scale from 0 to 4 with 0 being normal and 4 being the most severe or life threatening. Severe side effects can cause a delay in therapy or a dose modification of drug(s), or cessation of therapy (Table 10–4; see Chapter 6).

       (ii) Chemotherapy in the metastatic setting: Metastatic breast cancer is an incurable disease, making quality of life during treatment a primary concern. Systemic treatment is palliative in nature, and the goals

TABLE 10–3 Common Adjuvant Chemotherapeutic Regimens

CMF (Milan regimen)	Cyclophosphamide 100 mg/m² p.o. qd days 1 to 14
	Methotrexate 40 mg/m² IV day 1 and day 8
	5-fluorouracil 600 mg/m² IV day 1 and day 8
	Cycle is repeated every 28 days for six treatments.
AC	Doxorubicin 60 mg/m² IV
	Cyclophosphamide 600 mg/m² IV
	Cycle is repeated every 21 days for a total of four treatments.
	May be given every 2 weeks (dose dense) with growth factor support.
Taxol	Paclitaxel 175 mg/m² IV
	Cycle is repeated every 21 days for four treatments after four treatments with AC.
	May be given every 2 weeks (dose dense) with growth factor support.
	Or
	Paclitaxel 80 to 100 mg/m² IV weekly for 12 treatments
CEF	Cyclophosphamide 400 mg/m² IV
	Epirubicin 60 mg/m² IV
	5-Fluorouracil 500 mg/m² IV on days 1 and 8
	Cycle is repeated every 21 days for a total of six treatments.
CAF	Cyclophosphamide 600 mg/m²
	Doxorubicin 60 mg/m²
	Fluorouracil 600 mg/m²

of treatment include improving quality of life and prolongation of life. Median survival with metastatic breast cancer has been reported to be 18 to 24 months; however, some patients experience long-term survival.

  d. Systemic hormonal therapy: There are a number of exciting advances in hormonal therapy for the treatment of breast cancer in both the adjuvant and metastatic settings. The goal of hormonal therapy is to prevent breast cancer cells from receiving stimulation from estrogen. Hormonal therapy is recommended for women whose breast cancer tissue stains positive for estrogen receptor (ER) by immunohistochemistry. There is a small subset of women whose tumors lack ER but contain progesterone receptor (PR), who appear to benefit from hormonal therapy. The 2000 International Breast Cancer Consensus Conference recommended that hormonal therapy be given to women whose breast tumors contain HR protein, regardless of age, menopausal status, involvement of axillary lymph nodes, or tumor size.

    (1) Tamoxifen for 5 years continues to be the hallmark hormone treatment for HR-positive breast cancers. Tamoxifen is an antiestrogen that binds with the ER in breast cancer cells and interferes with DNA synthesis. Two major studies were conducted by the NSABP, B-14 and B-20, which established a 47%

reduction in recurrence and mortality with 5 years of use at 10 years. Tamoxifen has been extensively studied, and the side effects are well established (Fisher et al., 1998; Table 10–5).

(2) Aromatase inhibitors, such as letrozole and anastrozole, are newer agents that inhibit the aromatase enzyme from converting androgens into estrogens in postmenopausal women. These drugs are well established in the metastatic setting. Research evaluating their use in the adjuvant setting suggests they may be better than tamoxifen in preventing recurrence of the disease in some women. These results are preliminary. The current guidelines from the American Society of Clinical Oncologists recommend long-term follow-up before a major practice change will take place. Tamoxifen is still the drug of choice, but this new information does provide physicians with options, especially for those who cannot tolerate or who have a contraindication to tamoxifen. The side-effect profile of anastrozole is different than tamoxifen (Table 10–6).

(3) Ovarian ablation
   (a) Studies suggest that ovarian ablation should be offered to premenopausal women with stage I and II, receptor-positive breast cancer. An Austrian study (Jakesz, 2002) suggests that ovarian ablation in combination with tamoxifen is equal to CMF (see Table 10–3) chemotherapy.
   (b) This practice is widely used in Europe; however, it is not standard practice in the United States.

   e. Immunotherapy: HER2/neu is an oncogene that encodes a growth factor receptor. This gene is overexpressed in 10% to 40% of primary breast cancers. Trastuzumab is a monoclonal antibody that binds to the HER2 receptor and has significant activity in advanced breast cancer. In patients whose tumors overexpress HER2/neu, administration of trastuzumab as a single agent resulted in a response rate of 21%. Trastuzumab has been studied in combination with taxanes and vinorelbine. Patients treated with chemotherapy plus trastuzumab had an overall survival advantage as compared to those receiving chemotherapy alone. Trastuzumab is well tolerated by patients and offers another noncytotoxic option. Side effects may include fever, chills, headache, abdominal pain, and back pain. The incidence is low and generally occurs only with the first dose. Patients should be premedicated with acetaminophen and diphenhydramine, and close observation is required during and after the infusion.

E. Nursing Diagnosis and Related Interventions and Outcomes
   1. Knowledge deficit related to diagnosis and treatment
      a. *Problem:* Multiple interventions and sources of information may cause confusion and may inhibit decision making.
      b. *Interventions*
         (1) Begin teaching at the time of detection, and encourage the participation of a support person.
         (2) Provide an overview of treatment, but limit detailed information to the next intervention. (See Chapters 6, 8, and 9 for treatment details.)

TABLE 10–4 Side Effects of Chemotherapy

Side Effect	Cause	Nursing Interventions
Alopecia	Most chemotherapeutic agents cause some degree of alopecia. This depends on the dose, half-life of drug, and duration of therapy. Adriamycin causes 100% total hair loss. Patients receiving CMF have about a 50% chance of total hair loss. Usually begins 2 weeks after administration of chemotherapy. Re-growth takes about 3 to 5 months.	Use of scalp hypothermia and tourniquets for prevention is highly controversial because it has not been proven to be effective.
Taste changes	Chemotherapy changes the reproduction of taste buds. Absent or altered taste can lead to a decreased food intake. However, most women gain weight on chemotherapy due to decreased activity.	Consult with nutritionist for suggestions.

Fatigue	The cause of fatigue is generally unknown, but can be related to anemia, emotional stress, and altered sleep patterns.	Careful monitoring of hemoglobin levels is appropriate and may require intervention with erythropoietin if it falls below 9.0%. There has been some evidence to suggest that moderate exercise may help reduce chemotherapy-related fatigue.
Nausea and vomiting	Caused by the stimulation of the vagus nerve by serotonin released by cells in the upper GI tract.	Premedicate with a 5-HT$_3$ inhibitor (ondansetron, granisetron, dolasetron), and dexamethasone. Include a prn antiemetic such as metoclopramide (Reglan), droperidol, compazine, dexamethasone, or lorazepam (Ativan).
Mucositis	Caused by the destruction of the oral mucosa, causing an inflammatory response.	Patient education to avoid infection. Local comfort measures.
Neutropenia	Caused by suppression of the stem cell. Risk of infection is greatest with an ANC less than 500/mm^3. Usually occurs at 7 to 14 days after administration of chemotherapy.	Patient education. Patients need to be monitored and treated promptly for fever or other signs of infection.
Peripheral neuropathies (taxanes)	Caused by peripheral neurodegeneration.	May require dose modification if severe.
Hypersensitivity reaction (taxanes)	Exact cause unknown. Related to preservative, cremaphor.	Premedication with steroid, antihistamine, and H2 blocker.

TABLE 10–5 Side Effects of Tamoxifen

Side Effect	Nursing Considerations
Menopausal symptoms: hot flashes and vaginal dryness	Because the use of hormone replacement is controversial at best, and the research in management of hot flashes is limited, nurses need to be sensitive to this issue and explore options to minimize the symptoms and help patients cope with these symptoms. Behavioral strategies such as relaxation, dietary changes, and physical exercise may help reduce the severity of hot flashes. In addition, some antidepressants, such as clonidine and venlafaxine, have been shown to alleviate hot flashes. The use of soy and other supplements to alleviate hot flashes is being studied.
Increased risk of endometrial carcinoma and thrombo-embolic events	Risk seems to be limited to postmenopausal women, and the risk is about 1%. Women with a history of blood clots or who are currently on warfarin should not take tamoxifen.
Hair thinning, menstrual irregularities, and memory loss have also been observed.	Pregnancy should be avoided. Premenopausal women should continue barrier types of birth control.
May prevent bone loss and osteoporosis	Encourage routine bone density screening, calcium intake, and weight-bearing exercise.

(3) Provide multiple forms of education (eg, video, printed material, demonstration).
(4) Validate learning with patient and support persons.
(5) Review as needed.
c. *Desired outcome:* The patient and support person will understand treatment interventions and make informed decisions.

TABLE 10–6 Side Effects of Aromatase Inhibitors

Side Effect	Nursing Consideration
Menopausal symptoms: hot flashes and vaginal dryness	Usually not as pronounced as with tamoxifen
GI effects: mild nausea and vomiting	Uncommon and usually improves with time
Myalgias/arthralgias	Uncommon, but can be severe, requiring discontinuation of the drug
Osteoporosis and bone loss	There is an 8% increased risk of developing fractures while on aromatase inhibitors. Annual bone density is recommended for careful evaluation.
Hair loss	Rare. Usually mild and improves with time.

2. Potential for altered tissue perfusion related to treatment or disease
   a. *Problem:* Axillary node dissection and radiation therapy contribute to lymphedema. The frequency of the problem is decreasing with the trend toward sentinel node dissection, but the result may be immediate or delayed, temporary or chronic lymphedema.
   b. *Interventions*
      (1) Limit risk of infection: avoid trauma, invasive procedures, and excessive pressure or constriction on the ipsilateral arm.
      (2) Promote venous return: exercise as instructed, elevate arm when possible, use therapeutic massage or compression garments as ordered.
      (3) Refer to therapist as soon as edema is identified.
      (4) Ensure patient knowledge of safety precautions, monitoring, and reporting symptoms of redness, swelling, or pain.
   c. *Desired outcome:* Lymphedema and infections will be avoided or limited.
3. Pain related to disease or treatment
   a. *Problem:* Tumor, surgery, or radiation therapy may damage skin, muscle, or nerves, resulting in acute or chronic pain.
   b. *Interventions* (see Chapter 30)
   c. *Desired outcome:* Pain will be eliminated or controlled.
4. Body image disturbances related to disease or treatment
   a. *Problems*
      (1) Surgery and radiation alter the appearance of the breast.
      (2) Outpatient interventions require the patient and family to view the affected area immediately.
      (3) Patients and others may have misconceptions about breast conservation or reconstruction.
      (4) Side effects of chemotherapy or hormonal therapy cause visible changes such as weight gain and hair loss (see Tables 10–4 and 10–5).
   b. *Interventions*
      (1) Assess expectations of body changes.
      (2) Correct misconceptions using photographs of treated or reconstructed breasts.
      (3) Ensure that image concerns are recognized and addressed when therapy decisions are discussed.
      (4) Refer to counseling, support groups, plastic surgeons, nutritionists, exercise, or image consultants to maximize or improve body image.
   c. *Desired outcomes*
      (1) The patient and significant others will have realistic expectations of body changes related to disease and treatment.
      (2) The patient and family will be aware of resources to promote and maximize body image.
5. Ineffective coping related to diagnosis, recurrence, or treatment
   a. *Problems*
      (1) Diagnosis and disease recurrence are stressful times.
      (2) Coping responses to treatment are less effective in patients without support and a history of successful coping.

   b. *Interventions* (see Chapter 31)
     (1) Assess coping skills and history, and encourage use of successful past intervention.
     (2) Initiate psychosocial testing and skills education as indicated.
     (3) Refer to social work, clergy, or psychiatry if coping skills are not successful.
   c. *Desired outcome:* The patient and family will demonstrate effective coping and ability to function during diagnosis and treatment.
   6. Potential sexual dysfunction related to disease or treatment
     a. *Problem:* Breast cancer or treatment may result in physical and psychological changes that alter sexual function or intimacy.
     b. *Interventions*
       (1) Assess sexual function by taking a sexual history and identifying concerns about intimacy and sexual function.
       (2) Teach about interventions for side effects (see Chapter 31).
       (3) Refer for sexual therapy if appropriate.
     c. *Desired outcome:* The patient and partner will have a satisfactory intimate relationship.
F. Discharge Planning: Most therapy for breast cancer is provided in the ambulatory setting, and the discharge interventions are treatment specific. Ensure that patients and families are aware of follow-up appointments and have a plan to address emergent and nonemergent issues.
   1. Surgery
     a. Refer outpatients to home care for follow-up on day of surgery.
     b. Ensure patient and family have equipment and education needed for care at home of pain, drains, and incisions.
     c. See Chapter 9.
   2. Radiation
     a. See Chapter 8.
     b. Address issues of skin care, fatigue, and other side effects of therapy.
   3. Chemotherapy
     a. Needs differ with goals of therapy and agents used.
     b. Educate patients and families about common side effects and interventions.
     c. Ensure that prescriptions are provided for management of side effects.
     d. See Chapter 6.

REFERENCES

American Joint Committee on Cancer (Greene, F. L., et al. [Eds]). (2002). *AJCC cancer staging manual* (6th ed.). Philadelphia: Lippincott Williams & Wilkins.

Barse, P. M. (2000). Issues in the treatment of metastatic breast cancer. *Seminars in Oncology Nursing, 16*(3), 197–205.

Baum, M. (1999). Use of aromatase inhibitors in the adjuvant treatment of breast cancer. *Endocrine Related Cancer, 6*, 231–234.

Byers, T., et al. (2002). American Cancer Society guidelines on nutrition and physical activity for cancer prevention: Reducing the risk of cancer with healthy food choices and physical activity. *CA: A Cancer Journal for Clinicians, 52*(2), 92–119.

Buzdar, A. (2000). Exemestane in advanced breast cancer. *Anticancer Drugs, 11*(8), 609–616.

Carlson, R.W., Anderson, B.D., Bensinger, W., et al. (2000). National Comprehensive Cancer Network (NCCN) practice guidelines for breast cancer. *Oncology, 11A*, 33–49.

Carpenter, J. S. (2000). Hot flashes and their management in breast cancer. *Seminars in Oncology Nursing, 16*(3), 214–225.

Casciato, D. A., & Lowitz. B. L. (2000). *Manual of clinical oncology* (4th ed.). Philadelphia: Lippincott Williams & Williams.

Citron, M., Berry, D. A., Cirrincione, C., Hudis, C., Winer, E. P., Gradishar, W., Davidson, N., Martino, S., Livingston, R., Ingle, J. N., Perez, E., Carpenter, J., Hurd, D., Holland, J. F., et al. (2003). Randomized trial of dose dense versus conventionally scheduled and sequential versus concurrent combination chemotherapy as postoperative adjuvant treatment of node-positive primary breast cancer: First report of intergroup trial C9741/Cancer and Leukemia Group B Trial 9741. *Journal of Clinical Oncology, 21*, 1431–1439.

Cloutier, A. R. (2000). Advanced breast cancer: Recent developments in hormonal therapy. *Seminars in Oncology Nursing, 10*(3), 206–213.

Donegan, W., & Spratt, J. (2002). *Cancer of the breast* (5th ed). Philadelphia: W. B. Saunders.

Fisher, B., Dignam, J., Bryant, J., et al. (1996). Five versus more than five years of tamoxifen therapy for breast cancer patients with negative lymph nodes and estrogen receptor-positive tumors. *Journal of the National Cancer Institute, 88*(21), 1529–1542.

Fisher, B., Dignam, J., & Wolmark, N. (1997). Tamoxifen and chemotherapy for lymph node-negative, estrogen receptor-positive breast cancer. *Journal of the National Cancer Institute, 89*(22), 1673–1682.

Fisher, B., et al. (2002). Twenty-five year follow-up of a randomized trial comparing radical mastectomy, total mastectomy, and total mastectomy followed by irradiation. *New England Journal of Medicine, 347*(8), 567–575.

Fisher, B., et al. (1998). Tamoxifen for prevention of breast cancer: Report of the National Surgical Adjuvant Breast and Bowel Project P-1 Study. *Journal of the National Cancer Institute, 90*(18), 1371–1388.

Gail, M.H., Gostantino, J.P., Vogel, V., et al. (1999). Weighing the risks and benefits of tamoxifen treatment for preventing breast cancer. *Journal of the National Cancer Institute, 91*, 1829–1846.

Goldberg, R. M., Loprinzi, C. L., O'Fallon, J. R., et al. (1994). Transdermal clonidine for ameliorating tamoxifen-induced hot flashes. *Journal of Clinical Oncology, 12*(1), 155–158.

Goodman, M., & Chapman, D. (1997). Breast cancer. In S. C. Groenwald, M. H. Frogge, M. Goodman, & C. H. Yarbro (Eds.), *Cancer nursing: Principles and practice* (3rd ed., pp. 903–958). Boston: Jones & Bartlett. AQ

Honig, S. F. (1996). Hormonal therapy and chemotherapy. In J. R. Harris, M. Morrow, M. E. Lippman, et al. (Eds.), *Diseases of the breast* (pp. 669–734). Philadelphia: Lippincott-Raven.

Hortobagyi, G. N. (2000). Developments in chemotherapy of breast cancer. *Cancer, 15*(88 [12 Suppl]), 3073–3076.

Jakez, R., Hausmaninger, H., et al. (2002). Randomized adjuvant trial of tamoxifen and goserelin versus cyclophosphamide, methotrexate, and flurouracil: Evidence for superiority of treatment with endocrine blockade in premenopausal patients with hormone-responsive breast cancer—Austrian Breast and Colorectal Cancer Study Group—Trial 5. *Journal of Clinical Oncology, 20*(24), 4621–4627.

Jemal, A., Thomas, A., Murray, T., et al. (2002). Cancer statistics, 2002. *CA: A Cancer Journal for Clinicians, 52*(1), 23–47.

Knobf, M. T. (1991). Breast cancer. In S. B. Baird, et al. (Eds.), *Cancer nursing: A comprehensive textbook* (pp. 425–451). Philadelphia: W. B. Saunders.

Krag, D., et al. (1998). The sentinel node in breast cancer—A multicenter validation study. *New England Journal of Medicine, 338*(14), 941–946.

Lambe, M., et al. (1994). Transient increase in the risk of breast cancer after giving birth. *New England Journal of Medicine, 331*(1), 5–9.

Loprinzi, C. L., Pisanski, T. M., Foneseca, R., et al. (1998). Pilot evaluation of venlafaxine hydrochloride for the therapy of hot flashes in cancer survivors. *Journal of Clinical Oncology, 16,* 3277–3281.

Magnusson, C., et al. (1999). Breast cancer risk following long term estrogen and estrogen-progestin replacement. *International Journal of Cancer, 81,* 339–344.

Marchbanks, P. A., et al. (2002). Oral contraception and the risk of breast cancer. *New England Journal of Medicine, 346,* 2025–2032.

Mock, V., Burke, M. B., Sheehan, P., Creaton, E. M., Winningham, M. L. McKenney-Tedder, S., Schwager, L. P., & Liebman, M. (1994). A nursing rehabilitation program for women with breast cancer receiving adjuvant chemotherapy. *Oncology Nursing Forum, 21*(5), 899–907.

Mock, V., Dow, K. H., Meares, C. J., Grimm, P. M., Dienemann, J. A., Haisfield-Wolfe, M. E., Quitasol, W., Mitchell, S., Chakrayarthy, A., & Gage, I. (1997). Effects of exercise on fatigue, physical functioning, and emotional distress during radiation therapy for breast cancer. *Oncology Nursing Forum, 24*(6), 991–1000.

National Institutes of Health. *Consensus development program: Adjuvant breast cancer.* Available: www.nih.gov/consensus.

_____. (2003). *What you need to know about breast cancer.* No 00–1556. Available: www.cancer.gov/cancer.

Overgaard, M., et al. (1997). Post operative radiotherapy in high risk premenopausal women with breast cancer who receive adjuvant chemotherapy: Danish Breast Cancer Cooperative Group 826 trial. *New England Journal of Medicine, 337*(14), 949–955.

Ragaz, J., Jackson, S. M., et al. (1997). Adjuvant radiotherapy and chemotherapy in node positive premenopausal women with breast cancer. *New England Journal of Medicine, 337,* 956–962.

Reicht, A., et al. (2001). Postmastectomy radiotherapy: Guidelines of the American Society of Clinical Oncology. *Journal of Clinical Oncology, 19*(5), 1539–1569.

Rossouw, J. E., Anderson, G. L., Prentice, R. L., LaCroix, A. Z., Kooperberg, C., Stefanick, M. L., Jackson, R. D., Beresford, S. A., Howard, B. V., Johnson, K. C., Kotchen, J. M., Ockene, J., Writing Group for the Women's Health Initiative Investigators. (2002). Risks and benefits of estrogen plus progestin in healthy postmenopausal women: Principal results from the Women's Health Initiative randomized controlled trial. *Journal of the American Medical Association, 288,* 321–333.

Shapiro, C. L., & Recht, A. (2001). Side effects of adjuvant treatment of breast cancer. *New England Journal of Medicine, 344*(26), 1997–2008.

Slamon, D., et al. (2001). Use of chemotherapy plus monoclonal antibody against HER2 for metastatic breast cancer that overexpresses HER2. *New England Journal of Medicine, 344*(11), 783–792.

Stadtmauer, E. A., O'Neill, A., Goldstein L. J., et al. (2000). Conventional-dose chemotherapy compared with high dose chemotherapy plus autologous hematopoietic stem-cell transplantation for metastatic breast cancer. *New England Journal of Medicine, 342,* 1069–1076.

Taylor, C. W., Green, S., Dalton, W. S., et al. (1998). Multicenter randomized clinical trial of goserelin versus surgical ovariectomy in premenopausal patients with receptor-positive metastatic breast cancer: An intergroup study. *Journal of Clinical Oncology, 16*(3), 994–999.

Veronesi, U., et al. (2002). Twenty year follow-up of a randomized study comparing breast conserving surgery with radical mastectomy for early breast cancer. *New England Journal of Medicine, 347*(16), 1227–1232.

Winer, E. P. (2002). American Society of Clinical Oncology technology assessment on the use of aromatase inhibitors as adjuvant therapy for women with hormone receptor-positive breast cancer—Status report 2002. *Journal of Clinical Oncology, 20*(15), 3317–3327.

Wolff, A. C., & Davidson, N. E. (2000). Early operable breast cancer. *Current Treatment Options in Oncology, 1,* 210–220.

Yahlom, J., Petrek, J. A., Biddinger, P.W. et al. (1992). Breast cancer in patients irradiated for Hodgkin's disease: A clinical and pathological analysis of 45 events in 37 patients. *Journal of Clinical Oncology, 10,* 1674–1681.

11 Central Nervous System Cancers

Pendleton P. Powers

I. Definition: Central nervous system (CNS) malignancies occur in the brain or spinal cord; they may be primary or metastatic.

  A. Incidence: Approximately 18,300 people will be diagnosed with new cases of primary CNS malignancies each year in the United States, and over 13,000 will die. More than 100,000 new cases of metastatic CNS tumors are diagnosed each year in the United States. CNS tumors are more common in whites and, except for meningiomas, occur more often in men than women. The incidence of CNS tumors appears to be increasing in the elderly population; improved techniques are responsible for much of the increase in diagnoses over the last 30 years.

  B. Primary brain tumors include more than 100 histologic classifications and grades (Figure 11–1).

    1. The most common are gliomas (astrocytomas, oligodendrogliomas, ependymomas).

    2. Astrocytomas, the most common glial tumor, are graded from I to IV, low to high grade. High-grade astrocytomas, anaplastic astrocytomas, and glioblastoma multiforme occur most frequently and carry the worst prognosis.

    3. Survival and prognosis in adults are more favorable if patients have a low-grade tumor, are under age 40, have a high performance status (70% on the Karnofsky scale), and receive a good surgical resection.

  C. Metastatic tumors

    1. The brain is a common site of metastases for many cancers, including lung, breast, colon, renal, and melanoma.

    2. Signs and symptoms are the same as primary brain lesions.

    3. Prognosis is best for patients with solitary lesions, good performance ratings (70% on the Karnofsky scale), age <60 years, and primary tumor in remission.

    4. Metastatic lesions are treated with surgery, whole brain radiation, or stereotactic radiosurgery. The number, size, and location of the lesions, as well as the patient's condition and primary disease status, will determine which modality is used.

  D. Spinal cord tumors are less common than other CNS tumors. Symptoms depend on the location of the lesion. Surgery or radiation therapy or both are used to cure, control, or palliate disease.

II. Etiology: Although the causes of some CNS tumors are unknown, many genetic and environmental factors are being considered. Factors such as previous exposure to ionizing radiation and chemicals, viral infections, and low-frequency electromagnetic fields are possible; however, questions still prevail. Similarities in environmental exposure are thought to explain clustering of CNS tumors in families.

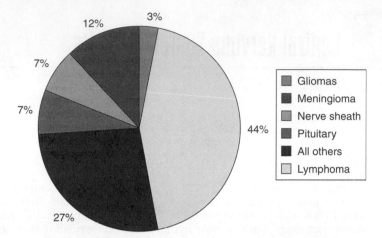

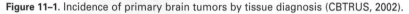

Figure 11–1. Incidence of primary brain tumors by tissue diagnosis (CBTRUS, 2002).

III. Patient Management

A. Assessment: Signs and symptoms of CNS tumors depend on the type of tumor, size, location in the brain, and the extent of increased intracranial pressure (ICP). Symptoms are caused by the disturbance or destruction of brain tissue secondary to tumor invasion, infiltration, and compression.

1. Many patients with CNS tumors present with similar general nonfocal symptoms such as cognitive changes, headaches, or seizures caused by increased ICP.

2. Other patients present with localizing signs, specific to the location of the tumor (Table 11–1).

3. A complete history and physical, neurologic examination, and family history are required to identify symptoms and establish baseline function. If cognitive ability is impaired, someone who knows the patient well can often assist in identification of specific symptoms and time of onset.

B. Diagnostic Parameters

1. Magnetic resonance imaging (MRI) detects brain and spinal abnormalities and reveals abnormalities in the nature and extent of tumor blood flow. The scan can last from 45 minutes (brain only) to 3 hours (cranial-spinal axis). Patients are required to lie in a loud, confined space, which may be problematic for claustrophobics, although open scanners address this issue. Intravenous (IV) contrast (gadolinium) is usually given. In contrast-enhanced scans, the disrupted tumor vasculature allows contrast dye to cross the blood–brain barrier (BBB) and is clearly visible on the scan. MRI is the standard evaluation for brain cancers; advantages include greater sensitivity than the computed tomography (CT) scan without ionizing radiation. Disadvantages include expense, potential patient anxiety, rare but possible reactions to contrast, and inability

▓ TABLE 11–1   **CNS Tumor Signs**

Anatomic Location	Deficit/Abnormality
Frontal	Personality/behavior changes, emotional lability, short-term memory deficits, impaired intellect and judgment, expressive aphasia, contralateral motor weakness, seizures, and urinary incontinence
Temporal	Hearing changes, hallucinations, memory loss, receptive aphasia, visual field changes, temporal lobe seizures
Parietal	Contralateral sensory disturbances (hyperesthesia, paresthesia, astereognosis, autotopagnosia); visual field defects; left-right discrimination; difficulty with language, writing, and calculations; and seizures
Occipital	Visual field deficits (vision loss in half of each visual field on side opposite the lesion), blindness, visual hallucinations, seizures, and difficulty naming objects
Cerebellum	Problems with gait, balance, and coordination; nystagmus; signs of increased ICP caused by obstruction of CSF flow
Hypothalamus	Endocrine dysfunction, temperature control malfunction, abnormal thirst and appetite, emotional lability
Intraventricular	Increased ICP, abnormal gait, cognitive impairment, urinary incontinence
Brain stem	Decreased level of consciousness; abnormal heart rate, respirtions, blood pressure, swallowing, vomiting; sensory motor impairment, cranial nerve deficits

to scan patients with metal foreign bodies (due to effects of the magnet).

2. CT scans have replaced more invasive diagnostic tests due to safety and accuracy. The CT scan can detect brain and spine abnormalities, including masses and edema. When the procedure is done on a high-speed multislice scanner, it requires several minutes to complete and IV contrast is usually given. Advantages include three-dimensional pictures viewed with special computers and the ability to visualize bony abnormalities and blood. Risks include the use of ionizing radiation and reactions to contrast media, although the new contrast agents are safer and produce fewer reactions.

3. Positron emission tomography (PET) measures regional brain metabolism and blood flow by tracing positron-emitting radionuclides. The procedure requires about 2 hours and an arterial line. PET scans are used to try to differentiate between active recurrent tumor and tumor necrosis by measuring the rate of glucose metabolism. Disadvantages include possible arterial line complications.

4. Single photon emission computed tomography (SPECT) is used to differentiate tumor growths from benign or necrotic lesions. The procedure is similar to a bone scan and requires about 1 hour. SPECT uses conventional radio tracers.

5. MRI spectroscopy (MRS) is functional MRI that studies numerous brain metabolites. Like PET, MRS can differentiate between necrotic tissue and active tumor. It is a useful diagnostic tool, and recent technologic advances have simplified its use in a clinical setting. No contrast agents are used; scanning parameters and postprocessing determine which metabolites are imaged. Disadvantages are that a spectroscopic scan adds about 20 minutes to the standard MRI examination.

6. Definitive diagnosis is determined by obtaining tissue, either during craniotomy or by biopsy. In certain areas of the brain where it is not safe to obtain tissue, diagnosis is presumed by evaluating imaging, patient history, and clinical assessment.

C. Treatment: Multimodal treatment of adult primary brain tumors usually includes surgery, with the addition of radiation therapy, chemotherapy, or all three for more aggressive tumors (Table 11–2). Chapters 6, 8, and 9 review common side effects and general management of patients treated with these therapies.

1. Surgical debulking of primary brain tumors defines pathology, decreases tumor mass and ICP, and may relieve neurologic symptoms.
   a. Surgery of accessible tumors is a safe procedure and usually well tolerated.
   b. Potential surgical complications include increased ICP leading to herniation, hemorrhage, local/regional brain damage, and cranial nerve injury. Complications are secondary to tissue damage and related to the area of tumor location.
   c. Potential postoperative complications include postoperative hematomas, infection, spinal fluid leaks, meningitis, deep venous thrombosis (DVT), and pulmonary embolism.

2. Radiation therapy is a localized treatment and requires individualized planning. External beam radiation is used to treat primary and metastatic brain tumors and some histologically benign brain tumors.
   a. Treatment planning considers histology, grade, location, radio responsiveness, intent, and patient status.
   b. Specialized techniques (eg, interstitial brachytherapy, stereotactic radiosurgery, gamma knife and proton beam particle delivery) allow radiation to be delivered with precision to the tumor.

TABLE 11–2 Chemotherapy Used to Treat High-Grade Astrocytomas

Drug	Route	Treatment Schedule
Carmustine (BCNU)	IV, intratumoral	One treatment q 6 weeks At the time of surgical resection
Temozolomide (Temodar)	PO	Daily × 5 days q 4 weeks
PCV regimen Procarbazine Lomustine (CCNU) Vincristine	PO and IV	

As a result, limited exposure of normal cells results in fewer complications and side effects. These techniques are not appropriate for all tumor types.

 c. Side effects of brain radiation may be acute (during therapy), subacute (from weeks up to 3 months after treatment), or long term. Side effects are related to the specific tissue treated, dose, treatment delivery, and individual patient factors.

  (1) Acute effects may include fatigue, alopecia in treatment area, cerebral edema, scalp reactions, taste disturbances, and hearing difficulties.

  (2) Radiation somnolence, characterized by excessive sleepiness, is a subacute side effect occurring 6 to 12 weeks after treatment and lasting up to 2 weeks.

  (3) Long-term side effects may include radiation necrosis, cognitive changes, decreased hormone production, and, in rare cases, radiation-induced neoplasms.

3. Chemotherapy has a role in the treatment of high-grade gliomas, CNS lymphomas, and leptomeningeal metastases. It may be part of the initial treatment plan or given at the time of tumor recurrence, depending on the tumor type.

 a. Oral, IV, intraarterial, and intrathecal routes of administration are used, as well as intratumoral implants of biodegradable BCNU polymers.

 b. The BBB ordinarily protects the brain by restricting access. In brain tumors, alterations in the BBB allow delivery of drugs to areas that would otherwise be blocked.

 c. The most frequently used drugs to treat high-grade gliomas are BCNU, temozolomide, procarbazine, and vincristine, which are not highly effective in this disease (Table 11–3). Chemotherapy may be given as an adjuvant to radiation therapy or preserved for use at the time of tumor recurrence.

 d. In some centers, primary CNS lymphomas are being treated with chemotherapy, as the initial treatment, rather than radiation therapy. Regimens that include high-dose methotrexate are providing more durable responses than radiation therapy, without the associated dementia.

4. Novel chemotherapy agents, chemotherapy resistance modifiers, radiation sensitizers, antiangiogenesis agents, immunotherapy, gene therapy, cell signaling modifiers, and differentiation agents are all being investigated as potential treatments. Clinical trials are underway for both systemic and local treatments that are delivered directly into the tumor.

D. Nursing Diagnosis and Related Interventions and Outcomes

 1. Alteration in cerebral perfusion related to cerebral edema

  a. *Problem:* Cerebral edema may occur with any brain tumor, regardless of the tumor location. It is caused by increased permeability of the capillaries, which allows extracellular leakage of plasma. When the size of the tumor, and any surrounding edema, exceed the compensatory mechanisms of the intracranial space, increased ICP will result. If untreated, ICP can lead to herniation and death.

TABLE 11–3   Treatment of Primary Brain Tumors

Tumor Type			
Astrocytoma: low-grade	Surgery	Observation	
		Consider radiation	Chemotherapy
Astrocytoma: high-grade	Surgery	Radiation	Chemotherapy in some cases
Ependymoma	Surgery	Radiation in some cases	Chemotherapy for anaplastic lesions
Oligodendroglioma	Surgery	Radiation for residual, recurrent lesions	Chemotherapy in some cases
Medulloblastoma	Surgery	Radiation	Consider chemotherapy for malignant meningioma
Meningioma	Surgery	Consider radiation if surgery is incomplete	
CNS lymphoma	Surgery	Radiation if not responsive to chemotherapy	Chemotherapy
Acoustic neuromas	Surgery or	Radiation	
Chordoma	Surgery	Radiation	
Germ cell tumors	Surgery	Radiation	Chemotherapy for some
Pituitary adenoma	Surgery—technique depends on size of lesion	Consider radiation for residual/recurrent tumor	

Adapted from Bohan, E. (2002). Brain tumors. In E. Barker (Ed.), *Neuroscience nursing: A spectrum of care* (2nd ed., pp. 269–301). St Louis, MO: Mosby.

b. *Interventions*
   (1) Assess for symptoms of increased ICP, including decreased level of consciousness, headache, confusion, lethargy, restlessness, nausea and vomiting, papillary edema, motor/sensory deficits, and changes in vital signs.
   (2) Monitor neurologic signs, fluids and electrolytes, and ICP, as ordered; document and report any changes.
   (3) Administer corticosteroids (dexamethasone) as ordered, to reduce cerebral edema. Teach patients about and monitor for steroid side effects, which include gastrointestinal (GI) irritation (if oral form is used), mood swings, diabetes mellitus, proximal myopathies, and immunosuppression. Steroids may mask normal symptoms of infection; any potential site of infection should be monitored and cultured if infection is suspected.
   (4) Elevate the patient's head (20 to 30 degrees).
   (5) Ensure a safe environment. (see III.D.4 below).
c. *Desired outcome:* Cerebral edema will be identified and managed.
2. Knowledge deficit related to diagnosis, treatment, and symptom management
   a. *Problem:* From the time of initial diagnosis, patients and families are required to make treatment decisions and manage symptoms.
   b. *Interventions*
      (1) Provide patients with adequate information about the natural history of their disease and treatment options.
      (2) Develop an individual treatment plan based on patient's clinical condition and the wishes of the patient and family. Ensure that the patient and caregivers are able to identify and comply with the treatment and follow-up plan.
      (3) Educate patient and caregivers about potential complications of the disease and side effects of medications and treatments.
         (a) Seizure (see III.D.4 below)
         (b) Cerebral edema (see III.D.1)
         (c) DVT
         (d) Immunosuppression
      (4) Teach patient and caregivers how to identify signs and symptoms of an emergency (eg, prolonged seizure, increased ICP, symptoms of DVT). Verify that they have a plan of action to follow in the event of emergency.
      (5) Assist patient and caregivers in identifying and contacting community resources to meet current and anticipated needs.
3. Impaired cognitive function related to symptoms of disease or treatment
   a. *Problem:* Difficulty reasoning and solving problems and memory deficits may result from edema or damage to brain tissue in the frontal lobe. Inability to concentrate or discipline one's behavior is often difficult for patients and others to anticipate or understand.

b. *Interventions*

(1) Repeat neurologic assessment to identify changes in cognitive function over time. Tools, such as the Mini Mental Status, should be administered and documented routinely. The patient, or someone who knows the patient well, is frequently aware of more subtle changes in behavior and other high-level functions and should be questioned about these symptoms.

(2) Orient the patient to date, place, and time as necessary. Provide a calendar, clock, and other orientation materials.

(3) Ensure that the patient has adequate supervision if the deficit is significant. If patient is at home, assist the family to find community resources to facilitate appropriate patient supervision. In medical care settings, patients should be placed near the nursing station or in an area where they can be easily observed.

c. *Desired outcome:* Cognitive function and appropriate behaviors are improved or maintained after treatment.

4. Risk for injury related to seizures or falls

a. *Problem:* Incidence of falls and injury increases for populations with seizures and motor, sensory, and perception deficits.

(1) Seizures are common in patients with intracranial tumors; 30% of adults with supratentorial tumors present with focal or generalized seizures at the time of diagnosis. During their lifetime, over half of brain tumor patients will experience seizures as a result of increased ICP or cerebral tissue compression or damage. The use of anticonvulsants as treatment of known seizures or for prophylaxis is common.

b. Interventions

(1) Interventions to decrease injury from seizures

(a) Assess for history of seizures and preconvulsive symptoms.

(b) Administer anticonvulsives as prescribed. Phenytoin, phenobarbital, valproic acid, and carbamazepine are commonly used anticonvulsants.

(c) Monitor serum anticonvulsant levels (when available) to maintain therapeutic dosing. Assess for anticonvulsant side effects and signs and symptoms of toxicity.

(d) Initiate seizure precautions per institution protocol if the patient is at risk for seizures. If the patient is at home, instruct the family concerning what to do in the event of a seizure.

(e) Give patient and family information about seizures and driving restrictions, as specified by state law.

(2) Tumors in the areas of the brain that control sensory and motor functions impact the ability to walk, climb steps, respond to stimuli, feel pain, maintain balance, and see. These deficits may be temporary or permanent and require interventions that limit the risk of injury. Assess for presence of sensory or motor deficits.

(3) Interventions to ensure patient safety

(a) Make environment safe with adequate lighting, removal of rugs and small objects from the floor, and padding on hard or slippery surfaces.

(b) Provide patient with adequate rest and supervision (if required) when walking, climbing stairs, cooking, and so on.

(c) Encourage and teach use of walkers, braces, eyeglasses, or other appliances that aid balance and stability.

(d) Teach about side effects of medications that could contribute to the risk of injury.

   c. *Desired outcome:* Risk for injury from falls and seizures will be minimized.

5. Impaired communication related to motor and memory deficits

   a. *Problem:* Tumors that impinge on areas of the brain that control hearing, vision, speech, interpretation, and memory impact on one's ability to give and receive communication.

   b. *Interventions*

   (1) Assess for impaired communication. Verbal responses to questions should be appropriate, timely, and clear. The ability to read and write should be appropriate for age and level of education.

   (2) Refer patient to a speech therapist for evaluation, consultation, and intervention if speech is affected.

   (3) Assist the patient to compensate for memory and motor compromise by using alternative communication methods (eg, writing, computers, pictures).

   c. *Desired outcome:* The patient demonstrates a satisfactory method of understanding and communicating thoughts and needs.

6. Self-care deficits related to symptoms of disease or treatment

   a. *Problem:* Fatigue, muscle weakness and deficits, and sensory or cognitive impairment may result from CNS tumors or treatment with surgery, chemotherapy, radiation, or medications. Impairment may be temporary or permanent. The ability to drive, walk, stand, or complete routine tasks may be altered. To maximize independence, patients must learn to adapt activities of daily living (ADL) to limitations.

   b. *Interventions*

   (1) Assist the patient and family in developing a plan of care that incorporates desires, needs, abilities, and limitations. Ensure that rest and safety are considered.

   (2) Identify and refer patient to programs that maximize independence (eg, physical and occupational therapy, home health care).

   c. *Desired outcome:* The patient will be able to achieve ADL and other desired activities with assistance appropriate to level of function.

7. Impaired mobility related to symptoms of disease or treatment

   a. *Problem:* Fatigue, pain, muscle weakness, and motor and sensory deficits may limit mobility and commonly occur as a result of CNS or spinal cord tumors or tumor treatment.

    b. *Interventions*

      (1) Assess the extent of impairment or refer patient to the appropriate specialty discipline for assessment and intervention (eg, physical therapy, occupational therapy, ophthalmology).

      (2) Assist the patient to maintain mobility by providing a safe environment, rest, pain medications, and assistance as needed for ambulation or ADL.

      (3) Teach range-of-motion exercises to maximize muscle strength.

      (4) Encourage brief, frequent periods (10 to 15 minutes per hour) of mobility when possible (see Chapter 25).

      (5) Assess for lower extremity thrombosis (pain, swelling, redness).

    c. *Desired outcome:* The patient will improve or maintain mobility appropriate to physical ability.

8. Impaired skin integrity related to poor nutrition, injury, or immobility

    a. *Problem:* Injury, poor nutrition, decreased bowel or bladder control, and immobility are potential complications of CNS tumors and their treatments. Each of these factors increases the risk that skin breakdown will occur as a result of trauma, pressure, cellular damage, inadequate skin care, or decreased flow of blood and nutrients.

    b. *Interventions*

      (1) Assess skin for evidence of breakdown, irritation, or pressure. Document assessments for basis of comparison. Evaluate factors that increase risk.

      (2) Institute the following:

        (a) Safety precautions (see III.D.4.b).

        (b) Skin care protocol or care plan to keep skin clean, dry, lubricated, and free of irritation. Provide for collection or absorption of urine if the patient is incontinent. Avoid perfumed or drying soaps and lotions. Gentle massage increases blood flow to high-pressure areas. Encourage mobility and ensure frequent change of position. Institute a pressure relief bed/mattress if indicated.

        (c) Adequate fluids and nutrition. Refer patient for nutrition consultation if nutrition is compromised (see Chapter 28).

        (d) Wound care protocol if indicated

        (e) Appropriate intervention if skin integrity is compromised due to treatment (see Chapters 6, 8, and 9).

    c. *Desired outcome:* Skin will be healthy and intact, or show evidence of healing, throughout the course of disease and treatment.

9. Pain related to damage by tumor or treatment

    a. *Problem:* Patients with CNS tumors may experience pain secondary to surgery, radiation therapy, trauma, increased ICP, or pressure of the tumor on nerves or within a confined space. The pain may be acute or chronic.

    b. *Interventions:* Follow recommendations in Chapter 30. If pain is due to increased ICP, steroids are administered to decrease cerebral edema.

    c. *Desired outcome:* The patient will be free of pain or achieve pain control that allows a good quality of life.

10. Altered body image related to effects of tumor and treatment

    a. *Problem:* Treatment or symptoms of CNS tumors may result in temporary or permanent changes in body characteristics. Surgery can damage nerves and tissue, causing noticeable functional deficits and scars. Alopecia is a side effect of cranial radiation and some chemotherapy. Steroids can cause weight gain, fluid retention, acne, and moon face.

    b. *Interventions*

       (1) Assess impact of change in appearance on social interactions, self-concept, ADL, and intimate relationships.

       (2) Encourage participation in activities valued by the patient.

       (3) Refer for counseling, body image consultation, physical or occupational therapy, or social work support.

    c. *Desired outcome:* Patient will adapt to or compensate for changes in appearance and function.

REFERENCES

Belford, K. (2000). Central nervous system cancers. In C. H. Yarbro, M. Goodman, M. H. Frogge, & S. C. Groenwald (Eds.), *Cancer nursing: Principles and practice* (5th ed., pp. 1048–1096). Boston: Jones & Bartlett.

Bohan, E. (2002). Brain tumors. In E. Barker (Ed.), *Neuroscience nursing: A spectrum of care* (2nd ed., pp. 269–301). St. Louis, MO: Mosby.

Central Brain Tumor Registry of the United States (CBTRUS). (2002). *Statistical report: Primary brain tumors in the United States, 1995–1999.* Chicago, IL: Author.

Eyre, H. J. (2003). Cancer statistics. CA: *Cancer Journal for Clinicians, 53*(1),7.

Hickey, J. V., & Armstrong, T. (1997). Brain tumors. In J. V. Hickey (Ed.), *The clinical practice of neurological and neurosurgical nursing* (4th ed., pp. 501–526). Philadelphia: J. B. Lippincott.

Lang, F. F., Wildrick, D. M., & Sawaya, R. (2000). Metastatic brain tumors. In *Neuro-oncology: The essentials* (pp. 329–337). New York: Thieme Medical.

Lesser, G. J., & Grossman, S. A. (1993). The chemotherapy of adult primary brain tumors. *Cancer Treatment Reviews, 19,* 270.

Rabbitt, J. E., & Page, M. S. (1998). Selected complications in neuro-oncology. *Seminars in Oncology Nursing, 14,* 53–60.

Sheidler, V., & Bucholtz, J. D. (1996). *Central nervous system tumors—Cancer nursing: A comprehensive textbook* (2nd ed., pp. 826–839). Philadelphia: W. B. Saunders.

Strickler, R. (2000). Astrocytomas: The clinical picture. *Clinical Journal of Oncology Nursing, 4,* 153–158.

CHAPTER

12 Gastrointestinal Cancers

JoAnn Coleman

I. Gastrointestinal (GI) Cancers—An Overview
  A. The GI tract has the highest incidence of malignant tumors.
    1. Cancers of the GI tract include parts of the bowel lumen—gastric, colorectal, rectal cancers.
    2. Cancers of the GI accessory organs—hepatic, biliary, bile duct, pancreas.
    3. Although the esophagus is a part of the GI system, it is viewed and managed as a tumor of the head and neck region.
  B. More than 25% of cancer deaths every year in the United States are attributed to cancer of the GI tract.
  C. The problems common to all GI cancers stem from the delay in clinical presentation.
    1. GI tumors proliferate insidiously and extend locally.
    2. Presenting signs and symptoms may be misdiagnosed or self-treated for a long time.
    3. As the tumor grows, it can exceed the distensible capacity of the GI lumen and result in obstruction.
  D. Most tumors of the GI tract are adenocarcinomas.
  E. The metastasis of GI tumors occurs by all three mechanisms of metastasis—local spread, blood vessel invasion, and dissemination through the lymphatic system. This diversity means these tumors metastasize to a large variety of sites outside the GI system.
  F. Prognosis of the GI malignancy depends on:
    1. Tumor type and site(s) of metastasis
    2. Tumor size
    3. Degree of cellular differentiation
    4. Extent of metastases
    5. Availability of effective treatments
    6. Person's general health
  G. Diseases have very different prognostic implications and are treated as separate disease processes.
  H. Table 12–1 provides an overview of the clinicopathophysiologic features of the GI malignancies (gastric cancer, hepatobiliary cancer, pancreatic cancer, colorectal cancer).

II. Etiology
  A. Diseases have variable genetic, environmental, dietary risk factors.
  B. Specific risk factors are discussed within Table 12–1.

III. Patient Management
  A. Assessment (Specific assessment findings for each type of malignancy are included in Table 12–1.)

1. Patient history
   a. Family history may be important in some of these disorders that are associated with familial genetic abnormalities (eg, colorectal cancer, pancreatic cancer).
   b. Diet and social history may provide information about carcinogen exposure (eg, esophageal cancer, hepatic cancer) or known dietary risk factors.
   c. History of infectious diseases. Viral illnesses or GI infections are known to predispose patients to certain GI malignancies (eg, hepatic cancer, gastric cancer, colorectal cancer).
2. Patient complaints
   a. Most patients have subtle changes in eating or bowel habits that are largely ignored or attributed to other medical problems (eg, reflux, change in stool characteristics).
   b. Abdominal pain is a common finding in many GI malignancies, although the localization of pain differs with each of the disorders.
      (1) Pain localization may be helpful in determining the area of the GI tract that is affected.
      (2) Low back pain or epigastric/substernal pain may also represent GI disease.
      (3) Pain that is "rebound" or worse with lifting the hand rather than pressing downward signals an acute abdominal crisis and possible surgical candidate.
   c. Bleeding from the GI tract is a cardinal symptom of malignancy. Any blood, such as old blood in emesis or stool, or smearing of blood on defecation is important to evaluate for the presence of malignancy.
3. Physical findings
   a. All patients with suspected GI malignancy should have a thorough abdominal assessment.
      (1) Bowel contours, bulges, pulsations
      (2) Bowel sounds for abnormalities
      (3) Light and deep palpation for areas of tenderness or masses
   b. Signs of abnormal fluid balance, nutrition, and metabolic regulation are common with all GI malignancies.
      (1) Dehydration and orthostasis occur due to fluid shifts into the peritoneal space when inflammation is present.
      (2) Nutrient absorption is often compromised before a diagnosis of malignancy is made. Symptoms may include dry, flaky skin; taste changes; alopecia; oral tenderness; bruising.
      (3) Symptoms may relate to the degree of constipation or diarrhea the patient has experienced.
B. Diagnostic Tests (Unique and specific diagnostic tests for each type of GI malignancy are included in Table 12-1.)
   1. *Screening guidelines.* The only GI cancer for which there are screening guidelines for early detection is colorectal cancer. Colorectal cancer detected in its early stages has an excellent prognosis, and screening tests are adequately sensitive and specific to provide this information. Controversy exists regarding the age at which to start screening (40 versus 50 years of age), best test, and frequency of

(Text continues on page 158)

TABLE 12–1 **Overview of Gastrointestinal (GI) Malignancies**

Key Feature	Gastric Cancer	Pancreatic Cancer
Definition/ epidemiology	• Incidence declining in the United States due to food preparation and preservation • Arises from the mucosa or inner lining of the stomach • Average age of onset is 50–70 years of age • Males have greater incidence than females • More prevalent in minority populations in United States • Proximal or GE-junction tumors now account for half of all stomach tumors and are associated with a poor prognosis • Most present with advanced disease • Overall 5-year survival rate is approximately 5% to 15%	• Fourth most common cause of cancer-related death in the United States • Arises in the lining of the pancreatic ducts • Average age of onset is 60–80 years of age • Equal incidence among males and females • Higher incidence in African Americans • Most tumors arise in the head of the pancreas • Overall 5-year survival rate is approximately 5%
Risk factors/ etiologies	• Dietary intake of nitroso-compounds and salts convert nitrates to carcinogenic nitrosamines in the stomach • *Helicobacter pylori* infection • Low socioeconomic status • Prior gastric resection for peptic ulcer disease • Patients with blood group A • Pernicious anemia	• Cigarette smoking is a major risk factor • No clear dietary factors, but fat content and an increased body mass index are associated with increased risk • Occupational exposure to chemicals may be a risk factor • Relationship among diabetes mellitus and chronic pancreatitis as precursors for pancreatic cancer uncertain at this time

Hepatobiliary Cancer	Colorectal Cancer
• Hepatobiliary cancers have low incidence in the United States • Gallbladder cancer is most common hepatobiliary malignancy, diagnosed in persons between the ages of 70 and 75 with a predilection for females over males • Hepatocellular cancer is seventh most common cancer in the world. Average age of onset is 50 to 55 years • Increased incidental finding of gall-bladder malignancy at the time of elective laparoscopic cholecystectomy	• Most common GI malignancy and the second leading cause of cancer death in the United States • Colon cancer is more common than rectal cancer • Screening and early detection are methods for reducing morbidity and mortality from colorectal cancer • Average age of onset is 60 to 70 years • Equal incidence in males and females of colon cancer, with rectal cancer more prevalent in men • One fourth of colorectal cancers are found
• Majority of gallbladder and bile duct cancers are adenocarcinomas • Five-year survival for stage I tumors after cholecystectomy is greater than 85%; for stage II, III, and IV tumors, 5-year survivals are 25%, 10%, and 2% • Cholangiocarcinomas or bile duct cancers can be diagnosed throughout the biliary tree and are classified as intrahepatic or extrahepatic (most common). Bile duct tumors arise from the epithelium of the bile ducts. Intrahepatic tumors tend to present as solitary masses. Extrahepatic tumors encompass hilar carcinomas, in the region of the junction of the right and left hepatic ducts and in the common hepatic and common bile ducts. These tumors occur in conditions where bile is stagnant, infected, or both. • Average age of onset of bile duct tumors is between 60 and 70 years of age and equal between males and females	in the rectum; remainder are located in some other part of the colon. Most colon cancers are found in the right colon. • Overall 5-year survival rate is approximately 50% to 55%.
• Cirrhosis associated with hepatitis B or C is a common precursor to hepatocellular malignancy. • Exposure to carcinogens such as aflatoxin, found in a number of grains • Gallstones associated with chronic cholecystitis is the greatest risk factor for gallbladder cancer, followed by a calcified gallbladder, gallbladder polyps, typhoid carriers, and carcinogens	• Sedentary lifestyle leads to decrease in in-testinal tract transit time allowing for poten-tial carcinogens to be in contact longer with colorectal mucosa • Diet high in fat • Inflammatory bowel disease • Obesity • Radiation exposure • Heavy alcohol consumption • Occupational exposure to carcinogens

(continued)

TABLE 12–1 **Overview of Gastrointestinal (GI) Malignancies**
(Continued)

Key Feature	Gastric Cancer	Pancreatic Cancer
Risk factors/ etiologies		• Familial pancreatic cancer is rare, but a genetic predisposition may be present in up to 5% of cases.

Signs and symptoms	• Complaints similar to peptic ulcer disease or other GI ailments
	• Reflux
	• Indigestion
	• Early satiety
	• Nausea and vomiting
	• Abdominal pain just above the umbilicus
	• Weight loss
	• Loss or decrease in appetite
	• Bloating after meals
	• Advanced disease findings include:
	  • Ascites
	  • Hepatomegaly
	  • Palpable epigastric mass or nodules around the umbilicus
		• Initial signs and symptomsdepend on the site and extent of tumor
		• Head of pancreas: jaundice; pain, deep and boring and/or radiating around to the back; weight loss; anorexia; steatorrhea or diarrhea; weakness; indigestion
		• Body and tail of the pancreas: pain, dull and vague, localized to epigastrium or back, or episodic and related to meals or constant and severe; weight loss; early satiety; indigestion; vomiting; GI bleed; splenomegaly
		• Palpable gallbladder (Courvoisier's sign) seen in obstruction of the distal common bile duct
		• Advanced disease presents with ascites, supraclavicular lymph nodes, a periumbilical mass, or a rectal mass
		• Diabetes of recent onset in elderly patients with vague GI symptoms may be from an underlying pancreatic tumor
		• Migratory thrombophlebitis (Trousseau's sign) may be seen in advanced disease
		• Depression may also be diagnosed in a number of patients before the diagnosis of a pancreatic tumor

Diagnostic tests	• CT scan is most common study for staging the extent of disease, detecting extragastric extension, lymph node involvement or metastatic disease • Barium swallow/upper GI series only shows anatomy of stomach	• CT scan is most common study for staging the extent of disease and lymph nodes and metastases • Ultrasound may be included in initial examination • MRI has not been shown to add any information but may be used if an iodine contrast allergy

Hepatobiliary Cancer	Colorectal Cancer
• Bile duct cancer risk factors include hepatolithiasis, ulcerative colitis, sclerosing cholangitis, choledochal cysts, chemical carcinogens, and liver fluke infections	• Genetic polyposis syndromes such as familial adenomatous polyposis (FAP), hereditary nonpolyposis colorectal cancer (HNPCC), hamartomatous polyposis syndromes (Peutz-Jeghers) and Gardener's syndrome • Anal cancer has been associated with infection with the human immunodeficiency virus (HIV)
• Similar for hepatocellular, bile duct and gallbladder tumors • Jaundice • Dark urine • Clay-colored stools • Anorexia • Weight loss • Malaise • Abdominal pain • Fever or cholangitis	• Vary depending on location: Ascending colon presents with anemia; a palpable mass on the right side; vague, dull pain; weakness; weight loss; fatigue; palpitations Transverse colon presents with a change in bowel habits and blood in stool Descending and sigmoid colon may exhibit constipation alternating with diarrhea, abdominal pain, nausea, vomiting, melena or perforation Rectal tumors may present as changes in bowel movement, rectal fullness, urgency, frequency, bleeding, tenesmus, malaise, occult blood, pelvic pain
• For hepatocellular tumors, a CT scan or MRI to define extent and number of primary liver lesions, vascular anatomy, blood vessel involvement, involvement with tumor and extrahepatic disease. • Alpha-fetoprotein (AFP) levels in the blood are elevated in approximately 60% to 90% of patients	• Clinical presentation is useful for identifying potential colorectal cancer in a given patient • CT scan • MRI used to detect recurrent rectal cancer and tumors too small to be evaluated on CT scan. • Colonoscopy • Air contrast barium enema

(continued)

TABLE 12–1 Overview of Gastrointestinal (GI) Malignancies
(Continued)

Key Feature	Gastric Cancer	Pancreatic Cancer
Diagnostic tests	• Upper endoscopy (EGD) allows direct visualization of mucosa and mechanism for biopsy of lesions. Accurately detects more than 95% of gastric cancers • Endoscopic ultrasound (EUS) can be performed during endoscopy to image and evaluate tumor depth through the layers of the stomach and any lymph node involvement • *H pylori* diagnosis by endoscopy and biopsy, rapid urease test, or carbon-labeled breath test	• Cholangiography to define site of biliary obstruction. Use of ERCP visualizes both biliary and GI tracts. • Endoscopic ultrasound (EUS) useful in staging tumors for size of tumor, extension into adjacent structures, lymph node involvement and any blood vessel involvement • Laparoscopy may be used for staging of the tumor and can identify liver and peritoneal metastases not seen by other studies • Percutaneous fine needle aspiration (FNA) biopsy may be performed for unresectable tumors to help direct palliative or neoadjuvant chemoradiation • The carbohydrate antigen 19-9 (CA 19-9) is tumor-associated, not tumor-specific, and may be used in conjunction with other studies to help diagnose pancreatic tumor. It is most useful in assessing patients being treated for pancreatic cancer
General management strategies	• Depending on the stage and location of a gastric tumor a partial or total gastrectomy may be performed (see Table 12-2) • Chemotherapy is given as adjuvant therapy after surgery and as palliative (primary) therapy for advanced disease (see Table 12-2)	• Surgical resection is the best therapeutic option and only opportunity for cure • Pancreaticoduodenectomy, the Whipple procedure, is the surgery most often performed for treatment of pancreatic cancer (see Table 12-3) • Adjuvant therapy with chemotherapy and radiation therapy is usually administered to prevent recurrence of disease (see Table 12-3)

Hepatobiliary Cancer	Colorectal Cancer
• Gallbladder and bile duct tumors are best detected by CT scan or MRI. For patients presenting with jaundice further workup should include an ERCP or magnetic resonance cholangio-pancreatography (MRCP). Percutaneous transhepatic cholangiography may also be performed to assess level of biliary obstruction and as a guide for the placement of percutaneous transhepatic biliary stents as needed for palliation of jaundice.	• Endoscopic ultrasound (EUS) to stage rectal tumors.
• Both carcinoembryonic assay (CEA) and CA 19-9 levels may be elevated in gallbladder and bile duct tumors.	
• Percutaneous needle aspiration biopsy, brush or scrape biopsy, or cytological exam of bile may aid in determining diagnosis.	
• Surgery remains the only curative modality for hepatobiliary tumors (see Table 12-4, Table 12-5, Table 12-6)	• Surgery is the primary treatment for colon cancer (see Table 12-7 and 12-8). Goals of rectal surgery are cure, local control, restoration of intestinal continuity, preservation of anorectal sphincter function, and preservation of sexual and urinary function.
• Alternative therapies for unresectable disease include ablative therapy, chemo-embolization, chemotherapy plus radiation for hepatocellular tumors.	
• Palliation includes surgical, endoscopic and interventional radiographic procedures for unresectable gallbladder and bile duct cancers.	• Neoadjuvant, adjuvant, and palliative radiation therapy are used for colorectal cancer (see Table 12-7).
	• Adjuvant chemotherapy is recommended for early rectal cancer and in advanced colon cancer (see Table 12-8).

(continued)

TABLE 12–1 **Overview of Gastrointestinal (GI) Malignancies**
(Continued)

Key Feature	Gastric Cancer	Pancreatic Cancer
General management strategies	• Radiation therapy is reserved for palliation of symptoms such as pain, bleeding, or obstruction by tumor (see Table 12-2)	• Chemotherapy may be given for palliation (see Table 12-3) • Radiation therapy may be given as palliation for pain or bleeding (see Table 12-3) • Surgical interventions for palliative relief of biliary and gastric obstruction as well as nerve blocks for pain management have been shown to improve quality of life (see Table 12-3). • Nonoperative palliation of obstructive jaundice by either percutaneous or endoscopic stents is effective. Duodenal obstruction may be palliated by a percutaneous gastrostomy tube for stomach decompression or by insertion of a duodenal stent to maintain patency of the lumen

testing. These guidelines are the recommendations of the Centers for Disease Control (CDC, 2002).

a. For healthy people starting at age 50 years without significant risk factors (see III.B.1.b for description of significant risk factors.)

  (1) Fecal occult blood test yearly AND

  (2) Flexible sigmoidoscopy or double contrast barium enema once every 5 years

  (3) Some advise a colonoscopy every 10 years after age 50 years for a more thorough inspection for polyps or suspicious lesions, but insurance reimbursement for this may be limited.

b. For people at any age with a significant risk factor (immediate family member with colorectal polyps or cancer, or a personal history of inflammatory bowel disease)

  (1) Fecal occult blood test and flexible sigmoidoscopy annually OR

  (2) Colonoscopy every year

c. For anyone with abnormal basic screening tests, the usual gold standard for follow-up assessment and detection of polyps or GI tumors is the colonoscopy.

Hepatobiliary Cancer	Colorectal Cancer
• Chemotherapy and radiation therapy as appropriate therapy remain controversial due to small number of patients and no definitive treatment with proven survival benefit	• Metastatic disease in the liver or lung should be considered for resection. This can then be followed by adjuvant therapy.

2. *Laboratory tests.* Few laboratory tests are exclusively diagnostic for any GI malignancy, although some tests that may be ordered for diagnosis or monitoring of response to treatment may include tests for:
   a. Genetic abnormalities
   b. Tumor markers
   c. Serum comprehensive chemistry profile, hepatic panel
3. Evaluation for potential GI malignancy often involves radiologic procedures (x-rays, computed tomography [CT] scans) to detect masses.
4. Many patients will also require an endoscopic procedure to visualize and possibly obtain a histopathologic specimen for diagnosis.
C. Treatment is individualized for patients depending on their clinical stage and type of disease. An overview of treatment options is provided in Tables 12–1 through 12–8. Basic concepts of treatment planning for patients with GI malignancies include the following:
   1. Surgical resection for cure is always the preferred treatment when an option.
   2. Adjuvant therapies have proven beneficial to prevent early recurrence in some of these patients.

(Text continues on page 171)

TABLE 12–2 Gastric Cancer Staging and Treatment

Stage	Surgery	Radiation Therapy	Chemotherapy
Stage I Tumor is confined to the first or second layers of the stomach wall. Tumor has not spread to lymph nodes or tumor is in the first layer of the stomach wall and has spread to lymph nodes very close to the tumor.	Partial gastrectomy removes the portion of the stomach that contains tumor including lymph nodes. Total gastrectomy removes the entire stomach and part of the esophagus, small intestine, and other tissues near the tumor including nearby lymph nodes. This is done for tumor in the proximal stomach or gastroesophageal junction.	Not shown to be effective as adjuvant or primary therapy.	Not shown to be effective as adjuvant therapy. May be used in disease recurrence.
Stage II Tumor is in the first layer of the stomach wall and has spread to lymph nodes further away from the tumor; tumor is only in the second layer of the stomach and has spread to lymph nodes very close to the tumor; tumor is only in the third layer of the stomach wall.	Partial gastrectomy removes the portion of the stomach that contains tumor including lymph nodes. Total gastrectomy removes the entire stomach and part of the esophagus, small intestine, and other tissues near the tumor including nearby lymph nodes. This is done for tumors in the proximal stomach or gastroesophageal junction.	Not shown to be effective as adjuvant or primary therapy.	Combination chemotherapy regimens containing 5-FU based therapy, mitomycin and doxorubicin for advanced disease, with or without surgery.

Stage III

Tumor is in the second layer of the stomach wall and has spread to lymph nodes further away from the tumor; tumor is in all three layers of the stomach wall and has spread to lymph nodes close to or further away from the tumor; tumor is in all four layers of the stomach wall and has spread to nearby tissues.

Not considered as initial therapy unless there is bleeding or a lesion that could cause a gastric outlet obstruction that may be relieved prior to chemotherapy.

Adjuvant treatment with chemotherapy (5-FU) in locally advanced, unresectable tumors.

Regimens containing 5-FU based therapy, mitomycin based therapy and doxorubicin-containing combination chemotherapy for advanced disease, with or without surgery. The use of cisplatin-based combination therapy is under investigation.

Stage IV

Tumor has spread to nearby tissues and to lymph nodes further away from the tumor, or has spread to other parts of the body.

Not considered as initial therapy unless there is bleeding or a lesion that could cause a gastric outlet obstruction that may be relieved before chemotherapy.

May be used as palliation for control of symptoms such as bleeding or pain.

Regimens using single agents or containing 5-FU based therapy, mitomycin based therapy, and doxorubicin-containing combination chemotherapy for advanced disease. The use of cisplatin-based combination therapy is under investigation.

TABLE 12-3 Pancreatic Cancer Staging and Treatment

Stage	Surgery	Radiation Therapy	Chemotherapy	Other
Stage I Tumor confined to the pancreas.	Classic pancreaticoduodenectomy (Whipple procedure) includes a hemigastrectomy along with excision of the distal bile duct, head of the pancreas, and duodenum. A pylorus-preserving pancreaticoduodenectomy includes all of the above but the hemigastrectomy, allowing retention of the entire stomach and the pyloric valve. For tumors in the body or tail of the pancreas a distal pancreatectomy and splenectomy is performed. A total pancreatectomy and splenectomy may be performed for tumor found throughout the pancreas.	External beam radiation in addition to chemotherapy as adjuvant therapy to surgery to prevent local recurrence.	Single or combination regimens alone or in combination with external beam radiation as adjuvant therapy to surgery to prevent local recurrence. Active agents include gemcitabine and 5FU.	Vaccines are being used in clinical trials to prevent recurrence.
Stage II Tumor extends directly to duodenum, bile duct, or peripancreatic tissues.	Classic pancreaticoduodenectomy (Whipple procedure) includes a hemigastrectomy along with excision of the distal bile duct, head of the pancreas, and duodenum. A pylorus-preserving pancreaticoduodenectomy includes all of the above but the hemigastrectomy, allowing retention of the entire stomach and the pyloric valve. A total pancreatectomy and splenectomy may be performed for tumor found throughout the pancreas.	External beam radiation in addition to chemotherapy as adjuvant therapy to surgery to prevent local recurrence.	Single or combination regimens alone or in combination with external beam radiation as adjuvant therapy to surgery to prevent local recurrence. Active agents include gemcitabine and 5FU	Vaccines are being used in clinical trials to prevent recurrence.

Stage III

Tumor confined to pancreas but with metastases to regional lymph nodes or tumor extends to duodenum, bile duct, or peripancreatic tissues with metastases to regional lymph nodes.

Classic pancreaticoduodenectomy (Whipple procedure) includes a hemigastrectomy along with excision of the distal bile duct, head of the pancreas, and duodenum. A pylorus-preserving pancreaticoduodenectomy includes all of the above but the hemigastrectomy, allowing retention of the entire stomach and the pyloric valve. A total pancreatectomy and splenectomy may be performed for tumor found throughout the pancreas.

External beam radiation in addition to chemotherapy as adjuvant therapy to surgery to prevent local recurrence or as therapy without surgery.

Single or combination regimens alone or in combination with external beam radiation as adjuvant therapy to surgery to prevent local recurrence or as therapy without surgery.

Stage IV

Tumor extends to stomach, spleen, colon, or adjacent large blood vessels with or without lymph node metastasis.

Palliative surgery for symptom management may be performed. A biliary bypass (choledochojejunostomy) for relief of jaundice and/or a gastric bypass (gastrojejunostomy) for gastric outlet obstruction. An alcohol block to the celiac nerve plexus is also performed for pain management.

Neoadjuvant therapy in combination with chemotherapy for tumors confined to the pancreas but encasing major blood vessels to help shrink tumors for possible surgical resection. May be used as palliation for symptoms such as bleeding and pain.

Neoadjuvant therapy in combination with radiation therapy for tumors confined to the pancreas but encasing major blood vessels to help shrink tumors for possible surgical resection. Single agent (5-FU, or gemcitabine) regimens may be used as palliation of symptoms. Combination chemotherapy regimens (5-FU and gemcitabine based) are being used in clinical trials.

TABLE 12–4 Hepatic Cancer Staging and Treatment

Stage	Surgery	Radiation Therapy	Chemotherapy
Stage I Single tumor of the liver that measures 2 cm or less and does not invade blood vessels.	Removal of lobe of the liver where tumor located or a non-anatomic wedge resection or anatomic resection of a specific segment of the liver. In patients with cirrhotic liver, the smallest resection that will remove all gross tumor is performed to reduce the chance of postoperative liver failure. Liver transplantation may be considered.	Not shown to be effective as adjuvant therapy	Not shown to be effective as adjuvant therapy. Clinical trials looking at developing adjuvant therapy directed at microscopic residual disease after surgery to prevent recurrence.
Stage II Single tumor of the liver more than 2 cm with blood vessel involvement, or multiple tumors (each less than 2 cm) limited to one lobe with blood vessel involvement or multiple tumors limited to one lobe (more than 2 cm) with or without blood vessel involvement.	Removal of lobe of liver where tumor located. May also have an extended resection, called a trisegmentectomy to remove involved liver and blood vessels. Liver transplantation may be considered for patients with fewer than three tumors and no blood vessel involvement.	Not shown to be effective as adjuvant therapy	Not shown to be effective as adjuvant therapy. Ablative therapies may be used to destroy tumor cells within the liver. Percutaneous ethanol injection may be performed directly during surgery or laparoscopy or percutaneously using ultrasound guidance. Cryosurgery is the repeated freezing and thawing of tissues to produced tissue destruction and usually is performed at the time of surgery. Radiofrequency ablation is the process of using heat generated by a radiofrequency electrode to kill tumors. This may be performed during surgery, laparoscopically, or percutaneously.

Stage			
Stage III Any of the above with lymph node involvement.	Removal of lobe of liver where tumor located. May also have an extended resection, called a trisegmentectomy, to remove involved liver and blood vessels.	Not shown to be effective as adjuvant therapy	Not shown to be effective as adjuvant therapy.
Stage IV Multiple tumors in more than one lobe or the tumor(s) involve major blood vessels or invasion of adjacent organs with or without lymph node involvement.	Surgery is not considered for treatment.	Not shown to be effective as adjuvant therapy. Three-dimensional conformal radiation therapy reduces radiation to the normal liver and may produce regression of tumor.	Chemoembolization for large hypervascular tumors. May be combined with percutaneous ethanol injection for tumors smaller than 3 cm or in patients with liver failure for whom surgery is not an option. Hepatic arterial embolization may be used for painful, unresectable tumors or tumors that have ruptured.

TABLE 12–5 Bile Duct Cancer Staging and Treatment

Stage	Surgery	Radiation Therapy	Chemotherapy
Stage I Tumor is confined to the bile duct mucosa or muscular layer.	Intrahepatic tumors are managed by appropriate liver resection. Distal tumors are treated by a pancreaticoduodenectomy (Whipple procedure). Extrahepatic tumors require excision of the entire extrahepatic biliary tree and reconstruction with a hepaticojejunostomy (with or without the placement of internal-external biliary stents).	Adjuvant therapy for distal tumors combined with chemotherapy (same as pancreatic cancer) Adjuvant therapy for extrahepatic tumors (external beam and/or intraluminal brachytherapy)	Used investigationally with radiation therapy but not shown to be effective as adjuvant therapy.
Stage II Tumor invades the periductal tissue.	Intrahepatic tumors are managed by appropriate liver resection. Distal tumors are treated by a pancreaticoduodenectomy (Whipple procedure). Extrahepatic tumors require excision of the entire extrahepatic biliary tree and reconstruction with a hepaticojejunostomy (with or without placement of internal-external biliary stents). A liver resection may also be performed along with a hepaticojejunostomy.	Adjuvant therapy for distal tumors combined with chemotherapy (same as pancreatic cancer) Adjuvant therapy for extrahepatic tumors (external beam or intraluminal brachytherapy)	Not shown to be effective as adjuvant therapy.

Stage III

Tumor may be confined to the bile duct mucosa or muscular layer with lymph node involvement or tumor invades the periductal tissues with lymph node involvement.

Intrahepatic tumors are managed by appropriate liver resection. Distal tumors are treated by a pancreaticoduodenectomy (Whipple procedure). Extrahepatic tumors require excision of the entire extrahepatic biliary tree and reconstruction with a hepaticojejunostomy (with or without biliary stents). A liver resection may also be performed along with a hepaticojejunostomy.

Adjuvant therapy for distal tumors combined with chemotherapy (same as pancreatic cancer)
Adjuvant therapy for extrahepatic tumors (external beam or intraluminal brachytherapy)

Not shown to be effective as adjuvant therapy.

Stage IV

Tumor invades adjacent structures such as liver, pancreas, duodenum, gallbladder, colon, stomach with or without lymph node involvement.

Palliation for biliary obstruction with a choledochojejunostomy

May be used as palliation for relief of obstructive symptoms.

Not shown to be effective as therapy.

TABLE 12–6 Gallbladder Cancer Staging and Treatment

Stage	Surgery	Radiation Therapy	Chemotherapy
Stage I Tumor invades lamina propria or muscle layer	Simple cholecystectomy	Not shown to be effective as adjuvant therapy.	Not shown to be effective as adjuvant therapy.
Stage II Tumor invades perimuscular connective tissue but no extension beyond serosa into the liver	Radical or extended cholecystectomy with a wide resection of the liver around the gallbladder bed and a wide lymph node dissection.	Not shown to be effective as adjuvant therapy.	Mitomycin C and 5-FU either alone or in combination are most commonly used agents, but results are poor.
Stage III Tumor invades lamina propria or muscle layer with metastases to lymph nodes or tumor perforates serosa or invades an adjacent organ, or both, with or without lymph node involvement.	Radical or extended cholecystectomy with a wide resection of the liver around the gallbladder bed and a wide lymph node dissection.	Not shown to be effective as adjuvant therapy.	Mitomycin C and 5-FU either alone or in combination are most commonly used agents, but results are poor.
Stage IV Tumor extends into the liver or into two or more other adjacent organs (stomach, duodenum, colon, pancreas, extrahepatic bile ducts) with or without lymph node involvement.	Aggressive therapy may be considered. Radical or extended cholecystectomy with a wide resection of the liver around the gallbladder bed and a wide lymph node dissection.	Palliative therapy with or without chemosensitization for relief from obstruction and pain. A form of radiotherapy (external beam or intraoperative radiation) may be offered as adjuvant therapy as it has a low morbidity.	Not shown to be effective as adjuvant therapy.

TABLE 12-7 Colon Cancer Staging and Treatment

Stage	Surgery	Radiation Therapy	Chemotherapy
Stage I Tumor invades submucosa or muscularis propria of bowel wall.	Bowel resection with a wide margin of normal bowel including the lymph nodes draining the area. Resections are performed according to location of the tumor, the blood supply and lymph nodes in the region. (Right or left hemicolectomy, transverse colectomy, sigmoid colectomy. Low anterior resection, subtotal colectomy and total abdominal colectomy).	Not shown to be effective as adjuvant therapy.	Usually not recommended.
Stage II Tumor invades through the bowel wall.	Bowel resection with a wide margin of normal bowel including the lymph nodes draining the area.	Not shown to be effective as adjuvant therapy.	Usually not recommended.
Stage III Tumor invades through the bowel wall along with lymph node involvement.	Bowel resection with a wide margin of normal bowel including the lymph nodes draining the area.	Not shown to be effective as adjuvant therapy.	Combination with 5-FU and leucovorin.
Stage IV Tumor has spread to other organs or structures.	Palliation for symptoms such as bleeding or bowel obstruction which may require diverting cstomy or bowel bypass.	Palliation for symptoms such as bleeding.	As primary or adjuvant therapy. Combination regimens using 5-FU and leucovorin, 5-FU, leucovorin and irinotecan, 5-FU, leucovorin and oxaliplatin or continuous 5-FU or capecitabine. Hepatic artery infusion therapy may be given for liver metastases. Anti-angiogenesis agents are under investigation.

TABLE 12-8 Rectal Cancer Staging and Treatment

Stage	Surgery	Radiation Therapy	Chemotherapy
Stage I Tumor is confined to the rectal wall.	Local transanal resection or total mesorectal excision	Neoadjuvant therapy in combination with chemotherapy to shrink tumor. Adjuvant therapy to decrease the risk of recurrence.	Neoadjuvant therapy in combination with radiation therapy to shrink tumor. Adjuvant therapy to decrease the risk of recurrence.
Stage II Tumor extends through the muscularis propria.	Depending on tumor location in the rectum. Middle and upper rectal tumors may be treated with a low anterior resection. Lower rectal tumors may be treated with an abdominal perineal resection and ostomy or removal of the rectum with a colon-to-anal anastomosis.	Adjuvant therapy to decrease the risk of recurrence.	5-FU based chemotherapy in combination with radiation therapy.
Stage III Tumor extends beyond the rectal wall and into regional lymph nodes.	Depending on tumor location in the rectum. Middle and upper tumors require a low anterior resection. Lower rectal tumors may be treated with an abdominal perineal resection and ostomy or removal of the rectum with a colon-to-anal anastomosis.	Combination therapy with 5-FU based chemotherapy.	5-FU based chemotherapy in combination with radiation therapy.
Stage IV Tumor has spread to other organs or structures.	Palliative therapy to relieve obstruction with a diverting ostomy.	Palliative therapy to control pain and bleeding.	Continuous or bolus 5-FU infusion.

3. New tumor-associated antigens have been identified on the cells of many patients with GI malignancies and may serve as future targets for antineoplastic agents (eg, epidermal growth factor receptor, tyrosine kinase c-Kit receptors).
4. Multimodal therapy regimens for many patients with advanced disease are a reflection of how few standard effective therapies exist for these patients.

D. Nursing Diagnoses
  1. Potential for altered bowel patterns related to surgical changes in anatomy and sexual dysfunction related to altered body structure
    a. *Problem:* Changes in the normal anatomy and function of the GI tract affect digestion and elimination. The need to alter eating patterns is affected by gastric surgery to prevent dumping. The presence of gastrostomy or jejunostomy feeding tubes is a constant reminder to the patient of the diagnosis. Placement of percutaneous biliary tubes for relieving biliary obstruction is a palliative measure. Pancreatic insufficiency from either tumor or pancreatic resection causes steatorrhea and makes the patient dependent on oral enzyme replacement with meals. Colorectal tumors may cause major alterations in elimination. The creation of an ostomy for the elimination of stool is a major alteration in body structure. Tubes, drains, and stomas from ostomies create a need for the patient to learn to care for the appliance and perform necessary tasks to maintain patency and security of tubes and drains.
    b. *Interventions*
      (1) Monitor frequency of bowel movements and consistency of stools.
      (2) Administer antidiarrheal agents as ordered to decrease stool frequency.
      (3) Use dietary fiber and bulking agents to absorb fluid and add firmness to stool to help with retention and control.
      (4) Involve an enterostomal therapy nurse in education and consultation.
      (5) Educate the patient and family about ostomy care.
        (a) The type of ostomy will determine the type of covering needed. Ileostomies drain intermittently and unpredictably, requiring a bag and special skin care. An ostomy in the sigmoid colon is the exact opposite; patients may never wear a bag, and stools are stimulated on a planned interval basis by instilling fluid into the ostomy.
        (b) Stool training will vary with location of the ostomy.
        (c) The degree of fluid and electrolyte imbalance will depend on the ostomy location. Ileostomies cause more electrolyte and nutritional disturbances.
        (d) Some colostomies are permanent; others can be reversed after healing of the resected bowel. Most temporary colostomies are reversed approximately 2 to 5 months after the initial surgery.
      (6) Assess patients for signs and symptoms of bowel obstruction or perforation from tumor or adhesions: severe intractable

abdominal pain, rebound tenderness, distention, absence of stool, absent bowel sounds, nausea/vomiting, hypertension, tachycardia, confusion, increased lactate, increased amylase.

c. *Desired Outcomes*
   (1) The patient will positively adapt his or her lifestyle to GI and genitourinary changes caused by the cancer.
   (2) Adverse effects are minimized by self care.
   (3) Bowel elimination schedule is normalized for the patient's physiologic limitations.

2. Alteration in nutrition, less than body requirements, related to nausea, anorexia, early satiety, abdominal distention, disease process, treatment, and increased metabolic demands
   a. *Problem:* Patients with GI cancer may experience a decrease in appetite as a result of the tumor and its invasion into structures or lumen obstruction, or as a consequence of treatment (surgery, chemotherapy, and/or radiation therapy) or abdominal pressure from ascites. This can make it difficult to maintain adequate nutrition.
   b. *Interventions:* Follow recommendations in Chapters 27 and 28.
   c. *Desired outcomes:* Improvement or maintenance of nutritional status as described in Chapter 28, and elimination or control of nausea and vomiting as described in Chapter 27.

3. Pain related to disease, its sequelae, or treatments
   a. *Problem:* Pain is frequently a symptom exhibited by patients with a GI cancer. Growth of the tumor can cause obstruction, or pressure on nerves, blood vessels, or other organs. Pain can also be associated with various treatments.
   b. *Interventions:* Follow recommendations in Chapter 30.
   (1) Pancreatic cancer is often refractory to traditional pain management therapies, but responsive to nerve blocks.
   c. *Desired outcome:* The patient will report that discomfort is adequately controlled (see Chapter 30).

4. Risk for fluid volume deficit related to anorexia, nausea, vomiting, diarrhea, or constipation and increased loss of fluids and electrolytes from the GI tract from tubes for decompression of an obstructed lumen
   a. *Problem:* Any obstructed area in the GI tract can interfere with a patient's ability to maintain normal ingestion, digestion, and elimination. Tumors can cause obstruction of the gastric outlet into the duodenum, in the distal common bile duct causing obstructive jaundice, in the head of the pancreas preventing passage of pancreatic enzymes, and tumors can impede the flow of stool (partial or complete bowel obstruction).
   b. *Interventions*
   (1) Assess for signs of dehydration, such as poor skin turgor and dry mucous membranes.
   (2) Assess abdomen for bowel sounds and presence of distention, flatus, and bowel movements.

(3) Monitor fluid status using vital signs, weights, intake (from any intravenous [IV] fluids, enteral or parenteral nutrition), and output (from urine, tubes, and drains).

(4) Provide patients with specific information about GI drains such as biliary stents.

    (a) Stents may be "internalized" and simply bypass an obstructed area or "externalized" and require tube care (flushing, dressing care).

    (b) Tube care is usually a "clean" procedure for patients at home, but a sterile procedure for nurses in the hospital.

    (c) Although studies are limited, biliary stents are usually flushed with preservative-free sterile water or saline because preservatives may have an unknown effect when instilled into the body cavities.

    (d) Stents may be a source of lost fluids and electrolytes.

    (e) Patients should be taught to recognize early symptoms of stent obstruction or dysfunction, such as difficulty flushing, reduced output, abdominal pain, increasing jaundice.

    (f) Biliary stent upsizing, downsizing, or adjustment of position may require frequent CT scans, and possible same-day surgical visits to the interventional radiology suite. Patients must also be aware of the high risk of fever and sepsis after stent adjustment.

(5) Monitor serum electrolytes.

(6) Maintain patency of any tubes, drains, IV access.

(7) Administer IV hydration and electrolyte supplements as well as any enteral or parenteral nutrition as ordered.

(8) Follow recommendations in Chapters 23, 27, and 28.

    c. *Desired outcome:* Patient will maintain adequate hydration.

5. Activity intolerance related to fatigue, lethargy, and malaise

    a. *Problem:* Patients may experience liver failure from primary liver cancer (rare in the United States) or metastatic disease because malignant tumors are likely to reach the liver by way of the portal system or lymphatic channels, or liver failure may be a result of adjuvant therapy (chemotherapy or radiation therapy), dehydration, surgery, infection, fever, excessive diuresis, and some medications. The liver is not able to detoxify and convert ammonia into urea. The ammonia accumulates in the bloodstream as a result of its inadequate absorption from the GI tract. The increased ammonia concentration in the blood causes brain dysfunction and damage, ultimately resulting in hepatic encephalopathy.

    b. *Interventions*

      (1) Assess level of activity tolerance and degree of fatigue, lethargy, and malaise when performing activities of daily living (ADL).

      (2) Assist with activities and hygiene when fatigued.

      (3) Encourage rest when fatigued.

(**4**) Assist with selection and pacing of desired activities and exercise.

(**5**) Restrict dietary protein as prescribed.

(**6**) Provide frequent, small feedings of carbohydrates.

(**7**) Give supplemental vitamins (A, B complex, C, and K).

c. *Desired outcomes:* The patient will report increased strength and well-being. This may be an irreversible condition for which the family will need explanation as to its cause and limited treatment. The failure of the liver to perform its necessary functions may eventually lead to the demise of the patient.

6. Impaired skin integrity related to pruritus from jaundice, compromised immunologic status, edema, and poor nutrition. Skin integrity also is altered due to surgical procedures or around tubes, drains, and ostomies.

a. *Problem:* Multiple problems exhibited by the patient with a GI cancer predispose to changes in the skin as a protective mechanism.

b. *Interventions*

(**1**) Assess skin integrity; instruct patient and family in this activity.

(**2**) Assess degree of discomfort related to pruritus and edema.

(**3**) Record extent of edema; elevate dependent extremities whenever possible.

(**4**) Keep patient's fingernails short and smooth.

(**5**) Instruct patient to avoid the use of soaps and alcohol-based lotions; may use emollients.

(**6**) Apply skin protectants around drains or ostomies that may irritate the skin.

c. *Desired outcome:* Patient will report no breaks in skin integrity.

7. Risk for injury and bleeding related to altered clotting mechanisms and altered level of consciousness

a. *Problem:* The liver plays an important role in protein metabolism and synthesizes blood-clotting factors. Prothrombin time and other blood clotting factors may be prolonged in liver failure. The blood clotting times are influenced by the supply of vitamin K.

Altered level of consciousness is related to deterioration of liver function and increased serum ammonia level.

b. *Interventions*

(**1**) Prevent injury from bleeding by implementing bleeding precautions (see Chapter 22).

(**2**) Assess for symptoms of anxiety, epigastric fullness, weakness, and restlessness, which may indicate GI bleeding.

(**3**) Observe stools and emesis for color, consistency, and amount, and test for occult blood.

(**4**) Administer vitamin K as prescribed.

(**5**) Encourage intake of foods with high content of vitamin C to enhance absorption of vitamin K.

(**6**) Promote improved thought processes.

(7) Assess level of consciousness and reorient as needed.

(8) Provide a safe environment and frequent surveillance.

(9) Restrict high protein from diet and monitor ammonia levels.

(10) Monitor fluid intake and output and serum electrolyte levels to prevent dehydration and hypokalemia.

   c. *Desired outcome:* Patient will have reduced risk of injury and bleeding.

8. Ineffective breathing pattern related to restriction of thoracic excursion, ascites, or hyperammonia with altered consciousness

   a. *Problem:* Damage to liver parenchymal cells caused by primary liver cancer, metastatic cancer, any obstruction of bile flow or derangement of hepatic circulation places patient at risk for liver failure and ascites. This can lead to discomfort from abdominal distention and dependent edema or altered breathing pattern from hyperammonia or pleural effusions. Patients may also experience impaired ventilatory capacity if the abdominal distention interferes with lung expansion by forcing the diaphragm upward.

   b. *Interventions*

     (1) Assist the patient with identifying comfortable positions. Patients may be more comfortable sitting in semi-Fowler's or reverse-Trendelenburg positions.

     (2) Assist the patient in maintaining maximal mobility and planning rest periods.

     (3) Monitor the patient's respiratory status and administer oxygen therapy as indicated.

     (4) Explain the paracentesis procedure to the patient and provide emotional support.

       (a) Patient must be supine for the procedure.

       (b) Limited movement is essential to prevent bowel perforation.

       (c) A special blunt-tipped needle called a Caudwell needle is recommended to reduce the incidence of perforation.

       (d) Noncollapsible tubing and vacuum bottles may be used to remove large quantities of fluid.

       (e) Obtain baseline vital signs, and check frequently if removing large amounts of fluid. Intravascular fluid shifts and hypotension may occur with large volume removal.

       (f) Obtain abdominal x-ray after procedure.

     (5) See Chapter 30 for suggestions on management.

   c. *Desired outcome:* Patient will report that discomfort is adequately controlled.

9. Risk for infection/impaired skin integrity related to poor nutrition, presence of wounds, tubes and drains related to interventional invasive treatment and/or GI surgery. Reduced immunoglobulin levels also occur with hepatic failure and predispose patients to infection.

   a. *Problem:* Patients having any invasive GI procedure or surgery are at risk for developing infections because the presence of normal intestinal flora may contaminate the surgical area, leading to infection. This risk can be compounded by the use of treatments, such as chemotherapy and radiation therapy, that can suppress immune function.

    b. *Interventions*

        (1) Instruct the patient in administration of any preprocedural or bowel preparation according to the type of procedure or surgery, patient's anatomy, and surgeon's preference.

        (2) Patients with ostomies may have a modified bowel preparation.

        (3) Frail patients may be unable to tolerate a bowel preparation and may require preoperative hospitalization to obtain an adequate bowel cleansing.

        (4) Monitor the patient after surgery for early signs of infection. This includes assessing for respiratory and urinary tract infections, redness and drainage from wounds or any invasive device (tubes, drains, IV sites), and checking for deep vein thrombosis.

        (5) Follow recommendations in Chapter 9.

    c. *Desired outcomes:* The patient does not experience any pneumonia, urinary tract infection, wound infection, fistula, or deep vein thrombosis or systemic sepsis.

  10. Body image disturbance related to surgical changes in anatomy, presence of tubes, drains, and/or stomas

    a. *Problem:* Treatment for GI malignancies may require changes in the functioning and route of exit for bowel contents as well as other GI fluids such as bile. Feeding gastrostomy or jejunostomy tubes may be placed for nutritional access, and gastrostomy tubes may be placed to decompress the stomach for gastric outlet obstruction. It may be difficult for patients to adjust to these changes in their appearance.

    b. *Interventions*

        (1) Before any interventional or surgical procedure, review/explain the procedure or surgery and what to expect after the procedure or surgery, the need for any devices/appliances, along with a brief review of how the patient will maintain the device/appliance.

        (2) Encourage the patient to verbalize any fears or anxieties. Incorporate patient and family into care to provide a sense of control.

        (3) Refer to support groups or mental health professionals as appropriate.

    c. *Desired outcomes:* Patient displays positive adaptive coping to changes in physical appearance and GI functions.

IV. Discharge Planning and Patient Education

  A. All Cancers

    1. Discuss implications of the disease and its treatment options.

    2. Provide information related to specific surgical procedure and the need to alter dietary/eating habits.

3. Educate patient and family about the importance of trying to maintain optimal nutrition.
4. Teach care of feeding tubes, venous access devices, ostomy appliances.
5. Initiate home referrals, as needed.

B. Gastric Cancer
1. Nutritionist referral for dietary plan, and nutritional goal setting.
2. Teach reportable signs and symptoms that may signal complications or recurrent/progressive disease, including:
   a. Decreased appetite or weight loss.
   b. Nausea and vomiting after ingestion of food or fluids.
   c. Presence or increase in abdominal pain.

C. Pancreatic Cancer
1. Instruct in appropriate use of supplemental pancreatic enzymes, as needed.
2. Teach reportable signs and symptoms that may signal complications or recurrent/progressive disease.
   a. Recurrence or increase in abdominal pain.
   b. Abdominal distention.
   c. Nausea, vomiting, weight loss, lethargy, and fatigue.
   d. Signs and symptoms of liver failure including increase in bleeding tendencies, easy bruising, ascites, jaundice, lethargy, failure to respond to painful stimuli.
   e. Discuss long-term pain-relief measures.
   f. Teach biliary stent care, signs and symptoms of obstruction or infection, and assessment for complications post manipulation.
   g. Develop a plan to assess and manage acute depression, which is highly associated with this cancer.

D. Hepatobiliary Cancers
1. Teach management of any biliary tubes placed for management of obstructive jaundice.
   a. Flushing of biliary tube to maintain patency
   b. Maintaining tube securely to abdomen
   c. Signs of malfunction
2. Teach reportable signs and symptoms that may signal complications or recurrent/progressive disease.
   a. Recurrence of jaundice
   b. Presence of ascites and abdominal distention
   c. Shortness of breath related to ascites, pleural metastases, or effusions
   d. Increase in bleeding tendencies, easy bruising, lethargy, malaise, failure to respond to painful stimuli as seen in liver failure

E. Colorectal Cancer
1. Closely monitor for response to treatment and for recurrence of disease. Colorectal cancer most commonly spreads to the lymph nodes, liver, and lungs. Recurrence of disease is greatest in the first few years after diagnosis.
2. Assess and refer the patient with a new ostomy, wound, or tube care need to appropriate home health care.

3. Provide information on support groups and referrals.
4. Emphasize the importance of follow-up with health care provider for disease monitoring (eg, periodic colonoscopy, annual fecal occult blood testing, and carcinoembryonic antigen (CEA) test).
5. Teach reportable signs and symptoms that may signal complications or recurrent/ progressive disease.
   a. Weight loss, fatigue
   b. Rectal bleeding
   c. Abdominal pain/abdominal distention
   d. Change in bowel habits
   e. Shortness of breath related to ascites, pleural metastases, or effusions.

REFERENCES

Ahrendt, S. A., Nakeeb, A., & Pitt, H. A. (2001). Cholangiocarcinoma. *Clinical Liver Disease, 5*(1), 191–218.

Barone, M., Ettore, G. C., Ladisa, R., et al. (2003). Transcatheter arterial chemoembolization (TACE) in treatment of hepatocellular carcinoma. *Hepatogastroenterology, 50*(49), 183–187.

Cameron, J. L. (Ed.). (2001). *Atlas of clinical oncology: Pancreatic cancer.* Hamilton, BC: Decker.

_____ (Ed.). (2001). *Current surgical therapy* (7th ed.). St. Louis: Mosby.

Centers for Disease Control (CDC). (2002). Screen for life. National Colo-rectal Cancer Action Campaign. Available: www.cdc.gov/cancer/screeningforlife/pdf/fs-patient.pdf.

Coutinho, A. K., & Rocha Lima, C. M. (2003). Metastatic colorectal cancer: Systemic treatment in the new millennium. *Cancer Control, 10*(3), 224–238.

Dawes, L. G. (2001). Gallbladder cancer. *Cancer Treatment Research, 109,* 145–155.

DiMaio, M., DeMaio, E., Perrone, F., et al. (2002). Hepatocellular carcinoma: Systemic treatments. *Journal of Clinical Gastroenterology, 35*(5 Suppl.), S109–S114.

Dunn, G. P. (2002). Surgical palliation in advanced disease: Recent developments. *Current Oncology Reports, 4*(3), 233–241.

Fong, Y., & Malhotra, S. (2001). Gallbladder cancer: Recent advances and current guidelines. *Advances in Surgery, 35,* 1–20.

Hohenberger, P., & Gretschel, S. (2003). Gastric cancer. *Lancet, 362*(9380), 305–315.

Jarnagin, W. R. (2000). Cholangiocarcinoma of the extrahepatic bile ducts. *Seminars in Surgical Oncology, 19*(2), 156–176.

Lenhard, R. E., Osten, R. T., & Gansler, T. (Eds.). (2001). *Clinical oncology.* Atlanta, GA: American Cancer Society.

Macdonald, J. S. (2002). Advances in the therapy of gastric cancer. *Gastric Cancer, 5*(Suppl. 1), 35–40.

Meyerhardt, J. A., & Mayer, R. J. (2003). Follow-up strategies after curative resection of colorectal cancer. *Seminars in Oncology, 30*(3), 349–360.

Nakeeb, A., Pitt, H. A., Sohn, T. A., et al. (1996). Cholangiocarcinoma. A spectrum of intrahepatic, perihilar, and distal tumors. *Annals of Surgery, 224*(4), 463–473.

National Comprehensive Cancer Network. (2003). NCCN clinical practice guidelines in oncology. Available: www.nccn.org.

Nicum, S., Midgley, R., & Kerr, D. J. (2003). Colorectal cancer. *Acta Oncology, 42*(4), 263–275.

Romeo, R., & Colombo, M. (2002). The natural history of hepatocellular carcinoma. *Toxicology, 27,* 181–182.

Sarmiento, J. M., & Nagorney, D. M. (2002). Hepatic resection in the treatment of perihilarcholangiocarcinoma. *Surgical Oncology Clinics of North America, 11*(4), 893–908.

Scaife, C. L., & Curley, S. A. (2003). Complications, local recurrence, and survival rates after radiofrequency ablation for hepatic malignancies. *Surgical Oncology Clinics of North America, 12*(1), 243–255.

Shoup, M., & Fong, Y. Surgical indications and extent of resection in gallbladder cancer. *Surgical Oncology Clinics of North America, 11*(4), 985–994.

Yarbro, C. H., Frogge, M. H., Goodman, M., & Groenwald, S. L. (Eds.). (2000). *Cancer nursing: Principles and practice* (5th ed.). Boston, MA: Jones & Bartlett.

Yeo, T. P., Hruban, R. H., Leach, S. D., et al. (2002). Pancreatic cancer. *Current Problems in Cancer, 26*(4), 176–275.

Yu, A. S., & Keeffe, E. B. (2003). Management of hepatocellular carcinoma. *Reviews of Gastroenterology Disorders, 3*(1), 8–24.

13 Genitourinary Cancers

Victoria J. Wah Sinibaldi

I. Genitourinary Malignancies (see Table 13–1 for an overview of the features of testicular, bladder, prostate, and kidney cancers)
   A. Includes malignancies of the male and female genitourinary tract.
   B. Diseases are variable in genetic, environmental, and social risk factors.
   C. Treatment and prognosis are unique to each diagnosis.

II. Nursing Diagnoses, Interventions, and Outcomes for Testicular Cancer (Table 13-2)
   A. Knowledge deficit related to early detection of testicular cancer
      1. *Problem:* Testicular cancer is a treatable disease that is often 100% curable in early stages. Clinical studies demonstrate that few men practice testicular self-examination or undergo physical examination by their physicians. Increased rates of early detection would result in improved outcomes for men with testicular cancer.
      2. *Interventions*
         a. Teach patients, families, and the public the importance of early detection.
         b. Provide information (discussions, pamphlets, seminars, media) about incidence, risk factors, screening, symptoms, diagnosis, prognosis, and treatment options.
         c. Instruct all males, age 15 and older, in the correct technique and time for performing testicular self-examination (Box 13–1).
         d. Provide support and encourage compliance with testicular self-examination and act as an advocate and liaison to ensure follow-up.
      3. *Desired outcome:* The patient will demonstrate adequate knowledge of screening and early detection of testicular cancer as evidenced by:
         a. Stating risk factors for the disease.
         b. Demonstrating testicular self-examination and stating importance of monthly examination.
         c. Returning for routine annual examinations.
         b. Encourage patients to ask questions and express concerns.
         c. See Chapters 6, 8, and 9 for details on chemotherapy, radiation, and surgical treatment.
   B. Anxiety related to a diagnosis of testicular cancer and the potential for side effects of therapy
      1. *Problem:* The diagnosis of cancer can produce anxiety about sexuality, fertility, survival, remission, and quality of life (QOL). All these factors can affect one's self-concept.
      2. *Interventions*

    a. Educate about the disease, treatments, side effects (particularly sexuality and infertility), and overall prognosis.

    b. Allow the patient to identify concerns and provide information accordingly.

    c. Discuss potential alterations in sexual potency and fertility.

    d. Discuss alternate ways of providing sexual gratification (see section on Prostate Cancer).

    e. Discuss family planning and sperm banking if appropriate.

        (1) Concerns about family planning may be subjugated to issues of treatment and prognosis; however, medical treatment may result in infertility. Accurate information helps the patient and partner consider alternative family planning.

        (2) Sperm banking is a costly procedure (approximately $100.00 to $130.00 for initial counseling and sperm analysis, approximately $120.00 for each additional cryopreservation, in addition to monthly fees for storage). Patients are instructed to abstain from sex 3 to 7 days before providing a specimen for analysis. If sperm are of good quality, three specimens may be banked. Analysis takes approximately 7 to 10 days (see Box 13–2 for available resources).

3. *Desired outcomes*

    a. Patient is able to cope with the diagnosis of testicular cancer as evidenced by:

        (1) Participation in own care.

        (2) Participation in treatment and follow-up.

    b. Patient states that he feels a lessening sense of fear regarding diagnosis of testicular cancer and its implications.

    c. Patient states that he is familiar with sperm banking and other reproductive technologies.

C. Pain related to disease or treatment of testicular cancer

    1. *Problem:* Pain is frequently a problem in patients with testicular cancer. Growth of the tumor can cause pressure on nerve fibers, blood vessels, or other organs. Pain can also be associated with various treatments.

    2. *Interventions:* Follow recommendations in Chapter 30.

    3. *Desired outcome:* Pain is eliminated or controlled as described in Chapter 30.

D. Body image disturbance related to development of gynecomastia and scrotal changes

    1. *Problem:* The body image of men with testicular cancer can be affected by breast enlargement or removal of one or both testicles (orchiectomy). Treatment may also alter sexual function (changes in ejaculation, orgasm, and libido). Young men may be particularly sensitive to these changes.

    2. *Interventions*

    a. Assess the patient's perception of scrotal and breast changes.

    b. Encourage open discussion about changes in body image between patient and partner.

    c. Provide information about etiology of changes and treatment options.

▨ TABLE 13–1 Overview of Genitourinary (GU) Cancers

Key Feature	Testicular Cancer	Bladder Cancer
Definition	Rare cancer <2% of all male cancers, most common solid malignancy in males 20–34 years old Cure rate almost 100% in early-stage disease Arise from testes as germ cell or non-germ cell tumors (see Table 13-2) Metastatic spread through lymphatics to lung, liver, viscera, bone, and brain	Second most common GU malignancy (6% of all male, 2% of female cancers in the US) Spreads by direct extension through submucosa and bladder wall Metastasis to lungs, liver, and bone
Risk factors/ etiologies	Etiology unknown Risk factors: family history of testicular cancer Cryptorchidism (failure of testicles to descend to scrotal sac) Exposure to estrogen in utero Trauma Inguinal hernia Klinefelter syndrome (congenital endocrine condition) Hermaphroditism (coexisting ovarian and testicular tissue) Degeneration, atrophy or torsion of testicles Vasectomy African-American descent Higher socioeconomic status	Cigarette smoking Exposure to arylamine used in dye, rubber, and leather industries and hair dye Excessive use of coffee, alcohol, saccharin, phenacetin Hypercholesterolemia Cyclophosphamide chemotherapy Pelvic irradiation Chlorination in water Exposure to *Schistosoma hematobium* (rare in US, common in Africa)
Signs and symptoms	Painless enlargement of testicle; heaviness in scrotum, inguinal area, or lower abdomen Testicular nodule/mass Lumbar, abdominal, groin pain Weight loss secondary to metabolic changes Gynecomastia caused by elevation in serum human chorionic gonadotropin hormone (beta HCG)	Hematuria (gross or microscopic) Dysuria and urinary frequency and urgency Urinary hesitancy and decrease in force and caliber of stream Hydronephrosis Pain in suprapubic region, rectum, back or flank. Bone pain with skeletal metastases Lymphadenopathy Abdominal mass or hepatomegaly from metastasis

Prostate Cancer	Kidney Cancer
Most common male cancer of all male cancers: 33% incidence, 10% mortality in US	~3% of all male cancers, and <2% of all female cancers
Incidence increases in men over age 65, with median age at diagnosis 72 years	Average age at diagnosis is 55–70 years
Incidence is highest in African Americans, lowest in Japanese	Prognosis is best in early stages
Prognosis is good for early-stage disease	Two classifications: cancers of the renal pelvis and ureters (~4% to 5% of all GU cancers), renal cell carcinomas of the kidney parenchyma (~85% of all kidney cancers)
Screening and detection recommendations are not universally standard (see Table 13-7)	Metastasizes by direct extension to lung, liver, bone, lymph nodes, adrenal gland and contralateral kidney
Tumors arise from prostate and are adenocarcinomas	
Locally spreads to seminal vesicles, bladder, and perineum; distant spread is through lymphatics or hematologic routes	
Metastasizes to bone, lymph nodes (supra-clavicular, scalene, retroperitoneal, pelvic, and periaortic); rare sites are mediastinum, lung, kidneys, or liver	
Etiology is unknown	Etiology is unknown
Risk factors: age >65 years, family history of prostate or breast cancer	Cigarette smoking
African-American heritage	Cadmium, asbestos, and lead exposure
Increased testosterone	Excessive use of analgesics (aspirin, phenacetin, or acetaminophen)
Sexually transmitted infections	Obesity (in females)
Cadmium exposure (used in welding, electroplating, alkaline battery production)	Estrogen
High-fat diet	History of adenomas
Vasectomy	Excessive use of caffeine or diuretics
Assess for prostate mass or nodule (asymmetry, induration), weight loss, back pain, urinary frequency, nocturia, dysuria, slow urinary stream, hematuria	Change in bowel patterns due to obstruction or compression
	Hematuria (gross or microscopic)
	Pain: flank pain, urethral pain related to obstruction or clots, metastatic pain
	Abdominal mass
	Fevers may be secondary to obstruction and infection or paraneoplastic syndrome
	Weight loss

(continued)

▨ TABLE 13–1 **Overview of Genitourinary (GU) Cancers (continued)**

Key Feature	Testicular Cancer	Bladder Cancer
Signs and symptoms	Supraclavicular mass due to lymph node metastases Cough, dyspnea, or hemoptysis from pulmonary metastases	Weight loss and decreased appetite Lower extremity edema due to obstruction Mental status changes and focal neurologic findings from brain metastases
Diagnostic tests	Serum tests: elevated HCG, alpha-fetoprotein (AFP), lactic acid dehydrogenase (LDH) Assess for enlargement of testes, scrotum, and lymph nodes Testicular ultrasound to detect a mass Excretory urogram (IVP) to assess displacement of ureter or kidney from a mass Chest radiographs to assess for pulmonary metastases CT scan of abdomen and pelvis to assess metastatic disease Liver, brain, and bone scans to evaluate metastases Surgical inguinal exploration with biopsy for tissue pathology	Serum tests: elevated carcinoembryonic antigen (CEA) Urine cytology to detect genetic or chromosomal changes Flow cytometry Cystoscopy to assess for a mass Transurethral resection (TUR) to assess for mass CT scan of abdomen, pelvis Magnetic resonance imaging (MRI) of abdomen/pelvis Chest x-ray to assess for metastases Bone scan to assess for metastasis Excretory urogram (IVP) to assess for tumor or obstruction
Treatment/ Management	Prognosis and treatment depend on stage (see Tables 13-2 and 13-3) Radical orchiectomy (removal of one or both testes, epididymis, vas deferens, some lymphatics and blood supply) Radical lymph node dissection is stage dependent Chemotherapy or radiation therapy are dictated by type and stage of disease (see Table 13-3)	Prognosis and treatment depend on the depth of invasion into the bladder mass and histologic grade of the tumor (see Table 13-6)

Prostate Cancer	Kidney Cancer
	Anemia secondary to bone marrow depression, bleeding, or suppressed erythropoietin production secondary to renal dysfunction
	Acute dyspnea and edema secondary to obstruction of vena cava
Serum tests: CBC (anemia may indicate bone marrow involvement), elevated acid phosphatase, elevated prostatic acid phosphatase, elevated alkaline phosphatase, elevated prostate specific antigen (PSA)	Serum tests: low serum iron and total iron binding capacity (TIBC) with anemia secondary to bleeding
Urine tests: cytology may show cancer cells, flow cytometry may show DNA changes	Elevated calcium secondary to paraneoplastic syndrome or bone metastases
Biopsy of prostate	Elevated liver function tests secondary to paraneoplastic syndrome
Cytology of prostate fluid, may show tumor cells	Elevated lactic acid dehydrogenase (LDH) with renal cell carcinoma
Bone scan for skeletal metastasis (bone e-rays may show lytic vs blastic lesions)	Elevated renin in renal cell carcinoma
CT scan of abdomen and pelvis for lymph node and visceral involvement	Urine tests: urinalysis may reveal hematuria, bacteria, or pus. Cytology may reveal malignant cells. Flow cytometry for DNA content of cells
MRI to evaluate extent of disease and metastases	Kidney, ureter, and bladder radiograph to assess for mass
Chest x-ray to evaluate pulmonary or pleural involvement	Excretory urogram (IVP) to assess for mass
Transrectal ultrasound (TRUS) to assess palpable mass	Retrograde urogram to assess for urethral obstruction
Excretory urogram (IVP) may show hydro-ureteronephrosis related to obstruction	Nephrotomograms to assess extra renal mass
	Renal ultrasound to assess mass
	MRI to assess mass/lymph node involvement
	CT of abdomen, chest, brain to assess for metastasis
	Cystoscopy, ureteroscopy, or nephroscopy with biopsy for definitive diagnosis
Treatment depends on stage of disease: surgery, radiation therapy, hormonal therapy, chemotherapy or combinations of therapy (see Tables 13-7, 13-8, and 13-9)	Primary therapy is surgery with/without radiation therapy. Chemotherapy, hormonal therapy, and biotherapy may be used in advanced or recurrent disease (see Tables 13-11 and 13-12)

▨ **TABLE 13–2 Classification of Testicular Cancers**

Germ Cell Tumors	Non–Germ Cell Tumors
Represent approximately 95% of all testicular malignancies	Represent <5% of all testicular malignancies
Seminomas	Leydig cell tumors
Classic seminoma	Sertoli cell tumors
Anaplastic seminoma	Gonadoblastomas
Spermatocystic seminoma	
Nonseminomas	
Embryonal cell carcinoma	
Endodermal sinus tumor	
Teratoma	
Choriocarcinoma	
Mixed cell type	

▼ **BOX 13-1** | **Testicular Self-Examination Procedure**

TESTICULAR SELF-EXAMINATION [ACS RECOMMENDATIONS]:
All males age 15 and older should perform testicular self-examination every month.
Perform testicular self-examination during or immediately after a warm shower.

1. Observe and compare each side of the scrotum. Note size and any differences in shape.
2. Hold scrotum in one hand. With the other hand, place the index and middle fingers on top of the scrotum and the thumb underneath. Gently roll each testicle between the fingers, noting any lumps or areas that seem hard or enlarged.
3. Locate the epididymis and note that it is soft and slightly tender. Examine the space between the front of the testis and back of the epididymis. Note any lumps.
4. Locate the spermatic cord and note that it is smooth, firm, and movable. Note any lumps.
5. Notify health care provider if any lumps or changes are noted.

▼ **BOX 13-2** | **Available Resources for Sperm Banking**

Washington Fertility Study Center (phone: 202-333-3100)
American Cancer Society (ACS) (www.cancer.org/docroot/home/index.asp)
Cancer Information Service (phone: 1-800-4-CANCER)
Sperm Bank Directory (www.spermbankdirectory.com)

TABLE 13–3 **TNM Staging Classification for Testicular Cancer**

Primary Tumor (T)
Extent of tumor is assessed after radical orchiectomy.

PTX	Unable to assess primary tumor
PT0	No evidence of tumor
PTis	Intratubular tumor: preinvasive cancer
PT1	Tumor limited to the testis, including rete testis
PT2	Tumor invades beyond the tunica albuginea or into the epididymis
PT3	Tumor invades the spermatic cord
PT4	Tumor invades the scrotum

Regional Lymph Nodes (N)

NX	Unable to assess regional lymph nodes
N0	No regional lymph node metastasis
N1	Metastasis in a single lymph node, ≤2 cm in greatest dimension
N2	Metastasis in a single lymph node, >2 cm but <5 cm in greatest dimension
N3	Metastasis in a lymph node >5 cm in greatest dimension

Distant Metastasis (M)

MX	Unable to assess distant metastasis
M0	No distant metastasis
M1	Distant metastasis

Stage Grouping

Stage I	Any pT	N0	M0
Stage II	Any pT	N0–3	M0
Stage III	Any pT	Any N	M1

American Joint Committee on Cancer, 1998.

    d. Discuss alternative ways of sexual gratification (see section on Prostate Cancer in this chapter).
    e. Provide emotional support.
    f. Refer to sexual counselor if appropriate.
  3. *Desired outcomes*
    a. Patient states that he understands the etiology of his bodily changes.
    b. Patient communicates with partner his feelings on sexuality.
    c. Patient is able to express sexuality within capabilities.
 E. Discharge Planning and Patient Education for Men With Testicular Cancer
  1. Discuss health care needs and concerns.
  2. Encourage patient to visit his physician annually for a thorough examination.
  3. For patients diagnosed with testicular cancer, ensure referral to an oncologist and emphasize the need for continued medical evaluation.
  4. Discuss the signs and symptoms for complications of treatment.

TABLE 13-4 Testicular Cancer Treatment Modalities and Estimated Survival

Stage	Treatment	Survival
Seminoma		
Stage I (tumor confined to the testicles)	Radical orchiectomy with postoperative radiation	Estimated 5-year survival: 95% to 99%
Stage II (tumor involving the testis and the retroperitoneal or para-aortic lymph nodes)	Tumors < 5 cm on CT: See stage I Tumors > 5 cm on CT: Radical orchiectomy with postoperative chemotherapy (see stage III for cisplatin combinations) or followed by radiation treatment to the lymph nodes	Estimated disease-free survival: 85% to 95%
Stage III (tumor has spread beyond the retroperitoneal nodes)	Radical orchiectomy with postoperative chemotherapy (cisplatin combinations with vinblastine and bleomycin *or* etoposide and bleomycin) Radiation therapy may be given if there is evidence of progression after chemotherapy	Same as for stage II
Nonseminoma		
Stage I	Radical orchiectomy plus retroperitoneal lymph node dissection	Estimated 5-year survival: 96%
Stage II–stage III	Radical orchiectomy plus chemotherapy (see above) If residual disease is present, salvage retroperitoneal lymph node dissection or resection of all disease may be employed. If progression of disease is seen, alternative regimens or new investigational approaches may be considered.	Estimated 5-year survival: 55% to 80%

Note: Based on information from PDQ Editorial Board, 1996.

  a. *Surgery:* Pain, infection, fatigue
  b. *Radiation therapy:* Fatigue, myelosuppression, infection, diarrhea
  c. *Chemotherapy:* Myelosuppression, infection, nausea, vomiting, nephrotoxicity, neurotoxicity, appetite changes, fatigue, temporary hair loss, bowel changes (diarrhea or constipation)
  5. Instruct patient to notify health care provider if unusual symptoms occur (such as fever, chills, excessive weakness, or increased scrotal edema).
  6. Discuss family planning and sperm banking if appropriate.

III. Nursing Diagnoses, Interventions, and Outcomes for Bladder Cancer

  A. Pain related to growth and treatment of bladder cancer
   1. *Problem:* Pain can be caused by growth of the tumor pressing on nerve fibers, blood vessels, or other organs. It can also be associated with treatments.
   2. *Interventions:* Follow recommendations in Chapter 30.
   3. *Desired outcome:* Elimination or control of pain, as described in Chapter 30.
  B. Alteration in urinary patterns related to disease or treatment
   1. *Problem:* Increased frequency, urgency, hematuria, and dysuria are symptoms commonly seen in patients with bladder cancer (usually secondary to invasion of the tumor into the bladder wall or inflammatory changes in the bladder epithelium or both). Chemotherapy may cause cystitis, and surgical treatment in many of these patients will require a urinary diversion.
   2. *Interventions*
    a. Assess patient's symptoms and provide information regarding the etiology and ways to alleviate symptoms.
    b. Instruct patient to avoid intake of substances that are bladder irritants (alcohol, tobacco, tea, spices).
    c. Provide information pertaining to urinary diversion, including explanation of the surgical procedure, changes in elimination, required self-care activities, and potential complications (Table 13–5).
    d. Discuss treatment plan and complications related to intrabladder chemotherapy or biotherapy as appropriate.
    e. Allow patient to express fears, concerns, and anxiety about the procedure and the lifestyle changes that accompany it.
   3. *Desired outcomes*
    a. Patient will maintain an acceptable urinary elimination pattern, evidenced by absence of bladder irritation and by normal laboratory tests.
    b. Patient will state the causes of bladder irritation and perform self-care activities to promote urinary elimination.
    c. Patient will describe the urinary diversion procedure and identify signs and symptoms of complications.
  C. Altered body image related to urinary diversion

TABLE 13–5 Urinary Diversions and Complications

Diversion	Complication
Ileal Conduit (Bricker Procedure): A piece of terminal ileum is used as the conduit (stoma is created); constant drainage of urine into the conduit and through the stoma, requiring an external appliance.	Complications of urinary diversions: Leakage of the anastomosis site leading to sepsis; stomal edema, stenosis, necrosis, ureteral reflux with resultant kidney damage, frequent urinary tract infections, skin problems, wound infections, and dehiscence (especially if placement of stoma is in creases or on bony prominences)
Kock Pouch: Continent urinary diversion: Distal ileum fashioned into a "U" to create an intra-abdominal pouch; two nipple valves created (one to prevent reflux and one to maintain continence).	Complications of continent diversions: Pouchitis, leakage, incomplete emptying, reflux, and incompetent continence mechanisms may occur
Indiana Pouch: Continent urinary diversion: A segment of right colon serves as the reservoir and a section of terminal ileum narrowed over a catheter provides continence mechanism along with disruption of the tubular nature of the bowel segment to counteract strong contractions. Ureters anastomosed through natural muscular tunnel to prevent reflux.	

1. *Problem:* Treatment choices for bladder cancer often include radical surgery with urinary diversion. The psychological impact of a stoma and external appliance as well as changes in sexuality may all contribute to an alteration in body image.
2. *Interventions:* Follow recommendations in Chapter 31.
3. *Desired outcome:* Patient will learn to adapt to physical changes, as described in Chapter 31.

D. Discharge Planning and Patient Education for Patients With Bladder Cancer
1. Provide patient with follow-up plan and discuss importance of compliance.
2. Emphasize need for adequate fluid intake, exercise, and rest.
3. Reinforce avoidance of bladder irritants (alcohol, tobacco, tea, spices).
4. Encourage intake of foods that are not irritating to the bladder (fruits, vegetables, and milk).
5. Address pain-relieving measures.
6. Instruct patient on care of urinary diversion.

TABLE 13-6 Bladder Cancer Treatment Modalities and Estimated Survival

Stage	Treatment	Survival
Stage TaN0M0: Superficial tumors	Transurethral resection of the bladder (TURB) and cauterization of lesions After surgery, intravesicular instillation of bacillus Calmette-Guérin (BCG), thiotepa, mitomycin-C, doxorubicin, or interferons	Estimated 5-year survival rate: 55–80%[*]
Stage T1N0M0: Tumor has invaded subepithelial but has not spread to lymph nodes	Large single lesions: TURB Extensive superficial involvement: Radical cystectomy; however, interstitial implants sometimes used; surgery often combined with preoperative or postoperative external beam radiation	Estimated 5-year survival rate: 75%[†]
Stage T2N0M0: Tumor has invaded the inner half of the superficial muscle	Radical cystectomy with or without preoperative radiation, or radiation therapy alone	Estimated 5-year survival rate: 20–40%[†]

Stage T3N0M0: Tumor has invaded deep muscle and may penetrate the perivesical fat	Radical cystectomy, postoperative radiation, and chemotherapy followed by cystectomy or radiation; radiation treatment may also be given preoperatively followed by cystectomy
	Chemotherapy
	  Various cisplatin-based regimens; MVAC (methotrexate, vinblastine, doxorubicin, cisplatin); MVC (methotrexate, vinblastine, cisplatin)
	  Single agents: Methotrexate, doxorubicin, vinblastine, cisplatin, paclitaxel, gemcitabine
	Neoadjuvant before radiation or surgery
		See stage T2N0M0

Stage T4N0M0: Tumor has metastasized to adjacent organs, bone, or lymph nodes	Chemotherapy: See above, or investigational regimens Palliative treatments: Cystectomy with urinary diversion or external beam radiation	5-year survival uncommon[†]

[*]Hudson & Herr, 1995.
[†]Thrasher & Crawford, 1993.

7. Provide information on support groups and refer as appropriate.
8. Provide information on the implications of treatment options chosen.

IV. Nursing Diagnoses, Interventions, and Outcomes for Prostate Cancer (Table 13-7)

A. Knowledge deficit related to screening and early detection of prostate cancer
   1. *Problem:* Patients need to understand the risk factors, screening, and disease process to make informed decisions about participating in screening and detection.
   2. *Interventions*
      a. Assess patient and family understanding of disease, screening, and detection.
      b. Provide information concerning risk factors, signs and symptoms, and screening and diagnostic tests.
      c. Supply the patient with materials from the American Cancer Society and the National Cancer Institute and Internet.
         (1) American Cancer Society. (1999). *Prostate cancer: What every man and his family should know* (rev. ed.). Atlanta, GA: American Cancer Society.
         (2) Ellsworth, P., Heaney, J., & Gill, O. (2002). *100 questions and answers about prostate cancer.* Boston, MA: Jones & Bartlett.
         (3) Fincannon, J., & Bruss, K. (2003). *Couples confronting cancer: Keeping your relationship strong.* Atlanta, GA: American Cancer Society.
         (4) Internet sites
            (a) www.cancer.org. American Cancer Society information on cancer and cancer treatment
            (b) www.cancereducation.com. Cancer education, news, and information for health care providers
            (c) www.cancerwise.com. Resources, news, facts, and statistics; includes nutrition, prevention, and links to support groups
            (d) www.oncology.com. Forum on needs of the cancer community; support for patients and families
            (e) www.cancer.gov. National Cancer Institute and other government organizations addressing the needs of the public, patients, and health care providers
      d. Encourage compliance with individualized decisions for screening and follow-up procedures.
   3. *Desired outcomes*
      a. Patient can state risk factors, screening recommendations, signs and symptoms, and diagnostic tests.
      b. Patient will state the potential risk versus benefits of routine screening and make an informed decision as to whether he will proceed with screening.
      c. Patient will participate in decisions related to his care.
B. Altered sexuality patterns related to the cancer and treatment (decrease in libido, erectile dysfunction, absence of emission or ejaculation)

TABLE 13-7 **Prostate Cancer Treatment by Stage**

Stage	Treatment	Nursing Considerations
Surgery		
Stage A2: Tumor not palpable but detectable microscopically; > 3 foci or 5% well, moderately, or poorly differentiated tumor cells Stage B: Tumor is palpable; confined to the prostatic capsule	Radical retropubic prostatectomy Laparoscopic pelvic lymph node dissection	Bleeding, infection, impotence, urinary and fecal incontinence
Stage D (palliation): Tumor has metastasized to regional lymph nodes, bone, or other organs	TURP for obstruction	Retrograde ejaculation, incontinence
Radiation Therapy		
Stage A: Tumor not palpable but detectable microscopically	External beam	Irritative bladder symptoms, bladder spasms, hematuria, rectal bleeding, cystitis, proctitis, diarrhea, bowel obstruction, bowel perforation, fistula, edema, dermatitis, and impotence
Stage B Stage C: Tumor extends beyond the prostate, with or without invasion of nearby organs; no distant metastasis		
Stage A: Tumor not palpable but detectable microscopically Stage B1: Palpable nodule confined to the prostate; involving less than one lobe Stage B2: For patients who refuse surgery or for whom surgery is contraindicated	Brachytherapy Radioactive iodine Radioactive gold Iridium	As for external beam radiation
Hormonal Therapy		
Stage D	Bilateral orchiectomy	Impotence, decreased libido, hot flashes, infection, pain, psychological impact (grief and depression)
	Estrogen therapy	Gynecomastia, edema, myocardial infarction, hypertension, cerebrovascular accident, thrombophlebitis, pulmonary embolus, nausea, vomiting, abdominal cramping, impotence, decreased libido

(continued)

▓ **TABLE 13-7 Prostate Cancer Treatment by Stage** *(Continued)*

Stage	Treatment	Nursing Considerations
Hormonal Therapy		
Stage D	Antiandrogens	Gynecomastia, diarrhea, impotence, abnormal elevation in liver function tests
	Luteinizing hormone releasing hormone (LHRH) agonists	Flare phenomenon, edema, nausea, vomiting, decreased testicular size, hot flashes, sweats, erectile dysfunction, anorexia, lethargy
	Adrenalectomy	Bleeding, infection
	Glucocorticoids	Euphoria, insomnia, psychotic behavior, hypertension, edema, cataracts, peptic ulcer, hypokalemia, hyperglycemia, muscle weakness, osteoporosis, increased susceptibility to infections
	Ketoconazole	Nausea, vomiting, hepatotoxicity, gynecomastia, pruritus, abdominal pain, diarrhea, constipation
	Aminoglutethimide	Lethargy, ataxia, hypotension, nausea, hypothyroidism
Chemotherapy		
Stage D3 (palliation): Progression of tumor despite hormonal treatment for metastatic disease	Estramustine phosphate + vinblastine (Velban)	Be aware of various side effects of chemotherapeutic agents
	Estramustine phosphate + etoposide	
	Suramin	
	Most regimens remain investigational	

1. *Problem:* Sexual dysfunction may occur as a result of medical/surgical castration, or damage to the nerves or muscular tissue surrounding the prostatic capsule caused by surgery or radiation.
2. *Interventions*
    a. Discuss patient/partner concerns.
    b. Provide accurate information concerning planned treatment and potential for sexual dysfunction.
        (1) Radical retropubic prostatectomy
            (a) Erection sufficient for penetration may not occur for 6 months or more.
            (b) No change in orgasmic feeling.
            (c) Dry orgasm.
        (2) Orchiectomy

▮ TABLE 13-8 Screening for Prostate Cancer

Three major organizations and their recommendations are as follows:

American Cancer Society (ASC): Recommends annual screening with digital rectal examination (DRE) and PSA for all men age 50 years and older, whose life expectancy is ≥10 years. Men at high risk (African descent and those with a first-degree relative with a diagnosis of prostate cancer) should begin testing at age 45. Men with history of multiple first-degree relatives with prostate cancer should begin testing at age 40. All patients with abnormal DRE or elevated PSA should be further evaluated with transrectal ultrasonography (TRUS).

American Urological Association: Recommends that men be offered screening for detection of cancer of the prostate beginning at age 50 if life expectancy is ≥10 years. They also recommend that men at high risk (ie, men with first-degree relative with history of prostate cancer and African-American men) be offered testing for screening at an earlier age.

U. S. Preventive Services Task Force (USPSTF) has not endorsed screening. In their report, they state that they "found good evidence that PSA screening can detect early stage prostate cancer but mixed inconclusive evidence that early detection improves health outcomes. Screening is associated with important harms, including frequent false-positive results and unnecessary anxiety, biopsies, and potential complications of treatment of some cancer that may never have affected a patient's health."

    (a) Loss of ability to produce sperm.
    (b) Sperm banking before surgery (see II).
    (c) Discuss alternative sexual activities that are compatible with patient's lifestyle (touching, masturbation).
    (d) Refer to sexual counselor, if appropriate.
  3. *Desired outcomes*
    a. Patient will express concerns regarding sexual functioning, satisfaction, and physical appearance.
    b. Patient will explore ways to enhance sexual gratification and achieve a satisfactory level of intimacy (hugging, kissing, touching, watching erotic movies, sharing sexual fantasies, bathing together).

▮ TABLE 13-9 Prostate Cancer: Gleason's Grading System

Assesses the potential aggressiveness of the tumor. The more poorly differentiated the cells, the more aggressive the tumor.

Grades	Definition
2–4	Well differentiated
5–6	Moderately differentiated
6	Moderately to poorly differentiated
8–10	Poorly differentiated

TABLE 13-10 **Staging Systems for Prostate Cancer**

Whitmore-Jewett	TNM (AJCC)*	Definition
A	T1	Clinically inapparent; tumor nonpalpable
A1	T1a	Tumor incidental histologic finding in <5% of sampled tissue
A2	T1b	Tumor incidental histologic finding in >5% of sampled tissue
B	T2	Clinically palpable tumor confined within the prostate
B1	T2a	Tumor ≤half of a lobe of the prostate
B2	T2b	Tumor in > half a lobe, but not both lobes of prostate
B2	T2c	Tumor involves both lobes
C	T3	Tumor extends through the prostate capsule
C1	T3a	Tumor extension through the capsule unilaterally
C1	T3b	Tumor extension through the capsule bilaterally
C1	T3c	Tumor involves seminal vesicles
C2	T4	Tumor is fixed (ie, pelvic wall) and/or invades adjacent tissues (ie, bladder neck, levator muscles, or rectum)
D	N/M	Metastatic disease
D1	N1	Regional lymph node involvement; microscopic pelvic lymph node metastasis; involvement of single lymph node, ≤2 cm in greatest dimension
D1	N2	Regional lymph node involvement; involvement of single lymph node, > 2 cm ≤ 5 cm in greatest dimension
D2	M1	Distant metastasis (ie, bones, lung, liver, brain)

Adapted from American Joint Committee on Cancer, 1998.

C. Altered pattern of urinary elimination related to disease and treatment of prostate cancer
1. *Problem:* Increased frequency, urgency, hematuria, dysuria, dribbling, and urinary incontinence are symptoms commonly seen in patients with prostate cancer because of tumor growth and various treatments (Table 13–6). These changes from normal elimination patterns may require the use of a urinary collection device (ie, indwelling Foley or condom catheter, or intermittent catheterization). Body image may also be affected.
2. *Interventions*
   a. Assess baseline and current elimination pattern.
   b. Evaluate the patient's emotional response to changes in elimination patterns.
   c. Monitor for edema.
   d. Monitor serum electrolytes (BUN, creatinine).
   e. Encourage a balance of adequate rest and exercise.
   f. Teach patient and caregiver how to manage the urinary collection device if indicated.
   g. Teach nephrostomy tube care.
3. *Desired outcomes*

      a. Patient will maintain a tolerable pattern of urinary elimination without unacceptable symptoms.

      b. Patient will discuss his emotional response to the changes in his elimination pattern.

  D. Pain related to disease and treatment of prostate cancer

      1. *Problem:* Pain can be caused by growth of the tumor pressing on nerve fibers, blood vessels, or other organs. It can also be associated with treatment.

      2. *Interventions:* Follow recommendations in Chapter 30.

      3. *Desired outcome:* Elimination or control of pain as described in Chapter 30.

  E. Discharge Planning and Patient Education for Patients With Prostate Cancer

      1. Provide information concerning implications of disease and therapy.

      a. Biopsy: Hematuria may be noted for up to 24 hours.

      b. Radical retropubic prostatectomy.

      c. Radiation therapy: External beam, brachytherapy, or interstitial implants (see Chapter 8).

      d. Hormone therapy.

      e. Instruct patient on treatment and side effects.

      f. Advise about body image changes (loss of libido, impotence, and decreased sperm production).

      g. Provide information about testicular prosthesis as appropriate.

      h. Teach patient signs of disease progression and to notify physician should they occur.

      i. Discuss pain-relieving measures.

      j. Discuss alternate expressions of sexuality and the availability and potential value of sexual counseling.

V. Nursing Diagnoses, Interventions, and Outcomes for Kidney Cancer

  A. Pain related to tumor growth and treatment

      1. *Problem:* Pain can be caused by growth of the tumor pressing on nerve fibers, blood vessels, or other organs. Pain can also be associated with various treatments.

      2. *Interventions:* Follow recommendations in Chapter 30.

      3. *Desired outcome:* Elimination or control of pain, as described in Chapter 30.

  B. Alteration in pattern of urinary elimination related to disease and treatment

      1. *Problem:* Kidney cancers often present with gross hematuria or hydronephrosis secondary to tumor growth. Treatment generally involves radical nephrectomy, leaving only one functioning kidney. Meeting the body's total need for elimination is essential.

      2. *Interventions*

      a. Encourage patient to express concerns about changes in elimination pattern.

      b. Provide information regarding etiology of symptoms.

      c. Teach patient to maintain an adequate fluid intake.

TABLE 13-11 **TNM Staging for Kidney Cancer**

Primary Tumor (T)

TX	Not able to assess primary tumor
T0	No evidence of primary tumor
T1	Tumor ≤2.5 cm in greatest dimension, limited to kidney
T2	Tumor >2.5 cm in greatest dimension, limited to the kidney
T3	Tumor extension to major veins, adrenal gland, or perinephric tissues, but not beyond

Gerota's fascia

T4	Tumor invades beyond Gerota's fascia

Regional Lymph Nodes (N)

NX	Unable to assess regional lymph nodes
N0	No regional lymph node metastasis
N1	Metastasis in a single lymph node, ≤2 cm in greatest dimension
N2	Metastasis in a single lymph node >2 cm in greatest dimension, but <5 cm, or multiple lymph nodes, none more than 5 cm in greatest dimension
N3	Metastasis in a lymph node >5 cm in greatest dimension

Distant Metastasis (M)

MX	Unable to assess distant metastasis
M0	No distant metastasis
M1	Distant metastasis

Stage Grouping

Stage I	T1	N0	M0
Stage II	T2	N0	M0
Stage III	T1	N1	M0
	T2	N1	M0
	T3a	N0–1	M0
	T3b	N0–1	M0
	T3c	N0–1	M0
Stage IV	T4	Any N	M0
	Any T	N2	M0
	Any T	N3	M0
	Any T	Any N	M1

American Joint Committee on Cancer, 1998.

    d. Monitor the patient's urine output.
    e. Maintain preoperative/postoperative care for nephrectomy (see Chapter 9).
  3. *Desired outcomes*
    a. Patient will state understanding of symptoms and changes and demonstrate adequate management.
    b. Patient will maintain adequate function of remaining kidney.

TABLE 13–12 Treatment Modalities for Kidney Cancer

Classification and Stage	Treatment
Renal Cell	
Stage I: Tumor confined to the kidney	Radical nephrectomy with or without lymphoidectomy External beam radiation (palliative) Bilateral disease: Nephrectomy of larger tumor and partial nephrectomy for smaller lesion Bilateral nephrectomies with peritoneal dialysis Investigational therapies
Stage II: Tumor involves peri-renal tissue or adrenals; within Gerota's fascia	Radical nephrectomy with or without lymphoidectomy Preoperative or postoperative external beam radiation and nephrectomy
Stage III: Tumor invading renal vein or inferior vena cava or lymph nodes	Investigational therapies See stage II
Stage IV: Tumor invading adjacent organs other than adrenals; distant metastasis	Prognosis: Very poor Treatment: Palliative Chemotherapy generally yields poor response rate: <10% for any given regimen Hormonal therapy: Progestational agents, testosterone, antiestrogens Biologic response modifiers: Alfa-interferons, interleukin-2, retinoids in combination with alfa-interferon
Renal Pelvis	
Tumor of the renal pelvis	Nephrectomy Radiation: Not proven to be effective Chemotherapy: Doxorubicin, cisplatin, methotrexate, vinblastine (Velban). For urothelial cancers, see Table 13-5.

C. Discharge Planning and Patient Education for Patients With Kidney Cancer

1. Provide patient with information concerning the extent of disease, prognosis, implications of therapies, symptoms necessitating medical attention, and required follow-up.
2. Be aware of the physical and psychological limitations and offer support and referral as appropriate.
3. Teach patients self-care techniques to manage side effects of treatment.

REFERENCES

Abel, L., Dafoe-Lambie, J., Butler, W. M., & Merrick, G. S. (January/February 2003). Treatment outcome and quality-of-life issues for patients treated with prostate brachytherapy. *Clinical Journal of Oncology Nursing, 7*(1), 48–54.

Abraham, J., & Allegra, C. J. (Eds.). (2001). *Bethesda handbook of clinical oncology.* Philadelphia: Lippincott Williams & Wilkins.

American Cancer Society, Inc. (2003). Internet site: www.cancer.org.

American Joint Committee on Cancer. (1998). *Handbook for staging of cancer* (5th ed.). Philadelphia: J. B. Lippincott.

American Urological Association. (February 2000). Prostate-specific antigen (PSA) best practice policy. *Oncology, 14*(2), 267–286.

Chung, L. W. K., Isaacs, W. B., & Simons, J. W. (2001). *Prostate cancer: Biology, genetics and the new therapeutics.* Totowa, NJ: Humana Press.

Dreicer, R., Manola, J., Roth, B. J., Cohen, M. B., Hatfield, A. K., & Wilding, G. (2000). Phase II trial of cisplatin and paclitaxel in advanced carcinoma of the urothelium: An Eastern Cooperative Oncology Group Study. *Journal of Clinical Oncology, 18*(5), 1058–1061.

Gaston, K. E., & Ornstein, D. K. (2002). Pharmacotherapy for biochemical recurrences after therapy for localized prostate cancer. *Pharmacotherapy, 3*(6), 657–669.

Held, J. L., Osborne, D. M., Volpe, H., & Waldman, A. R. (1994). Cancer of the prostate: Treatment and nursing implications. *Oncology Nursing Forum, 21*(9), 1517–1529.

Hudson, M. A., & Herr, H. W. (1995). Carcinoma in situ of the bladder. *Journal of Urology, 153*(3, Part 1), 564–572.

Jemal, A., Taylor, M., Samuels, A., Ghafoor, A., Ward, E., & Thun, M. J. (2003). Cancer statistics, 2003. *CA: Cancer Journal for Clinicians, 53*(1), 5–26.

Kantoff, P. W., Carroll, P. R., & D'Amico, A. V. (Eds.). (2002). *Prostate cancer: Principles and practice.* Philadelphia: Lippincott Williams & Wilkins.

Kaufman, D., Raghavan, D., Carducci, M., Levine E. G., Murphy, B., Aisner, J., Kuzel, T., Nicol, S., & Oh, W. (2000). Phase II trial of gemcitabine plus cisplatin in patients with metastatic urothelial cancer. *Journal of Clinical Oncology, 18*(9), 1921–1927.

Kelly, L. P., & Miaskowski, C. (1996). An overview of bladder cancer: Treatment and nursing implications. *Oncology Nursing Forum, 23*(3), 459–468.

Lind, J. (1998). Nursing care of the client with cancer of the urinary system. In J. K. Itano & K. N. Taoka (Eds.), *Core curriculum for oncology nursing* (3rd ed.). Philadelphia: W.B. Saunders.

McCaffrey, J. A., Hilton, J. A., Mazumdar, M., Sedan, S., Kelly, W. K., Scher, H. I., & Bajorin, D. F. (1997). Phase II trial of docetaxel in patients with advanced or metastatic transitional cell carcinoma. *Journal of Clinical Oncology, 15*(5), 1853–1857.

Moore, M. J., Tannock, I. F., Ernst, D. S., Huan, S., & Murray, N. (1997). Gemcitabine: A promising new agent in the treatment of advanced urothelial cancer. *Journal of Clinical Oncology, 15*(12), 3441–3445.

O'Rourke, M. E. (2001). Genitourinary cancers. In S. E. Otto (Ed.), *Oncology nursing* (4th ed.). St. Louis, MO: Mosby.

Partin, A. W., Mangold, L. A., Lamm, D. M., Walsh, P. C., Epstein, J. I., & Pearson, J. D. (2001). Contemporary update of prostate cancer staging nomograms (Partin tables) for the new millennium. *Urology, 58*(6), 843–848.

Pound, C. R., Partin, A. W., Eisenberger, M. A., Chan, D. W., Pearson, J. D., & Walsh, P. C. (1999). Natural history of progression after PSA elevation following radical prostatectomy. *Journal of the American Medical Association, 281*(17), 1591–1597.

Reilly, N. J. (1995). Cancer of the bladder. In K. A. Karlowicz (Ed.), *Urologic nursing principles and practice.* Philadelphia: W. B. Saunders.

Roth, B. J., Dreicer, R., Einhorn, L. H., Neuberg, D., Johnson, D. L., Smith, J. L., Hudes, G. R., Schultz, S. M., & Loehrer, P. J. (1994). Significant activity of paclitaxel in advanced transitional cell carcinoma of the urothelium: A phase II trial of the Eastern Cooperative Oncology Group. *Journal of Clinical Oncology, 12*(1), 2264–2270.

Smith, R. A., Cokkinides, V., & Eyre, H. (2003). American Cancer Society guidelines for early detection of cancer, 2003. *CA: Cancer Journal for Clinicians, 53*(1), 27–43.

Sperm Banking Directory.com. (2003). Internet site: www.spermbankingdirectory.com.

Thrasher, J. B., & Crawford, E. D. (1993). Current management of invasive and metastatic transitional cell carcinoma of the bladder. *Journal of Urology, 149*(5), 957–972.

Wilkes, G. M., Ingwersen, K., & Barton-Burke, M. (2003). *Oncology nursing drug handbook.* Sudbury, MA: Jones & Bartlett.

U. S. Preventive Services Task Force. (2000–2003). Screening for prostate cancer: Recommendations and rationale. In *Guide to clinical preventive services* (3rd ed.). Available: http://www.preventiveservices.ahrq.gov.

Vogelzang, N. J., Shipley, W. U., Scardino, P. T., & Coffey, D. S. (Eds.). (1996). *Comprehensive textbook of genitourinary oncology.* Baltimore, MD: Williams & Wilkins.

14 Gynecologic Cancers

Sharon D. Thompson

I. Gynecologic malignancies (see Table 14–1 for an overview of the clinicopathophysiologic features of each of the gynecologic malignancies [uterine cancer, ovarian cancer, cervical cancer, vulvar cancer])
   A. Comprise malignancies involving female genitalia of the pelvic region
   B. Diseases have variable genetic, environmental, and social risk factors.
   C. Diseases have very different prognostic implications and are treated as separate disease processes.
   D. See Tables 14–2, 14–3, 14–4, and 14–5 for specific cancer staging and treatments.

II. Nursing Diagnosis and Related Interventions and Outcomes
   A. Body image disturbance related to loss of female reproductive organ function, alopecia and weight changes
      1. *Problem:* Treatment for gynecologic malignancies includes hysterectomy or other radical changes in the functioning or physical appearance of reproductive organs and related structures. Treatment for ovarian cancer may also involve chemotherapy, which can cause temporary hair loss. It can be difficult for patients to adjust to these changes in their appearance.
      2. *Interventions*
         a. Before the procedure, teach the patient the impact on reproductive organ function to facilitate anticipatory grieving and decrease the risk of body image disturbances.
         b. Encourage grieving by the patient and family for the loss of patient's femininity after changes have occurred.
         c. Incorporate patient and family into care to provide sense of control.
         d. Report critical changes in behavior to the physician immediately (ie, suicidal ideation, self-destructive behavior, self-neglect).
         e. Facilitate referral for psychological counseling as indicated by patient's level of distress.
         f. Dispel falsehoods related to hysterectomy (eg, cervix is necessary for orgasm, postsurgical weight gain, loss of sexual interest, mental deterioration).
      3. *Desired outcomes*
         a. Patient will express any feelings related to loss of femininity.
         b. Patient will identify and employ effective coping mechanisms.
   B. Sexual dysfunction related to changes in female reproductive organ function
      1. *Problem:* Patients may experience changes in sexuality as a result of the gynecologic cancer and its treatment. Patients with endometrial, ovarian, and cervical cancers may experience decreased vaginal

(*text continues on page 213*)

TABLE 14–1 Overview of Gynecologic Malignancies

		Definition		
Endometrial Cancer	*Ovarian Cancer*	*Cervical Cancer*		*Vulvar Cancer*
• Most common gynecologic malignancy • Arises from the epithelial lining of the uterus • Primarily affects postmenopausal women 55 to 70 years of age • Most present with early-stage disease • Overall 5-year survival rate about 85% • See Table 14-2 for staging of endometrial cancer.	• Arises from the surface epithelium of the ovaries • Accounts for about one third of all cancers of the female reproductive tract and a little more than half of all deaths from gynecologic cancers • Overall 5-year survival rate is approximately 44%, with a greater than 90% 5-year survival rate for early-stage disease. • Epithelial tumors account for 80% to 90% of all malignant ovarian neoplasms. • See Table 14-3 for staging of ovarian cancer.	• Progressive disease, beginning with neoplastic cells in the epithelial layer of the cervix, that spread into the stromal tissue causing invasive cervical cancer. • Incidence has steadily decreased as a result of the Pap smear, which can detect the disease in a preinvasive state. • Comprises approximately one third of all gynecologic malignancies • Overall 5-year survival rate for all stages is close to 70%. • See Table 14-4 for staging of cervical cancer.		• Accounts for only 3% to 4% of all gynecologic cancers and has a 70% to 75% 5-year survival rate • Lesions can develop anywhere on the vulva, 70% occurring on the labia. Tumors can also arise on the clitoris, Bartholin's glands, and the perineum. • Usually remains a localized disease with definite margins • 90% are squamous cell malignancies, and the remaining are Bartholin's gland, sarcoma, basal cell, Paget's, and verrucous cancer. • See Table 14-5 for staging of vulvar cancer.

(continued)

TABLE 14-1 Overview of Gynecologic Malignancies *(Continued)*

Risk Factors/Etiologies

Endometrial Cancer	Ovarian Cancer	Cervical Cancer	Vulvar Cancer
• Obesity • Hypertension • Diabetes • History of infertility, breast or ovarian cancer • Irregular menses or failure to ovulate • Prolonged estrogen replacement therapy • Endometrial hyperplasia	• Nulliparity • First pregnancy after age 35 • High-fat diet • Family history of ovarian cancer • Late menopause • Early menarche • Hormonal therapy • Exposure to environmental toxins, such as coal, tar, and talc	• Infection with human papilloma virus (HPV) or herpes simplex virus 2 (HSV2) • Sexual intercourse before age 17 • Multiple sexual partners • History of smoking • Spouse whose previous wife had cervical cancer • Maternal use of diethylstilbestrol (DES). • Immunosuppression • Multiparity • Lower socioeconomic status • African-American or Hispanic descent • A spouse with penile cancer	• Age > 60 years • Chronic vulvar irritation • History of other lower genital tract malignancy • History of infection with HSV2, HPV, or other STDs • Exposure to coal tar derivatives

Signs and Symptoms

Endometrial Cancer	Ovarian Cancer	Cervical Cancer	Vulvar Cancer
• Postmenopausal vaginal bleeding is the classic presenting symptom. • Tumors arising in the epithelium and spreading to the myometrium may cause bleeding within the uterine cavity.	• No typical symptoms have been correlated with early-stage ovarian cancer, and lack of specific symptoms usually leads to diagnosis at a later stage of disease.	• Watery vaginal discharge may be experienced by women with cervical cancer in a preinvasive state, although most cervical cancers are asymptomatic. • Postcoital bleeding, bleeding between menstrual cycles, and heavy menstrual flow are later symptoms.	• Mass or growth in the vulvar area is most common symptom. • Some vulvar cancers are asymptomatic with lesions detected only during annual examinations. • Vulvar bleeding may occur

Endometrial Cancer	Ovarian Cancer	Cervical Cancer	Vulvar Cancer
• Irregular or heavy menstrual flow may be a symptom in the premenopausal patient. • Pain, particularly in the lumbosacral, hypogastric, or pelvic regions, and an enlarging nonpregnant uterus can be signs of advanced disease.	• GI complaints such as abdominal discomfort, bloating, indigestion, dyspepsia, increased flatulence, changes in bowel habits, loss of appetite, and pelvic pressure may be experienced as the tumor grows within the pelvis. GI work-up is usually negative. • Genitourinary symptoms such as burning, urgency, and frequency may occur. • Palpable mass, ascites, and shortness of breath are signs of late disease but may be the first symptoms experienced.	• Malodorous, serosanguineous, or yellowish vaginal discharge from necrotic tissue is often a complaint in advanced stages. • Pain in the pelvis, hypogastrium, flank, or leg is a symptom of late disease secondary to involvement of the pelvic sidewall, lymph nodes, ureters, or nerves. • Urinary or rectal symptoms, such as urgency, frequency, or rectal pressure, may indicate invasion of the bladder or bowel by tumor. • Lower-extremity edema may develop in late-stage disease due to lymphatic or venous obstruction.	due to irritation by the tumor. • Vulvar pain may also be experienced.

Diagnostic Tests

Endometrial Cancer	Ovarian Cancer	Cervical Cancer	Vulvar Cancer
• Bimanual pelvic examination allows the evaluation of the shape, size, and consistency of the uterus. • Endometrial biopsy is 90% effective in detecting cancer, indicated with suspicious abnormal bleeding. It may also be used to screen women who are at increased risk of the disease (eg, women on estrogen replacement therapy).	• Pelvic examination usually reveals a large pelvic mass in late-stage disease and is effective in detection of early-stage disease in only a small number of asymptomatic women. • Ultrasound (US), CT, or MRI evaluates the size and location of a pelvic mass and may help diagnose lymph node involvement.	• Pap smear is the most accurate, convenient, and cost-effective technique used to detect cervical cancer. American Cancer Society recommends that women who are sexually active or who are 18 years of age or older have a Pap smear and pelvic examination annually. Pap smears can identify numerous infections, reactive changes, and cellular abnormalities. If a Pap smear is abnormal, other	• Physical examination of the external genitalia may reveal a mass or other lesion. Vulvar biopsy of a palpable mass or observable lesion is the most definitive method of diagnosing vulvar cancer. Colposcopy is sometimes used to pinpoint the areas to be biopsied. • Pap smear of the cervix is *(continued)*

TABLE 14–1 Overview of Gynecologic Malignancies *(Continued)*

Diagnostic Tests

Endometrial Cancer	Ovarian Cancer	Cervical Cancer	Vulvar Cancer

• Dilatation and curettage may obtain additional tissue for diagnosis if an endometrial biopsy is negative or contains suspicious cells that are not diagnostic
 	
• Cystoscopy or intravenous. pyelogram (IVP) may be performed if urologic involvement is suspected.
 	
• MRI, CT, hysterography, hysteroscopy, ultrasonography, and lymphangiography may be used to evaluate the size of the tumor and to determine nodal involvement.
	• CA-125 serum testing may determine if the antigen specific for epithelial ovarian cancer is detectable in the patient's bloodstream.
	
	• Exploratory laparotomy with complete surgical staging is performed for definitive diagnosis and to determine the extent of the disease.
	
	• IVP can determine the location of the pelvic mass in relation to the ureters.
	
	• Tests to rule out other malignancies or detect metastatic disease:
	  —Proctoscopy, sigmoidoscopy, or barium enema
	  —Chest x-ray
		tests are necessary to diagnose the problem.
		
		• Colposcopy is a diagnostic test used to evaluate the cervix after an abnormal Pap smear. A 3% acetic acid solution is applied to the cervix which allows the examiner to visualize and biopsy abnormal areas.
		
		• A cervical biopsy may be performed for definitive diagnosis of abnormal areas seen during colposcopy.
		
		• Cystoscopy or IVP may be performed to rule out bladder or renal involvement.
		
		• Chest x-ray is done to rule out metastases in the pleural cavity.
		
		• Proctoscopy, sigmoidoscopy, or barium enema may be performed if bowel involvement is suspected. MRI or CT scan may be used to evaluate the size of the tumor and extent of the disease, including lymph node, bowel, or bladder involvement.
		
		• A supraclavicular lymph node biopsy is done if any of these nodes are palpable.
			also performed because a small number of women diagnosed with vulvar cancer will also have preinvasive or invasive cervical cancer.
			
			• Chest x-ray is performed to rule out metastatic disease in the pleural cavity.
			
			• Colonoscopy, proctosigmoidoscopy, or barium enema may be performed to rule out bowel involvement.
			
			• Cystoscopy or IVP may be performed to rule out bladder or renal involvement.
			
			• CT scan or MRI may be useful in diagnosing lymph node involvement and disease spread.

General Management Strategies

Endometrial Cancer	Ovarian Cancer	Cervical Cancer	Vulvar Cancer
• Total abdominal hysterectomy and bilateral salpingo-oophorectomy (TAH-BSO) with pelvic and paraaortic lymph node dissection is the initial treatment for all stages of endometrial cancer (see Table 14-2). • Intracavitary or external beam radiation therapy may be initiated after surgery for stages III and IV to prevent local recurrence of the disease or in earlier stages if the patient is not a surgical candidate (see Table 14-2).	• Initial treatment—total abdominal hysterectomy and bilateral salpingo-oophorectomy (TAH-BSO) with pelvic and paraaortic lymph node dissection, along with cytoreductive surgery and adequate surgical staging. • Optimal cytoreductive surgery with less than 1 cm residual tumor volume is a favorable prognostic indicator for both response to chemotherapy and survival. • Systemic chemotherapy after initial surgery is required for stages Ic through IV using a combination regimen of cisplatin or carboplatin with paclitaxel for at least six courses. • Hormone therapy may be used to stabilize disease in patients who have failed chemotherapy regimens, but it usually does not promote tumor regression.	• Depending on the degree of cervical invasion and the staging, treatment may include total abdominal hysterectomy (TAH), total vaginal hysterectomy (TVH), or radical abdominal hysterectomy (RAH). • These may be performed as initial treatment or after the tumor volume is reduced by intracavitary or external beam radiation therapy (see Table 14-4).	• Initial treatment is surgical removal of the tumor. Depending on the stage of disease, surgery may include a simple vulvectomy, radical vulvectomy, or total pelvic exenteration. • Radiotherapy may be used preoperatively as neoadjuvant therapy, or to treat groin or pelvic lymph node disease.

TABLE 14–2 Endometrial Cancer Staging and Treatment

Stage	Surgery	Radiation Therapy	Chemotherapy	Hormonal Therapy
Stages I and II—Tumor confined to the uterus	Total abdominal hysterectomy (TAH) and bilateral salpingo-oopherectomy (BSO), with pelvic and paraaortic lymph node dissection if patient is a surgical candidate.	Localized Intracavitary or external beam radiation therapy in addition to surgery to prevent local recurrence in selected patients with minimal invasion. Primary therapy if patient is not a surgical candidate.	Not shown to be effective as adjuvant therapy. May be used in disease recurrence.	Not shown to be effective as adjuvant therapy. May be used in disease recurrence.
Stage III—Tumor extends to fallopian tubes, ovaries, vagina, or pelvic/paraaortic lymph nodes; ascites present or positive peritoneal washing	TAH and BSO, with pelvic and paraaortic lymph node dissection if patient is a surgical candidate.	Regional Intracavitary or external beam radiation therapy in addition to surgery to prevent local recurrence. Primary therapy if patient is not a surgical candidate.	Not shown to be effective as adjuvant therapy. May be used in disease recurrence.	Not shown to be effective as adjuvant therapy. May be used in disease recurrence.
Stage IV—Involvement of bladder, rectum, or bowel; or distant metastasis, most commonly to lungs, liver, bone, or brain; positive inguinal lymph nodes	TAH and BSO, with pelvic and paraaortic lymph node dissection if patient is a surgical candidate.	Distant External beam radiation therapy in addition to surgery for local control of disease in pelvis. Primary therapy if patient is not a surgical candidate.	Doxorubicin or high-dose platinum-based agent/taxol or both for advanced or recurrent disease, with or without surgery.	Synthetic progestational agents (megestrol acetate) or antiestrogen agents (tamoxifen) may be used in distant or recurrent disease.

TABLE 14-3 Ovarian Cancer Staging and Treatment

Stage	Surgery	Radiation Therapy	Chemotherapy	Hormonal Therapy
Stage I—Tumor confined to one or both ovaries; ascites present or positive peritoneal washings	TAH and BSO with pelvic and paraaortic lymph node dissection, omentectomy.	Localized Abdominally instilled radioactive chromic phosphate (P32) after surgery or whole abdominal external beam radiation therapy	Usually not recommended for stage 1 disease without ascites or positive washings. Cisplatin-based therapy usually given if positive ascites or peritoneal washings.	Not shown to be effective as adjuvant therapy
Stages II and III—Tumor spread beyond ovaries to the pelvis and other intraperitoneal structures, including lymph nodes	TAH and BSO with pelvic and paraaortic lymph node dissection, possible omentectomy. Major goal—Less than 1 cm residual tumor.	Regional Possible external beam radiation therapy to the whole abdomen after surgery if there is residual disease less than 1 cm (significant morbidity)	Combination regimens using cisplatin or carboplatin with cyclophosphamide or paclitaxel are usually given (most effective form of adjuvant therapy).	Tamoxifen and megestrol acetate used when first-line treatment fails. Usually does not produce tumor regression, although some patients may exhibit stabilization of disease.
Stage IV—Distant metastases, most commonly to pleura, lungs, or liver parenchyma	TAH and BSO with pelvic and paraaortic lymph node dissection, possible omentectomy. Major goal—less than 1 cm residual tumor.	Distant Possible external beam radiation therapy to the whole abdomen after surgery if there is residual disease less than 1 cm (significant morbidity)	Combination regimens using cisplatin or carboplatin with cyclophosphamide or paclitaxel are usually given. Topotecan is also an active anti-cancer agent. Intraperitoneal antineoplastic therapy may also have a future role in management of advanced disease.	Tamoxifen and megestrol acetate used when first-line treatment fails. Usually does not produce tumor regression, although some patients may exhibit stabilization of disease.

TABLE 14–4 Cervical Cancer Staging and Treatment

Stage	Surgery	Radiation Therapy	Chemotherapy	Hormonal Therapy
Stages I and IIa— Tumor involving cervix or uterus	*Minimal/early invasion:* Total abdominal hysterectomy (TAH) or total vaginal hysterectomy (TVH) in selected patients. *Invasive disease:* Radical abdominal hysterectomy (RAH; removal of the uterus, upper third of vagina, entire uterosacral and uterovesical ligaments, and entire parametrium) and pelvic lymph node dissection.	Localized Possible intracavitary radiation or external beam radiation alone or in combination with surgery	Usually not recommended	Usually not recommended
Stages IIb and III— Tumor spreads to parametrial tissue, pelvic sidewall, lower vagina, or compresses ureters producing hydronephrosis	Surgery alone is not primary treatment; RAH may be done after initial radiation therapy.	Regional Whole pelvis external beam radiation therapy with parametrial boosts or extended fields along with intracavitary radiation	May be used as a radiation sensitizer (cisplatin, 5-fluorouracil, or hydroxy-urea together with radiation).	Usually not recommended

Stage IV—Bladder, bowel, or distant metastasis, most commonly to lungs, liver, bone, mediastinal, or supraclavicular lymph nodes	RAH or total pelvic exenteration (removal of entire pelvic viscera, requiring a colostomy and diversion of urinary drainage) may be necessary in selected patients as primary therapy for recurrence	Distant Whole pelvis external beam radiation therapy with parametrial boosts or extended fields along with intracavitary radiation	May be used as a radiation sensitizer (cisplatin, 5-fluorouracil, or hydroxyurea together with radiation) or as a systemic regimen. Minimal response rates generally seen—usually only considered in patients with recurrent or persistent disease. Other active agents that may be administered with a platinol drug include ifosfamide, vinorelbine, and mitomycin	Usually not recommended

TABLE 14–5 Vulvar Cancer Staging and Treatment

Stage	Surgery	Radiation Therapy	Chemotherapy	Hormonal Therapy
Stages I and II—Tumor confined to the vulvar region and/or perineum. Stage I is less than 2 cm in its greatest dimension.	Wide local excision or radical vulvectomy with groin dissection depending on size, extent of lesion, and depth of stromal invasion	Localized¹ Generally not indicated as primary treatment of vulvar cancer	Not shown to be effective as adjuvant therapy	Not shown to be effective as adjuvant therapy
Stage III—Tumor of any size spread to lower urethra, anus, vagina, or unilateral regional lymph node metastasis	Radical vulvectomy (en bloc dissection of the tumor, contiguous skin, subcutaneous fat, regional inguinal and femoral lymph nodes, labia majora, clitoris, and perineal body); pelvic lymph node dissection is performed if positive groin nodes are found.	Regional May be useful for patient who is a poor surgical risk. May be used to treat groin or pelvic lymph node disease	Not shown to be effective as adjuvant therapy	Not shown to be effective as adjuvant therapy
Stage IV—Metastases to upper urethra, bladder, rectal mucosa, pelvic bone, regional or distant lymph nodes, or distant metastatic disease	Radical vulvectomy, total pelvic exenteration, or both may be indicated if the bladder or rectum is involved.	Distant May be used to shrink non-resectable tumor to operable size. May be used to treat groin or pelvic lymph node disease.	May be used as palliation or in combination with radiation as a sensitizer; active agents include bleomycin, CCNU, and methotrexate	Not shown to be effective as adjuvant therapy

lubrication and alterations in orgasm. Patients with cervical cancer may also experience shortening of the vagina after radical hysterectomy. Patients who undergo radical procedures for vulvar cancer can experience loss of clitoral arousal and orgasm, as well as significant changes in their external genital structure.

2. *Interventions*
   a. Preoperatively review normal anatomy, physiology, and sexual functioning and inform the patient of anticipated physical changes.
   b. Review anticipated changes in sexual functioning related to treatment and decreased estrogen levels.
   c. Dispel falsehoods related to hysterectomy (eg, cervix is necessary for orgasm, postsurgical weight gain, loss of sexual interest, mental deterioration).
   d. Provide specific suggestions that may assist the patient in adapting to changes in sexuality, such as using a lubricant for vaginal dryness and planning intercourse during times of the day when the patient has the most energy. Patients with a shortened vagina may need to try different positions for intercourse. Patients who have undergone radical procedures for vulvar cancer may need to be given specific suggestions about alternative methods of sexual arousal and expression, even though sexual intercourse is usually still possible.
   e. See Chapter 31 for more interventions.

3. *Desired outcomes:* Patient and significant other will adapt to changes in sexual functioning and, if necessary, employ alternative methods of sexual expression.

C. Increased risk of infection related to surgical wounds
   1. *Problem:* Wounds created during surgical procedures increase a patient's risk of developing infection. This risk can be compounded by the use of treatments, such as chemotherapy and radiation therapy, that can suppress immune function.
   2. *Interventions:* Follow recommendations in Chapters 9 and 22.
   3. *Desired outcomes:* See Chapters 9 and 22.

D. Altered nutrition, less than body requirements, related to anorexia, nausea, or vomiting
   1. *Problem:* Patients with endometrial and ovarian cancer can experience a decrease in appetite as a consequence of chemotherapy, radiation therapy, or abdominal pressure from ascites or a pelvic mass. The decrease in appetite makes it difficult for patients to consume adequate food and fluids.
   2. *Interventions:* Follow recommendations in Chapters 27 and 28.
   3. *Desired outcomes:* See Chapters 27 and 28.

E. Ineffective, compromised family coping related to increased anxiety and depression in response to cancer diagnosis and treatment
   1. *Problem:* Cancers of the reproductive tract often cause stress within the family unit. The patient or family may experience unexpected changes in thought, feeling, and behavior in response to cancer diagnosis and treatment.
   2. *Interventions:* Follow recommendations in Chapter 31.
   3. *Desired outcomes:* See Chapter 31.

F. Gas exchange: potential for impairment related to pleural effusions

    1. *Problem:* One of the more common sites for metastasis in endometrial and ovarian cancers is the pleural cavity. This places the patient at an increased risk of developing pleural effusions.

    2. *Interventions:* Follow recommendations in Chapter 36.

    3. *Desired outcomes:* See Chapter 36.

G. Deficit in fluid status related to nausea and vomiting from bowel dysfunction (ovarian cancer)

    1. *Problem:* Patients with ovarian cancer may develop bowel dysfunction when tumor encases the bowel or from external compression of the bowel wall by a pelvic mass. This dysfunction can interfere with the transit of bowel contents, leading to nausea and vomiting.

    2. *Interventions*

        a. Assess for abdominal distention, bowel sounds, flatus, and bowel movements.

        b. Assess for signs of dehydration, such as poor skin turgor and dry mucous membranes.

        c. Monitor fluid status using vital signs, weights, intake, and output from kidneys and nasogastric tube (if applicable).

        d. Monitor serum electrolytes.

        e. Maintain patency of the nasogastric or intestinal drainage tube, as indicated.

        f. Administer intravenous (IV) hydration and electrolyte supplements as ordered.

        g. Follow recommendations in Chapter 27.

    3. *Desired outcomes:* Patient will maintain adequate hydration until resolution of the bowel dysfunction.

H. Alteration in elimination, urinary or gastrointestinal

    1. *Problem:* Malignancies involving the gynecologic organs within the pelvic region often invade into or externally compress genitourinary structures and the bowel. Obstruction of the bowel, ureters, bladder, and urethra produce infection and organ failure that may lead to life-threatening crises. Additionally, surgical and radiation treatments for gynecologic malignancies may cause inflammation, adhesions, or infections affecting elimination.

    2. *Interventions*

        a. Assess intake and output on a regular basis, comparing expected with actual, and correlating to abdominal and pelvic symptoms.

        b. Assess the abdomen every shift for the presence of pain, distention (general abdominal or bladder), bowel sounds, lymph nodes, and masses. Report intractable pain, rebound tenderness, inability to void, fever, confusion, and vital sign changes.

        c. Assess vital signs and clinical symptoms for evidence of infection every shift or outpatient visit (e.g., fever, rigors, low diastolic blood pressure, headache, elevated WBC count).

        d. Monitor laboratory tests that will detect signs and symptoms of genitourinary (increased blood urea nitrogen, increased creatinine) or gastrointestinal obstruction (increased hepatic transaminases, hyperammonemia).

        e. Maintain therapies designed to provide palliative support for bowel or urinary obstruction.

(1) Nasogastric tubes reduce the amount of fluid and gas that must pass through the gastrointestinal tract, alleviating the symptoms of partial small bowel obstruction. Nurses must assess position and patency at least every shift or with medication administration.

(2) Gastrointestinal stimulants (e.g., cholinergic agents) may be used to enhance bowel motility, especially with small bowel obstruction.

(3) Provide information about potential for bowel or genitourinary obstruction in nurse-to-nurse report, so that early symptoms can be detected.

(4) Externalized nephrostomy stents or surgical urinary diversions require specialized nursing care (e.g., flushing, dressings) dictated by institutional policies.

   3. *Desired outcomes*

     a. Normal urine and stool output

     b. Absence of fever

     c. Normal blood chemistry, hepatic profile, and urinalysis results

I. Alteration in comfort related to pelvic ascites

   1. *Problem:* Women with ovarian cancer may develop malignant peritoneal effusions (ascites) due to tumor seeding in the peritoneum, which may result in obstruction of the abdominal lymphatics. This can lead to discomfort from abdominal distention and dependent edema. Patients may also experience impaired ventilatory capacity if the abdominal distention interferes with lung expansion by forcing the diaphragm upward.

   2. *Interventions*

     a. Assist the patient with identifying comfortable positions. (Patients may be most comfortable sitting in a semi-Fowler's or high-Fowler's position.)

     b. Assist the patient in maintaining maximal mobility and planning rest periods.

     c. Monitor the patient's respiratory status and administer oxygen therapy as indicated.

     d. Explain the paracentesis procedure to the patient. Provide emotional support during the procedure.

     e. See Chapter 30 for suggestions on management.

   3. *Desired outcomes:* The patient will report that her discomfort is adequately controlled.

III. Discharge Planning and Patient Education

A. Provide therapy-specific patient education that incorporates expected outcomes and possible adverse effects.

B. Refer to mental health professional for altered body image or coping difficulties.

C. Provide patient education regarding care of external diversional devices (stents, urinary diversions) and home care referral for supervision, continued education, or supplies.

D. Assess need for home or ambulatory management of nutritional or fluid imbalances. Refer as appropriate.

REFERENCES

Ahmedin, J., Murray, T., Samuels, A., Ghafoor, A., Ward, E., & Thun, M. J. (2003). Cancer statistics, 2003. *CA: A Cancer Journal for Clinicians, 53,* 5–26.

Daud, A., Munster, P., Munster, P., et al. (2001). New drugs in gynecologic cancer. *Current Treatment Options in Oncology, 2*(2), 119–128.

Door, A. (2002). Less common gynecologic malignancies. *Seminars in Oncology Nursing, 18*(3), 207–222.

Greene, F. L., Page, D. L., Balch, C. M., Fleming, I. D., & Morrow, M. (Eds.). (2002). *AJCC: Cancer staging manual* (6th ed.). New York: Springer-Verlag.

Neto, A. G., Deavers, M. T., Silva, E. G., et al. (2003). Metastatic tumors of the vulva: A clinicopathologic study of 66 cases. *American Journal of Surgical Pathology, 27*(6), 799–804.

Olt, G. J. (2003). Fatigue and gynecologic cancer, *Current Women's Health Reports, 3*(1), 14–18.

Otto, S. E. (Ed.). (2001). *Oncology nursing* (4th ed.). Philadelphia: Mosby.

Ozols, R. F. (2002). Update on the management of ovarian cancer. *Cancer Journal, 8*(Suppl. 1), S22-S30.

Porter, S. (2002). Endometrial cancer. *Seminars in Oncology Nursing, 18*(3), 200–206.

Salom, E., Almeida, Z., & Mirhashemi, R. (2002). Management of recurrent ovarian cancer: Evidence-based decisions. *Current Opinions in Oncology, 14*(5), 519–527.

Sigimura, K., & Okizuka, H. (2002). Postsurgical pelvis: Treatment follow-up. *Radiology Clinics of North America, 40*(3), 659–680.

Tabano, M., Condosta, D., & Coons, M. (2002). Symptoms affecting quality of life in women with gynecologic cancer. *Seminars in Oncology Nursing, 18*(3), 223–230.

Tewari, K. S., & DiSaia, P. J. (2002). Radiation therapy for gynecologic cancer. *Journal of Obstetrics and Gynaecologic Research, 28*(3), 123–140.

Yarbro, C. H., Frogge, M. H., Goodman, M., & Groenwald, S. L. (Eds.). (2000). *Cancer nursing: Principles and practice* (5th ed.). Boston: Jones & Bartlett.

15 Head and Neck Cancer

Nancy D. Tsottles

Anita M. Reedy

I. Definition: Cancers of the head and neck are characterized by alterations or mutations of the cells of the mucous membranes lining structures in this region. This results in uncontrolled cell growth or cancer.
   A. Incidence
      1. Ninety percent of these cancers are of the squamous cell type. Head and neck cancers are categorized by location. The regions are the face, the nasal cavity and paranasal sinuses, the oral cavity, the pharynx, the larynx, and the thyroid.
      2. Head and neck cancers account for 5% of total cancers or 60,000 new cases per year. Fifty percent of these cancers are located in the oral cavity (25%) and larynx (25%).
   B. Epidemiology: The majority of people who contract the disease are over 50 years old, with men being two and one half times more likely to develop it than women. The incidence in women, however, has been increasing due to their increased use of tobacco products and alcohol.
   C. Morbidity and Mortality
      1. Stage I and II tumors are small and have a 5-year survival rate of 80% or more. Tumors are more difficult to detect at this stage.
      2. Stage III and IV tumors may involve surrounding tissue or lymph nodes. The 5-year survival is 40% or less. Detection at later stages is not uncommon, but distant metastases are not usually present.
      3. Most relapses occur locally in the head and neck.
      4. Distant metastases usually involve the lung, bone, and liver.
      5. There is a 20% to 40% chance of developing a second cancer of the head and neck, lung, or esophagus, possibly due to exposure to precipitating carcinogens, such as alcohol and tobacco.

II. Etiology: The development of head and neck cancers has been linked to several factors.
   A. Oral, pharyngeal, and laryngeal cancers have been linked to tobacco, including the smokeless variety, and alcohol use.
   B. Nasopharyngeal cancers have been linked to exposure to the Epstein-Barr virus and to being of Chinese ancestry.
   C. Exposure to the human papilloma virus, occupational hazards (eg, materials used in the furniture and textile industries), and vitamin deficiencies (vitamins B, C, and riboflavin, among others) may also play a role in the development of head and neck cancers.
   D. Genetic predisposition to cancer, such as mutations of the p53 tumor-suppressor gene, may also contribute to the development of head and neck cancers.

III. Patient Management

A. Assessment: Head and neck cancers may be hard to detect because of location.

1. Asymptomatic or silent in the early stages. This is particularly the case in the regions of the nasopharynx, paranasal sinuses and nose, oropharynx, hypopharynx, and cervical or upper esophagus.

2. Leukoplakia (white plaques) or painless erythroplasias (red, smooth areas) are often present in the oral cavity in the early stages of head and neck cancers. These lesions may be precancerous.

3. Sore throats and coldlike symptoms are also considered early signs.

4. Dysphagia, hoarseness, stridor, wheezing, and a lump in the neck are serious, late symptoms caused by tumors of the hypopharynx, larynx, thyroid, and parathyroid glands.

5. Dysphasia and bloody sputum result from tumor growth in the pharynx or esophagus.

6. Persistent earache may be caused by tumors in the nasopharynx and oral cavity.

7. Hearing loss, pain, tinnitus, and nasal obstruction may be caused by tumor growth in the nasopharynx.

8. Metastasis can result if the tumor invades the vascular system. The lungs and bones are the most frequent sites of metastasis.

B. Diagnostic parameters: Usually a combination of some or all of these procedures is used to diagnose head and neck cancers.

1. Physical examination is the best method of detection of tumors in the head and neck region.

   a. The mouth needs to be thoroughly examined using a light.

   b. The neck needs to be palpated to check for masses and lymph nodes. Although a thyroid nodule is not diagnostic, a rapidly growing mass, especially when associated with pain, does cause a high level of suspicion for a thyroid malignancy.

2. Elevated thyroid function tests and serum calcitonin levels may be a sign of cancer of the thyroid.

3. Imaging tests include computed tomography (CT) scans and magnetic resonance imaging (MRI) for screening as well as diagnosis of head and neck cancers, especially of the sinuses and soft tissue of the neck. MRI has superior capabilities for imaging soft tissue and may reveal small masses. Dental imaging or Panorex studies may be used to evaluate the teeth and to look for bone invasion. Positron emission tomography (PET) scans are also sometimes used to further evaluate the extent of disease and to assist in detecting metastatic disease.

4. Endoscopies can view primary tumors as well as metastasis. Endoscopy can also be used to biopsy places that are difficult to view, such as the nasopharynx, larynx, and esophagus.

5. Biopsy is the only definitive diagnostic procedure and should be performed when cancer is suspected. All sites except the larynx and esophagus are accessible to biopsy using local anesthetics; however, laryngoscopy under anesthesia may be necessary to obtain a thorough examination. The tumor is then staged as to size and the presence of regional or distant metastasis.

C. Treatment: Treatment for head and neck cancers depends on the type of tumor, the staging of the tumor, and the general condition of the patient. There are single and multiple modality treatment approaches. Single modality treatment with surgery or radiation therapy is generally recommended in stage I or II disease. For stage III or IV disease, multiple treatments are utilized (Table 15–1) and may include combinations of chemotherapy, radiation therapy, and surgery. When the disease is advanced, evaluation should include a multidisciplinary team (ie, surgeon, medical oncologist, radiation oncologist, nutritionist, dentist, and rehabilitation specialists in speech and swallowing). Clinical trials are being conducted to evaluate the effectiveness of giving chemotherapy as a first-line treatment to decrease the size of the tumor before surgery or radiation. The goal is to preserve organ function.

  1. Chemotherapy may be given in inpatient, outpatient, or home settings. It is usually given in combination with other treatment modalities. Chemotherapy may be used before, during, or after surgery or radiation therapy. Some commonly used agents include cisplatin, carboplatin, paclitaxel, docetaxel, 5-fluorouracil, gemcitabine, and methotrexate. These may be used in combination or as single agents.

  a. Patients and families need to be taught what side effects to expect, such as nausea, vomiting, diarrhea, loss of appetite, alopecia, fatigue, peripheral neuropathy, and bone marrow suppression.

  b. Patients and families need to be taught how to manage these side effects, including instructions for use of an antiemetic regimen (see Chapters 22, 23, 25, 27, and 28).

  c. Patients need to be taught how to take their temperatures to assess for fevers during times when their white blood cell counts are low and to use safety precautions (eg, electric razors for shaving) when their platelet counts are low.

  d. Patients and families need to know about troubleshooting problems with infusion pumps and the resources available to them.

  e. Home nursing needs to be in place for patients receiving chemotherapy or supportive care at home.

  f. Some chemotherapeutic drugs (eg, cisplatin, carboplatin, 5-fluorouracil, and bleomycin) can cause severe nausea and vomiting and are toxic to the kidneys. Patients need to be hydrated with intravenous (IV) fluids and encouraged to take in oral fluids to minimize renal toxicity (see Chapter 6).

  g. Teaching should include symptoms and side effects that should be reported immediately (eg, fever, uncontrolled nausea and vomiting).

  2. Radiation may be given alone or in combination with other treatment modalities.

  a. Patients and families need to know the side effects of radiation therapy, such as fatigue, nausea, vomiting, diarrhea, loss of appetite, loss of taste, mucositis, xerostomia, alopecia, irritation and swelling to the area of treatment, and skin changes.

TABLE 15-1 Treatment Modalities Used in Head and Neck Cancers

Location	Signs/Symptoms	Stage	Treatment
Lip	Slow-growing mass or ulcerative lesion, pain, bleeding	Usually detected early (Stage I or II)	Simple surgical removal of tumor or radiation
Oral cavity	Exophytic mass or infiltrating tumor, pain, bleeding, loose teeth or ill-fitting dentures, difficulty chewing and talking	Stage I or II Stage III or IV	Transoral resection; radiation. May include surgical procedures such as mandibulectomy and unilateral or bilateral neck dissection; radiation; chemotherapy
Oropharynx	Dysphagia, pain, weight loss, neck mass	Stage I or II Stage III or IV	Radiation; surgery (neck dissection) Surgery; radiation; chemotherapy (often in combination)
Nasopharynx	Nasal obstruction, pain, otitis media, tinnitus, neck mass	Stage I or II (rarely diagnosed at this stage) Stage III or IV (especially with metastasis to areas such as the cranium or brain where surgery is not an option)	Radiation is the primary treatment; may be followed with surgery Radiation in combination with chemotherapy
Nasal cavity and paranasal sinuses	Unilateral nasal obstruction, dental pain, loose teeth, ill-fitting dentures, trismus, headache, diplopia, nonhealing ulcer, bleeding	Stage I or II Stage III or IV (often diagnosed as a more advanced tumor)	Surgical removal of lesion Extensive surgical procedures (eg, orbital exenteration) may be needed along with radiation and, possibly, chemotherapy. It is important to consider the emotional and physical condition of the patient and especially the prognosis before employing extensive surgical procedures.

Larynx	Hoarseness, dyspnea if airway involved	Stage I or II	Definitive radiation or surgical removal of the tumor, usually with partial laryngectomy, may include modified or radical neck dissection
		Stage III or IV	Organ preservation using induction chemotherapy followed by definitive radiation +/− surgery depending on response or surgery usually requiring total laryngectomy (loss of function when total laryngectomy done), partial thyroidectomy and modified or radical neck dissection, may be followed by adjuvant radiation.
Hypopharynx	Pain, otalgia, neck stiffness, neck mass, irritation, and retention of mucus	Stage I or II (usually not diagnosed in these stages)	Surgical removal of tumor with modified or radical neck dissection; radiation
		Stage III or IV	Surgery (may require laryngectomy); radiation; chemotherapy; organ preservation using induction chemotherapy and definitive radiotherapy may be used as an alternative to surgery for patients with T2-T3 disease.
Thyroid	Asymptomatic thyroid nodule	Stage I or II	Sub- or total thyroidectomy and radiation
		Stage III or IV	Radiation

    b. Patients need to know how to manage side effects (eg, methods to maintain adequate nutrition, use of nutritional supplements, feeding tubes, mouth care, skin care, and energy conservation; see Chapter 28).

    c. Patients receiving radiation therapy to the head and neck area should have a dental evaluation before starting treatment and should receive prophylactic fluoride because they are at high risk for tooth decay secondary to xerostomia.

    d. Patients need to be aware of the importance of keeping follow-up appointments and where to call for any problems or questions.

  3. Surgery may be used alone or in combination with other treatment modalities. The type of surgery depends on the site of disease, size of tumor, and structures involved. Lymph nodes (LN) in the neck may be removed due to the risk of nodal metastasis. Surgery may be a radical, modified radical, or selective LN dissection, depending on the tumor site and degree of cervical LN involvement.

    a. Patient and families need to know about the management of surgical sites (which may include tracheostomies, radical neck dissections, or facial surgeries) and resources available to assist them. Wound healing may be delayed if prior radiation therapy has been given.

    b. Home nursing or physical, occupational, swallowing, or speech therapy may be necessary. Maintaining adequate nutrition may require the use of a feeding tube. Patients and families will require instruction regarding care of the tube and the procedure for feeding.

    c. Potential emergency situations, such as carotid artery rupture, should be discussed, and a plan for intervention should be identified.

D. Nursing Diagnosis and Related Interventions and Outcomes

  1. Alteration in health maintenance related to lifestyle, which may include tobacco and alcohol use, and lack of knowledge about the prevention and detection of head and neck cancers

    a. *Problems*

      (1) Certain lifestyles put patients at greater risk for developing head and neck cancers. There is a strong correlation between smoking, alcohol use, and head and neck cancer. Patients who stop smoking (Ostroff et al., 1994) and who stop drinking alcohol (Deleyiannis, Thomas, Vaughan & Davis, 1996) have a longer survival rate after treatment for head and neck cancers and are less likely to experience tumor recurrence or secondary tumors. It can be difficult for patients to stop smoking or drinking alcohol because the use of either substance involves a complex dependency issue and the diagnosis of cancer increases life stress.

      (2) Routine examination is essential for early detection of head and neck cancers.

    b. *Interventions*

      (1) Gather the patient's history, including alcohol and tobacco use as well as radiation and chemical exposure.

(2) Educate the patient about the association between alcohol and tobacco use and the development and recurrence of head and neck cancer. Encourage the patient to stop the use of tobacco and alcohol. Refer the patient to support groups or therapists for help in this process.

(3) Assess the oral cavity areas for leukoplakia, erythroplasia, and poor oral hygiene. Educate the patient about the importance of assessing his or her own mouth for leukoplakia or erythroplasia. The patient can do this while brushing teeth. Educate the patient about maintaining good oral hygiene. Assess the frequency of the patient's dental visits, because routine oral examinations are often conducted at this time.

(4) Palpate the neck for masses and the presence of enlarged lymph nodes.

  c. *Desired outcomes*

(1) The patient will state the risk factors associated with the development of head and neck cancer and the resources available to decrease these risk factors (smoking cessation programs and so forth).

(2) The patient will state the signs and symptoms of head and neck cancer and a plan to monitor for tumors.

2. Knowledge deficit related to disease process and treatment

  a. *Problem:* Fear, anxiety, and uncertainty are emotions that accompany the diagnosis of head and neck cancer. One way to help patients deal with this is to teach them about the disease process and treatment. This helps the patient to gain some control over decisions regarding treatment options.

  b. *Interventions*

(1) Begin instructional sessions with simple explanations about the patient's diagnosis and planned treatments. Assess response to learning. The patient may not be able to assimilate complicated information right away due to fear, anxiety, or denial; therefore, plan on more than one instructional session with the patient and family.

(2) Reinforce information on the treatment options appropriate for the patient.

(3) Discuss possible side effects of specific treatments, and assure the patient that there are methods to manage side effects.

(4) Use a variety of methods for teaching (eg, pamphlets, handouts, and audiovisuals). Discussions with other patients who have had similar treatment may be helpful.

(5) Provide emotional and advocacy support for decisions made by the patient.

  c. *Desired outcomes*

(1) The patient will state risk factors of alcohol and tobacco use in the development and recurrence of head and neck cancer.

(2) The patient will identify resources to help with the cessation of tobacco and alcohol use.

(3) The patient will state the warning signs of head and neck cancer and demonstrate how to assess for signs of head and neck cancer.

(4) The patient will be able to state the importance of good oral hygiene and the importance of routine visits to the dentist.

3. Body image disturbance related to presence of cancer and its treatment

    a. *Problem:* Depending on the extent of tumor growth at diagnosis and on required treatment, the patient may experience significant changes in physical appearance. Surgical procedures may result in a tracheostomy, loss of muscle mass, and damage to some of the nerves in the neck. Treatment with radiation may result in damage to surrounding internal tissue and to the skin, causing changes such as redness, dryness, and peeling. Chemotherapy may result in skin changes and hair loss. Poor appetite, dysphagia, nausea, and vomiting may result in weight loss. All these can contribute to a drastic change in appearance and require many emotional adjustments.

    b. *Interventions*

        (1) Prepare the patient ahead of time for changes that may occur.

        (2) Assure the patient that most of these changes (skin alterations, hair and weight loss) are temporary and that tracheostomy stoma shrinkage, restrengthening of muscle mass, and regeneration of nerves will improve over time.

        (3) Encourage the patient to discuss feelings about these changes.

        (4) Discuss the use of wigs, hats, and turbans and the locations where these can be purchased. Discuss the use of loose clothing and scarves that can be placed around the neck to help conceal the stoma.

        (5) Initiate a social work consult for patients who seem withdrawn or depressed, or who would benefit from group support or individual therapy.

    c. *Desired outcomes*

        (1) The patient and family will be able to describe expected changes in physical appearance and some interventions that can help minimize them.

        (2) The patient will discuss feelings related to changes in the body and body image.

4. Fear and anxiety related to cancer diagnosis and possible recurrence or spread of the disease.

    a. *Problem:* Early-stage (local) tumors have a better rate of cure, but more advanced disease increases the possibility of metastasis and recurrence. Prognosis is based primarily on the type of tumor, staging of the tumor, and the general condition of the patient. The condition of the patient at the time of diagnosis impacts on ability to tolerate treatment. Specific information about treatment and prognosis may reduce anxiety.

    b. *Interventions*

        (1) Recognize the fears and concerns of the patient as valid and include the patient's priorities in treatment decisions.

        (2) Openly discuss and encourage verbalization of these feelings.

(3) Balance feelings of fear with reasonable hope so that a realistic set of expectations can be obtained.

(4) Give the patient all the information available to help make the best decisions and to promote a feeling of control.

c. *Desired outcomes*

(1) The patient and family will express fears and concerns related to diagnosis and fear of recurrence.

(2) The patient and family will have realistic expectations of treatment.

5. Less than adequate nutrition to meet body requirements, related to such symptoms as dysphagia, nausea, vomiting, diarrhea, and poor appetite.

a. *Problem:* Both tumor and treatment can interfere with many bodily functions. This can make it difficult to maintain adequate nutrition. Dysphagia is a late symptom of tumor presence that can interfere with the patient's ability to swallow anything more than liquids. Nausea, vomiting, diarrhea, and decreased appetite, all of which limit the patient's nutrition, are associated with treatment. Xerostomia (dry mouth) may be associated with some chemotherapy agents, radiation therapy, or surgery that may involve the salivary glands. In some instances, the xerostomia may be permanent, and may be mild to severe.

b. *Interventions*

(1) Assess ability to maintain adequate nutrition by such measures as weights and calculation of intake and output.

(2) Initiate a dietary consult, at which time a calorie count can be started. Patient preferences can be solicited. A liquid or soft diet with dietary supplements may be necessary if there is obstruction or damage to the gastrointestinal (GI) tract.

(3) Maintain nutrition status through a feeding tube (gastrostomy or jejunostomy) or IV feeding if necessary. Assess and maintain the catheter site as needed. Teach patient and family how to administer nutrition through a feeding tube. Home nursing visits may be needed to assess proper maintenance of nutrition and fluid intake, as well as use and care of the catheter.

(4) Monitor nausea, vomiting, xerostomia, and diarrhea because they can inhibit adequate nutrition (see Chapter 28).

(5) Chronic xerostomia may interfere with many activities of daily living including eating (taste, chewing, swallowing, dentures), speaking, sleeping, physical exercise, and social activities. This condition has been associated with an increase in dental caries, periodontal disease, oral stomatitis, and gastroesophageal reflux. In addition to interventions listed in Chapter 29, pilocarpine may be used to stimulate residual function of the salivary glands but is contraindicated for people with uncontrolled asthma, acute iritis, or narrow-angle glaucoma.

c. *Desired outcomes*

(1) The patient will maintain adequate nutrition and hydration.

(2) The patient and family will state the factors interfering with proper nutrition and the methods to maintain adequate nutrition.

(3) The patient and family will administer adequate nutrition through a feeding tube when the patient is unable to maintain adequate oral intake. The patient and family will state the importance of contacting the primary caregiver if adequate nutrition and hydration cannot be maintained.

(4) The patient and family will state methods to control nausea, vomiting, diarrhea, and other side effects of disease or treatment.

6. Potential for ineffective airway clearance related to thick secretions in tracheostomy or the presence of a tumor

  a. *Problem:* Neck masses can impinge on the integrity of the airways, causing shortness of breath, tachypnea, wheezing, and stridor. In the presence of a tracheostomy, the airway has been shortened and is easily dried out, causing thickened mucus that is difficult to clear by coughing, possibly leading to respiratory distress. Both of these conditions are potentially life threatening.

  b. *Interventions*

  (1) Assess respiratory rate, shortness of breath, dyspnea, the use of accessory muscles, and lung sounds, with particular attention to wheezing and stridor. Respiratory distress in the presence of a neck mass may require emergency procedures to protect the airway.

  (2) Assess expectorated mucus for thickness. Encouraging or providing adequate fluid intake can often prevent thickened respiratory secretions. Humidified air can also be helpful in keeping the secretion liquefied. In the presence of respiratory distress where the patient has a tracheostomy and thickened secretions, lavaging the tracheostomy with normal saline and suctioning the secretions until clear is usually effective. Keep an extra tracheostomy tube at the bedside.

  (3) If the patient goes home with a tracheostomy tube, instruct the patient and family on the care of the tube. Home nursing may also be needed to continue with teaching, assessing continued maintenance of the airway, and supporting the patient and family.

  c. *Desired outcomes*

  (1) A patent airway will be maintained.

  (2) The patient and family will be able to state the importance of maintaining a patent airway; routine care, if appropriate; and the interventions needed should the patient have difficulty breathing.

7. Fatigue related to radiation therapy or chemotherapy

  a. *Problem:* Fatigue is a common side effect of the treatment modalities used to treat head and neck cancer. Fatigue can interfere with the patient's ability to work, to maintain the home and family, and to continue receiving treatments.

  b. *Interventions:* Follow the recommendations in Chapter 25.

  c. *Desired outcomes:* See Chapter 25.

8. Pain related to side effects of treatment or local or metastatic tumor invasion of soft tissue and bone

    a. *Problem:* Treatment for head and neck cancer can result in painful side effects, such as mucositis. Tumors can press against or invade nerve fibers present in body tissue, causing pain. Pain decreases the patient's quality of life and can make it difficult to carry on most normal activities. Pain is also irritating and distracting for the patient. Most pain can be managed with a variety of techniques.

    b. *Interventions:* Follow the recommendations in Chapter 30.

    c. *Desired outcomes*

       (1) Patient and family will be able to state strategies for the control of pain.

       (2) Pain will be controlled or eliminated.

E. Discharge Planning and Patient Education

    1. Provide education specific to the treatment received and condition of the patient. Provide information, teaching, and support related to pain and symptom management, tracheotomy care, nutritional support, feeding tube care, dental care, xerostomia, smoking cessation, and social integration.

    2. Provide the patient and family with information about plans for follow-up and emergency care. Patients should have a complete head and neck examination every 1 to 3 months during the first year after treatment, and every 2 to 4 months during the second year. The intervals between examinations can then be lengthened to 3 to 6 months during years 3 to 5, and 6 to 12 months thereafter. The risk of relapse is highest in the first 2 years after treatment.

    3. Assess and refer the patient and family to appropriate home care or rehabilitation programs. Individual counseling or participation in support groups may provide additional psychosocial support. Provide information regarding community and Internet resources such as Support for People with Oral and Head and Neck Cancer (SPOHNC), International Association of Laryngectomees (IAL), and the American Cancer Society's Cancer Survivor Network.

REFERENCES

Deleyiannis, F. W. B., Thomas, D. B., Vaughan, T. L., & Davis, S. (1996). Alcoholism: Independent predictor of survival in patients with head and neck cancer. *Journal of the National Cancer Institute, 88*(8), 542–549.

Fang, B., & Forastiere, A. (2001). Head and neck cancer. In J. Abraham & C. Allegra (Eds.), *Bethesda handbook of clinical oncology.* Philadelphia: Lippincott Williams & Wilkins.

Gluckman, J., Gullane, P., & Johnson, J. (1994). *Practical approach to head and neck tumors* (pp. 1–16). New York: Raven Press.

Iwamoto, R. R. (1996). Xerostomia. In S. L. Groenwald, M. H. Frogge, M. Goodman, & C. H. Yarbro (Eds.), *Cancer symptom management.* Boston: Jones and Bartlett.

National Comprehensive Cancer Network. (2001). *Practice guidelines in oncology: Head and neck cancers.* Version 1.

Ostroff, J. S., Jacobsen, P. B., Moadel, A. B., Spiro, R. H., Shah, J. P., Strong, E. W., et al. (1994). Prevalence and predictors of continued tobacco use after treatment of patients with head and neck cancer. *Cancer, 75*(2), 569–576.

Snow, G. B. (1992). Evaluating and staging. In G. B. Snow & J. R. Clark (Eds.), *Multimodality therapy for head and neck cancer* (pp. 4–22). New York: Thieme Medical.

16 Leukemia

Aiko M. Kodaira

I. Definition

A. Leukemia accounts for about 4% of all new cancer cases in the United States and is generally perceived as a fatal disease (Jemal et al., 2003). Leukemia is a group of hematopoietic malignancies characterized by both quantitative and qualitative alteration in circulating leukocytes affecting the bone marrow and lymphatic system. It is believed that leukemia may be caused by the arrest of one or more of the following normal cell functions: cell differentiation (maturation), proliferation (reproduction), and/or apoptosis (programmed natural cell death). Leukemia is a malignant disease associated with diffuse abnormal and uncontrolled proliferation of immature leukocyte precursors in the bone marrow. The malignant cell replaces normal elements in all areas of hematopoietic bone marrow. Leukemia is described by a particular cell type of origin. Most types originate in the white blood cell lines, but leukemia can also begin in the erythroid (red blood) or megakaryoid (platelet) cell line. Leukemias are classified by the extent of differentiation or by the maturity of the cells. The acute leukemias are minimally or poorly differentiated and are characterized by the presence of immature cells called blasts. The chronic leukemias show a greater degree of differentiation or maturation. An overview of the common subtypes of leukemia, classifications, and characteristics is included in Table 16–1. Some institutions use the French-American-British (FAB) classification system for acute leukemia. This is presented in Figure 16–1.

B. Different types of leukemia affect different age groups. The majority of acute lymphocytic leukemia (ALL) cases are seen in children, whereas chronic lymphocytic leukemia (CLL) is typically a disease of the elderly. Remissions are often obtained with current therapies; however, relapse is common and probable, especially in adults. The two most common causes of death in leukemic patients are infection and bleeding. The accumulation of dysfunctional cells limits available nutrients and space in the bone marrow. This restricts the production of normal hematopoietic cells and their ability to differentiate, mature, and function normally. Failure to manage the consequences of this loss of functional leukocytes, red blood cells, and platelets often results in death. The etiology of leukemia remains unclear; however, recent advances in molecular genetic analysis have provided critical insights into the nature of leukemia. Although there are still many questions to be answered, there is no doubt that molecular genetic analysis will change the future of leukemia treatment.

II. **Etiology:** The definitive etiology of leukemia is unknown, although a number of causative factors have been identified.

  A. Immune Response Factors

  1. The first theory is the immune competence theory, which states that having any immune deficiency predisposes a person to a hematologic malignancy. This is supported by an increased incidence of leukemia after solid organ transplantation.

  2. A second theory is that genetic predisposition abnormalities may cause leukemia. There is an increased incidence of acute leukemia in children with Down syndrome and Fanconi's anemia. Additionally, people with a family member diagnosed with leukemia have four- to sevenfold increased risk for leukemia (Yarbro, Frogge, Goodman & Groenwald, 2000).

  3. The viral theory links some viruses to the development of leukemia. The most significant supporting factor is the human T-cell leukemia virus (HTLV-I) associated with adult T-cell leukemia in Japan and the Caribbean. HTLV-II is associated with a rare form of hairy cell leukemia and is prevalent in intravenous drug abusers.

  B. Risk Factors: Two clear risk factors exist for the development of leukemia, especially the acute form.

  1. Exposure to ionizing radiation (survivors of the atomic bomb or nuclear accidents have an increased incidence of acute leukemia).

  2. Exposure to known cytotoxic chemicals (cytotoxic drugs are often used to treat other malignancies or autoimmune diseases). Acute myelogenous leukemia (AML) is the most frequently reported treatment-related secondary cancer.

III. **Patient Management**

  A. Assessment: The following are signs and symptoms of leukemia:

  1. *Granulocytopenia-related symptoms:* Fevers, persistent infections (common sites are lung and sinus, urinary tract, abdomen, oral cavity, and perirectal area), prolonged wound healing. These symptoms often indicate malignant changes in both quality and quantity of leukocytes.

  2. *Thrombocytopenia-related symptoms:* Petechiae, rashes, easy bruising, bleeding gums, epistaxis, hemoptysis. Uncontrolled bleeding or intracranial bleeding may occur secondary to disseminated intravascular coagulation (DIC), a common complication associated with acute promyelocytic leukemia (APL or M3 AML).

  3. *Anemia-related symptoms:* Fatigue, malaise, and decreased tolerance for exercise or activities of daily living (ADL), pallor, dyspnea, chest pain, cold intolerance.

  4. *Leukemia infiltrate-related symptoms:* Splenomegaly, lymphadenopathy, pain or swelling in bones and joints, inflammation of the gums. In severe cases, renal failure or respiratory distress may be observed. Headache, mental status change, nausea and vomiting, and cranial nerve palsies are occasionally exhibited as signs of central nervous system (CNS) infiltration by leukemia cells and most frequently occur in patients with ALL.

TABLE 16–1 Leukemia Overview

Leukemia Type (FAB classification)	Defining Characteristics	Prognosis
Acute nonlymphocytic leukemia	Cell maturation arrested along the myeloid cell line	Prognosis of leukemia is highly dependent on the type of cytogenetic abnormality involved. Cytogenetic abnormalities are divided into three groups: normal, favorable, and poor.
Acute leukemia—minimally differentiated (M0 AML)	Age at onset: 18–25 years and 45–60 years, low to high WBC count at presentation. Splenomegaly, hepatomegaly, and lymphadenopathy are usually not seen.	No abnormality, +8, 11q23, +21, del(9q) are normal t(8;21), inv(16) are favorable, and complex, −7, −5 are poor. M4 and M5 AML often involve MLL gene (11 gene) abnormalities, such as t(11;17)(q23;q21) or t(6;11)(q27;q23). 65% to 80% achieve remission with therapy, relapse is common. Median survival with treatment is 10–15 months.
Acute leukemia—undifferentiated myelocytic (M1 AML)		
Acute myelocytic leukemia AML (M2 AML)		
Acute myelomonocytic leukemia AM ML (M4 AML)	Often high WBC at presentation, with organ infiltration, such as gum hypertrophy, cutaneous leukemia, splenomegaly, hepatomegaly and lymphadenopathy. High incidence of central nervous system (CNS) involvement.	
Acute monocytic leukemia AMoL (M5 AML)		
Erythroleukemia EL (M6 AML)	Complicated diagnosis, hard to distinguish from MDS, poor response to chemotherapy	Poor prognosis
Megakaryocytic leukemia (M7 AML)	Extremely rare type of AML. Large organs (liver, spleen), accumulation of sclerotic tissue in bone marrow	Poor prognosis
Acute promyelocytic leukemia APL (M3 AML)	Normal to moderately high WBC at presentation, high risk for DIC	APL with t(5;17) with PML/RARα fusion protein is highly responsive to ATRA therapy and approximately 85% of patients achieve complete remission.

Acute lymphocytic leukemia

Erythroleukemia EL (M6 AML)

Cell maturation arrested along the lymphoid cell line

T-cell disease has a favorable prognosis

Childhood acute lymphocytic leukemia (L1 ALL)

Leukemia is most common form of cancer in children, and 75% of those are ALL. Age of onset: 2–3 years.

Patient with t(9;22), t(1;19), infant with t(4;11), high WBC count, age <1 year or >10 years, CNS involvement, and longer time to achieve remission are associated with poor prognosis.

Splenomegaly, hepatomegaly, lymphadenopathy, CNS involvement are prevalent.

Adult acute lymphocytic leukemia (L2 ALL)

Philadelphia chromosome (t(9;22)) is the most common cytogenetics abnormality in adults. Splenomegaly, hepatomegaly, lymphadenopathy, CNS involvement are prevalent.

Poorer prognosis than childhood ALL. Poor prognosis with t(9;22) involving 11q23 and t(1;19). Age >50 years, high WBC, longer time to achieve remission are associated with poorer prognosis.

Burkitt's type leukemia (L3 ALL)

Age at onset: after 65 years, mature B-cell ALL, high CNS involvement and high tumor burden, high risk for TLS, rapid clinical course

Worst prognosis in ALL, involve t(8;14)(q24;q11). High LDH associated with poor prognosis.

Chronic myelocytic leukemia (CML)

7% to 15% of adult leukemia, median age at onset 45–55 years, 90% of patients have + Philadelphia chromosome (t(9;22)), characterized by a chronic phase followed by an accelerating and blastic phase.

Treatment is most effective in chronic phase. Accelerating and blastic phases are often refractory to treatment. 3 years of median survival with treatment.

Chronic lymphocytic lymphoma (CLL)

Age at onset: after 60 years, most common type of leukemia in adults, may be familial, prone to viral infection, patients with low-risk CLL often do not require treatment for many years.

4–6 years of median survival rate. Low-risk patients mostly die of other causes, whereas the high-risk CLL patients die from disease-related complications within a few months of diagnosis.

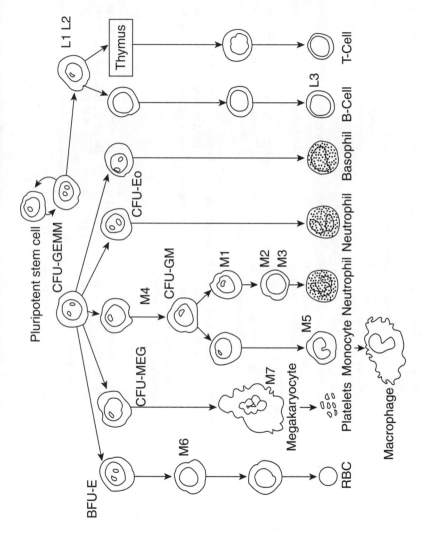

Figure 16-1. Hematopoietic cascade and FAB classification.

B. Diagnostic Parameters
   1. Laboratory tests
      a. Complete blood count (CBC) reflects anemia, thrombocytopenia, and neutropenia.
      b. Differential white blood cell (WBC) count will indicate the main cell type involved and reveal the number of absolute neutrophil cells (ANC). This helps to determine the body's infection fighting potential.
   2. Other tests
      a. Bone marrow aspirate typically shows the highest concentration of blast (immature) WBC. This specimen provides information such as flow cytometry analysis and cytogenetics. It allows physicians to make a preliminary reading for the diagnosis. Peripheral blood may be used for flow cytometry in the case of an unsuccessful bone marrow aspirate or biopsy. Flow cytometry identifies the cluster of differentiation (CD) on leukocytes' surface and is used to determine the maturation of cells, which aids in the diagnosis.
      b. Morphology, molecular genetic analysis, and fluorescence in situ hybridization (FISH testing) are also commonly used in the specific diagnosis of the type of leukemia.
      c. Bone marrow biopsy provides information such as bone marrow cellularity, architecture, fibrosis, and immunohistochemistry.
      d. Peripheral blood smear can be used for preliminary diagnosis, but a full examination of the bone marrow is required for the final diagnosis.
C. Treatment (see Table 16–2 for common leukemia treatments): Remissions are frequently obtained with chemotherapy, but relapse is common. Patients with "poor prognostic" leukemia, such as refractory disease, poor cytogenetic abnormalities, or secondary or myelodysplastic syndrome (MDS)-related leukemia may benefit from blood and marrow transplantation (BMT). BMT offers the greatest chance for disease-free survival or cure in these patients. Children have the best survival and cure rates with BMT (see Chapters 5 and 6).
D. Nursing Diagnoses
   1. Alteration in protective mechanisms related to disease and treatment
      a. *Problem:* The combination of bone marrow failure, overproduction of malignant hematopoietic cells, the presence of dysfunctional WBC, and treatment-induced granulocytopenia often leads to the development of bacterial, fungal, and viral infections in leukemia patients. Unresolved infection can result in sepsis and death. The state of low WBC counts is called neutropenia (ANC <1000).
      b. *Interventions* (see Chapter 22)
        (1) Assess potential sites for early detection of infection. Central access devices, oropharynx, lung, and perineal and rectal areas are common sites of infection. Implement infection prevention precautions.
        (2) Recognize signs of infection in the aplastic patient. Fever is often the first sign of infection in a leukemic patient due to the absence of leukocytes.

TABLE 16-2 Treatment of Common Types of Leukemias

Diagnosis	Treatment	Treatment-Related Common Issues
Acute myelogenous leukemia (AML)	Induction therapy: Cytosine arabinoside continuous infusion + daunorubicin, idarubicin, doxorubicin, etoposide, mitoxantrone, amsacrine Consolidation therapy: High-dose cytosine arabinoside boluses only or + etoposide Blood or marrow transplantation (BMT) Relapse: Gemtuzumab, same drugs as induction	Moderate to high-dose cytosine arabinoside (>200 mg/m^2), especially if given as contentious IV infusion, can cause severe pulmonary capillary leak syndrome and may result in ARDS. High-dose cytosine arabinoside, especially if given as boluses, can cause cerebellar toxicity. Maximum anthracycline doses may be reached after multiple relapses.
Acute promyelocytic leukemia (APL, M3AML)	Induction therapy: All-trans-retinoic acid (ATRA) + daunorubicin Maintenance therapy: ATRA Relapse: Arsenic	During induction therapy, ATRA increases the number of circulating WBC and may cause ATRA syndrome. The symptoms include fever, fluid retention, pleural infiltrates and effusion. Hydroxyurea and steroids are given to patients with high WBC count at diagnosis to prevent ATRA syndrome. Leukapheresis is strictly contraindicated in APL secondary to the high risk for DIC.
Acute lymphocytic leukemia (ALL)	Induction therapy: Vincristine, prednisone, asparaginase, daunorubicin, 6-mercaptopurine, cyclophosphamide, cytosine arabinoside, may include etoposide, mitoxantrone. CNS prophylaxis: Intracranial radiation and intrathecal methotrexate Postremission therapy: Induction drugs + methotrexate, and thioguanine Relapse: Same drugs as induction + ifosfamide	Asparaginase may increase ammonia level. Intrathecal treatment can be given by way of lumbar puncture or through ommaya reservoir. CNS prophylaxis can cause side effects such as somnolence, chemical arachnoiditis, cranial nerve paresis.

234

| Chronic myeloid leukemia (CML) | Chronic phase: Interferon alfa, imatinib mesylate, hydroxyurea, busulfan
Accelerating phase: Same as chronic phase
Blast crisis phase: Similar to that used in AML induction therapy.
Allogeneic bone marrow transplantation | Myelosuppression is a serious side effect of busulfan.
Long-term side effects include pulmonary or retroperitoneal fibrosis.
Heavy pretreatment increases risk of hepatic veno-occlusive disease (VOD) with marrow transplantation. |
| Chronic lymphocytic leukemia (CLL) | Asymptomatic patients: Observation only
Symptomatic patients: Rituxan, fludarabine, chlorambucil, cyclophosphamide, corticosteroids to treat leukocytosis and cytopenia, alemtuzumab
Radiation to treat lymphadenopathy or painful splenomegaly.
Advanced disease: Cyclophosphamide, vincristine, doxorubicin, and prednisone or fludarabine | Chronic and opportunistic infections are common problems. |

(3) Maintain patient on universal precautions and take additional precautions when other patients have severe or resistant infections that could be fatal to the patient with neutropenia.

(4) Reduce exposure to pathogens by limiting visitors with known infections and by having the patient wear a mask while in crowded areas.

(5) Obtain diagnostic cultures, x-rays, and computed tomography (CT) scans to identify infection.

(6) Administration of antimicrobial agents within the first hour of a new onset of fever is critical for neutropenic patients to prevent sepsis. Undetected gram-negative infection may result in rapidly developing sepsis and death. Monitor antimicrobial levels for normal range. Some institutions administer norfloxacin for gut decontamination to decrease gram-negative infection by way of the gastrointestinal (GI) tract.

(7) The use of hematopoietic colony stimulating factors, such as GCSF or GM-CSF, is not common practice during the AML induction therapy due to the theoretical concern of potentially enhancing the growth of residual myeloid leukemia. However, research indicates that the use of colony stimulating factors does not negatively affect the outcome of the AML treatment (Glaspy, 2001; Heil, 1997).

  c. *Desired outcome:* Infections will be prevented or successfully treated.

2. Alteration in protective mechanisms related to disease and treatment

  a. *Problem:* Thrombocytopenia occurs due to disease and treatment. Bleeding often occurs despite transfusion support.

  b. *Interventions*

  (1) Monitor daily blood counts and coagulation studies to determine if patient is at risk.

  (a) Spontaneous bleeding occurs at platelets $< 20,000/mm^3$.

  (b) DIC is a common complication of acute promyelocytic leukemia (APL/M3), although it may occur in other types of acute leukemia. APL cells are rich in procoagulants, and release of this substance into the bloodstream alters the normal coagulation cascade, leading to DIC. Management of DIC is critical because this remains a source of significant morbidity and mortality in the early stage of treatment in APL. Leukapheresis is strictly contraindicated in this population because it increases the risk of massive DIC (see Chapter 33).

  (2) Assess frequently the potential bleeding sites, such as oral cavity, IV access sites, urologic tract, GI tract, or any wounds. Test specimens for blood if bleeding is suspected (eg, emesis, urine, and stool).

  (3) Menstruation coexisting with thrombocytopenia and anemia can lead to life-threatening bleeding. Medications such as birth control pills are often used to cause cessation or absence of menstruation. Assess any vaginal blood loss by pad per day usage if patient continues to menstruate.

(4) Educate patient and family about bleeding potential, symptoms, reportable conditions, and interventions.

(5) Implement bleeding precautions (see Chapter 22). Avoid trauma and provide a safe environment. Limit invasive procedures when possible.

(6) Administer platelets, fresh frozen plasma, or cryoprecipitate as ordered.

c. *Desired outcome:* Patient will be successfully supported through the period of thrombocytopenia, as evidenced by minimal or no bleeding.

3. Fatigue related to disease and treatment

a. *Problem:* Disease and treatment may cause anemia, inability to rest/sleep, inadequate nutrition, and many other factors that result in fatigue.

b. *Interventions:* Follow recommendations in Chapter 25.

c. *Desired outcome:* Patient will manage fatigue to participate in self-care and optimize well-being.

4. Altered gas exchange related to disease process

a. *Problem:* Hypoxemia or hypercarbia occurs when excess WBC obstruct the pulmonary vasculature preventing the normal RBC circulation, altering gas exchange. Chemotherapy, especially cytosine arabinoside given as a continuous infusion, causes pulmonary capillary leak syndrome, resulting in fluid accumulation in the lungs. Pancytopenia and poor nutritional status result in a low vascular osmolality, which causes "third spacing" of fluid. Infection and vasodilation occurring with sepsis alter ventilatory exchange. ATRA, a drug used in APL treatment, may cause a rapid increase in the leukocyte count, which results in a number of symptoms (ATRA syndrome) that ultimately can cause acute respiratory distress syndrome (ARDS).

b. *Interventions*

(1) Assess risk for compromised pulmonary status: high WBC counts, treatment with cytosine arabinoside or ATRA, respiratory tract infection, sepsis, pancytopenia, or low blood osmolality.

(2) Monitor baseline and trends of arterial blood gases and oxygen saturations if indicated.

(3) Assess breath sounds every 8 hours and prn for crackles, bronchial sounds, or diminished breath sounds.

(4) Encourage coughing, turning, deep breathing, and ambulation. Encourage use of incentive spirometry to fully inflate lungs periodically.

(5) Monitor intake and output; ensure adequate urine output if aggressive hydration is needed.

c. *Desired outcomes:* Patient will maintain or achieve adequate pulmonary status as evidenced by (1) clear lung sounds, (2) Po_2 above 75%, (3) Sao_2 above 90%.

5. Alteration in fluid volume related to disease, treatment, or renal insufficiency

a. *Problem:* Increased fluid volume results from altered renal function and inadequate fluid excretion secondary to chemotherapy toxicity, antibiotic administration, and diuretics. Leukostasis (WBC > 100,000 cells/mm^3) causes sluggishness of blood and decreases glomerular filtration rate, which also results in decreased urine output. The uric acid produced by leukemic cell death may cause uric acid crystallization and kidney tubule obstruction. Aggressive hydration with inadequate urine output can worsen this condition. Lastly, capillary permeability or impaired cardiac function will increase fluid retention, although the fluid may not be in the vascular space.

b. *Interventions*
   (1) Assess population at risk, which includes patients receiving chemotherapy, aminoglycosides, amphotericin, or diuretics, and patients with high tumor burden, which may result in severe tumor lysis (see Chapter 40).
   (2) Monitor fluid volume status by strict intake and output measurements, frequent weights, and central venous pressures. Establish a goal weight and give diuretics as ordered to limit fluid retention.
   (3) Administer allopurinol, as ordered, with chemotherapy to prevent renal dysfunction from increased uric acid. Electrolyte imbalance can occur due to multiple causes (eg, antifungal therapy; see Chapter 22).
   (4) Monitor closely the respiratory status, check O_2 saturation every 4 hours, and auscultate breath sounds for crackles.
   (5) Assess for appearance of pitting edema in extremities.
   (6) Assess effects of hydration given in conjunction with diuretics.
   (7) Give renal doses of dopamine (1 to 2 μg/kg/min), as ordered, to increase renal perfusion.

c. *Desired outcomes:* Patient will maintain optimal fluid balance and renal function as evidenced by:
   (1) Maintenance of goal weight.
   (2) Normal blood urea nitrogen (BUN) and creatinine.
   (3) Adequate urine output.
   (4) Absence of crackles and edema.

6. Alterations in elimination related to chemotherapy or infection
   a. *Problem:* Diarrhea is a side effect of both chemotherapy and infection.
   b. *Interventions*
      (1) Recognize population at risk, which includes patients who are receiving chemotherapy or who are neutropenic.
      (2) Assess for potential causes of diarrhea, such as gastric toxic chemotherapy (see Chapter 6) or *Clostridium difficile* infection.
      (3) Obtain three successive stool cultures to rule out infectious etiology.
      (4) Assess perirectal area for breakdown and implement perirectal wound care recommendations.
      (5) Encourage use of bulk-forming foods or agents if diarrhea is not secondary to infection (see Chapter 23).

(6) Administer antidiarrheal medications, as ordered (only in the absence of infection). With recurrent diarrhea, give antidiarrheal only after negative results are confirmed from a new culture.

(7) Place patient on contact precautions according to institutional protocol, if potentially infected.

c. *Desired outcomes:* Patient will prevent or manage diarrhea and rectal breakdown.

E. Discharge Planning and Patient Education

1. Teach patients and family to avoid exposure to infection (eg, avoid large crowds and sick people) and recognize signs of infection and hemorrhage (see Chapter 22).

2. Educate patient and family members about the importance of optimal nutrition after discharge. Encourage foods high in calories to maintain adequate caloric intake, and magnesium and potassium to replace excreted electrolytes.

3. Refer the patient and family for social work/psychiatric consultation or follow-up if indicated.

4. Teach care of venous access devices.

5. Initiate home care referrals, as needed.

6. Teach the patient to recognize and report symptoms requiring immediate intervention (ie, fever, bleeding, sudden change or onset of symptom). Patient should verbalize a plan and have written instructions for emergency situations.

7. Review the plan of follow-up care and provide return appointments and appropriate referrals, such as evaluation for bone marrow transplantation, hospice, or home care.

REFERENCES

Applebaum, F. R. (1999). Molecular diagnosis and clinical decisions in adult acute leukemia. *Seminars in Hematology, 36*(4), 401–410.

Applebaum, F. R., et al. (2001). Acute myeloid leukemia. *Hematology, 2001,* 62–86.

Brain, B. (1998). Classification of acute leukemia: The need to incorporate cytogenetic and molecular genetic information. *Journal of Clinical Pathology, 51*(6), 420–423.

Cataland, S. R., et al. (2001). Genetic subtyping of adult acute leukemias and implications for treatment. *Oncology Spectrums, 2*(9), 617–625.

Courtens, A. M., et al. (1998). Nursing diagnosis in patients with leukemia. *Nursing Diagnosis, 9*(2), 49–61.

DeVita, V. T., et al. (2001). *Cancer: Principles & practice of oncology* (6th ed., pp. 2389–2509). Philadelphia: Lippincott Williams & Wilkins

Glaspy, J. A. (2001). Hematopoietic growth factors for patients with cancer. *Clinical Oncology, 4*(1), 1–13.

Heil, G. (1997). A randomized, double-blind, placebo-controlled, phase III study of filgrastim in remission induction and consolidation therapy for adult with de novo acute myeloid leukemia. *Blood, 90*(12), 4710–4718.

Jemal, A., Taylor, M., Samuels, A., Ghafoor, A., Ward, E., & Thun, M. J. (2003). Cancer statistics, 2003. *CA: Cancer Journal for Clinicians, 53*(1), 5–26.

Rowley, J. D. (1999). The role of chromosome translocations in leukemogenesis. *Seminars in Hematology, 36*(4), 59–72.

Rowley, J. D. (2000). Cytogenetic analysis in leukemia and lymphoma: An introduction. *Seminars in Hematology, 37*(4), 315–319.

Stoltsfus, P. K., et al. (2001). Molecular cytogenetics and gene analysis: Implication for oncology nurses. *Clinical Journal of Oncology Nursing, 5*(5), 201–206.

Swayers, C. L. (1999). Chronic myeloid leukemia. *The New England Journal of Medicine, 340*(17), 1330–1340.

Tallman, A. S., et al. (2002). Acute promyelocytic leukemia: Evolving therapeutic strategies. *Blood, 99*(3), 759–767.

Yarbro, C. H., Frogge, M. H., Goodman, M., & Groenwald, S. L. (Eds.). (2000). *Cancer nursing: Principles and practice* (5th ed., pp. 1244–1268). Boston, MA: Jones & Bartlett.

17 Lung Cancer

Jan Wemmer

I. Definition
  A. Pathology
    1. Lung cancer can arise from any tissue in the lungs.
    2. It can spread by direct extension into surrounding structures or by metastasizing through the lymphatic or hematogenous systems.
  B. Epidemiology
    1. Most common form of cancer among men and women in the United States.
    2. Leading cause of cancer death for both genders.
    3. Overall survival for all lung cancers remains poor, with less than 15% of patients alive 5 years after diagnosis.
    4. Prognosis is best with early-stage diagnosis, when treatment can lead to a 60% to 90% chance of cure. However, once the disease has spread beyond the early-stage tumor, curative treatment is unlikely.
  C. Classification of lung cancer is based on cell histopathology.
    1. Small-cell lung carcinomas (SCLC)
      a. Account for about 20% to 25% of all lung cancers.
      b. Tend to metastasize early in the course of the disease and commonly spread rapidly to bone, liver, central nervous system, lymph nodes, and pleura.
      c. Further divided into the following subtypes:
        (1) Oat cell
        (2) Intermediate grade
        (3) Mixed (small cell combined with another lung carcinoma cell type)
    2. Non-small-cell lung carcinomas (NSCLC)
      a. Account for 70% to 80% of lung cancers.
      b. Usually spread by direct extension and compression of surrounding structures, but can metastasize to bone, liver, brain, adrenals, and pericardium.
      c. Further differentiated into the following subtypes:
        (1) Epidermoid or squamous cell carcinoma
        (2) Adenocarcinoma (most commonly occurring lung cancer among nonsmokers and in women)
        (3) Large-cell carcinoma (lowest incidence overall)
    3. Pleural mesothelioma arise from the pleural lining of the lung.
      a. About 75% of tumors are diffuse and usually malignant.
      b. The remaining 25% are localized and usually benign.

II. Etiology

A. Tobacco smoke exposure is the main causative factor in both SCLC and NSCLC.

  1. Tobacco smoke is a potent carcinogen, and it also promotes the carcinogenic effect of other substances.

  2. Risk of lung cancer increases with the number of years of smoking, the number of cigarettes smoked, and the tar content of the cigarettes.

  a. Cigarette smoking risk is quantified in pack-years, which is the number of packs smoked per day multiplied by the number of years of smoking.

  b. At 10 pack-years, the number of deaths from lung cancer among smokers exceeds those among nonsmokers.

  c. Risk of lung cancer starts to decrease 5 years after smoking cessation.

B. Asbestos exposure has been implicated in the development of lung cancers (especially mesothelioma) in miners, shipyard workers, and pipe fitters.

C. Radon exposure is considered a risk factor for lung cancers, particularly in uranium miners. It is uncertain at this time whether environmental exposure to radon constitutes significant risk for lung cancer.

D. Other substances may play a role in the development of lung cancer.

  1. Arsenic

  2. Coal

  3. Chloromethyl methyl ether (CMME)

  4. Chromium

  5. Copper

  6. Hydrocarbons

  7. Ionizing radiation

III. Patient management: is determined by cell type, stage of disease, and symptomatology.

A. Assessment: The following signs and symptoms of lung cancer may be due to local tumor effects, metastasis, or systemic effects caused by paraneoplastic syndromes (Gerber, Mazzone & Arroliga, 2002; Mazzone & Arroliga, 2003; Messori, Lanza, Serio & Salvolini, 2003; Wen & Schiff, 2003). (See Table 17–1 for paraneoplastic syndromes associated with lung cancer.)

  1. Cough is the most common presenting symptom, occurring in up to 75% of patients.

  a. Centrally located tumors (ie, mainstem bronchi) are most often seen in small cell and squamous cell cancers, and are likely to cause bronchial obstruction, or atelectasis, that stimulates the cough reflex.

  b. Peripherally located tumors may also lead to coughing by creating pressure on the J receptors within the lung.

  c. Cough is frequently intractable and exhausting.

  d. Sputum production is usually indicative of a concomitant pulmonary infection due to airway obstruction and retained secretions.

  2. Wheezes are present with airway obstruction or bronchospasm related to coughing.

TABLE 17-1 Paraneoplastic Syndromes Associated With Lung Cancer

Syndrome	Primary Symptoms	SCLC	NSCLC
Cushing's syndrome	Ectopic secretion of adrenocorticotropic hormone, edema, proximal myopathy, elevated plasma and urinary cortisol levels, hyperglycemia, hypokalemic alkalosis	X	
Syndrome of inappropriate antidiuretic hormone (SIADH)	Hyponatremia, serum hypo-osmolality, urine hyperosmolality, elevated urine sodium, normal creatinine	X*	X
Hypercalcemia	Ectopic parathyroid hormone production and bone metastases are causes; serum calcium >11 mg/dL, anorexia, N/V, constipation, lethargy, irritability, confusion, coma, dehydration	X	X*
Lambert-Eaton myasthenic syndrome (LEMS)	Impairment of acetylcholine release from cholinergic terminals, muscle weakness, and hyperreflexia (especially lower extremities), autonomic dysfunction; symptoms may appear 2 to 4 years before tumor is diagnosed	X*	X
Encephalomyelitis	Dementia, cerebellar degeneration, brainstem encephalitis, myelitis; may occur months to years before tumor is diagnosed; may be associated with autoimmune mechanism	X*	X
Trousseau's syndrome	Hypercoagulable state; migratory venous thrombophlebitis and thromboembolism; unresponsive to oral anticoagulants	X	X

An asterisk in a column indicates higher prevalence of that complication.

3. Loud wheezes or stridor is most likely caused by obstruction of the large airways.
4. Hemoptysis can occur when tumors erode into the blood vessels in the lung.
5. Dyspnea may have multiple tumor-related etiologies, including compression of airways, atelectasis, pleural effusion, and pulmonary embolism.
6. Hoarseness is due to vocal cord paralysis resulting from tumor impingement on the laryngeal nerve.
7. Pain
   a. Chest wall pain caused by lung tumors may be described as an intermittent ache on one side, may be pleuritic in nature, or may be subscapular.
   b. Large tumors in the apex of the lung (Pancoast tumor) may cause pressure on the brachial plexus and result in shoulder pain (one of the symptoms of Horner's syndrome).

    c. Pain located elsewhere may be due to bone metastasis.

  8. Horner's syndrome, associated with apical tumors, causes nerve compression with shoulder or arm pain, ptosis, and weight loss.

  9. Weight loss is most commonly a symptom of late-stage disease, but may occur at any time.

    a. Well-established negative prognostic factors for patients with lung cancer include weight loss, poor performance status, presence of systemic symptoms, and a later stage at diagnosis.

    b. Weight loss bears such prognostic significance with this disease that many treatment protocols have significant weight loss as an exclusion criteria.

  10. Altered mental status is a common occurrence and may be due to various etiologies.

    a. Hypoxia can affect mental status and judgment.

    b. Most often an indicator of brain metastasis.

    c. Hypercalcemia should be considered in susceptible patients.

B. Diagnostic Parameters: Studies are performed to determine cell type and stage of disease (Tables 17–2, 17–3, and 17–4) and their prognostic implications (Table 17–5).

  1. Staging

    a. SCLC may be staged using two categories:

      (1) Limited stage (tumor confined to one hemithorax and regional lymph nodes and can fit into one radiation portal)

      (2) Extensive stage (outside of limited stage) metastatic

    b. NSCLC is most commonly classified using TNM (tumor, node, metastasis) classifications (see Table 17–3) and stage I-IV grouping (see Table 17–4).

  2. Diagnostic tests (see Table 17–2 for nursing interventions related to these pulmonary tests)

    a. Cytologic specimens may be obtained by several different techniques:

      (1) Sputum cytology

      (2) Fiberoptic bronchoscopy with brush washings

        (a) Ensure platelets >50,000 to 100,000/mm³ before procedure (exact count may vary with planned procedure or physician preference).

        (b) Establish a normal international normalized ratio (INR).

      (3) Mediastinoscopy with biopsy is especially useful if lymph nodes are visualized on positron emission tomography (PET) or computed tomography (CT).

      (4) Percutaneous needle biopsy may be used alone or in combination to determine cell type.

    b. Radiography (CXR), CT, magnetic resonance imaging (MRI), and PET are used to ascertain the location and size of the primary tumor and to determine sites of metastasis within and outside the thorax.

      (1) CXR may show a space-occupying, enhancing mass, although this test has proven too insensitive for early detection to be used as a screening tool, even in high-risk people.

      (2) CT scan (especially spiral/helical CT) is helpful in identifying suspicious masses and their exact location.

TABLE 17-2 Diagnostic Tests Used for Assessment/ Management of Lung Cancer

Procedure/ Description	Potential Complication	Nursing Management
Bronchoscopy: To Localize or Perform a Biopsy on a Lesion		
Local anesthetic (duration 2–8 hours)	Loss of gag reflex	• Give patient nothing by mouth before the procedure and until the gag reflex has returned. • Light sedation is also often used to reduce anxiety and distress during the procedure. • Maintain flat or semi-Fowler's position. • Administer bronchodilator.
Hyperextended neck	Tension on neck muscles and vertebrae	• Apply ice collar first 24 hours, then heat. • Provide lozenges and gargles when gag reflex returns. • Administer analgesics if pain is severe.
Insertion of bronchoscope	Laryngeal edema Possible laryngospasms or bronchospasms	• Observe for and report respiratory distress. • Obtain topical corticosteroid spray for the airway or racemic epineph-rine as ordered by the physician. • Administer oxygen.
Brush or needle biopsy	Possible bleeding	• Observe and report: – Hemoptysis.
	Possible infection	– Symptoms of upper respiratory infection—fever, cough, haziness on chest x-ray. – Dyspnea, decreased breath sounds, cyanosis.
	Possible pneumothorax	– Pneumothorax is often a slow-developing occurrence after pro-cedure due to a slow air leak, so it may present as dyspnea, chest discomfort, unequal chest excur-sion, diminished breath sounds on the lung where biopsy was per-formed, tympany of chest on side where biopsy was per-formed. • Administer oxygen.
Mediastinoscopy: To evaluate lymph node involvement		
General anesthetic	Aspiration	• Give client nothing by mouth before the procedure and until the gag reflex has returned.

(continued)

TABLE 17–2 Diagnostic Tests Used for Assessment/ Management of Lung Cancer *(Continued)*

Procedure/ Description	Potential Complication	Nursing Management
Mediastinoscopy: To evaluate lymph node involvement		

Insertion of scope into the intercostal space	Manipulation of the trachea
	Possible air leaks into the skin
	Possible pneumothorax
	Possible bleeding
	Possible mediastinitis
		• Administer analgesics as needed.
		• Assess for subcutaneous emphysema
		• Observe and report:
		  – Hemoptysis.
		  – Symptoms of upper respiratory infection—fever, cough, haziness on chest x-ray.
		  – Dyspnea, decreased breath sounds, cyanosis.
		  – Pneumothorax is often a slow-developing occurrence after procedure due to a slow air leak, so it may present as dyspnea, chest discomfort, unequal chest excursion, diminished breath sounds on the lung where biopsy was performed, tympany of chest on side where biopsy was performed.
		• Administer oxygen.

Postoperative recovery period	Two to three small incisions with sutures	• Administer mild analgesics as needed. • Clean and dress the exit wounds to prevent infection. • Assess for the presence of subcutaneous emphysema at the surgical sites and report to physician if present.
	Possible chest tube remaining postoperatively	• Observe drainage, exit site, respiratory fluctuations in the tubing, and presence or absence of an air leak. • Patients with an air leak should not be transported without suction unless specifically ordered by the physician. • Provide education, home care consultation, and follow-up visit plans for patients who go home with tubes in place.
Radiologic/nuclear imaging studies: To localize lesion or detect node involvement		
Chest x-ray	Radiologic exposure	• Instruct the patient of the need to take a deep breath and hold it for several seconds.

(continued)

TABLE 17–2 Diagnostic Tests Used for Assessment/ Management of Lung Cancer *(Continued)*

Procedure/ Description	Potential Complication	Nursing Management
Radiologic/nuclear imaging studies: **To localize lesion or detect node involvement**		
Computed tomography (CT) scan—Serial x-ray examination of sectional planes of the thorax and computer analysis to provide three-dimensional studies of the tissue	Noninvasive and a very short procedure if a spiral CT scanner is used, but patient must remain still and the machine surrounds the body and makes noises.	• Advise the patient when results may be available. • Instruct the patient of the need to take a deep breath and hold it for several seconds. • Advise the patient when results may be available.
CT scan with contrast media containing iodides or radioactive materials	Intravenous administration Possible hypersensitivity to contrast media (rare) Renal challenge of contrast media with subsequent renal insufficiency	• Warn patient of immediate sensations of warmth, flushing, bitter or salty taste, nausea/vomiting, and itching, and pain at the insertion site. • Perform emergency procedures as needed. • Assess baseline renal status with blood urea nitrogen (BUN), creatinine, and possibly creatinine clearance. • Provide hydration before and after procedure as ordered.
Positron emission tomography (PET) scanning	Intravenous administration Possible hypersensitivity to contrast	See above for implications.
Percutaneous CT- or Ultrasound-Guided Needle Biopsy: **To Obtain Histopathologic Specimen**		
CT scan or ultrasound with skin marking to note the location of a mass, nodule, or enlarged lymph node.	Pain at injection site and the discomfort of maintaining a specified position for a period of time. If particularly difficult, the scan or ultrasound may be simultaneous to the biopsy.	• Teach patient importance of histologic diagnosis. • Provide specific education about diagnostic test.

(continued)

▨ TABLE 17–2 **Diagnostic Tests Used for Assessment/ Management of Lung Cancer** (Continued)

Procedure/ Description	Potential Complication	Nursing Management
Sputum Cytology: To Collect and Assess Shedding Endobronchial Tissue for Histologic Diagnosis		
Three containers with fixative given to the patient for collection of sputum and saliva for cytology	None	• Instruct patient to collect daily specimens upon arising and before oral intake or brushing of teeth. • Inform patient about time required to analyze tissue and complete report.

Adapted from Lind, J. (1998). Nursing care of the client with lung cancer. In J. Itano & K. Taoka (Eds.), *ONS core curriculum for oncology nursing* (3rd ed., pp. 448–458). Philadelphia: W. B. Saunders.

(3) MRI may be used to differentiate tumor from vascular abnormalities.

(4) PET scan is especially helpful in conjunction with CT to more precisely define abnormalities in density that may indicate occult metastatic disease. The incidence of inaccurate early staging of NSCLC is significant enough that performing a PET scan before taking patients to the operating room for presumed curative surgery has become a standard of care (Silvestri, Tanoue, Margolis, Barker & Detterbeck, 2003).

   c. Bone scan is used to definitively diagnose bone metastasis.

   d. Hematology studies and blood chemistries are used to determine general health status and to identify paraneoplastic syndromes.

C. Treatment

  1. Surgery is the preferred treatment modality for limited-stage disease.

   a. Surgical procedures may be curative, controlling, or used for palliative symptom management.

   b. Newer surgical techniques have permitted minimally invasive procedures with more rapid recovery.

    (1) Video-assisted thoracoscopic surgery (VATS)

    (2) Ng laser endobronchial tumor resection (Morris et al., 2002)

   c. Common procedures

    (1) Lobectomy: Removal of affected lobe of lung

    (2) Wedge resection: Removal of larger portion of affected lung

    (3) Pneumonectomy: Removal of entire affected lung

    (4) Selective metastatic lesion excision (eg, solitary brain metastasis)

  2. Chemotherapy is the treatment of choice for patients with SCLC and with stage III and stage IV NSCLC. Table 17–6 lists chemotherapeutic regimens and drugs commonly used in the treatment of SCLC, NSCLC, and mesothelioma (see Chapter 6).

TABLE 17–3 Lung Carcinoma TNM Grading System

T = Primary Tumor

TX	Primary tumor cannot be assessed, or tumor proven by presence of malignant cells in sputum or bronchial washes but not visualized with imaging or bronchoscopy
T0	No evidence of primary tumor
TIS	Carcinoma in situ
T1	<3 cm diameter, surrounded by lung or pleura without invasion of mainstem bronchus
T2	Any of the following: >3 cm diameter, involves the mainstem bronchus 2 cm or more distal to the carina, invades visceral pleura, associated with atelectasis or obstructive pneumonitis extending to the hilar region but not involving the entire lung
T3	Any tumor size with direct extension into the chest wall, diaphragm, mediastinal pleura, parietal pericardium; tumor in the main bronchus <2 cm distal to the carina without involving the carina, associated atelectasis or obstructive pneumonitis involving the entire lung
T4	Tumor of any size invading any of the following: mediastinum, heart, great vessels, trachea, esophagus, vertebral body, carina; or tumor with malignant pleural effusion

N = Nodal Involvement

NX	Regional lymph nodes cannot be assessed
N0	No regional lymph node metastasis
N1	Metastasis in ipsilateral peribronchial and/or ipsilateral hilar lymph nodes, including direct extension
N2	Metastasis in ipsilateral mediastinal and/or subcarinal lymph node(s)
N3	Metastasis in contralateral mediastinal, contralateral hilar, ipsilateral or contralateral scalene or supraclavicular lymph node(s)

M = Distant Metastasis

MX	Distant metastasis cannot be assessed
M0	No distant metastasis
M1	Distant metastasis (beyond ipsilateral supraclavicular nodes)

Occult Stage

TX, N0, M0	Bronchopulmonary secretions contain malignant cells on multiple samples but no other evidence of primary tumor, or metastasis to regional or distant lymph nodes

American Joint Committee on Cancer. (1998). *AJCC cancer staging handbook* (6th ed., pp. 191–203). New York: Springer.

3. Radiotherapy is used as the primary treatment of stage I and II NSCLC tumors in patients who are not surgical candidates. Cranial radiotherapy also may be administered on a prophylactic basis in patients with SCLC to prevent brain metastasis. In addition, radiotherapy is used in the palliative treatment of many sequelae of lung cancer, including pain due to bone or brain metastasis, hemoptysis, severe cough, dyspnea, hoarseness, spinal cord compression, and obstructive pneumonia.

■ TABLE 17–4 **Lung Carcinoma Stage Grouping**

Stage 0		
Tis	N0	M0
Stage IA		
T1	N0	M0
Stage IB		
T2	N0	M0
Stage IIA		
T1	N1	M0
Stage IIB		
T2	N1	M0
T3	N0	M0
Stage IIIA		
T1	N2	M0
T2	N2	M0
T3	N0	M0
T3	N1	M0
T3	N2	M0
Stage IIIB		
anyT	N3	M0
T4	N0	M0
T4	N1	M0
T4	N2	M0
Stage IV		
any T	any N	M1

American Joint Committee on Cancer. (2002). *AJCC cancer staging handbook* (6th ed., pp. 191–203). New York: Springer.

■ TABLE 17–5 **Approximate 5-Year Survival With Treatment**

Stage	TNM subset	Average 5-year survival
IA	T1 N0 M0	82%
IB	T2 N0 M0	68%
IIA	T1 M1 N0	52%
IIB	T2 N1 M0	40%
	T3 N0 M0	
IIIA	T3 N1 M0	10% to 15%
	T1–3 N2 M0	
IIIB	T4 N0-2 M0	<5%
	T1–4 N3 M0	
IV	any T, any N, M	<2%

American Joint Committee on Cancer. (2002). *AJCC cancer staging handbook* (6th ed., pp. 191–203). New York: Springer.

▉ TABLE 17-6 Chemotherapy Drugs Used to Treat Lung Cancer

Small Cell

CAV	Cyclophosphamide Doxorubicin Vincristine	CCMV	Cyclophosphamide Lomustine Methotrexate Vincristine
CAVE	Cyclophosphamide Doxorubicin Vincristine Etoposide	Taxanes Topotecan Irinotecan	Paclitaxel or docetaxel
VP-P	Etoposide/VP-16 Cisplatin	Gleevec Vinorelbine	
CAE	Cyclophosphamide Doxorubicin Etoposide/VP-16	**Non–Small Cell**	
CEV	Cyclophosphamide Etoposide Vincristine	CAP	Cyclophosphamide Doxorubicin Cisplatin
PCE	Carboplatin Cyclophosphamide Etoposide	CMV	Cisplatin Mitomycin-C Vinblastine
IMP	Ifosfamide (with Mesna) Carboplatin	MACC	Methotrexate Doxorubicin Cyclophosphamide Lomustine
VP	Vincristine Carboplatin	EP	Etoposide Cisplatin
EP	Etoposide Cisplatin	MVP	Mitomycin Vinblastine Cisplatin
CVP	Cyclophosphamide Etoposide/VP-16 Cisplatin	Cisplatin/VP-16 (etoposide)	
PACE	Cisplatin Doxorubicin Cyclophosphamide Etoposide	Cisplatin/gemcitabine Cisplatin/vindesine/ VP-16 Cisplatin/vindesine	
CAVP16	Cyclophosphamide Doxorubicin Etoposide/VP-16	Cisplatin/vinorelbine Vinorelbine Paclitaxel	
MOCA	Methotrexate Vincristine Cyclophosphamide Doxorubicin	Paclitaxel/cisplatin Mitomycin/vinblastine/ cisplatin Iressa	
High-dose CMC-VAP	Cyclophosphamide Methotrexate Lomustine Vincristine Doxorubicin Procarbazine	*Note:* Carboplatin may be substituted for cisplatin. *Mesothelioma* Cisplatin Carboplatin Gemcitabine	

4. The addition of chemotherapy to radiation therapy has been shown to improve survival in patients with stage III NSCLC over radiation therapy alone.

D. Nursing Diagnoses

1. Impaired gas exchange related to lung tumors or loss of lung tissue

a. *Problem:* Lung tumors can impinge on surrounding structures causing airway obstruction, pleural effusion, blockage of the superior vena cava (superior vena cava syndrome), or postobstructive pneumonia. Patients with lung cancer are also at increased risk for pulmonary embolism due to mechanisms that are not completely understood at this time. Patients may also lose portions of the lung because of surgical procedures, leaving less surface area for oxygen diffusion.

b. *Interventions*

(1) Assess for shortness of breath (dyspnea on exertion, wheezing, stridor, labored respirations, crackles, rhonchi, orthopnea, anxiety, restlessness).

(2) Assess for symptoms of pulmonary infection (fever, chills, productive cough).

(3) Assess oxygenation status (color of nailbeds and mucous membranes, pulse oximetry, arterial blood gas results).

(4) Administer humidified oxygen as prescribed for decreased oxygen saturation and to maintain sputum that can be expectorated.

(5) Administer bronchodilators by metered-dose inhaler or nebulizer as ordered for wheezing and airway obstruction. Monitor for tachycardia or hypertension indicative of adverse effects of therapy.

(6) Assist patient to optimal position for ease of breathing (usually upright, leaning forward slightly).

(7) Administer opioids and anxiolytics as prescribed to decrease the work of breathing.

(8) Administer antibiotics as prescribed for infection.

(9) Administer chemotherapy or radiotherapy or both as prescribed for tumor shrinkage or relief of symptoms.

(10) Prepare patient for pleural tap, if ordered for management of pleural effusions.

(11) Stay with patient and provide reassurance as needed.

c. *Desired outcomes:* Patient will demonstrate improved oxygenation, as evidenced by:

(1) Unlabored respirations.

(2) Respiratory rate less than 20.

(3) Pink mucous membranes and nailbeds.

(4) Brisk capillary refill.

(5) Oxygen saturation >95%.

(6) Clear lung sounds.

2. Potential alteration in cardiac output related to cardiac dysrhythmias

a. *Problem:* Lung disease, such as tumor, infection, or antineoplastic therapy toxicities, often causes cardiac irritability, particularly atrial dysrhythmias. This problem is exacerbated by anorexia and treatment-related adverse effects such as vomiting or diarrhea that may cause fluid and electrolyte imbalances. Cardiac compromise is also associated with tumor compression of the superior vena cava (see Chapter 38) or involvement of the pericardium (see Chapter 35).

  b. *Interventions*

    (1) Assess heart rate and rhythm with each clinic visit, or routinely if an inpatient.

    (2) Perform 12-lead electrocardiogram (ECG) as ordered for differential diagnosis of rhythm disturbances.

    (3) Maintain a vigilant awareness of intake and output, and need to replace fluid or electrolytes.

    (4) Assess heart rate baseline and in response to bronchodilator therapy.

    (5) Assess other medications or medical conditions that may exacerbate the risk of cardiac dysrhythmias (eg, chronic obstructive lung disease [COPD], diabetes mellitus).

    (6) Teach patient the importance of reporting physical signs and symptoms of dysrhythmias or cardiac compromise.

      (a) Dysrhythmias—palpitations, intermittent dizziness or syncope, intermittent sharp and sudden dyspnea

      (b) Cardiovascular compromise—edema, mottled or dusky skin

  c. *Desired outcomes*

    (1) Normal heart rate and rhythm

    (2) Normal blood pressure

    (3) Absence of edema

    (4) Normal skin color and temperature

3. Pain related to lung tumors or surgical procedures

  a. *Problem:* Lung cancer can cause pain by compressing surrounding structures by way of local invasion or distant metastasis to organs such as the bones and spine. Patients who undergo surgical procedures can also experience incision site pain.

  b. *Interventions:* Follow recommendations in Chapter 30.

    (1) Surgical sympathectomy may be used more commonly in these patients in whom nerve or nerve root compression is common.

    (2) Low back or leg pain may be a hallmark of spinal cord compression, a common complication associated with bone metastases of lung cancer.

  c. *Desired outcome:* Elimination or control of pain, as described in Chapter 30.

4. Impaired activity tolerance and fatigue related to decreased tissue oxygenation and toxicities of treatments

  a. *Problem:* Poor tissue oxygenation can occur when tumors impinge on or obstruct the ventilatory or circulatory structures of the lungs. The treatments for cancer can also contribute to fatigue.

  b. *Interventions:* Follow recommendations in Chapter 25.

  c. *Desired outcome:* Elimination or control of fatigue, as described in Chapter 25.

5. High risk for injury related to weakness or changes in mental status
   a. *Problem:* Lung tumors may directly or indirectly cause hypercalcemia, which can lead to weakness and changes in mental status. Lung tumors that metastasize to the bones can lead to compression and weakness of the spinal cord.
   b. *Interventions:* Follow recommendations in Unit V.
   c. *Desired outcome:* Elimination or control of risk factors, as described in Unit V.
6. High risk for infection related to airway obstruction, radiation injury, or myelosuppression from chemotherapy or radiation therapy
   a. *Problem:* Patients who undergo chemotherapy or radiation therapy are at significant risk for lowered white blood cell counts (leukopenia), increasing their risk for infection.
   b. *Interventions:* Follow recommendations in Chapter 22.
   c. *Desired outcome:* Elimination or control of leukopenia.
7. Nutrition: altered, less than body requirements related to anorexia and to nausea and vomiting
   a. *Problem:* Patients often experience anorexia with lung cancer as a consequence of their disease or treatments. Patients undergoing treatment for lung cancer can also experience nausea and vomiting, decreasing their ability to tolerate food.
   b. *Interventions:* Follow recommendations in Chapters 27 and 28.
   c. *Desired outcomes:* Improved or maintained nutritional status, as described in Chapter 28, and elimination or control of nausea and vomiting, as described in Chapter 27.
8. Knowledge deficit related to lung cancer risk factors, diagnosis, complications, and treatment
   a. *Problem:* Patients and families are usually unfamiliar with diagnostic procedures and treatment modalities for lung cancer and require this information to make informed choices and facilitate coping.
   b. *Interventions*
      (1) Teach the patient and family what they can expect with common diagnostic procedures. See Table 17–3 for a list of tests and procedures commonly used to diagnose lung cancer.
      (2) Teach the patient about surgery and postoperative care, including:
         (a) Placement of drains.
         (b) Optimum positioning after lobectomy, wedge resection, and pneumonectomy.
            (i) Lobectomy—Avoid positioning on surgical side.
            (ii) Wedge resection—Avoid positioning on surgical side.
            (iii) Pneumonectomy—Avoid Trendelenburg and positioning on nonoperative side.
         (c) Airway stenting procedures may be used to provide immediate and temporary airway opening while awaiting onset of effects from radiation or chemotherapy (Unger, 2003).
            (i) Tracheobronchial stents placed during an inflexible bronchoscopic anesthetized procedure.

        (ii) Bronchoscopies or helical CT scans are performed before and after procedure, and after antineoplastic therapy to assess whether tumor shrinkage has affected the fit of the stent (Ferretti et al., 2003).

        (iii) Patients must be taught signs and symptoms of misplaced stent (sudden onset of severe coughing, dyspnea, stridor, wheezing), which require immediate emergency management.

    (d) Prevention of thromboembolic complications.

        (i) Use of elastic stockings and pneumatic pressure devices

        (ii) Subcutaneous heparin injections, position changes, and early ambulation

  (3) Teach the patient and family about side effects expected with chemotherapy (see Chapter 6).

    (a) High risk of pneumonia in these patients may necessitate prophylactic administration of growth factors or antimicrobials.

    (b) Research suggests that concomitant oral anticoagulants or Cox2 inhibitors may be chemotherapy enhancers in this patient population.

  (4) Teach the patient and family side effects of radiotherapy.

    (a) Radiotherapy to lungs may cause inflammation and increased secretions that further impair oxygenation about 7 to 14 days after beginning therapy.

    (b) Radiation pneumonitis is possible due to inclusion of alveoli in the radiation port. Onset is about 3 weeks after the start of therapy.

    (c) Radiation to major airways may induce cough and hemoptysis, with the incidence peaking about 2 to 3 weeks after start of therapy. If patients are receiving multimodal therapy, platelet counts should be monitored carefully during this time period.

    (d) Innovative methods of delivering radiation directly to the tumor bed in major airway lesions include implanted radioactive seeds and endobronchial radiotherapy.

  c. *Desired outcomes:* The patient and family members will be able to identify side effects of chemotherapy, radiotherapy, and surgery, as appropriate, including self-care measures to use if toxicities or other problems occur.

E. Discharge Planning and Patient Education

  1. Give postoperative patients and their families detailed instructions for wound care, including signs and symptoms of infection.

  2. Arrange for home nursing care as needed to ensure safe recovery through prevention of infection and other complications.

  3. For patients receiving chemotherapy and radiotherapy, closely monitor and instruct for management of treatment-related toxicities, including myelosuppression, nausea and vomiting, diarrhea, constipation, stomatitis, esophagitis, fatigue, dyspnea, and peripheral neuropathies.

4. Initiate supplemental oxygen at home, if necessary. Instruct the patient and family in oxygen safety, especially avoidance of smoking and other combustion hazards when oxygen is in use.

5. Due to rapid progression of disease, especially in SCLC, identify and mobilize sources of emotional, physical, social, and financial support for the patient. Hospice care is often an appropriate referral choice for patients who are diagnosed with extensive or stage IV disease. Home hospice care continues to become increasingly available, and many organizations will accept patients who are undergoing treatment, especially if it is palliative in nature.

REFERENCES

Al Shanquetti, A., Kaplan, C., & Govindan, R. (2002). Lung cancer. In R. Govindan & M. Arquette (Eds.), *The Washington manual of oncology* (pp. 238–251). Philadelphia: Lippincott Williams & Wilkins.

American Joint Committee on Cancer. (2002). *AJCC cancer staging handbook* (6th ed., pp. 191–203). New York: Springer.

Auperin, A., Arriagada, R., Pignon, J. P., et al. (1999). Prophylactic cranial irradiation for patients with small-cell lung cancer in complete remission. *New England Journal of Medicine, 341,* 476–484.

Cleri, L. B., & Haywood, R. (2002). *Oncology pocket guide to chemotherapy* (5th ed., pp. 363–365). New York: Mosby.

Ferretti, G. R., Kocier, M., Calaque, O., Arbib, F., Righinim C., Coulomb, M., & Pison, C. (2003). Follow-up after stent insertion in the tracheobronchial tree: Role of helical computed tomography in comparison with fiberoptic bronchoscopy. *European Radiology, 13*(5), 1172–1178.

Gerber, R. B., Mazzone, P., & Arroliga, A. C. (2002). Paraneoplastic syndromes associated with bronchogenic carcinoma. *Clinics in Chest Medicine, 23*(1), 257–264.

Langerak, A., & Dreisbach, L. (2001). *Chemotherapy regimens and cancer care* (pp. 129–140). Georgetown, TX: Landes Bioscience.

Lind, J. (1998). Nursing care of the client with lung cancer. In J. Itano & K. Taoka (Eds.), *ONS core curriculum for oncology nursing* (3rd ed., pp. 448–458). Philadelphia: W. B. Saunders.

Mazzone, P. J., & Arroliga, A. C. (2003). Endocrine paraneoplastic syndromes in lung cancer. *Current Opinion in Pulmonary Medicine, 9*(4), 313–320.

Messori, A., Lanza, C., Serio, A., & Salvolini, U. (2003). Resolution of limbic encephalitis with detection and treatment of lung cancer: Clinical-radiological correlation. *European Journal of Radiology, 45*(1), 78–80.

Morris, C. D., Budde, J. M., Godette, K. D., Kerwin ,T. L., & Miller, J. I., Jr. (2002). Palliative management of malignant airway obstruction [including discussion]. *Annals of Thoracic Surgery, 74*(6), 1928–1933.

Silvestri, G. A, Tanoue, L. T., Margolis, M. L., Barker, J., & Detterbeck, F. (2003). American College of Chest Physicians. The noninvasive staging of non-small cell lung cancer: the guidelines. *Chest, 123*(1 Suppl), 47S–156S.

Tierney, L., McPhee, S., & Papadakis, M. (Eds.). (2003). Current medical diagnosis and treatment (42nd ed.). New York: Lange Medical Books.

Unger, M. (2003). Endobronchial therapy of neoplasms. *Chest Surgery Clinics of North America, 13*(1),129–147.

Wen, P.Y., & Schiff, D. (2003). Neurologic complications of solid tumors. *Neurologic Clinics, 21*(1), 107–140, viii.

18 Lymphoma

Janet Briel
Tracy T. Douglas

I. Definition: Lymphomas are a diverse group of malignancies that originate in the lymphoid system. This system includes the lymph nodes as well as extranodal sites, such as bone marrow, the spleen, the tonsils and adenoids, the thymus gland, and Peyer's patches in the small intestine. There are two major types of lymphoma: Hodgkin's disease (HD) and non-Hodgkin's lymphoma (NHL). HD makes up 15% of lymphomas and is characterized by the Reed-Sternberg cell. NHL diseases are very heterogeneous and consist of approximately 23 different histologic types (see Table 18–1 for types of lymphoma). Although each type of NHL is biologically different, there are two major categories of NHL: indolent and aggressive (see Table 18–2 for characteristics of uncommon NHL types).

A. Incidence: NHL is the sixth leading site of cancer among men and women. According to the American Cancer Society (2003), there were an estimated 53,400 new cases of NHL in 2003. The incidence of lymphoma has increased steadily since the 1970s. This rapid rise is in part due to the increase in human immunodeficiency virus (HIV) and subsequent NHL development in this patient population. A decrease in the incidence of HIV-related NHL may be seen as the use of highly effective antiretroviral therapy (HAART) increases. HAART increases the immunocompetence of people with HIV, thereby potentially lowering their increased cancer risk. Improved diagnostics and chronic immunosuppression (eg, organ transplantation patients) have also been implicated in the rising incidence of lymphoma. NHL is more common and the mortality rates are greater than those of HD. The American Cancer Society (2003) reports an estimated 7,600 new cases of HD in 2003. HD has a bimodal incidence that peaks in youth, between the ages of 18 and 24, and then peaks again at 50 to 70 years of age. NHL has a peak incidence of 50 years. Males are at greater risk of lymphoma than females.

B. Morbidity and Mortality Statistics: The American Cancer Society (2003) reports an estimated 1,300 deaths in 2003 from HD, and there will be an estimated 23,400 deaths in 2003 from NHL. HD is highly curable with chemotherapy. NHL is the fifth leading cause of death among men and the sixth leading cause of death among women. Many of the indolent NHL diseases have a natural course lasting 10 to 15 years, whereas the more aggressive NHL course can lead to death quickly if left untreated. Higher mortality is seen in urban and higher socioeconomic populations.

TABLE 18–1 Revised European-American Lymphoma (REAL)/World Health Organization (WHO) Classification of Lymphoid Neoplasms

Classification of NHL

B-cell Neoplasms

Precursor B-cell neoplasm
- Precursor B-lymphoblatic leukemia (precursor B-cells acute lymphoblastic leukemia)

Mature (peripheral) B-cell neoplasms
- B-cell chronic lymphocytic leukemia/small lymphocytic lymphoma
- B-cell prolymphocytic leukemia
- Lymphoplasmacytic lymphoma
- Splenic marginal zone B-cell lymphoma (with or without villous lymphocytes)
- Hairy cell leukemia
- Plasma cell myeloma/plasmacytoma
- Extranodal marginal zone B-cell lymphoma of MALT type
- Nodal marginal zone B-cell lymphoma (with or without monocytoid B-cells)
- Follicular lymphoma
- Mantle cell lymphoma
- Diffuse large B-cell lymphoma
- Burkitt lymphoma/Burkitt cell lymphoma

T-cell and NK-cell Neoplasms

Precursor T-cell neoplasm
- Precursor T-lymphoblatic/leukemia (precursor T-cell acute lymphoblastic leukemia)

Mature (peripheral) T/NK-cell neoplasms
- T-cell prolymphocytic leukemia
- T-cell granular lymphocytic leukemia
- Aggressive NK-cell leukemia
- Adult T-cell lymphoma/leukemia (HTLV1+)
- Extranodal NK/T-cell lymphoma, nasal type
- Enteropathy-type T-cell lymphoma
- Hepatosplenic T-cell lymphoma
- Subcutaneous panniculitis-like T-cell lymphoma
- Mycosis fungoides/Sezary syndrome
- Anaplastic large cell lymphoma, T/null cell, primary cutaneous type
- Peripheral T-cell lymphoma, not otherwise characterized
- Angioimmunoblastic T-cell lymphoma
- Anaplastic large cell lymphoma, T/null cell, primary systematic type

Harris, N. L., Jaffe, E. S., Diebold, J., et al. (1999). The World Health Organization classification of neoplastic diseases of the hematopoietic and lymphoid tissues. Report of the Clinical Advisory Committee meeting, Airlie House, Virginia.

TABLE 18-2 Characteristics of Uncommon NHL Types

Type	Characteristics
Small lymphocytic lymphoma	Morphologically indistinguishable from CLL 10% to 20% progress to CLL 5% transform to an aggressive form of lymphoma treated with fludarabine, cyclophosphamide, chlorambucil, prednisone, CVP
Gastric MALT lymphoma	Associated with chronic gastritis and *H pylori,* which is a bacteria that induces gastric ulcers May be treated with antibiotics, local radiation, gastrectomy, chemotherapy
Burkitt's lymphoma	Rapid doubling time ~1 day Need immediate treatment High risk for tumor lysis syndrome Patients often present with high LDH and bulky disease 20% to 30% risk of CNS disease IT prophylaxis High-risk patients may need blood or marrow transplantation if chemotherapy responsive
Mantle cell lymphoma	Presents in older patients >50 years of age Median survival 3 to 5 years 80% are males Difficult to treat Metastasizes to the liver, spleen, bone marrow, and GI tract Blood and marrow transplantation are under investigation
AIDS-related lymphoma	T-cell destruction leads to immunosuppression Poor survival Aggressive, present with advanced disease, more severe side effects from treatment Often need dose reductions in chemotherapy regimens 20% to 53% have bone marrow involvement 20% to 45% have CNS involvement Most are diffuse B-cell and Burkitt's ~50% may be EBV related Primary CNS lymphoma is more common in AIDS patients who have low CD4 counts Performance status and CD4 count at diagnosis are prognostic indicators
T-cell lymphomas	Lymphoblastic—aggressive, most present with large mediastinal masses, bone marrow, and CNS involvement Treatment is patterned after ALL +/− radiation Mycosis fungoides—cutaneous T-cell lymphomas Initial indolent course with wide dissemination Cure is uncommon Should be considered for clinical trials Poor prognosis if visceral and blood/marrow involvement

(continued)

▐ TABLE 18-2 **Characteristics of Uncommon NHL Types** *(Continued)*

Type	Characteristics
T-cell lymphomas	Treatment includes topical therapies, photopheresis, electron beam therapy, interferon A, psoralen plus ultraviolet A radiation (PUVA), monoclonal antibody treatments (eg, Ontak-CD 25 MAB)
	Skin eruptions, nodular/necrotic tumors, and visceral involvement occur
	Patients experience significant body image changes, depression
	Infection is a common cause of death in these patients
CNS lymphoma	Rare
	NHL confined to the central nervous system
	Most are high-grade, diffuse, B-cell type
	Incidence is on the rise
	25% of patients have ocular involvement
	Treatment includes whole brain radiation and/or high-dose methotrexate with leucovorin rescue

II. Etiology

A. Risk Factors

1. Immunodeficiency disorders such as rheumatoid arthritis and systemic lupus erythematosus are associated with lymphoma.
2. Patients who have undergone organ transplantation and who are on chronic immunosuppression have a higher risk of NHL.
3. Inherited immunodeficiency syndromes increase one's risk of developing a lymphoma (eg, Klinefelter's syndrome, telangiectasia, and ataxia).
4. Treatments for cancer, including chemotherapy and radiation therapy, can cause second malignancies, which often present as a lymphoma or leukemia.
5. Viral infections are known to be associated with the development of lymphomas.
   a. Epstein Barr virus (EBV) infection occurs earlier in childhood in underdeveloped countries and is associated with Burkitt's lymphoma in those areas. In developed countries, EBV is associated with post-transplantation lymphoproliferative disorders. Some scientists believe that HD is caused by EBV infection.
   b. The incidence of NHL in HIV-positive patients is approximately 60 times greater than that of the general population (Tulpule & Levine, 1999). HIV infection is also associated with HD but to a lesser extent.
   c. Human T-cell leukemia/lymphoma virus (HTLV-1) is associated with NHL. This virus is most common in Japan and the Caribbean; however, incidence is on the rise in some parts of the United States.
6. *Helicobacter pylori* is a bacteria associated with the development of primary gastric NHL.

7. There is some indication that benzene compounds, insecticides, and herbicides may increase the risk of lymphomas; however, the data are not yet conclusive.

III. Patient Management

A. Assessment: Symptoms are commonly associated with compression of structures adjacent to nodal groups, decreased lymphatic function, and systemic infiltration of the disease.

1. Complete history and physical examination are obtained with a special emphasis on lymphatic areas and extranodal sites that may be involved.

2. Performance status scales, such as the Karnofsky or Eastern Cooperative Oncology Group (ECOG) scale, have proven to be a key factor in prognosis of aggressive NHL. In 1993, a group of physicians developed the International Prognostic Index (IPI) to help determine therapy in aggressive lymphomas. The IPI includes age >60 years, LDH >1× normal, performance status 2–4, stage III or IV, and extranodal involvement >1 site. IPI levels of 4 or 5 are at high risk of relapse. (International Non-Hodgkin's Lymphoma Prognostic Factors Project, 1993)

3. Lymphadenopathy of the cervical, supraclavicular, axillary, inguinal, or mediastinal areas is the most common presenting symptom. This reflects the increased growth of cancer cells in the lymph nodes. Growth is often rapid; nodes are painless and may be unilateral or bilateral. About 20% of patients report pain of the enlarged lymph nodes after alcohol ingestion. HD spreads in a contiguous manner along lymph node chains, whereas NHL spreads in a less predictable manner to lymph nodes and to extranodal sites not adjacent to the original site.

4. Fever, fatigue, night sweats, pruritus, frequent infections, and weight loss are symptoms associated with altered immune response patterns and systemic involvement. The definition of "B symptoms" includes an unexplained fever for greater than 1 month, unintentional weight loss of >10%, and night sweats for more than 1 month. Pruritus is another presenting symptom in some lymphoma patients. The presence of B symptoms indicates a poor prognosis in HD patients, and these symptoms can also be a harbinger of relapse and advanced disease. "A symptoms" refers to the absence of "B symptoms."

5. Cough, dyspnea, dysphagia, and superior vena cava syndrome are symptoms that may result from the tumor causing pressure or obstructing an adjacent area. These symptoms are most often seen when mediastinal nodes are involved.

6. Abdominal pain in the left upper quadrant suggests enlargement of the spleen.

7. Jaundice can result from bile duct obstruction.

8. General abdominal pain and bowel or bladder dysfunction can be caused by retroperitoneal adenopathy.

9. Cytopenias are common, and it is important to differentiate between treatment-related aplasia, autoimmune disorders, and lymphoma infiltration of the bone marrow in order to direct treatment.

10. Confusion, lethargy and cranial nerve palsies are associated with central nervous system (CNS) NHL.

IV. Diagnostic Parameters

A. Lymph Node Biopsy: Lymphadenopathy can result from allergic reactions, infections, and other nonspecific causes. If the enlarged node persists for several weeks, a lymph node biopsy is indicated. Cervical lymph node excisional biopsies are more diagnostic than inguinal nodes, which often demonstrate benign reactivity instead of malignancy.

1. The Reed-Sternberg cell is a large, binucleated cell that is thought to be derived from a B-cell. This characteristic cell is required for the diagnosis of HD. See Table 18–3 for HD histopathologic classifications.

2. The pathologic diagnosis of NHL depends on the type of malignant lymphocyte found. In 1994, the International Lymphoma Study Group (ILSG) introduced a new classification system for lymphoid neoplasms called the Revised European-American Lymphoma Classification of Lymphoid Neoplasms (REAL). The World Health Organization (WHO) also updated its classification. The REAL/WHO classification is now the standard for classification in lymphoma. See Table 18–1 for the REAL/WHO classifications. Classification depends on the architecture of the lymph node, immunophenotype, and molecular characteristics. For example, affected lymph nodes in follicular lymphoma retain their follicular appearance, whereas lymph nodes affected by diffuse large cell lymphoma have no resemblance to a lymph node under the microscope. NHL can arise primarily from the B-cell (85%) and the T-cell (15%).

B. Laboratory Tests: For baseline monitoring purposes and to detect deviations from normal that indicate immunodeficiency or organ involvement, the following tests may be performed:

1. Complete blood count (CBC) and differential: A complete differential is useful to assess the degree of lymphocyte involvement, anemia, and infection risks. Coombs'-positive hemolytic anemia is sometimes present in lymphoma patients.

2. Liver function studies: Elevated transaminase levels may indicate hepatic involvement.

3. Tumor lysis labs: Serum uric acid, potassium and phosphorus elevations, and hypocalcemia may reflect cell destruction. Cell destruction can be seen in lymphomas that are rapidly growing at diagnosis and with treatment initiation. This syndrome is called tumor lysis syndrome (see Chapter 40 for patient management of this oncologic emergency).

4. Lactase dehydrogenase (LDH) elevation can be a general expression of tumor load and has prognostic implications as defined by the IPI.

5. HIV, HTLV-1, and EBV may be obtained. For those patients who are known to be HIV positive, a viral load and CD4 count will help assess immunocompetence. *H. pylori* testing in early-stage mucosa-associated lymphoid tissue (MALT) lymphomas by way of blood antigen testing or breath test is utilized for diagnosis.

6. Unilateral or bilateral bone marrow aspirates may be indicated to support or rule out disease in the marrow.

7. Immunophenotyping tumor cells by way of flow cytometry of the bone marrow or blood are important tests used to differentiate different lymphomas. CD-20, CD-45, CD-10, and CD-19 are common

TABLE 18-3 Revised European-American Lymphoma (REAL) Classification and Characteristics of Hodgkin's Disease

Histologic Subtype (Rye classification)	Pathologic Characteristics	Features
Nodular sclerosing (NSHD)	Classic Reed-Sternberg cells, variant lacunar cells, CD-15+, CD-30+, CD-45−	• Most common HD ~65% to 80% • Most common in young adults (15–25 years) • Incidence = women > men • B symptoms occur in 30% of patients • Mediastinal involvement is common
Mixed cellularity (MCHD)	Classic Reed-Sternberg cells, CD-15+, CD-30+, CD-45−	• Second most common type of HD • Age 25–45 years • Incidence = men > women • B symptoms are common at diagnosis • 50% of patients are diagnosed at stage III or IV
Lymphocyte predominant (LPHD)	Lymphocyte and histiocyte variant cells, nodular or diffuse subtypes include nodular: CD-19+, CD-20+, CD-45+, CD-15−, CD-30− and diffuse: CD-15+, CD-30+, CD-45−.	• Uncommon 5% to 10% of HD cases • Age 30–40 years • Slow growing • B symptoms uncommon at diagnosis • Incidence = men > women • Multiple recurrences can occur • Good prognosis
Lymphocyte depleted (LDHD)	Numerous Reed-Sternberg cells	• Rare 5% to 10% • Occurs in older patients >40 years • Metastatic at diagnosis • B symptoms are common • Poor prognosis

lymphoma tumor markers. Different combinations are considered immunophenotypes.

8. Chromosome analysis also contributes to the diagnosis and may be helpful in determining prognosis. Approximately 90% of follicular lymphomas have the BCL2 gene caused by translocation t(14;18); t(11;14) is common in mantle cell lymphomas. Burkitt's lymphoma commonly has translocations involving chromosome 8.

9. Computed tomography (CT) scans are important to identify the extent of disease. Lymphadenopathy in the mediastinum, periaortic, or retroperitoneal areas; hepatomegaly; and splenomegaly are evaluated. Involvement of organs and lymph systems above and below the diaphragm may be differentiated and will influence the choice of treatment.

10. Gallium scans or positron emission tomography (PET) scans may be performed as a baseline to evaluate response to therapy. The use

of PET scans is still controversial because of their expense, and the validity of these scans in lymphoma is still under evaluation. Gallium and PET scans look at the metabolic uptake of radionucleotides of masses and can differentiate a fibrotic mass from active tumor after therapy.

11. Magnetic resonance imaging (MRI) does not expose a person to ionizing radiation and provides a three-dimensional image of the body. MRI is useful for visualizing bones, vessels, and soft tissues. A lymphangiogram is done to identify the extent of nodal involvement. Dye is injected into the feet and traced to the first obstruction. MRI often replaces lymphangiograms because it is more accurate and better tolerated by patients.

12. Laparotomy, which includes splenectomy, and sampling of the liver and abdominal lymph nodes are rarely required today because of advances in diagnostic imaging. Less invasive testing establishes the extent of disease with much less patient morbidity.

13. Lumbar puncture is necessary for aggressive NHL, including Burkitt's lymphoma, where CNS disease is suspected or probable.

V. Treatment of Hodgkin's Disease: The Ann Arbor-Cotswold staging system for HD and NHL indicates prognosis and treatment (Table 18–4 and Box 18–1). Treatment of HD is determined by stage of disease. Some variation may occur with histopathology. Treatments include radiation therapy, chemotherapy, and blood and marrow transplantation. Combination therapy can cure 50% to 85% of HD patients.

  A. Radiation Therapy
   1. Fields
     a. Mantle irradiation (used for chest disease) includes the area from the mandible to the diaphragm. The lungs, spinal cord, and heart are shielded. A total dose of 3,500 to 4,400 cGy is usually given over 4 to 6 weeks. This field may be extended to include the top of the Y field, but not the pelvic area.
     b. The inverted Y field (used for abdominal disease) includes the area from the diaphragm to the ischial tuberosity and the spleen. The spinal cord, kidneys, bladder, rectum, and gonads are protected.
     c. Total nodal irradiation includes the mantle and inverted Y zones.
   2. Side effects are specific to the area treated (see Chapter 8).

TABLE 18–4 Treatment of Hodgkin's Disease

Hodgkin's Disease Stage	Treatment
I, II (A or B)	Subtotal lymphoid irradiation
I, II (A or B, with large mediastinal mass)	Combination chemotherapy, then radiation to involved field
IIIA1 (minimal abdominal disease)	Radiation to the involved field
IIIB	Combination chemotherapy
IV (A or B)	Combination chemotherapy, with or without BMT (if high risk)
Relapsed disease	Salvage chemotherapy, with or without BMT

▼ BOX 18-1 | **Ann Arbor–Cotswold Staging System for Hodgkin's and Non-Hodgkin's Lymphomas**

- Stage I Involvement of a single LN region or lymphoid structure
- Stage II Involvement of two or more LN regions on the same side of the diaphragm
- Stage III Involvement of LN regions or structures on both sides of diaphragm
- Stage IV Involvement of extranodal sites beyond that designated as E (see below)
- Further staging designations include the following:
  - Suffix A—No symptoms (any disease stage)
  - Suffix B—Fever (temperature >38°C); drenching sweats; unexplained weight loss (eg, 10% of body weight within preceding 6 months; any disease stage)
  - Suffix E—Involvement of a single extranodal site that is contiguous or proximal to the known nodal site (stages I–III)
- Cotswold modifications are as follows:
  - Suffix X—Denotes bulky disease (a widening of the mediastinum by more than one third or the presence of a nodal mass with a maximal dimension of >10 cm)
  - Subscripts—Used to indicate the number of anatomic regions
  - Stage III subdivisions—May be subdivided to include III(1), with or without splenic, hilar, celiac, or portal nodes and III(2), with paraaortic, iliac, or mesenteric nodes

Lister, T. A., Crowther, D., Sutcliffe, S. B., et al. (1989). Report of a committee convened to discuss the evaluation and staging of patients with Hodgkin's disease: Cotswolds meeting. *Journal of Clinical Oncology, 7*(11), 1630–1636.

B. Chemotherapy
1. Chemotherapy is indicated when extensive disease or systemic symptoms are present. Cells are usually highly sensitive, and response rates are high.
2. Combination chemotherapy is given in alternate cycles to prevent drug resistance and overlapping side effects. For common chemotherapeutic agents, see Table 18–5. (See Chapter 6 for appropriate nursing interventions.)

TABLE 18–5 Chemotherapy Regimens for Hodgkin's Disease

ABVD: Adriamycin, bleomycin, vinblastine, DTIC
MOPP: Methotrexate, vincristine, procarbazine, prednisone
BCVPP: BCNU, Cytoxan, vinblastine, procarbazine, prednisone

See Chapter 6 for specific side effects and management for each agent.

3. Blood and marrow transplantation (BMT) is used to treat HD that is relapsed or progressive through chemotherapy, if responsiveness to therapy is still present.

C. Treatment of NHL: NHL is often disseminated at the time of diagnosis and requires a treatment plan that addresses the aggressiveness of the tumor and the stage based on Ann Arbor-Cotswold staging system (see Table 18–4). The Ann Arbor-Cotswold staging system is not effective at determining stage of small lymphocytic lymphoma or chronic lymphocytic leukemia because these almost always have bone marrow involvement. The modified RAI classification (Table 18–6) is used to determine prognosis and treatment in this group.

1. Low-grade or indolent, early-stage lymphomas may be treated with a "watch and wait" approach if asymptomatic. Radiation therapy given in doses ranging from 2,500 to 4,000 cGy over 4 weeks and/or single-agent chemotherapy may also be an option. Advanced indolent lymphomas can be watched if symptoms are absent; however, single-agent or combination chemotherapy is often started in an attempt to obtain prolonged disease-free survival. Most patients with low-grade lymphomas present with advanced stage, which is considered incurable at this time. A number of indolent lymphomas undergo a histologic conversion to aggressive diffuse large-cell lymphoma. Once transformation occurs, the survival can be limited to approximately 12 months. These patients may be candidates for blood or marrow transplantation. Novel treatments using monoclonal antibodies alone and with radiation to directly attack the lymphoma cells have recently emerged for the treatment of indolent or transformed lymphomas.

a. Rituxan (rituximab) (IDEC Pharmaceuticals Corp.) is an unconjugated MAb that targets the CD-20 antigen and is widely used in CD-20+ lymphoma patients.

b. Zevalin Y-90 (ibritumomab tiuxetan) (IDEC Pharmaceuticals Corp.) is a radioimmunotherapy agent used in conjunction with Rituxan. It is FDA approved for the treatment of relapsed or refractory low-grade, follicular, or transformed B-cell non-Hodgkin's lymphoma.

c. Bexxar (tositumomab and iodine [131]I- tositumomab) (GlaxoSmithKline) is a monoclonal antibody that is conjugated with ^{131}I and is used in combination with tositumomab (without radiation). Bexxar is FDA approved for the treatment of patients

TABLE 18–6 RAI Classification System for SLL/CLL

Stage	Description	Risk Status
0	Lymphocytosis, lymphocytes in blood >15,000/mm³ and >40% lymphocytes in the bone marrow	Good
I	Stage 0 with enlarged lymph node(s)	Intermediate
II	Stage 0–I with splenomegaly, hepatomegaly, or both	Intermediate
III	Stage 0–II with hemoglobin <11.0 g/dL or hematocrit <33%	High
IV	Stage 0–III with platelets <100,000/mm³	High

Rai, K., R., Sawitsky, A., Cronkite, E. P., et al. (1975). Clinical staging of CLL. *Blood, 46*, 219–234.

with CD-20+, follicular, non-Hodgkin's lymphoma (NHL), with and without transformation who have failed Rituxan. (See Chapter 4 for side effects of these therapies.)

(1) Monoclonal antibodies used in conjunction with autologous blood and marrow transplantation are being studied in clinical trials in an attempt to enhance response rates in a disease that is presently incurable. (For side effects of specific chemotherapy drugs and radiation therapy, refer to Chapters 6 and 8 for recommendations.)

(2) High-grade lymphomas require immediate and aggressive combination chemotherapy (Table 18–7). Long-term remission, after six to nine monthly cycles, occurs in 35% to 45% of patients. Radiation therapy may be used in conjunction with other treatment modalities to involved areas. Biological response modifiers with or without conjugation may be useful adjuncts to therapy and are under investigation at this time. Rituxan combined with CHOP chemotherapy in CD-20+ lymphoma patients has become a standard treatment. Blood and marrow transplantation is a viable and potentially curative option for high-risk patients and those who relapse after standard therapy. Chemotherapy-responsive, aggressive, diffuse large-cell lymphoma (DLCL) is associated with a 50% to 60% response rate with autologous blood or marrow transplantation. (For side effects and nursing care, see Chapter 5.) Chemotherapy-resistant, aggressive DLCL has a response rate closer to 10%. Refractory patients can be treated with salvage regimens such as ESHAP or ICE. Patients with Burkitt's or

TABLE 18–7 Treatment Regimens for Non-Hodgkin's Lymphomas

Single Agents: Chlorambucil, 2-CDA, fludarabine, cyclophosphamide, prednisone, busulfan, Rituxan, Zevalin, Bexxar
(These agents may also be used in combination in various regimens.)

CHOP/ +/− Rituxan: Cyclophosphamide, doxorubicin, vincristine, prednisone +/− Rituxan

CVP: Cyclophosphamide, vincristine, prednisone

m-BACOD: Methotrexate, bleomycin, doxorubicin, cyclophosphamide, vincristine, dexamethasone

ProMACE-CytaBOM: Prednisone, methotrexate, doxorubicin, cytarabine, bleomycin, vincristine

MACOP-B: Methotrexate, leucovorin, doxorubicin, cyclophosphamide, vincristine, prednisone, bleomycin

ESHAP: Etoposide, cytosine arabinoside, cisplatin, methylprednisolone

BEAM: BCNU, etoposide, cystosine arabinoside, cyclophosphamide

MINE: Mesna, ifosfamide, mitoxantrone, etoposide

CNOP: Cyclophosphamide, doxorubicin, vincristine, prednisone

COPP: Cyclophosphamide, vincristine, procarbazine, prednisone

Hyper C-VAD: Fractionated cyclophosphamide, vincristine, Adriamycin, dexamethasone (alternating with high doses of methotrexate/cytarabine)

ACVB: Doxorubicin, cyclophosphamide, vindesine, bleomycin

See Chapter 6 for specific side effects and management for each agent.

Burkitt's-like aggressive lymphomas often are considered for blood or marrow transplantation or a leukemic regimen that consists of CNS prophylaxis because of the tendency of this disease to spread to the CNS. (See Table 18–7 for treatment regimens used in NHL.)

D. Nursing Diagnoses, Interventions, and Outcomes for HD and NHL

    1. Immediate and short-term side effects: Aplasia, nausea, fatigue, and hair loss related to chemotherapy and radiation treatment

        a. *Problem:* Radiation and chemotherapy treatments for HD and NHL result in the common side effects of the agents used (see Chapters 6 and 8).

        b. *Interventions:* Discuss side effects and specific management strategies with patient and caregivers before start of therapy. (See Chapters 6 and 8 for treatment-specific side effects.)

        c. *Desired outcome:* Patient will understand and manage the side effects of chemotherapy and radiation therapy.

    2. Long-term complications related to radiation treatment and chemotherapy (Table 18–8)

        a. *Problem:* Radiation therapy and chemotherapy alone or combined may result in long-term complications for survivors of lymphomas.

        b. *Interventions:* Complications should be treated symptomatically when they occur, but should be anticipated and prevented whenever possible.

        c. *Desired outcome:* Patient will anticipate, prevent, and control complications to ensure optimal quality of life.

    3. Knowledge deficit related to diagnosis and treatment

        a. *Problem:* Patients, especially adolescents and children, may not be knowledgeable about the disease or treatment.

TABLE 18–8 Long-Term Complications of Lymphoma Treatment

Causative Agents
Radiation therapy (RT) and chemotherapy

Complications
Hypothyroidism, pericarditis, cardiomyopathy, pneumonitis and pulmonary fibrosis, immunologic imcompetence, growth retardation in children, infertility, and dental caries, second malignancies (leukemia, lymphoma, and other solid tumors [eg, breast, lung, sarcoma, thyroid]).

Management
Appropriate shielding and technique to minimize RT exposure
Careful selection and monitoring of combination chemotherapy
Reproductive counseling and dental examination/care before treatment
Splenectomy, surgical therapy
Immunologic dysfunction, sepsis, and herpes zoster-varicella
Appropriate vaccinations and antibiotic prophylaxis
Conservative splenectomy
Antiviral therapy
Long-term follow-up yearly

b. *Interventions*
   (1) Assess knowledge and learning style.
   (2) Provide age-appropriate learning materials and education to the patient and family.
   (3) Evaluate patient and family mastery of information throughout the treatment period.
c. *Desired outcomes*
   (1) The patient will demonstrate age-appropriate knowledge of the disease and treatment.
   (2) The patient and family will make informed decisions concerning treatment.
   (3) The patient and family will participate in and comply with the plan of care.

4. Hypothyroidism related to radiation therapy
   a. *Problem:* Sixty to seventy percent of patients receiving high-dose radiation to the cervical lymph nodes experience symptoms of hypothyroidism as a late effect of therapy.
   b. *Interventions*
      (1) Teach signs and symptoms of hypothyroidism.
      (2) Monitor for symptoms of hypothyroidism and thyroid-stimulating hormone (TSH).
      (3) Monitor T3, T4, and thyroid-stimulating hormone (TSH) levels.
      (4) Initiate thyroid replacement therapy if hypothyroidism occurs.
   c. *Desired outcomes*
      (1) Patient will report signs and symptoms of hypothyroidism.
      (2) If the patient becomes hypothyroid, symptoms will be managed with thyroid replacement therapy.

5. Sterility related to combined therapy
   a. *Problem:* Drug treatments such as mechlorethamine, vinblastine, vincristine, procarbazine, and prednisone may cause infertility. Men show evidence of azoospermia after one to two courses of treatment. Women may have ovarian failure after six cycles but are less likely to become sterile.
   b. *Interventions*
      (1) Discuss the risks for sterility associated with treatment before treatment initiation.
      (2) If a woman is having a staging laparotomy, protect ovaries from radiation therapy.
      (3) Refer patient for sperm banking or egg harvesting, and reproductive and sexual counseling, as appropriate.
   c. *Desired outcomes*
      (1) Patient and significant other will understand the risk for treatment-associated sterility.
      (2) Patient and significant other will have a plan to address reproductive issues, if this is important to them.

6. Secondary malignancy related to combined therapy
   a. *Problem:* Combined modality therapies (chemotherapy and radiation) and some of the chemotherapeutic agents used to treat HD are known to result in the occurrence of secondary leukemia and NHL.

b. *Interventions*
    (1) Teach the patient to self-screen for signs and symptoms of leukemia and NHL.
    (2) Provide the patient with information regarding annual screening for leukemia and NHL and the importance of long-term follow-up.
c. *Desired outcomes*
    (1) Patient will comply with plans for long-term follow-up.
    (2) Patient is aware of and reports any signs or symptoms of leukemia or NHL as they occur.
E. Discharge Planning and Patient Education
  1. Patient and family will understand and comply with plans for outpatient therapy.
  2. Patient and family will be knowledgeable about and report signs and symptoms of complications of the disease or treatment in a timely manner.
  3. Patient and family will understand the long-term risks associated with treatment.

REFERENCES

Aleman, B. M. P., van den Belt-Dusebout, A. W., Klokman, W. J., et al. (2003). Long-term cause-specific mortality of patients treated for Hodgkin's disease. *Journal of Clinical Oncology, 21,* 3431–3439.

Batchelor, T., Carson, K., O'Neill, A., Grossman, S. A., Alavi, J., New, P., Hochberg, F., & Priet, R. (2003). *The treatment of primary central nervous system lymphoma with methotrexate and deferred radiotherapy: A report of NABTT 96–07* (Report No. NABTT 96–07). Baltimore, MD: CNS Consortium.

Callaghan, M. (2000). Nursing perspective on MALT lymphoma. *Clinical Oncology Updates, 1*(2).

Connors, J. M. (2003). Hodgkin's lymphoma: The hazards of success. *Journal of Clinical Oncology, 21*(18), 3388–3390.

DeAngelis, L. M., Seiferheld, W., Schold, S. C., Fisher, B., & Schultz, C. J. (2002). Combination chemotherapy and radiotherapy for primary central nervous system: Radiation Therapy Oncology Group study 93–10. *Journal of Clinical Oncology, 20,*(24), 4643–4648.

Greene, F., Page, D., Fleming, I., Fritz, A., Balch, C., Haller, D., & Morrow, M. (2001). Lymphoid neoplasms. In *American Joint Committee on Cancer cancer staging handbook* (6th ed.; pp. 427–448). New York: Springer.

The International Non-Hodgkin's Lymphoma Prognostic Factors Project. (1993). A predictive model of aggressive non-Hodgkin's lymphoma. *New England Journal of Medicine, 329,* 987–994.

Jemal, A., Thomas, A., Murray, T., et al. (2003). Cancer statistics, 2003. *CA: A Cancer Journal for Clinicians,* (53), 5–26.

Josting, A., Wiedenmann, S., Franklin, J., et al. (2003). Secondary myeloid leukemia and myelodysplastic syndromes in patients treated for Hodgkin's disease: A report from the German Hodgkin's Lymphoma Study Group. *Journal of Clinical Oncology, 21,* 3440–3446.

Yarbro, C. (2000). Malignant lymphomas. In Yarbro, C. H., Frogge, M. H., Goodman, M., & Groenwald, S. L. (Eds.), *Cancer nursing: Principles and practice* (5th ed.). Boston, MA: Jones & Bartlett.

Zelenetz, A., Appelbaum, F., Cabanillas, F., et al. (2003). *National Comprehensive Cancer Network clinical practice guidelines in oncology: Non-Hodgkin's lymphoma, Version 1.* Rockledge, PA: National Comprehensive Cancer Network Inc.

19 Multiple Myeloma

Kathy A. Shane
Brenda K. Shelton

I. Definition: Multiple myeloma is defined as a malignancy of the plasma cells or their immunoglobulins.

A. Multiple myeloma comprises only 1% of all cancers, and 10% to 12% of hematologic malignancies, with an estimated 14,000 cases per year.

B. Although not a malignancy of high incidence, the number of new cases has increased steadily over the past decade. Whether this reflects the more precise diagnostic criteria, earlier and more specific diagnostic methods, or an actual increase in incidence is unknown. The growing aged population may also contribute to the rising incidence of this disease.

C. Multiple myeloma affects males more commonly than females (3:2).

D. Less than 2% of cases occur before the age of 40, with peak incidence occurring in 50- to 70-year-old people; however, a trend toward disease presentation under the age of 55 has been observed in recent years, implying environmental causes.

E. African Americans develop multiple myeloma twice as commonly as other ethnic groups, although this may be attributable to higher baseline immunoglobulin levels, providing a larger base from which malignant cells can proliferate.

F. The prognosis for patients with multiple myeloma is poor, with 40% to 50% of the patients dying within 3 months of diagnosis, and 85% to 90% within 2 years. There is only a 3% 10-year survival rate despite more effective treatment regimens.

G. Pathophysiology

1. Plasma cells are antibody-forming cells derived from B lymphocytes and act as transcriptionists for the creation of specific antibodies or immunoglobulins.

2. The homogeneous antibody production or monoclonal gammopathy characteristic of multiple myeloma most commonly affects immunoglobulin G or A (52% and 21%, respectively).

3. When plasma cells become malignant, they proliferate uncontrollably, infiltrating the bone marrow, then the bone matrix, causing osteolytic bone lesions.

4. Myeloma cells proliferate outside the bone marrow in all lymphoid tissues where plasma cells normally reside.

5. Paraproteins (referred to as M, myeloma, or monoclonal protein) are secreted in excess by the abnormal plasma cells.

   a. May result in hyperviscosity of body fluids, affecting the function of all blood cell lines and many organs.

    b. The presence and/or degree of abnormal proteins accounts for the symptomatology, as well as the staging or classification of the disease.

    c. Paraproteins may also degrade to amyloid, a proteinaceous substance that deposits between cells; particularly in the heart, liver, spleen, and kidneys.

H. Multiple myeloma is a disease that varies from a smoldering abnormality of immunoglobulin without frank malignant cells, to a highly aggressive malignant disease (Zaidi & Vesole, 2001).

II. Etiology: The precise cause of multiple myeloma is unknown; however, some factors have been associated with the development of this cancer.

  A. Abnormal genetic karyotypes are observed in 50% to 70% of patients.

    1. Several chromosomes have been implicated, but the most common are chromosomes 11 and 13.

    2. Relapsing or treatment-refractory patients have a higher frequency of chromosomal abnormalities.

    3. Dysregulation of oncogenes and tumor suppressor genes controlling cellular proliferation, growth arrest, and apoptosis contribute to the pathogenesis of most malignancies, and multiple myeloma is no exception. The genes thought to be most often affected in multiple myeloma are the p53 tumor suppressor gene, Mip-1 alpha gene, monosomy 13, and IgH translocations (Ho et al., 2002; Magrangeas et al., 2003).

  B. The cytokines, interleukin 6 (IL-6), and tumor necrosis factor (TNF) are potent growth and survival factors for myeloma cells.

  C. A history of chronic infections or repeat allergic stimulation may place people at risk for the development of multiple myeloma because this cancer involves the antibody-producing cells of the body. In recent years, viruses, particularly hepatitis C and human immunodeficiency virus (HIV), have been identified as possible triggers in the development of multiple myeloma.

  D. Exposure to ionizing radiation is considered a risk factor for the disease because of the prevalence of this disease among people with significant exposure to radiation (eg, atomic blast) and those in occupations with chronic low-level radiation exposure.

  E. Other suspected risk factors include exposure to wood, rubber, textile, and petroleum processing, hair dye, and asbestos.

III. Patient Management

  A. Assessment

    1. Bony "tumor sites" are commonly palpable on the skull, jaw, scapulae, sternum, clavicles, vertebrae, pelvis, or ribs. Tumors are pink or reddish looking and fleshy feeling.

    2. Bone pain is the most common subjective complaint, occurring in 65% to 75% of patients presenting with multiple myeloma. The proliferation of plasma cells and crowding of the bone marrow produce intractable bone pain that is difficult to differentiate from pain that may be associated with pathologic fractures that can also occur with this disease. In fact, 25% to 35% of patients present with pathologic fractures.

3. Extraskeletal tumor sites (called plasmacytomas) are occasionally noted in the nasopharynx, paranasal sinuses, larynx, thorax, paravertebral or epidural tissues, lymph nodes, and gastrointestinal (GI) tract.

4. Fatigue is a common complaint of patients, occurring as the malignant cells crowd the bone marrow and produce anemia, or related to white blood cell (WBC) dysfunction and infections. Fatigue and muscle weakness are also manifestations of hypercalcemia, a common complication of this disease. At time of diagnosis, 25% to 30% of patients present with symptomatic hypercalcemia.

5. Easy bruising and bleeding occur when the bone marrow becomes crowded with malignant cells, resulting in thrombocytopenia.

6. Mental status changes occur in extensive or progressive disease, and can be due to hypercalcemia, renal dysfunction, hyperviscosity, or an infectious complication. Moderate changes in personality signal a metabolic disorder such as hypercalcemia. More serious focal deficits, such as unequal pupils or single-sided weakness, may be indicative of a thrombotic stroke due to hyperviscosity. Myeloma protein deposition on peripheral nerves can result in both motor and visual deficits and sensory neuropathies.

7. Spontaneous pathologic fractures occur due to bone invasion by myeloma cells. Fractures of long bones with minimal activity (eg, femur, humerus) are common, although vertebral collapse with spinal cord compression is also prevalent. Pathologic fractures and spinal cord compression impair patient mobility.

8. Oliguria and impaired renal function can result from damage to renal tubules by myeloma protein, and is a presenting symptom in 25% to 40% of patients.

9. Despite the wide array of symptoms that can signal a diagnosis of multiple myeloma, 30% of patients are diagnosed on routine examination.

B. Diagnostic Parameters
   1. Serum tests
      a. There is one specific serum test to diagnose multiple myeloma (serum protein electrophoresis) and the specific type of gammopathy. On electrophoresis, the abnormal immunoglobulin separates differently than normal immunoglobulins found in the serum.
      b. Serum immunofixation determines the type of myeloma protein, light or heavy chain.
      c. Tests to detect common complications of the disease (complete blood count, serum calcium)
         (1) The complete blood count is performed to detect the severity of bone marrow infiltration with malignant plasma cells. There are usually a large number of lymphocytes (40% to 50% of total WBC count) and not less than 3% plasma cells. In severe disease, anemia and thrombocytopenia are present.
         (2) Serum calcium levels are elevated above 10.5 mg/dL, or 4.5 mEq/L due to abnormal bone resorption when myeloma invades the bony matrix.

d. Tests to monitor the disease's response to therapy (eg, serum viscosity, erythrocyte sedimentation rate)

(1) Serum viscosity levels (plasma/saline ratio) are elevated above 1.9 due to excess immunoglobulin.

(2) Hyperuricemia (uric acid >4 mg/dL) is present when there is a large tumor burden and rapid cell turnover.

(3) The erythrocyte sedimentation rate (ESR) is increased due to inflammation and abnormal levels of immunoglobulin. This test may be used to monitor response to treatment.

e. Tests to assess severity of disease or disease progression (Beta 2 microglobulin, C-reactive protein, lactate dehydrogenase [LDH], plasma cell labeling index values, cytogenetics)

(1) Beta 2 microglobulin is a protein normally found on the surface of myeloma cells; a level >3 μg/mL indicates extensive disease.

(2) C-reactive protein is produced by the liver; a level >6 μg/mL is indicative of a poorer prognosis.

(3) LDH is a measure of tumor cell burden; increasing levels may indicate disease progression.

(4) Plasma cell labeling index is the percentage of plasma cells actively growing; a normal value is <1%.

(5) Cytogenetic testing assesses the number and normalcy of chromosomes.

2. Urine Tests

a. A 24-hour urine test for Bence Jones protein (the light chain of the immunoglobulin molecule) detects the presence of abnormal immunoglobulin. The kidneys normally resorb abnormal immunoglobulin, but when it is present in large amounts, it will spill into the urine. Its absence may not rule out disease, but its presence does confirm diagnosis.

b. On urinalysis, plasma cells may be present in urine sediment.

c. Hypercalciuria (any detectable urine calcium) is present when there is serum hypercalcemia, and it is present in many patients with multiple myeloma.

3. Other Tests

a. A bone marrow aspiration shows abnormal numbers of immature plasma cells, as well as decreased WBC, red blood cells (RBC), and platelets.

b. Computed tomography (CT) scans or magnetic resonance imaging (MRI) scans will demonstrate amyloid plaquelike lesions on the liver, spleen, lymph nodes, adrenal glands, kidneys, and GI tract.

c. X-rays initially show osteoporosis and eventually demonstrate multiple, sharply circumscribed osteolytic (punched out) lesions, particularly on the skull, pelvis, and spine.

C. Treatment: The three major considerations in staging multiple myeloma are the IgG or IgA levels, renal function, and isolation of discrete tumors. A summary of the staging criteria for multiple myeloma are noted in Box 19–1. Classifications of monoclonal gammopathies are noted in Table 19–1.

▼ **BOX 19-1** | **Myeloma Staging System**

Stage   Criteria

I   All of the following:
    Hgb value > 10 g/dL
    Serum calcium value normal (< 12 mg/dL)
    On roentgenogram, normal bone structure or solitary bone
        plasmacytoma only
    Low M-component production rates
        IgG value < 5 g/dL
        IgA value < 3 g/dL
        Urine light chain M-component on electrophoresis
            < 4 g/24 hr

II   Overall data not as minimally abnormal as shown for Stage I,
    and no single value as abnormal as defined for Stage III

III   One or more of the following:
    Hgb value < 8.5 g/dL
    Serum calcium value > 12 mg/dL
    Advanced lytic bone lesions
    High M-component production rates
        IgG value > 7 g/dL
        IgA value > 5 g/dL
        Urine light chain M-component on electrophoresis
            > 12 g/24 hr

Subclassification
A = relatively normal renal function (serum creatinine value
        < 2.0 mg/dL)
B = abnormal renal function (serum creatinine value
        > 2.0 mg/dL)

Examples
Stage IA = low cell mass with normal renal function
Stage IIIB = high cell mass with abnormal renal function

Source: Alexanian, R., Balcerzak, S., Bonnet, J. D., et al. (1975). Prognostic factors in multiple myeloma. *Cancer, 36,* 1192-1201. Copyright © 1975 American Cancer Society.
Reprinted by permission by Wiley-Liss, Inc., a subsidiary of John Wiley & Sons, Inc.

---

1. Patients with monoclonal gammopathy of undetermined significance (MGUS) or smoldering myeloma are usually not actively
treated but observed frequently for disease conversion.
2. Patients with indolent multiple myeloma are usually managed conservatively, receiving local radiation to specific lesions or oral
chemotherapy.

TABLE 19-1 Classification of Monoclonal Gammopathy

Classification	Characteristics	Management
Monoclonal gammopathy of undetermined significance (MGUS)	Serum M protein < 3g/dL Bone marrow plasma cells < 10% Absence of anemia, renal failure, hypercalcemia, and lytic bone lesions	Observation, with treatment beginning at disease progression
Smoldering multiple myeloma (SMM)	Serum M protein < 3g/dL and/or Bone marrow plasma cells ≥ 10% Absence of anemia, renal failure, hypercalcemia, and lytic bone lesions	Observation with treatment beginning at disease progression
Indolent or asymptomatic multiple myeloma (IMM)	Presence of serum/urine M protein Bone marrow plasmacytosis Mild anemia or few small lytic bone lesions Absence of symptoms	Monitoring every 3 months, with treatment beginning at disease progression Possible bisphosphonates and prednisone to reduce osteoclastic activity
Symptomatic multiple myeloma (MM)	Presence of serum/urine M protein Bone marrow plasmacytosis Anemia, renal failure, hypercalcemia, or lytic bone lesions Patients with primary systemic amyloidosis and bone marrow plasma cells ≥30% are considered to have both MM and amyloidosis.	Immediate treatment

MGUS does not always undergo malignant transformation; patients may present with a variety of symptoms related to monoclonal gammopathy such as polyneuropathy, hemolytic anemia, cryoglobulinemia, corneal keratopathy, xanthoderma, primary amyloidosis, and POEMS syndrome (coined to refer to a syndrome comprising polyneuropathy, organomegaly, endocrinopathy, M protein, and skin changes).
Waldenström's macroglobulinemia is a malignant monoclonal gammopathy of IgM with symptoms of hyperviscosity, which may progress to myeloma.
Multiple Myeloma Research Foundation. (2002). *Multiple myeloma: A disease overview*. New Canaan, CT: Author.

3. Prednisone is given to many patients, in addition to other therapies, because it stabilizes bone resorption and decreases the concentration of serum proteins, including the monoclonal proteins of multiple myeloma. Prednisone has the secondary benefit of stimulating RBC and WBC production, potentially improving the hematocrit and decreasing the complications of anemia.

4. About 50% of patients improve with oral alkylating agents such as melphalan (Alkeran), chlorambucil (Leukeran), cyclophosphamide, or carmustine (BCNU). Prolonged use of such agents can be mye-

loablative and may limit the success of future autologous transplant (Traynor, Noga & NCCN Multiple Myeloma Practice Guidelines Panel, 2001).

5. A standard regimen of vincristine, doxorubicin, and Decadron (VAD) has had comparable results to oral agents without the irreversible bone marrow suppression (Traynor, Noga & NCCN Multiple Myeloma Practice Guidelines Panel, 2001).

6. Plasmapheresis is used for palliative removal of monoclonal proteins and for prevention of renal failure. It is important for patients receiving plasmapheresis to have replacement fluid therapy to prevent worsening hyperviscosity.

7. In hopes of effecting longer-term response rates or cures, some clinicians advocate use of autologous or allogeneic bone marrow transplantation with the first remission (Pandit & Vesole, 2002).

8. Androgens may be administered to reduce hypercalcemia.

9. Patients usually require monthly infusions of bisphosphonates for life to prevent further osteoclastic activity and perhaps slight antimyeloma effect by inhibiting cell growth and angiogenesis (Lipton, Small, Saad, et al., 2002).

10. Thalidomide has been successfully used in refractory myeloma (Cool & Herrington, 2002; Thomas & Doss, 2002).
    a. Antiangiogenesis effects
    b. 100 to 200 mg orally daily up to a maximum of 800 mg daily
    c. Adverse effects: peripheral neuropathy, dizziness, drowsiness, GI distress

11. Bortezomib (Velcade) has recently been licensed for treatment of patients with multiple myeloma who have demonstrated disease progression despite receiving at least two prior therapies (Millennium Pharmaceuticals, 2003).
    a. Reverse inhibitor of chymotrypsinlike activity of the 26S proteasome
    b. Administration: 1.3 mg/m^2/dose twice weekly for 2 weeks, followed by 10 days' rest, up to eight treatment cycles
    c. Adverse effects: orthostatic hypotension during administration, peripheral neuropathy, nausea and vomiting, diarrhea or constipation, thrombocytopenia, reduced clearance with hepatic disease

12. Other agents (eg, PS 341, arsenic) have demonstrated some antitumor response (Ryoo, Cole & Anderson, 2002).

D. Nursing Diagnoses
   1. Knowledge deficit regarding multiple myeloma diagnosis and treatment
      a. *Problem:* Patients newly diagnosed with multiple myeloma need to understand the disease process and treatment options to make informed decisions about their care and plan for their future. Patients often have a poor prognosis despite therapy, because the tumor becomes resistant to treatment. The specific nursing care of patients receiving radiation therapy, chemotherapy, or bone marrow transplantation are addressed in Chapters 5, 6, and 8.
      b. *Interventions*
         (1) Provide patient with specific information about the prescribed therapy.

(2) Assess mental competence in hearing treatment options and making decisions about care. Hypercalcemia and hyperviscosity may interfere with the patient's ability to make decisions.

(3) Assist the patient and significant others in identifying their concerns and questions about the disease or treatment.

c. *Desired outcomes*

(1) The patient verbalizes understanding of the disease process and treatment options.

(2) The patient demonstrates appropriate information-seeking behaviors and decision-making skills.

(3) The patient is compliant in treatment regimen and the need for lifelong follow-up care.

2. Pain related to osteolytic bone lesions

a. *Problem:* Bone pain is the most common complaint of patients with multiple myeloma. Pain is predominantly located in the lower back and ribs. Pain is often exacerbated by movement but can be gradual or fluctuating.

b. *Interventions:* For generalized care of the patient, see Chapter 30.

(1) Administer nonsteroidal antiinflammatory agents to abrogate pain related to multiple myeloma. These agents' antiprostaglandin activity is especially helpful, because bone pain may be generated by prostaglandin release.

(2) Administer bisphosphonates (pamidronate [Aredia], zoledronic acid [Zoledronate]) to reduce osteoclastic activity, reducing osteolytic lesions and decreasing bone pain.

(3) Maintain maximal mobility with reasonable periods of rest to reduce bone pain.

c. *Desired outcomes*

(1) The patient will rate pain as < 2 out of ten.

(2) The patient verbalizes interventions helpful in management of bone pain.

3. Activity intolerance related to fatigue, pathologic fractures, and bone pain

a. *Problem:* Cancer itself, pain, and bone destruction can lead to altered activity tolerance and inability to perform activities of daily living (ADLs). These alterations are often due to functional impairments, such as pathologic fractures, but may also be sensory in nature.

b. *Interventions*

(1) Provide mild exercises interspersed with periods of rest to maximize the patient's ability to function in ADLs.

(2) Provide activity-assist devices, such as walkers, canes, and wheelchairs, as indicated.

(3) Refer patient to physical therapy to develop an exercise and rest regimen to maintain muscle tone.

(4) Refer patient to occupational therapy to assess patient's home care/self-care needs and modifications required in the home setting.

(5) Provide validation for needed home health aides or other resources (eg, Meals on Wheels) to assist patient with ADLs.

(6) Provide for patient safety to prevent pathologic fractures (eg, assistance when out of bed, open and clear hallways when walking, braked chairs).

c. *Desired outcomes*

(1) The patient will be able to independently perform some ADLs.

(2) The patient will be able to recognize and modify factors affecting activity intolerance.

(3) The patient will be free of pathologic fractures.

4. Altered fluid volume, less than required

a. *Problem:* Patients with multiple myeloma have hyperviscosity due to excess malignant immunoglobulin and are likely to exacerbate this condition due to hemoconcentration associated with hypercalcemic polyuria.

b. *Interventions*

(1) Assess intake and output records for excess fluid loss.

(2) Weigh the patient daily to assess total body fluid.

(3) Monitor central venous pressure when available to determine circulating volume.

(4) Assess orthostatic heart rate and blood pressure when the intake is less than output and there has been weight loss.

(5) Monitor for laboratory evidence of hyperosmolarity (osmolarity >285 mOsmol, Na >145 mEq/L) indicative of fluid loss.

(6) Encourage the patient to drink at least 2 L of fluid intake (preferably free water) per day. Provide intravenous (IV) hydration if oral intake is inadequate.

(7) Assess the patient's other organ systems for evidence of reduced perfusion (eg, mental status changes, chest pain, hypotension, oliguria, decreased bowel sounds).

c. *Desired outcomes*

(1) The patient will maintain central venous pressure between 5 and 15 cm water, or 2 to 6 mmHg.

(2) The patient will display no evidence of altered tissue perfusion due to hypovolemia (eg, oliguria, altered mental status, dyspnea, chest discomfort).

5. Altered elimination, urinary

a. *Problem:* The presence of high quantities of M-protein immunoglobulin causes increased uric acid production with potential renal damage. In addition, bone destruction associated with this disease causes increased osteoclastic activity, hypercalcemia, and renal tubular damage from high excretory levels of calcium.

b. *Interventions*

(1) Monitor intake and output every shift, or have the patient keep a log of fluid intake and voiding.

(2) Encourage consumption of at least 2 L of fluid daily to dilute immunoglobulins, reduce hypercalcemia, and decrease renal damage by hyperuricemia.

(3) When evaluating renal function with excretory urography, use iothalamate or diatrizoate instead of the usual contrast medium to avoid precipitation of calcium.

(4) Administer allopurinol daily to block production of methylxanthine oxidase, the toxic metabolite of urea. This medication protects the kidneys against uric acid crystallization and destruction of the kidney tubules.

(5) Limit medications and procedures known to challenge renal function (eg, IV contrast medium, antimicrobials) and administer hydration before and/or after renal toxic interventions.

(6) Monitor blood urea nitrogen, serum creatinine, and creatinine clearance routinely, and renally adjust medication dosages as indicated. Medications often requiring renal dose adjustment include antimicrobials, angiotensin-converting enzyme inhibitors, electrolyte supplements.

c. *Desired outcomes*

(1) The patient's urine output in 24 hours is >2000 mL and greater than intake by at least 200 mL.

(2) The patient's serum calcium remains within normal limits (between 8.5 and 10.5 mg/dL when corrected for albumin level).

(3) The patient's serum uric acid level remains <5 mg/dL.

6. Potential for injury related to fall, spontaneous fractures, leukopenia, and thrombocytopenia

a. *Problem:* Patients with multiple myeloma are at risk for general injury related to multiple etiologic factors. Patients who are hypovolemic are prone to falls. Bone demineralization from disease places patients at risk for fractures, and malignant bone marrow involvement causes bone marrow aplasia with potential for bleeding or infection.

b. *Interventions*

(1) Assist patients when out of bed or provide for home health assistants after discharge.

(2) Clear the floor area of obstructions or sources of injury.

(3) Assess the specific risk factors for injury and provide appropriate referrals.

(4) Provide the patient and family with a list of important reportable symptoms (fever >100.5° F, shortness of breath, difficulty arousing from sleep, inability to void, no urination for more than 8 hours, or a fall of any kind that results in ongoing discomfort).

c. *Desired outcomes*

(1) The patient will not fall or suffer injury.

(2) The patient and family will be able to identify symptoms that place the patient at greater risk for injury.

7. Fatigue

a. *Problem:* Bone marrow suppression with leukopenia, anemia, and thrombocytopenia depletes the patient's energy. Patients with multiple myeloma may be less able to use exercise as a strategy to abrogate fatigue, because bone injury is a high risk.

In addition, bone pain, infection, and hypercalcemia contribute to the presence of this symptom.

b. *Interventions:* For generalized interventions, see Chapter 25.

  (1) Provide frequent rest periods.

  (2) Assess the presence or severity of fatigue as a possible indication of the concomitant occurrence of hypercalcemia.

c. *Desired outcomes:* The patient verbalizes the ability to satisfactorily adjust lifestyle to the physical limitations of disease.

8. Potential altered mental status related to hypercalcemia

a. *Problem:* High serum calcium levels are the result of bone demineralization. These levels produce mental status changes that can cause airway incompetence, high risk of injury, and altered ability to care for self.

b. *Interventions:* Follow recommendations in Chapter 34.

c. *Desired outcomes*

  (1) The patient's serum calcium will be <10.5 mg/dL.

  (2) The patient will remain oriented to person, place, and time and will behave appropriately.

9. Potential for infection related to leukopenia

a. *Problem:* The malignant plasma cells of multiple myeloma crowd other WBCs and their normal development within the bone marrow, causing leukopenia. This WBC deficit, coupled with malignancy of the plasma cell, predisposes the patient to infection and its dissemination. The treatment of multiple myeloma is also systemic in nature, causing bone marrow suppression and increased risk of infection.

b. *Interventions:* Follow recommendations in Chapter 22.

c. *Desired outcomes*

  (1) The patient's body temperature will be <38° C.

  (2) The patient's WBC count returns to normal between cycles of therapy.

10. Potential altered tissue perfusion (less than required) related to anemia, or hypovolemia

a. *Problem:* Bone marrow suppression due to excessive production of malignant plasma cells leads to anemia that can be significant enough to compromise tissue oxygenation.

b. *Interventions*

  (1) Monitor complete blood count frequently.

  (2) Assess for potential benefit and administer erythropoietic growth factors or blood transfusions as needed.

  (3) Teach the patient energy conservation measures.

  (4) Administer or encourage fluid intake that enhances circulating blood volume.

c. *Desired outcomes*

  (1) Hemoglobin >12 mg/dL

  (2) No evidence of organ dysfunction attributable to poor perfusion

11. Potential alteration in mobility related to pathologic fractures and spinal cord compression

a. *Problem:* Patients with multiple myeloma develop osteolytic bone destruction with collapse of the bony matrix. This weakens the bones, predisposing them to fracture. Minimal or no injury may still result in pathologic fractures, particularly in the axial skeletal bones (eg, vertebrae, hips, femurs).

    b. *Interventions*

       (1) Encourage regular, mild exercise to maintain muscle strength for support of bony structures.

       (2) Advise the patient to avoid situations that may induce minimal trauma and bone fractures because of their high risk (eg, amusement park rides).

       (3) Provide supportive devices to decrease risk of stress fractures (eg, back brace, cervical collar).

       (4) Administer pamidronate as ordered to decrease hypercalcemia, relieve bone pain, and potentially decrease osteoclastic activity.

       (5) Make referrals to occupational therapy for assist devices (eg, walker, cane) as needed.

       (6) Be certain patient and significant others are knowledgeable about the signs and symptoms of spinal cord compression (see Chapter 37).

    c. *Desired outcomes*

       (1) The patient will be free of skeletal fractures on bone scan and x-ray.

       (2) The patient and significant others verbalize strategies to prevent bone fracture.

       (3) The patient and significant others can describe important reportable signs and symptoms of spinal cord compression.

E. Discharge Planning and Patient Education: Patients with multiple myeloma have a chronic incurable disease and suffer many exacerbations and remissions.

    1. Focus nursing care on both treatment of disease and minimizing complications. The disease results in multiple debilitating complications that require frequent clinical monitoring and diagnostic testing.

    2. Teach the patient about the medical follow-up required and have social support to enable attendance at these follow-up appointments.

    3. Provide the patient with information about ambulatory assist devices and assistance with ADLs. Home health care and social support are essential for comprehensive care of these patients.

REFERENCES

Alexanian, R., Balcerzak, S., Bonnet, J. D., et al. (1975). Prognostic factors in multiple myeloma. *Cancer, 36,* 1192–1201.

Cool, R. M., & Herrington, J. D. (2002). Thalidomide for the treatment of relapsed and refractory multiple myeloma. *Pharmacotherapy, 22*(8), 1019–1028.

Curtiss, C. P., Maxwell, T. L., & Swift, R. A. (2001). Comprehensive care of the patient with multiple myeloma: Physiology, chemotherapy, bisphosphonates, and psychosocial issues. *2001 Annual Congress Symposium Highlights* (pp. 9–12). Pittsburgh, PA: Medical Association Communications and the Oncology Nursing Society.

Durie, B.G. (2002). Low-dose thalidomide in myeloma: Efficacy and biologic significance. *Seminars in Oncology, 29*(6, Suppl. 17), 34–38.

_____. (2002). PS-341: The patient experience. *International Myeloma Foundation,*[AQ] 5(2), 1–2.

Ho, P. J., Campbell, L. J., Gibson, J., et al. (2002). The biology and cytogenetics of multiple myeloma. *Reviews in Clinical and Experimental Hematology, 6*(3), 276–300.

Hussein, M. A., Juturi, J. V., & Lieberman, I. (2002). Multiple myeloma: Present and future. *Current Opinions in Oncology,14*(1), 31–35.

International Myeloma Foundation. (2002). Multiple myeloma: Cancer of the bone marrow (pp. 5–14). North Hollywood, CA: Author.

Kaplan, A. A. (2001). Therapeutic apheresis for the renal complications of multiple myeloma. *Therapeutic Apheresis, 5*(3), 171–175.

Kaufmann, H., Urbauer, E., Ackerman, J., Huber, H., & Drach, J. (2001). Advances in the biology and therapeutic management of multiple myeloma. *Annals of Hematology, 80*(8), 445–451.

Lipton, A., Small, E., Saad, F., et al. (2002). The new bisphosphonate, Zometa (zoledronic acid), decreases skeletal complications in both osteolytic and osteoblastic lesions: A comparison to pamidronate. *Cancer Investigation, 20*(Suppl. 2), 45–54.

Magrangeas, F., Nasser, V., Avet-Loiseau, H., et al. (2003). Gene expression profiling of multiple myeloma reveals molecular portraits in relation to the pathogenesis of the disease. *Blood, 101*(12), 4998–5006.

Millennium Pharmaceuticals. (2003). Velcade™ (bortezomib) for injection. Prescribing information. Cambridge, MA: Millennium Pharmaceuticals.

Moehler, T. M., Neben, K., Ho, A. D., & Goldschmidt, H. (2001). Angiogenesis in hematologic malignancies. *Annals of Hematology, 80*(12), 695–705.

Multiple Myeloma Research Foundation. (2002). *Current and emerging trends in the treatment of multiple myeloma* (pp. 7–28). New Canaan, CT: Author.

Pandit, S., & Vesole, D. H. (2002). Multiple myeloma: Role of allogeneic transplantation. *Oncology, 16*(9), 1268–1274.

Pellat-Deceunynck, C. (2003). Tumour-associated antigens in multiple myeloma. *British Journal of Haematology, 120*(1), 3–9.

Ryoo, J. J., Cole, C. E., & Anderson, K. C. (2002). Novel therapies for multiple myeloma. *Blood Reviews, 16*(3), 167–174.

Thomas, M., & Doss, D. (2002). *Thalidomide Nursing Roundtable update* (pp. 8–36). Skillman, NJ: American Academy of CME.

Traynor, A. E., Noga, S. J., & NCCN Multiple Myeloma Practice Guidelines Panel. (2001). NCCN practice guidelines for management of multiple myeloma. *Cancer Control, 8*(6, Suppl 2), 78–87.

Wellington, K., & Goa, K. L. (2003). Zoledronic acid: A review of its use in the management of bone metastases and hypercalcemia of malignancy. *Drugs, 63*(4), 417–437.

Wilkes, G. M., Ingwersen, K., & Barton-Burke, M. (2002). Introduction to chemotherapy drugs. In *2002 Oncology Nursing Drug Handbook* (p. 3). Sudbury, MA: Jones & Bartlett.

Zaidi, A. A., & Vesole, D. H. (2001). Multiple myeloma: An old disease with new hope for the future. *CA: A Cancer Journal for Clinicians, 51*(5), 273–285.

20 Sarcomas

Beth L. Kozak Onners

I. Definition
A. Tumors Arising From Connective Tissues
1. Comes from the Greek word meaning "fleshy growth"
2. Types of sarcomas: Bone and soft tissue
   a. Bone sarcomas are malignant tumors arising from the skeletal system of the body. Malignant bone tumors represent 5% of all malignancies in children and 10% of all malignancies in adolescents. For specific types of bone sarcomas and the tissues from which they originate, see Table 20–1.
   b. Soft tissue sarcomas are malignant tumors arising from the extraskeletal connective tissue of the body. Soft tissues are those that connect, support, or surround other structures and organs in the body. The incidence of soft tissue sarcomas outnumbers bone sarcomas 3:1. For specific types of soft tissue sarcomas and the tissue from which they originate, see Table 20–1.
B. Incidence (American Cancer Society, 2003)
1. About 8,300 new cases yearly in the United States, and make up less than 1% of all newly diagnosed cancers.

TABLE 20–1 Types of Sarcomas

Type of Sarcoma	Tissue Origin
Bone Sarcomas	
Osteosarcoma	Bone
Chondrosarcoma	Cartilage
Ewing's sarcoma	Bone marrow
Fibrosarcoma of the bone	Spindle cell connective tissue
Soft Tissue Sarcomas	
Clear cell sarcoma	Bone marrow
Liposarcoma	Fat
Kaposi's sarcoma	Endothelial cells
Fibrosarcoma	Fibrous soft tissue (eg, tendons, ligaments)
Angiosarcoma	Blood vessels
Lymphangiosarcoma	Lymph vessels
Synoviosarcoma	Synovia
Leiomyosarcoma	Smooth muscle
Rhabdomyosarcoma	Striated/skeletal muscle

2. The morbidity rate of soft tissue cancer in 2003 is predicted to be 8,000, with the mortality estimate of 3,900.
3. Five-year survival rate is 90% in localized disease, but 10% to 15% when diagnosed after it has metastasized.
4. The diagnosis of most sarcomas is distributed equally among male and female with the incidence peaking during childhood and in the fifth decade of life.
5. The incidence is slightly higher in males than females and no racial preference except for Ewing's sarcoma, which is even more rare in African Americans.

C. Grading of sarcomas: Tables 20–2 and 20–3 review the grading system used for bone and soft tissue sarcomas.
   1. Clinical staging includes physical examination, clinical laboratory tests, and biopsy of the sarcoma for microscopic diagnosis and grading.

TABLE 20–2 Grading System for Bone Cancers

Primary Tumors (T)

TX Primary tumor cannot be assessed
T0 No evidence of primary tumor
T1 Tumor confined within the cortex
T2 Tumor invades beyond the cortex

Regional Lymph Nodes (N)

NX Regional lymph nodes cannot be assessed
N0 No regional lymph node metastasis
N1 Regional lymph node metastasis

Distant Metastasis (M)

MX Presence of distant metastasis cannot be assessed
M0 No distant metastasis
M1 Distant metastasis

Histopathologic Grade (G)

GX Grade cannot be assessed
G1 Well differentiated
G2 Moderately differentiated
G3 Poorly differentiated
G4 Undifferentiated
Note: Ewing's sarcoma is classified as G4.

Stage Grouping

Stage IA	G1,2	T1	N0	M0
Stage IB	G1,2	T2	N0	M0
Stage IIA	G3,4	T1	N0	M0
Stage IIB	G3,4	T2	N0	M0
Stage III	Not defined			
Stage IVA	Any G	Any T	N1	M0
Stage IVB	Any G	Any T	Any N	M1

American Joint Committee on Cancer, 1997.

TABLE 20-3 Grading System for Soft Tissue Sarcomas* in People ≥16 years of age

Primary Tumors (T)
TX Primary tumor cannot be assessed
T0 No evidence of primary tumor
T1 Tumor 5 cm or less in greatest dimension
T2 Tumor more than 5 cm in greatest dimension

Regional Lymph Nodes (N)
NX Regional lymph nodes cannot be assessed
N0 No regional lymph node metastasis
N1 Regional lymph node metastasis

Distant Metastasis (M)
MX Presence of distant metastasis cannot be assessed
M0 No distant metastasis
M1 Distant metastasis

Histopathologic Grade (G)
GX Grade cannot be assessed
G1 Well differentiated
G2 Moderately differentiated
G3 Poorly differentiated
G4 Undifferentiated

Stage Grouping

Stage IA	G1,2	T1	N0	M0
Stage IB	G1,2	T2	N0	M0
Stage IIA	G3,4	T1	N0	M0
Stage IIB	G3,4	T2	N0	M0
Stage III	Not defined			
Stage IVA	Any G	Any T	N1	M0
Stage IVB	Any G	Any T	Any N	M1

*With exception of Kaposi's sarcoma, dermatofibrosarcoma, desmoid type fibrosarcoma grade 1, sarcomas arising from the dura mater, brain, or parenchymatous organs or hollow viscera.
American Joint Committee on Cancer. (1997). *AJCC cancer staging handbook* (pp. 133-146). Philadelphia: Lippincott-Raven Publishers. (Reprinted with permission.)

2. Pathologic staging includes removal of the primary tumor, nodes, and suspected metastases.

II. Etiology: Little is known regarding the cause of primary bone and soft tissue tumors; however, a few risk factors have been identified. Table 20–4 shows the more common types of sarcomas and their incidence and etiology. The following have been identified as possible risk factors for the development of sarcomas:

   A. Prior cancer therapy, including high-dose irradiation
   B. Exposure to alkylating agents (ie, melphalan, procarbazine, nitrosureas, and chlorambucil) and chemicals (ie, vinyl chloride gas, arsenic, and dioxin, or Agent Orange).
   C. Chronic immunosuppressed patients, such as organ transplant recipients and patients who have acquired immunodeficiency syndrome (AIDS), are at high risk for soft tissue sarcomas.

▨ TABLE 20-4 Incidence and Etiology of Sarcoma

Type	Epidemiology	Etiology
Bone Sarcomas		
Osteosarcoma	• Most common type of bone cancer • Accounts for 34% of bone cancer • Incidence is greatest in people 1–25 years of age • Twice as common in males after the age of 13. In children younger than 13 years of age, the incidence is similar in males and females • Located primarily around the knee joint, either in the distal femur or proximal tibia	• Etiology of osteosarcoma is unclear • Increased incidence of osteosarcoma during adolescence, which has been correlated with skeletal growth patterns • People with Paget's disease have a higher affinity
Chondrosarcoma	• Second most common bone tumor • Accounts for about 13% of malignant bone cancers • Incidence is greatest in people 30–60 years of age • More common in males • Usually located in the pelvis or femur	• Development of chondrosarcoma has been associated with syndromes of skeletal maldevelopment • People with Ollier's disease (a syndrome of polyosteotic benign cartilage tumors) have a higher affinity
Fibrosarcoma of the bone	• Rare; accounts for fewer than 4% of primary bone tumors • Occurs in any age range, but is rare in children • No sex predominance • Generally originates in many mesenchymal sites; usually involves the abdominal wall or extremities • 50% occurrence in the femur and tibia • 10% are poorly differentiated with survival directly related to tumor grade	• Paget's disease • Chronic osteomyelitis • Fibrous dysplasia • Previous therapeutic irradiation
Ewing's sarcoma	• Accounts for 5% of malignant bone cancers, represents 1% of all childhood cancers • 80% of people diagnosed are under the age of 30, younger patient population than any other primary bone cancers. Ewing's is rarely seen before age 5 or after age 30. • 66% are males • Caucasians six times more likely to be diagnosed with Ewing's	• No specific etiologic factors, but may be genetic in origin given family predisposition

(continued)

TABLE 20–4 **Incidence and Etiology of Sarcoma** (Continued)

Type	Epidemiology	Etiology
	sarcoma than African Americans • Prognosis is poorer in males than females • More commonly found in the bones of the trunk than in long bones	

Soft Tissue Sarcomas

Type	Epidemiology	Etiology
Soft tissue sarcoma	• Occur over 50% of the time in the extremities, with the remainder in the head, neck, and the retroperitoneum regions	• Exposure to herbicides and other chemicals • Prior radiotherapy for cancers • Neurofibromatosis can lead to soft tissue sarcomas
Liposarcoma	• Most commonly diagnosed soft tissue tumor • These tumors usually originate in the deep fatty tissues of the thigh, behind the knee, the groin, the gluteal area, or behind the abdominal cavity (retroperitoneum) • Liposarcomas are most commonly found in adults between 30 and 60 years of age • Slightly more prevalent in males than females • Rarely metastasize (less than 10%) and are usually present as firm lumps which will aggressively invade the surrounding tissues	• Same as above
AIDS-related Kaposi's sarcoma	• More common in homosexual/bisexual males • 20,000 times more likely to occur in an HIV-infected person than the general population • Lesions or nodules can occur anywhere on the body	• HIV infection • Prolonged immunosuppression • African, Jewish, or Mediterranean descent with possible genetic predisposition
Clear cell sarcoma	• Now recognized as a form of malignant melanoma; however, incidence is rare • Affects adults younger than 40 years of age • Presents as painless, firm, spherical growths on tendon sheaths and aponeurotic structures of distal extremities • 5-year survival rate is approximately 50%	• Herbicides or other environmental carcinogen exposures

D. Family history of bone cancers, such as osteosarcoma, Ewing's sarcoma, and chondrosarcoma.
  1. Ewing's sarcoma is associated with abnormalities of the EWS gene and an ets transcription factor gene (Kovar, 2003).
  2. C-KIT gene abnormalities have been identified with osteosarcoma (Sandberg & Bridge, 2003)
E. Preexisting bone conditions (associated with malignant bone cancers). People with Paget's disease have a 0.8% chance of developing osteosarcoma and other rare cancers. Most osteosarcomas in people over age 40 years are associated with Paget's disease (Helman & Meltzer, 2003)
F. Tumor suppressor genes (noted in a few sarcomas; however, additional research is required in this area; Kovar, 2003; Sandberg & Bridge, 2003).

III. Patient Management
A. Assessment
  1. Bone sarcomas in general
     a. Sarcomas of the bone can have similar signs and symptoms. Unique features are listed below.
        (1) Localized pain
        (2) Presence of a tender mass with enhanced superficial vascularity
        (3) Edema of affected area
        (4) Functional deficit such as limited joint mobility
        (5) Pathologic fractures
     b. Osteosarcoma
        (1) Pain commonly worsens at night.
        (2) Weight loss is due to anorexia caused by the cancer or treatment.
        (3) Anemia is due to bone marrow suppression caused by the cancer or treatment.
     c. Ewing's sarcoma
        (1) Fever
        (2) History of severe persistent pain, and joint stiffness
        (3) Skin warmth over the affected area is common.
  2. Soft tissue sarcomas
     a. In the early stages of soft tissue sarcoma, no symptoms are experienced because soft tissue is relatively elastic and tumors can grow unchecked before they are felt or cause symptoms.
     b. In the later stages of soft tissue sarcoma, the signs and symptoms can include a painless mass, peripheral neuralgia, paralysis, ischemia, bowel obstruction, weight loss, fever, general malaise, and episodic hypoglycemia.
     c. Liposarcoma: Frequently occurs as a mass arising in soft tissues in the proximal lower extremities of adults (buttocks, thigh, groin, retroperitoneum).
     d. Rhabdomyosarcoma: Commonly presents as a painless mass arising in the muscle tissues of the head and neck region of children.
     e. Synovial sarcoma: Pain and swelling of the joints precedes appearance of a mass.
     f. Kaposi's sarcoma

        (1) Reddish black or purple cutaneous and subcutaneous nodules may appear anywhere on the body.

        (2) Found in patients with cytomegalovirus (CMV) and/or human immunodeficiency virus (HIV) type 1, or of African, Jewish, or Mediterranean descent.

B. Diagnostic Parameters

  1. Bone sarcomas

    a. Osteosarcoma

      (1) Serum tests

        (a) Low hemoglobin and hematocrit reflect inadequate production of red blood cells due to tumor in bones where blood products are formed.

        (b) Elevated serum calcium is due to bone destruction.

        (c) Elevated serum alkaline phosphatase levels represent osteoblastic activity. Serum alkaline phosphatase levels decline after tumor removal; however, can become elevated during recurrence or metastasis.

      (2) X-rays are useful in diagnosing osteosarcoma. Classic findings are:

        (a) Cortical bone destruction

        (b) Extension of the tumor into soft tissue

        (c) Periosteal bone formation that may appear in a perpendicular striated or "sunburst" pattern.

    b. Chondrosarcoma

      (1) Serum tests

        (a) Low hemoglobin and hematocrit reflect inadequate production of red blood cells due to the cancer.

        (b) Cytologic changes of the cartilage cells. Chondrosarcoma present with plump nuclei or clumps of chromatin.

      (2) Bone films of chondrosarcoma show a lobular pattern with or without calcification. Calcification is generally seen in a circular or semicircular pattern.

        (a) Central chondrosarcoma in the long bones may show thickening of the cortex because of edema.

        (b) Peripheral chondrosarcoma may show a vast, dense, blotchy appearance. Irregular radiopaque streaks extending away from the central part of the lesion may also be seen.

    c. Ewing's sarcoma

      (1) Serum tests: Low hematocrit/low hemoglobin, high erythrocyte sedimentation rates, and sometimes leukocytosis can be present at time of diagnosis. These changes are thought to be related to inflammation and similar to osteomyelitis.

      (2) X-rays show bone destruction that involves the shaft. Varying amounts of periosteal thickening may be present.

    d. Fibrosarcoma of the bone

      (1) Serum tests

        (a) Histologic changes: The degree of differentiation of the malignant fibroblasts, the cellular pattern, and the amount of collagen produced may vary.

        (b) Cytologic changes: Moderate anaplasia and cell irregularity may reflect fibrosarcomas.

        (c) Low hemoglobin/low hematocrit is due to tumor invasion into the bone marrow.

    (2) Computed tomography (CT) scan angiography is highly sensitive.

2. Soft tissue sarcomas

    a. Imaging and other tests

        (1) X-ray or CT scan identifies the size and location of the tumor, and are particularly useful when the malignancy is located in the chest, abdomen, or pelvis.

        (2) Magnetic resonance imaging (MRI) identifies the size and location of the tumor. MRI may be used to diagnose extremity soft tissue sarcomas (Fenstermacher, 2003).

        (3) Bone scan looks for bony invasion of a soft tissue sarcoma.

        (4) Arteriogram reveals the arterial insufficiency related to tumor compression of a vessel.

        (5) Open or closed biopsy of tissue identifies specific histologic patterns.

    b. Serum tests (only used for Kaposi's sarcoma): Abnormal values are seen with acquired immunodeficiency syndrome (AIDS)-related Kaposi's sarcoma; however, the abnormal values may be a result of HIV. These include

        (1) Elevated erythrocyte sedimentation rate.

        (2) Mild anemia.

        (3) Leukopenia.

        (4) Depressed cosyntropin stimulation.

        (5) Elevated serum transaminase levels.

        (6) Lowered platelet count.

C. Treatment

    1. Surgery: Low-grade sarcomas can be cured by surgical resection in 80% of the cases. Size, location, extent, and grade are considered before surgery is elected. Surgical procedures for sarcomas include:

    a. Radical resection with reconstruction.

    b. Radical resection without reconstruction (can be performed on the expendable bones, such as clavicle and sacrum).

    c. Amputation.

    d. Limb-sparing surgery.

    2. Chemotherapy: At the time of diagnosis, approximately 20% of patients present with distant metastases.

    a. Chemotherapy agents used to treat metastasis include doxorubicin, ifosfamide, vincristine, dacarbazine, and etoposide.

    b. New targeted therapies (directed at tyrosine kinase, kit receptors) may prove useful as characteristic genetic abnormalities are identified.

    c. Doxorubicin and ifosfamide are the most active single agents in soft tissue sarcomas. Individual side effects of the agents listed above are similar (see Chapter 5).

    d. Common adverse effects of chemotherapy regimens for sarcoma (for additional detail, review Chapter 5).

  (1) Granulocytopenia and thrombocytopenia occur 7 to 14 days after therapy (see Chapter 20).
  (2) Mucositis, esophagitis, and diarrhea are due to the destruction of epithelial cells lining the gastrointestinal (GI) tract.
  (3) Nausea and vomiting are anticipated, and prophylactic antiemetics should be prescribed (see Chapter 27).
  (4) Renal toxicity is a risk of ifosfamide. Mesna may be given to reduce this toxicity.
  (5) Cardiac toxicity may be avoided if the cumulative lifetime dose of doxorubicin does not exceed 550 mg/m^2.
  (6) Cognitive neurotoxicity presenting as disorientation, confusion, agitation, or somnolence may occur with ifosfamide. This dose-limiting toxicity is usually totally reversible.

3. Radiation therapy is used alone or in combination with other therapies to treat locally advanced, inoperable, recurrent, or metastatic disease. Radiation may cause tissue damage to areas in the treatment field.
  a. Delay of postoperative radiation therapy may be necessary to allow for surgical wound healing, but risk of relapse has led to rapid sequencing (2 to 4 weeks) between the two therapies (Ballo et al., 2003).
  b. Local erythema, edema, and pain are common adverse effects.
  c. Reopening of surgical wounds is a significant risk during radiation therapy.
4. Multimodality is being explored as a means of preventing early relapse.
  a. Operative procedures with "limb perfusion" allow intraoperative chemotherapy administration (Eggermont, 2003).
  b. Intraoperative radiation therapy has shown some promise (Domanovic, Ouzidane, Ellis, Kinsella & Beddar, 2003).
  c. Radiosensitization with chemotherapeutic agents is being used experimentally.
D. Nursing Diagnoses
  1. Knowledge deficit related to therapy (surgery, radiation therapy, chemotherapy)
    a. *Problem:* The patient and family require knowledge of therapeutic options and outcomes to participate in care.
    b. *Interventions*
      (1) Instruct the patient and family about therapy using various teaching approaches, based on the patient's level of knowledge and learning style.
      (2) Consider the psychological needs of the patient, particularly those facing amputation, or the implications associated with multimodality therapy.
      (3) Review the therapy plan (eg, surgical procedure, radiation plan). Instruct the patient about prevention of complications related to anesthesia and immobility, adverse effects of radiation or chemotherapy.

(4) Perform a complete baseline neurovascular assessment, because nerve injury (distal to the surgical site) may occur during the surgical management of sarcoma.

(5) Inform the patient that blood transfusions may be required during therapy. Patients with malignancies cannot bank their blood, but family members may donate blood.

(6) Explain position restrictions, such as limb elevation, or bed rest, depending on the extent of surgery and the physician's philosophy.

(7) Ensure patients are aware of reportable conditions that are related to the disease or therapy.

   (a) Fever, especially in the immediate postoperative period or after chemotherapy

   (b) Pain, swelling, or exudates at the site of tumor or surgical excision

(8) Initiate rehabilitation after surgery or initial therapy. Physical therapy should start during the patient's hospitalization and continue after discharge to home or rehabilitation facility.

(9) Initiate social work or occupational therapy consults to assist patient in dealing with potential social and economic losses.

  c. *Desired outcomes*

   (1) Patient will be able to state the type of therapy planned.

   (2) Patient will understand the potential risks and benefits of the therapy.

   (3) Patient will be able to state important pre- and posttherapy care and limitations.

   (4) Patient will be able to state the plan for rehabilitation.

2. Alteration in physical mobility

  a. *Problem:* Patients with sarcomas have tumor masses that may interfere with normal physical activities. These limitations are exacerbated after surgical interventions, in the presence of edema, with certain treatment, or when pain is present due to tumor or treatment-related adverse effects.

  b. *Interventions*

   (1) Assess need for physical, occupational, or psychological rehabilitation referral.

    (a) Assess personal physical goals.

    (b) Perform or refer for a family and home assessment.

   (2) Assist patients in home or work modifications, or disability applications that will permit them to adjust to any disease-related limitations.

   (3) Explore job retraining or family role modifications that may be the result of cancer or its therapy.

   (4) Provide contact information of associations that provide support for durable medical goods, or rehabilitation equipment.

  c. *Desired outcomes*

   (1) Absence of, or adaptive coping to physical limitations related to disease.

(2) Ability to become a productive and effective worker, family member, or friend despite disease-related limitations.

3. Alterations in comfort related to disease and treatments
   a. *Problem:* Pain is common in patients with sarcoma and may be related to any of the following:
      (1) Bone tumor pain often presents gradually and may take months before the patient seeks medical assistance.
      (2) Musculoskeletal tumor pain is often constant and worsens at night.
      (3) The patient may experience pain as a result of pressure of the sarcoma on surrounding tissue or because of treatment interventions.
      (4) Pain can be related to the location and size of the sarcoma, treatment damage, or phantom limb syndrome. The location of the sarcoma along nerve fibers, blood vessels, and viscera can cause intense pain.
      (5) The severity of sarcoma pain steadily increases as the tumor grows.
   b. *Interventions* (for additional interventions to aid in management of pain, consult Chapter 30)
      (1) Control early postoperative pain with an epidural catheter, and progress to oral opiates or antiinflammatory agents as healing occurs.
      (2) Teach the patient about the phenomenon of phantom limb sensations associated with amputations. (One third of people who have amputations experience this type of pain phenomenon.)
      (3) Teach patient about the types and symptoms of pain and the importance of reporting changes in pain because different pain syndromes may occur and respond differently to specific therapies.
      (4) Help the patient develop an activity and rest program to minimize pain.
   c. *Desired outcome:* Patient's pain will be controlled as evidenced by:
      (1) Ability to use pain relief measures and patient-controlled analgesics.
      (2) Pain rate of 3 or less on scale of 1 to 10.
      (3) Ability to perform ADL and participate in physical therapy with minimal discomfort.

4. Potential for infection related to surgery
   a. *Problem:* Surgery is a major risk factor for infection. Infection can result in delayed postoperative therapy, wound necrosis, and unplanned amputation.
   b. *Interventions*
      (1) Administer broad-spectrum intravenous (IV) antibiotics prophylactically for 48 hours after surgery. Prophylactic oral antibiotics may be continued after the resection.
      (2) Treat wound necrosis with débridement and frequent dressing changes. (Wound necrosis can occur if large flaps are used to close the wound. Plastic surgery may be required to

create a flap or split-thickness skin graft to close the wound if it does not heal properly.)

(3) Advise the patient regarding lifelong prevention of implant infection from a hematologic source. A simple infection can cause the implant to become infected when bacteria circulates in the bloodstream.

(4) Assess the surgical site every day, or as ordered. Assess for redness, drainage, odor, and skin warmth. Report any symptoms immediately, because they can indicate signs of infection. Remember that immune-suppressed patients may not present with these symptoms.

(5) Maintain proper antibiotic dosing.

c. *Desired outcomes*

(1) Patient will be afebrile.

(2) Patient's surgical site will heal properly and without infection.

5. Potential for ineffective coping related to amputation

a. *Problem:* The psychological and psychosocial needs of the patient undergoing amputation should be addressed pre- and postoperatively. Patients often fear dying, disability, and deformity. Loss of function may impact the patient's financial status and lifestyle. These fears and concerns can impede the ability to learn or participate in rehabilitation, and can lead to changes in self-esteem, manifested by anxiety and depression.

b. *Interventions*

(1) Initiate a social work consult to discuss financial status, personal relationships, and community resources.

(2) Initiate an occupational therapy consult to discuss the home environment.

(3) Discuss procedure, and give detailed information on what to expect postoperatively and during the recovery phase.

(4) Provide information about appropriate types of prosthesis.

(5) Initiate a physical therapy consult.

(6) If possible, suggest a preoperative meeting with a patient who has undergone a similar surgery.

(7) Encourage realistic expectations regarding level of mobility with or without prosthesis.

c. *Desired outcomes*

(1) Patient will state the postoperative plan of care.

(2) Patient will demonstrate a realistic understanding regarding the surgery.

(3) Patient will participate in rehabilitation regimen.

E. Discharge Planning and Patient Education

1. Determine discharge planning based on the type of treatment received by the patient.

2. Continue postoperative care in the home setting (ie, dressing changes, monitoring for signs of infection, and stump care).

3. Monitor or alter pain management if necessary. Phantom pain management may also necessitate ongoing, progressive intervention.

4. Assess and arrange home physical therapy, equipment, and nursing care.

5. Teach the patient the potential side effects and management of therapy.
6. Review discharge medications and ensure patient's compliance and understanding.
7. Assess the psychosocial and socioeconomic impact that the diagnosis and treatment of sarcoma will have on the patient's current way of life. Bone-jarring leisure activities, such as basketball and jogging, may have to be eliminated.
8. Initiate a social work consult, and encourage the patient to use community resources.

REFERENCES

American Cancer Society. (2003). *What are the key statistics for sarcoma?* Available: http://www.cancer.org/docroot/CRI_2_4_1x_what_are_the_key_statistics_for_sarcoma_28.asp?sitearea=.

American Joint Committee on Cancer. (1997). *AJCC cancer staging handbook* (pp. 133–146). Philadelphia: Lippincott-Raven.

Ballo, M. T., & Zagars, G. K. (2003). Radiation therapy for soft tissue sarcoma. *Surgical Oncology Clinics of North America,12*(2), 449–467, vii.

Ballo, M. T., Zagers, G. K., Cormier, J. N., Feig, B. W., Patel, S. R., & Pisters, P. W. (2003). The length of time between surgery and post-operative radiotherapy and local control for soft tissue sarcomas. *International Journal of Radiation Oncology, Biology, Physics, 57*(2 Suppl), S254.

Blazer, D. G., Sabel, M. S., & Sondak, V. K. (2003). Is there a role for sentinel lymph node biopsy in the management of sarcoma? *Surgical Oncology, 12*(3), 201–206.

Bramwell, V. H., Anderson, D., Charette, M. L., & Sarcoma Disease Site Group. (2003). Doxorubicin-based chemotherapy for the palliative treatment of adult patients with locally advanced or metastatic soft tissue sarcoma. *Cochrane Database Systematic Review, 3,* CD003293.

Carrubba, D. M., Jankowski, C. B., & Kunsman, J. (1999). Nursing management of soft tissue sarcomas of the extremities. *Clinical Journal of Oncology Nursing, 3*(4), 168–179.

Domanovic, M. A., Ouzidane, M., Ellis, R. J., Kinsella, T. J., & Beddar, A. S. (2003). Using intraoperative radiation therapy—a case study. *AORN Journal, 77*(2), 412–417.

Eggermont, A. M. (2003). Isolated limb perfusion in the management of locally advanced extremity soft tissue sarcoma. *Surgical Oncology Clinics of North America, 12*(2), 469–483.

Eilber, F. C., & Eilber, K. S. (2001). Soft tissue sarcoma. In J. L. Cameron (Ed.), *Current surgical therapy* (7th ed., pp. 1213–1217). St Louis, MO: Mosby.

Fenstermacher, M. J. (2003). Imaging evaluation of patients with soft tissue sarcoma. *Surgical Oncology Clinics of North America, 12*(2), 305–332.

Fraser, M., Marentay, P., & Bertha, R. (1999). A collaborative approach to isolated limb perfusion. *AORN Journal, 70*(4), 642–647, 649, 654–658 [quiz].

Gray, A. M., & Pollock, R. E. (2002). Management of soft tissue sarcomas: Extremity and chest wall. In K. I. Bland (Ed.), *The practice of general surgery* (pp. 1033–1040). Philadelphia: W. B. Saunders.

Helman , L. J., & Meltzer, P. (2003). Mechanisms of sarcoma development. *National Review of Cancer, 3*(9), 685–694.

Hwang, R. F., & Hunt, K. K. (2003). Experimental approaches to treatment of soft tissue sarcoma. *Surgical Oncology Clinics of North America, 12*(2), 499–521.

Khanfir, K., Alzieu, L., Terrier, P., Le Pechoux, C., Bonvalot, S., Vanel, D., & Le Cesne, A. (2003). Does adjuvant radiation therapy increase loco-regional control after optimal resection of soft-tissue sarcoma of the extremities? *European Journal of Cancer, 39*(13), 1872–1880.

Kline, N. E., & Sevier, N. (2003). Solid tumors in children. *Journal of Pediatric Nursing, 18*(2), 96–102.

Kovar, H. (2003). Ewing tumor biology: Perspectives for innovative treatment approaches. *Advances in Experimental Medicine and Biology, 532,* 27–37.

Kuiper, D. R., Hoekstra, H. J., Veth, R. P., & Wobbes, T. (2003). The management of clear cell sarcoma. *European Journal of Surgical Oncology, 29*(7), 568–570.

Micromedex Healthcare Series. (2003). *Drugdex drug evaluation*s. Available: http:jhmcis.jhmi.edu/mdxcgi/display.

Noy, A. (2003). Update in Kaposi sarcoma. *Current Opinion in Oncology, 15*(5), 379–381.

O'Sullivan, B., & Pisters, P. W. (2003). Staging and prognostic factor evaluation in soft tissue sarcoma. *Surgical Oncology Clinics of North America, 12*(2), 333–353.

O'Sullivan, B., Ward, I., & Catton, C. (2003). Recent advances in radiotherapy for soft-tissue sarcoma, *Current Oncology Reports, 5*(4), 274–281.

Potter, B. O., & Sturgis, E. M. (2003). Sarcomas of the head and neck. *Surgical Oncology Clinics of North America, 12*(2), 379–417.

Reid, R., Chandu De Silva, M. V., Paterson, L., Ryan, E., & Fisher, C. (2003). Low-grade fibromyxoid sarcoma and hyalinizing spindle cell tumor with giant rosettes share a common t(7;16)(q34;p11) translocation. *American Journal of Surgical Pathology, 27*(9), 1229–1236.

Sandberg, A. A., & Bridge, J. A. (2003). Updates on the cytogenetics and molecular genetics of bone and soft tissue tumors: Osteosarcoma and related tumors. *Cancer Genetics and Cytogenetics, 145*(1), 1–30.

Scaife, C. L., & Pisters, P. W. (2003). Combined-modality treatment of localized soft tissue sarcomas of the extremities. *Surgical Oncology Clinics of North America, 12*(2), 355–368.

Schuetz, B. (2002). Cutaneous angiosarcoma. *Dermatology Nursing, 14*(6), 400.

Znajda, T. L., Wunder, J. S., Bell, R. S., & Davis, A. M. (1999). Gender issues in patients with soft tissue sarcoma: A pilot study. *Cancer Nursing, 22*(2), 111–118.

21 Skin Cancer

Kathleen Burks
Constance R. Ziegfeld

I. Definition: In the United States, skin cancers are the most common of all cancers in Caucasians, occurring more frequently in males than females, and increasing with age. Due to ultraviolet (UV) radiation, people who live at higher altitudes or closer to the equator are at higher risk for skin cancers. Lesions occur most commonly in areas of the skin exposed to the sun. There are three types of skin cancer. Basal cell cancer (BCC) and squamous cell cancer (SCC) are often referred to as nonmelanoma skin cancers (NMSC) because of similarities in treatment and outcome. They often require extensive and recurrent treatment but have low metastatic and mortality rates. BCC and SCC account for less than 0.1% of patient deaths due to cancer. According to the American Cancer Society, 1.3 million cases of nonmelanoma skin cancer occur in the United States each year. Approximately 2,200 deaths occurred in 2002 due to nonmelanoma skin cancer. Nonmelanoma skin cancer has greater than a 95% cure rate when diagnosed in the early stages. Malignant melanomas (MM) have a higher mortality and metastatic rate but are less common.

  A. BCC is the most commonly occurring cancer, with almost 1 million new cases diagnosed annually in the United States. It begins in the epithelial tissue, most frequently on the head and neck. It is usually slow growing, and it invades and destroys surrounding tissues including bone, cartilage, and blood vessels.

  B. Approximately 200,000 new cases of SCC are diagnosed annually in the United States. SCC also begins in the epithelial tissue but is faster growing and more irregular in shape than BCC. It commonly appears on mucous membranes of the face (lower lip, tongue) or on the ears or back of the hands. Metastatic potential is greater than with BCC.

  C. MM arises from the melanocytes, which generate and transport melanin. These cells are in the basal epidermis, the eyes, meninges, lymph nodes, and alimentary and respiratory tracts. Incidence of MM has increased faster than any other cancer over the past 20 years. Although comprising only 4% of skin cancers, MM is responsible for about 75% of the deaths from skin cancer worldwide.

II. Etiology
  A. Risk Factors
    1. People with light skin and hair color or who are otherwise prone to sunburn are at increased risk for all skin cancers. A history of early sunburn or intense intermittent sun exposure increases the risk of MM.

2. Advanced age is a risk factor for both BCC and SCC.
3. History of skin trauma, overexposure to ionizing radiation, long-term arsenic ingestion, xeroderma pigmentosum, history of immunosuppression (organ transplantation, human immunodeficiency virus [HIV]), and scarring skin diseases (discoid lupus erythematosus, lupus vulgaris, chronic skin ulceration) also increase risk for BCC and SCC.
4. Nevoid BCC syndrome is a hereditary disorder characterized by development of BCC early in life. Affected people usually develop the disease by age 20 and may have over 100 BCC lesions.
5. Actinic keratoses (AK) due to chronic sun exposure have the potential to develop into SCC.
6. Several hereditary syndromes may be involved in development of a small percentage (5% to 12%) of MM: familial multiple mole melanoma syndrome (FAMMM), dysplastic nevus syndrome, and atypical mole syndrome.

B. Environmental Factors
1. Exposure to UV rays of the sun has been implicated in all types of skin cancer. Recommendations for avoiding UV exposure include use of sunscreens (SPF 15 or higher), wearing sun-protective clothing (long sleeves, hats), and avoiding sun exposure during peak times of 10 AM to 4 PM. It is not clear whether use of sunscreens actually reduces risk of MM because there is some evidence that it actually increases duration of sun exposure.
2. Mutations of the tumor suppressor gene p53 have been described in AK and skin cancers. In these instances, p53 mutations are most likely due to damage from UV rays of the sun, primarily UVB and UVC wavelengths, which are filtered by the stratospheric ozone layer.

III. Patient Management

A. Assessment: The following are signs and symptoms of skin cancer:
1. Basal cell carcinoma (BCC)
   a. White, pink, or skin-colored, waxy lesions are characteristic of the most common type of NMSC: Noduloulcerative BCC. The lesion appears as a firm, well-circumscribed, raised papule. It is commonly found on the face, head, or neck, and ulcerates and may bleed as it develops.
   b. Flat, red, or pink scaling is often the appearance of superficial BCC, which is also a common NMSC. It is usually well circumscribed and is most often found on the limbs or trunk.
   c. Black, brown, or blue lesions found on the face, head, or neck may be pigmented BCC. It is similar in appearance to MM but is like nodular BCC in growth.
   d. A flat, ivory, scarlike lesion on the head or neck may be morpheaform BCC. Although rare, it is more aggressive than other BCC.
   e. A hornlike growth in the postauricular sulcus may be a keratotic (or basosquamous) BCC. This is the most aggressive BCC and frequently recurs and metastasizes.
2. Squamous cell carcinoma (SCC)

    a. Keratinization and keratin pearl formation in the epithelium are typical in SCC but are less evident as the tumor becomes more advanced.

    b. Raised, firm papule, which is red or flesh colored, is usually the initial appearance.

    c. A crusted, ulcerated, and indurated lesion may appear as it spreads to surrounding tissue.

    d. Symptoms include pain in skin that has been exposed to UV rays.

    e. Tumors may be found in scar tissue of radiation, chemical, or thermal burns or in areas of chronic inflammation.

3. Malignant melanoma (MM): There are three precursor lesions of MM.

    a. Dysplastic nevi (DN) occur in familial and nonfamilial patterns. Familial DN are not common, but risk of people with DN developing MM is almost 100%. The general population risk of nonfamilial DN is 5% to 10%.

        (1) DN usually have some clinical features of MM, which may include color, asymmetry, or irregularity of shape. DN occur in clusters (100 or more) and are found on the face, trunk, arms, buttocks, groin, scalp, and female breasts.

        (2) Colors vary and may be tan to brown, black, red, or pink.

    b. Congenital nevi are present at birth and may be as small as 1.5 cm or may cover extensive areas of the body.

        (1) There is a lifetime risk of malignant conversion of about 7%.

        (2) Lesions are brown to black in color and may be slightly raised with regular borders and areas of nodularity.

    c. Lentigo maligna is similar to its counterpart lentigo maligna melanoma (see types of MM listed below).

4. Classification of MM: There are four major types of MM.

    a. Lentigo maligna melanoma is found on body areas with frequent sun exposure (face, neck, arms, legs). It grows slowly, in a radial pattern, for many years before beginning a vertical growth phase. It is characteristically large (about 10 cm) in size and may be tan or brown with irregular borders. In the vertical phase, nodules appear on the surface.

    b. Superficial-spreading melanoma accounts for about 70% of MM. In men, it is often on the trunk; whereas lesions in women are more commonly on the legs. The radial growth phase is about 1 to 5 years. Lesions appear flat and tan/brown with a scaly surface. In the more aggressive vertical phase, color may change to red, blue, or white and the lesion may be ulcerated.

    c. Nodular melanoma occurs commonly on the head, neck, or trunk, and begins with a rapid vertical growth phase. It appears as a dome shape with blue-black or red color, and it may ulcerate or bleed.

    d. Acral lentiginous melanoma is the least commonly occurring MM but is the most common type seen in dark-skinned people (35% to 60%). It occurs on the mucous membranes, soles of feet, palms of hands, and nail beds. The radial phase lasts 2 to 5 years and looks similar to lentigo maligna. The vertical phase has areas of nodularity and is more aggressive in growth. It has high potential to metastasize and has the poorest survival rate of the MM types.

B. Diagnostic Parameters

   1. Assessment of a lesion suspected as MM

      a. Establish when the lesion was first noticed and any change in appearance. (Note changes in color, size, or shape; personal and family history of skin cancers or DN; sun exposure; and skin injury or trauma.)

      b. Evaluate the lesion by the "ABCD" method. Assess for A, asymmetry; B, border irregularity; C, color changes; and D, diameter more than 0.6 cm.

      c. Palpate lymph nodes, with special attention to those regionally adjacent to the lesion.

   2. Cytogenetic analysis is being studied as a predictor of hereditary predisposition for MM. Although abnormalities are frequently found on chromosomes 1 and 6, clinical indications are not clear and more research is required.

   3. Biopsy is the only accurate diagnostic procedure for skin cancers. For suspected NMSC, three techniques are commonly used.

      a. *Punch biopsy* samples a thick section of the lesion with a special tool.

      b. *Incisional biopsy* removes a section of the lesion.

      c. *Excisional biopsy* removes the entire lesion.

   4. For suspected MM, a complete excisional biopsy provides the most information for a complete histopathologic diagnosis.

   5. Metastatic evaluation of MM

      a. Most common sites of MM metastasis are lymph nodes, lung, liver, brain, and bowel. However, because MM can metastasize to any organ, a careful review of systems and metastatic screening should be performed.

      b. Tests include chest x-ray, blood count, and serum chemistry with liver function studies. If tests or symptoms suggest the involvement of other organs, appropriate metastatic testing should follow.

C. Treatment of SCC and BCC: Choice of treatment should consider tumor growth pattern and location, age, health status, and desired cosmetic outcome.

   1. Staging for both SCC and BCC is done per the American Joint Committee on Cancer (AJCC) skin cancer staging guidelines. This TNM classification is used to stage both basal cell carcinoma and squamous cell carcinoma.

   2. Surgical excision is the most frequent curative therapy. It is often done under local anesthesia in an ambulatory setting. Advantages include decreased time and cost to the patient, rapid healing, and good cosmetic results for most lesions. Skin grafts or flaps may be required if the tissue is on a bony area, such as the head, nose, or scalp. Risks include infection and poor cosmesis in areas with little subcutaneous tissue.

   3. Mohs' micrographic surgery is the most conservative therapy. It involves sequential, thin, horizontal slicing of tissue, which are immediately stained and reviewed until all margins are clear. This is the most tissue-sparing procedure but is traumatic to the patient who experiences multiple procedures with intervals of waiting for histologic review. Because this technique is often used in areas with insufficient tissue for closure, flaps or grafts are often required.

4. Curettage and electrodesiccation are only appropriate for lesions less than 2 cm in size and superficial. The tumor is removed by curettage. The tumor base is then treated with low-voltage electrodes. This procedure heals fast and results in minimal trauma and discomfort.

5. Radiotherapy is used for inoperable or recurrent lesions, or when the patient is a poor candidate for surgery.
   a. Radiation may be the better treatment for lesions in difficult areas to treat (eyelid, lip, nose) but should be avoided for those under 45 years of age because treatment sites become more atrophic and erythematous with age.
   b. Doses are given in fractions to increase skin tolerance and may require 3 to 4 weeks of treatment.
   c. Although radiation may result in a better cosmetic outcome, it also increases the risk for NMSC at the treatment site.
   d. Direct application of radiation to the skin, in the form of radon molds, requires more research to establish how the mechanism is most effective.

6. Cryotherapy (BCC)
   a. Liquid nitrogen is applied to the lesion. This freezing and thawing process is repeated until the tissue is necrotic.
   b. The procedure is best for superficial, well-defined lesions.

D. Treatment of MM
   1. Staging of MM
      a. Although the traditional three-stage system is used (local, regional, distant), it does not include all of the important prognostic criteria.
      b. AJCC, World Health Organization (WHO), and the European Organization for Research and Treatment of Cancer (EORTC) approved a new four-stage system developed by the AJCC. AJCC identifies level of invasion (T) from no evidence to >4 mm thickness, with and without ulceration; and nodal involvement from 0 to ≥4. Metastases are characterized as distant skin, subcutaneous tissue, and lymph nodes; lung; and other visceral metastases (See section II.A for risk factors.)
      c. Ulceration of lesions is significant. Ulcerated lesions are more likely to metastasize and, thus, carry a poorer prognosis.
      d. Prognoses are improved for thin lesions (<0.5 mm), negative sentinel lymph node (SLN) status, younger age (<60 years), female gender, and presence of tumor-infiltrating lymphocytes.
   2. Excisional biopsy followed by wide excision surgery
   3. Surgery will be curative for 90% of patients
      a. Less radical surgery can be performed in select patients due to advancements in this treatment option.
      b. Surgery for cytoreduction may be an option for patients with metastasis.

4. WHO has declared sentinel lymph node (SLN) biopsy a standard of care for appropriate patients with MM.
   a. Which patients are deemed appropriate for SLN remains somewhat controversial, but it is generally indicated for patients with ulcerated lesions or lesions >1mm in thickness.
   b. Improves staging and prognostic accuracy
   c. Provides guidance for treatment decisions
5. Immunotherapy and biotherapy
   a. Based on observations that melanomas are highly immunogenic
   b. Goals are to make cancer cells appear more "foreign" to the immune system (vaccine therapies), increase the level of immune response (biotherapies), or a combination of both.
   c. Agents used include biotherapies interferon alfa 2b (IFN), interleukin 2 (IL-2), tumor-infiltrating lymphocytes, lymphokine-activated cells, granulocyte-macrophage colony stimulating factor (GM-CSF), and several types of immunotherapy vaccines (see Chapter 4).
   d. Adjuvant high-dose IFN is the only FDA-approved treatment for resected stage III MM.
      (1) Response rates from 15% to 20%, about one third of which may be durable.
      (2) Approximately 25% of patients unable to complete full course of prescribed therapy due to toxicities.
   e. Other approaches remain investigational.
6. Chemotherapy is used with limited success to treat metastatic MM. For chemotherapy administration, side effects, and management, see Chapter 6.
   a. Dacarbazine (DTIC) is the only FDA-approved chemotherapy agent for metastatic MM; however, response rates are low (5% to 20%).
   b. Other commonly used chemotherapy regimens include the "Dartmouth Regimen" (DTIC, BCNU, and cisplatin, with or without tamoxifen), and methyl-CCNU.
   c. High-dose chemotherapy with autologous bone marrow transplantation frequently has high morbidity and short duration of response. See Chapter 5 for management.
7. Biochemotherapy using combinations of chemotherapy drugs (commonly DTIC, vinblastine, and cisplatin with IFN and/or IL-2 and temozolomide with biotherapy) is under investigation as a possible approach to treating metastatic MM.
8. Vaccine therapy
   a. Tumor vaccines under investigation with or without chemotherapy/biotherapy
9. Loco-regional chemotherapy
   a. Isolated limb perfusion is a controversial adjuvant therapy.
      (1) Melphalan is most commonly used; however, other agents include thiotepa, dacarbazine, carmustine, cisplatin, and doxorubicin.
      (2) Complications may include tissue necrosis, edema in treatment extremity, infection, vein thrombosis, or neurologic changes.

     b. Intraarterial infusion is similar to limb perfusion but is less exact in distribution.

E. Nursing Diagnoses

  1. Body image changes related to disease or treatment

    a. *Problem:* Skin cancers are often on visible body parts, such as the face, head, and neck. Lesions, skin changes, or scarring from treatment may have a negative impact on body image.

    b. *Interventions*

      (1) Assess expectations and perceptions of the physical changes resulting from disease or treatment. Evaluate differences in intimacy and social interactions resulting from changes in appearance.

      (2) Assist the patient and significant other to form realistic expectations of cosmetic outcomes using photographs and other visual aids.

      (3) Cover lesions with a minimal dressing that is secure and functional (see Chapters 8 and 9 for care regarding radiation therapy and surgical therapy).

      (4) Refer patient for consultation to plastic surgeons, image consultants, or makeup experts (who may be associated with, or known to, burn treatment programs).

    c. *Desired outcomes*

      (1) Patient will maintain intimate relationships and social interactions during and after diagnosis and treatment.

      (2) Patient will verbalize realistic cosmetic expectations of treatment and a realistic plan to manage lesions or other physical changes resulting from treatment.

  2. Impaired skin integrity related to disease or treatment

    a. *Problem:* Lesions occurring on the skin may become ulcerated. Surgery, local chemotherapy, cryotherapy, and radiation therapy may also damage the integrity of the skin.

    b. *Interventions:* Teach about care and treatment of the skin as appropriate to the source of problem (see Chapters 6, 8, and 9).

    c. *Desired outcomes*

      (1) Skin integrity will be maintained, or healing will occur.

      (2) Patient will experience minimal discomfort due to skin lesions.

      (3) Patient will be free of infection.

  3. Noncompliance related to lifestyle habits

    a. *Problems:* Unprotected exposure to chemicals, radiation, and sun is the major factor in the development of NMSC. Exposures can be limited by precautions, which may require a change in lifestyle or personal habits. (Using sunscreen with a protection factor of 15 or greater, through age 18, may decrease the lifetime incidence of NMSC by 78%.)

    b. *Interventions*

      (1) Assess knowledge and compliance with protective behaviors: sunscreen, protective clothing, and preventive practices.

      (2) Educate about prevention and detection measures (see section II.A for risk factors).

(3) Assist patient to develop a plan to protect against exposure when possible.

c. *Desired outcome:* Patient will participate in behaviors and take appropriate precautions to limit or prevent exposure to agents that cause or promote skin cancer.

F. Discharge Planning and Patient Education
   1. Teach the patient and family interventions to care for skin during treatment.
   2. Assist the patient and family in development of technique for skin self-examination.
   3. Assist the patient to develop a plan to prevent or limit future exposures to high-risk agents or situations.
   4. Emphasize the importance of physician follow-up for care and detection of skin cancers. Close follow-up is essential after diagnosis and treatment of any skin cancer. Recurrent tumors and new primary tumors occur most commonly in the first 5 years after diagnosis.
   5. Emphasize importance of physician examination for siblings and children of patients diagnosed with MM.

REFERENCES

Balch, C. M., Buzaid, A. C., Soong, S-J., Atkins, M. B., Cascinelli, N., Coit, D. G., Fleming, I. D., Gershenwald, J. E., Houghton, A., Jr., Kirkwood, J. M., McMasters, K. M., Mihm, M. F., Morton, D. L., Reintgen, D. S., Ross, M. I., Sober, A., Thompson, J. A., & Thompson, J. F. (2001). Final version of the American Joint Committee on Cancer staging system for cutaneous melanoma. *Journal of Clinical Oncology, 19,* 3635–3648.

Bataille, V. (2000). Genetics of familial and sporadic melanoma. *Clinical and Experimental Dermatology, 25,* 464–470.

Essner, R. (2003). Surgical treatment of malignant melanoma. *Surgical Clinics of North America. 83*(1), 109–156.

Goldstein, A., & Tucker, M. A. (2001). Genetic epidemiology of cutaneous melanoma. *Archives of Dermatology, 137,* 1493–1496.

Hall, J. C. (2003). Tumors of the skin. In J. C. Hall (Ed.), *Sauer's manual of skin diseases* (Chap. 32). Philadelphia: Lippincott Williams & Wilkins.

Hart, P. H., Brimbaldeston, M. A., & Finlay-Jones, J. J. (2001). Sunlight, immunosuppression and skin cancer: Role of histamine and mast cells. *Clinical and Experimental Pharmacology and Physiology, 28,* 1–8.

Hollis, G., Recio, A., & Schuchter, L. (2003). Diagnosis and management of high-risk and metastatic melanoma. *Seminars in Oncology Nursing, 19*(1), 32–42.

Jemal, A., Murray, T., Samuels, A., Ghafoor, A., Ward, E., & Thun, M. J. (2003). Cancer statistics, 2003. *CA: A Cancer Journal for Clinicians, 53,* 5–26.

Kim, C. J., Dessureault, S., Gabrilovich, D., Reintgen, D. S., & Slingluff, C. L., Jr. (2002). Immunotherapy for melanoma. *Cancer Control, 9,* 22–30.

Lacour, J. P. (2002). Carcinogenesis of basal cell carcinomas: Genetics and molecular mechanisms. *British Journal of Dermatology, 146,* 17–19.

Langeman, A. (1996). Skin cancers. In R. McCorkle et al. (Eds.), *Cancer nursing: A comprehensive textbook* (2nd ed., pp. 860–869). Philadelphia: W. B. Saunders.

Loescher, S. (1997). Skin cancers. In S. C. Groenwald, M. H. Frogge, M. Goodman, & C. H. Yarbro (Eds.), *Cancer nursing: Principles and practice* (3rd ed., pp. 1355–1373). Boston, MA: Jones & Bartlett.

MacKie, R. M. (2000). Malignant melanoma: Clinical variants and prognostic indicators. *Clinical and Experimental Dermatology, 25,* 471–475.

McMasters, K. M., Reintgen, D. S., Ross, M. I., Gershenwald, J. E., Edwards, M. J.,

Sober, A., Fenske, N., Glass, F., Balch, C. M., & Coit, D. G. (2001). Sentinel lymph node biopsy for melanoma: Controversy despite widespread agreement. *Journal of Clinical Oncology, 19*(11), 2851–2855.

Ortonne, J. P. (2002). From actinic keratosis to squamous cell carcinoma. *British Journal of Dermatology, 146,* 20–23.

SUPPORTIVE CARE FOR COMMON COMPLICATIONS OF CANCER

22 Bone Marrow Suppression

Kathy A. Shane
Brenda Shelton

I. Definition

A. Bone marrow suppression is one of the most common problems experienced by patients with cancer.

B. Bone marrow suppression is defined as a reduction in the production and maturation of all blood cell lines of the bone marrow resulting in leukopenia, anemia, and thrombocytopenia of the peripheral blood.

C. Hematopoiesis Review (see Figure 16–1)

   1. Hematopoiesis begins in the yolk sac of the embryo by the third month, but by the end of the seventh month, the bone marrow throughout the body is the primary site of hematopoiesis.

   2. By adulthood, hematopoiesis is normally confined to the proximal ends of long bones, and flat bones such as the sternum, vertebrae, ribs, ileum, and skull where the red bone marrow resides.

   3. In certain disease states, the marrow can reexpand back into the long bones as well as the spleen and liver, known as extramedullary hematopoiesis.

   4. Adults have 1.7 L of bone marrow comprised primarily of reticular tissues and hemopoietic progenitor cells.

   5. The reticular tissue and hemocytoblasts form a framework of sinusoids that feed into the marrow drainage system and venous system of the body.

   6. The reticular tissue provides support and nutrition for developing blood cells and secretes several colony-stimulating factors.

   7. The hemocytoblast, or colony-forming unit, is the pluripotent stem cell.

   a. Pluripotent stem cells express a surface protein or antigen, CD34, and have receptors for stem cell growth factors, which promotes their proliferation.

   b. Once "committed," the hemocytoblast becomes a progenitor cell for a specific hematopoietic cell line.

   c. These cell lines are erythroid (red cells); granulocytic, monocytic, and lymphoid (white cells); and megakaryocytic (platelets).

   d. Commitment, or differentiation and maturation, occurs due to the acquisition or loss of specific growth factor receptors and the action of cytokines.

   8. Marrow function is tightly regulated to provide appropriate numbers and types of blood cells needed to meet the body's physiologic requirements.

a. Glycoprotein hormones, or growth factors, regulate the proliferation, differentiation, maturation, and activation of progenitor and mature blood cells, and prevent apoptosis of them.

b. Each growth factor has a specific receptor and their presence on the cell surface varies with cell lineage and stage of differentiation.

c. Some hematopoietic growth factors include interleukins 1, 3, 5, and 6, granulocyte-macrophage colony-stimulating factor (GM-CSF), granulocyte colony-stimulating factor (G-CSF), macrophage colony-stimulating factor (M-CSF), stem cell factor (SCF), thrombopoietin, and erythropoietin.

9. Normally, mature blood cells, except for platelets, enter the bloodstream by migrating through the epithelial lining of the sinusoidal walls. Platelets are released directly from megakaryocytes, which form part of the sinusoidal wall.

II. Etiology: More than 50% of cancer patients will experience bone marrow suppression during the course of their disease (Shelton, 2003). Like any rapidly dividing cell, the bone marrow is prone to injury. Bone marrow suppression can be related to the cancer itself, cancer treatment, comorbidities, other treatment modalities, or a combination of these factors.

A. Cancer-Induced Bone Marrow Suppression

1. Hematologic malignancies such as leukemias and multiple myeloma involve a defect of a specific blood cell type. Often, this results in overproduction of this cell type, usually with immature, poorly functioning cells; this overproduction results in overcrowding of the marrow compartment with suppression of other cell lines.

2. Lymphomas, which often present as extramedullary disease, can infiltrate the bone marrow leading to decreased function of the cell lines, particularly the lymphocytes.

3. Certain solid tumor malignancies infiltrate the bone marrow in the course of metastasis, most commonly breast and lung cancer.

B. Chemotherapy-Induced Bone Marrow Suppression

1. The organ most consistently and frequently affected by cancer chemotherapeutic agents is the bone marrow, and secondarily the peripheral blood cells.

2. The effect on stem cell lines is predictable based on the agent used.

3. The degree of bone marrow suppression desired or tolerated is a guide for what agent or combination of agents to use, as well as the dosage, the route of administration, and the frequency of administration.

4. A few chemotherapeutic agents affect the pluripotent stem cells, thereby affecting all cell lines; an example is the class of nitrosoureas. These agents tend to be noncycle active and result in the longest period of myelosuppression.

5. Most agents are cell-cycle active, phase nonspecific, such as anthracyclines and alkylators, resulting in a moderate degree of suppression; whereas others are phase specific, such as antimetabolites and vinca alkaloids. Such agents have the shortest degree of suppression.

6. The only chemotherapeutic agents that are completely nontoxic to bone marrow are steroidal hormones (Table 22–1).

7. The rate of proliferation of the three major cell lines, erythrocytes, platelets, and leukocytes, helps determine the severity of depression of that specific cell type.

TABLE 22-1 Myelosuppressive Chemotherapy Agents

Drug or Class	Type of Action	Degree of Myelosuppression	Nadir (days)	Duration of Myelosuppression (days)
Alkylating agents	Cell-cycle nonspecific	Moderate	10–21	18–40
Antimetabolites:	Cell-cycle specific			
Anthracyclines		Severe	6–13	21–24
Antifolates		Severe	7–14	14–21
Antipyrimidines		Severe	7–14	21–24
Antipurines		Moderate	7–14	14–21
Antitumor antibiotics	Cell-cycle nonspecific	Moderate		
Camptothecins	Cell-cycle specific	Moderate	4–7	6–12
Epipodophyllotoxins	Cell-cycle specific	Moderate	5–15	22–28
Nitrosureas	Cell-cycle nonspecific	Severe	26–60	35–85
Miscellaneous:				
Busulfan	Cell-cycle nonspecific	Severe	11–30	24–54
Carboplatin	Cell-cycle nonspecific	Severe	16	21–25
Dacarbazine	Cell-cycle nonspecific	Severe	21–28	28–35
Hydroxyurea	Cell-cycle specific	Moderate	7	14–21
Mitomycin	Cell-cycle nonspecific	Moderate	28–42	42–56
Mithramycin	Cell-cycle nonspecific	Mild	5–10	10–18
Nitrogen mustard	Cell-cycle nonspecific	Severe	7–14	28
Procarbazine	Cell-cycle nonspecific	Moderate	25–36	35–50
Plant alkaloids	Cell-cycle specific	Mild to moderate	4–9	7–21
Taxanes	Cell-cycle specific	Moderate	8–12	15–21

Adapted from Perry, M. C. (Ed.). (2001). *The chemotherapy source book* (3rd ed., p. 562). Philadelphia: Lippincott Williams & Wilkins.

8. Typically, erythrocytes have a half-life of 120 days, platelets have a half-life of 5 to 7 days, and granulocytes have a half-life of 6 to 8 hours.
   a. Generally, leukopenia is the earliest indicator of bone marrow suppression but the quickest to recover.
   b. Platelets have the longest nadir.
   c. Red cells, with their long half-life, rarely present a serious problem unless a bleeding problem also exists.
9. In the past decade, use of hematopoietic growth factors (colony stimulating factors) has resulted in an earlier recovery of bone marrow cell lines. Their basic mechanism of action is to enhance stem cell differentiation and maturation (Shelton, Ashenbrenner & Shane, 2002).

C. Radiation-Induced Bone Marrow Suppression
   1. Occurs after radiation therapy when:
      a. The treatment field involves marrow-producing tissue.
      b. Patients have received doses greater than 1,500 rads.

D. Miscellaneous reasons for bone marrow suppression, such as other disease states and treatment modalities, will be covered in the following sections on leukopenia, anemia, and thrombocytopenia.

III. Patient management varies depending on the cell line predominantly affected.

Leukopenia

I. **Definition:** Leukopenia is defined as a reduced number of circulating leukocytes (white blood cells [WBC]).
   A. The two major types of WBC are granulocytes and agranulocytes. Granulocytes include neutrophils, eosinophils, and basophils. Agranulocytes include lymphocytes and monocytes. (See Table 22–2 for specific functions of white cells.)

TABLE 22-2 Types and Functions of Leukocytes and Complications That Present When Their Numbers Are Reduced

Type of Cell	Function	Complication When Reduced or Absent
GRANULOCYTES		
Neutrophils	Phagocytosis	Bacterial infections
Eosinophils	Allergic reactions, defense against parasites	Inadequate inflammatory responses, parasitic infections, dermatologic or pulmonary infections
Basophils	Allergic reactions, inflammatory reactions	Inadequate inflammatory responses
AGRANULOCYTES		
Lymphocytes	Immunity (T cells and B cells)	Viral or opportunistic infections, cancer
Monocytes	Phagocytosis	Fungal infections

B. Neutropenia is defined as a decrease in the number of neutrophils in the blood.

  1. Neutropenia most often occurs in diseases involving bone marrow production, as a result of excess destruction by autoimmune mechanisms or certain marrow toxic treatments, or increased consumption during chronic illness. (See Box 22–1 for specific etiologies.)

  a. A diminished number of neutrophils alters the body's defenses against bacterial invaders.

  b. There is some disagreement as to what constitutes neutropenia. Some argue that the condition occurs when the absolute neutrophil count (ANC) is less than 2,500 cells/mm³. Others define it as an ANC less than 1,000 cells/mm³. In patients with normal WBC counts, the higher, more conservative number is used to trigger infection precautions (Shelton, 2003).

C. Lymphocytopenia is defined as a reduction in the number of lymphocytes in the blood.

  1. The suppression of T-lymphocyte function results in reduced ability to recognize foreign tissue, malignant cells, and viruses.

  2. Lymphocytopenia is seen most commonly in acquired immunodeficiency syndrome (AIDS).

  a. The CD4 molecules destroyed by the human immunodeficiency virus (HIV) are reflected in the helper lymphocyte count (also called T4 count, or absolute lymphocyte count).

▼ BOX 22-1 | Etiologies of Neutropenia

Malnutrition
Protein deficiency
Calorie deficiency
Vitamin B deficiency

Health States
Chronic fever
Chronic illness
Diabetes mellitus
Elderly

Medications
Alkylating agents (antineoplastic and immunosuppressive; eg, cyclophosphamide)
Antidysrhythmics (eg, procainamide, quinidine)
Antimetabolites (eg, methotrexate, azathioprine)
Antiretroviral agents (eg, zidovudine)
Antitumor antibiotics (eg, bleomycin, Adriamycin)
Plant alkaloids (eg, vincristine, vinblastine, paclitaxel)
Trimethoprim-sulfamethoxazole (Bactrim)
Zyloprim (allopurinol)

    b. AIDS is classified by the CD4 count and the presence of other defining clinical syndromes.

   3. Other etiologies of lymphocytopenia:

    a. Therapeutically induced to suppress rejection of a transplanted organ before, during, and after transplantation (see Chapter 5)

    b. Certain medications, such as corticosteroids

    c. Acquired phenomenon from other physical disorders, such as intravenous (IV) drug use

    d. Genetic abnormalities, such as congenital T-lymphocyte suppression

    e. Hodgkin's disease, which has been linked to familial tendencies, history of viral infection, or unknown congenital causes

    f. Acquired specific immune system dysfunctions, such as viral-induced lymphoproliferative disorders. These syndromes may also cause T-cell non-Hodgkin's lymphoma.

II. Patient Management

  A. Assessment: The following are signs and symptoms of leukopenia:

   1. Fever is the cardinal symptom of infection.

   2. Other inflammatory symptoms (eg, swelling, erythema, pus formation) may not occur due to the lack of WBC.

   3. Fatigue with or without infectious complications.

   4. Organ-specific signs and symptoms of infection (Table 22–3) are the prevalent clinical presentations for leukopenia. Virtually all who are leukopenic for 21 days become infected, often being colonized by normal body flora.

  B. Diagnostic Parameters: Serum tests are the only tests that can be used to detect leukopenia.

   1. Total WBC count and differential determine whether there is an adequate number of WBCs to combat infection and mount inflammatory responses to injury. A low WBC count signals the probability of reduced neutrophil efficacy.

    a. Normally, the total WBC count is 5,000 to 10,000 cells/mm^3.

    b. About 35 % to 75% of these cells are neutrophils.

   2. The ANC is indicative of the number of neutrophils available to combat infection

    a. It is calculated by using the WBC differential with the following formula:

$$\text{Total number of WBC} \times \% \text{ neutrophils} = \text{ANC}$$

     Example:

$$5,000 \times 0.20 = 1,000$$

   3. CD4 count reflects the absolute number of CD4 molecule-containing cells, which are primarily helper T lymphocyte cells, but also include monocytes (Shelton, 2001).

    a. CD4 counts lower than 500/mm^3 are considered significant.

    b. CD4 counts are used to diagnose, plan treatment, and evaluate therapeutic response to treatment for AIDS.

  C. Treatment: Leukopenia is best treated by reversing the underlying cause, if known, and by the administration of growth factors, cytokines, immune globulin, or granulocyte transfusions (Boxes 22–2, 22–3, and 22–4).

  D. Nursing Diagnoses

▨ TABLE 22-3 Organ-Specific Signs and Symptoms of Infection

Body System	Complication	Signs and Symptoms
Neurologic	Encephalitis	Confusion, lethargy, difficulty arousing, headache, visual difficulty/photosensitivity, nausea, hypertension
	Meningitis	Lethargy and somnolence, confusion, nuccal rigidity
Head/neck	Conjunctivitis	Reddened conjunctiva, excess tearing of eye, puslike exudates from eye, blurred vision, swelling of eyelid, eye itching
	Otitis media	Earache, difficulty hearing, itching inner ear, ear drainage
	Sinusitis	Discolored nasal mucus, nasal congestion, face pain, blurred vision
	Oropharyngeal infection	Oral ulcerations or plaques, halitosis, reddened gums, abnormal papillae of the tongue, sore throat, difficulty swallowing
	Lymphadenitis	Swollen neck lymph glands, tender lymph glands, lump felt when swallowing
Pulmonary	Bronchitis	Persistent cough, sputum production, gurgles in upper airways, wheezes in upper airways, hypoxemia, hypercapnia
	Pneumonia	Chest discomfort pronounced with inspiration, persistent cough, sputum production, diminished breath sounds, crackles or gurgles, asymmetric chest wall movement, labored breathing, nasal flaring with breathing, hypoxemia
	Pleurisy	Chest discomfort pronounced with inspirtion; sides of chest painful to palpation, usually bilateral; splinting with deep breathing
Cardiovascular	Myocarditis	Dysrhythmias, murmurs or gallops, elevated jugular venous pulsations, weak thready pulse, hypotension, point of maximal impulse shifted laterally
	Pericarditis	Aching, constant chest discomfort unrelieved by rest or nitrates, pericardial rub, muffled heart sounds
	Endocarditis	Dyspnea, chest discomfort, gallops, murmurs, altered mental status, septic emboli in the extremities.
Gastrointestinal	Gastritis	Nausea, vomiting within 30 minutes of eating, heme positive emesis, aching stomach that is initially improved by eating
	Infection	Greater than six loose stools per day, clay-colored stools, foul-smelling stools, abdominal cramping, abdominal distention
	Pancreatitis	Epigastic discomfort, intolerance to high-fat meal, clay-colored stools, nausea and vomiting, hyperglycemia, hypocalcemia, hypoalbuminemia, increased lipase and amylase

(continued)

TABLE 22-3 Organ-Specific Signs and Symptoms of Infection *(Continued)*

Body System	Complication	Signs and Symptoms
	Hepatitis	Jaundice, right upper quadrant discomfort, hepatomegaly, elevated transaminases and bilirubin, fatty food intolerances, nausea and vomiting, diarrhea
Genitourinary	Urethritis	Painful urination, difficulty urinating, itching of feeling genitourinary orifice
	Cystitis	Small frequent urination (urinary urgency), of fullness of the bladder, suprapubic tenderness
	Nephritis	Flank discomfort, oliguria, protein in urine
	Vaginitis	Itching of vaginal area, vaginal discharge
Musculoskeletal	Arthritis	Joint discomfort, swollen and warm joints
	Myositis	Aching muscles, weakness
Dermatologic	Superficial skin infection	Rashes; itching; raised or discolored skin lesions; open, draining skin lesions; patterns are unique to specific microorganism
	Cellulitis	Redness, warmth, and swelling of subcutaneous tissue area; radiating pain from area toward middle of body
Hematologic immunologic	Bacteremia	Low diastolic BP, headache, confusion, oliguria, decreased bowel sounds, warmth, flushing, positive blood cultures, adenopathy

Signs and symptoms presented here are unique features of each process and do not include the common constitutional signs and symptoms seen with all infections (eg, fever, chills, malaise, leukocytosis, positive tissue culture for microorganisms, increased erythrocyte sedimentation rate, adenopathy).

Shelton, B. K. (1996b). Immunologic disorders. In J. Hebra & M. M. Kuhn (Eds.). *Manual of critical care nursing* (pp. 221–225). Boston, MA: Little, Brown.

▼ **BOX 22-2** | **Cell Line Stimulating Factors**

Granulocyte colony stimulating factor (GCSF, filgrastim, pegfilgrastim)

Dose

Single daily (filgrastim) IV or SQ dose of 5–10 µg/kg every day for up to 2 weeks based on postchemotherapy nadir. Administer slowly SQ, over 1 minute. Administer over 30 minutes IV.

Should not be used 24 hours before to 24 hours after the administration of antineoplastic chemotherapy.

Therapy should be continued within this 2-week time frame until the WBC count reaches 10,000 cells/mm^3.

Pegfilgrastim is administered as a single 6 mg IV or SQ injection once per cycle or no more frequently than every 21 days. It is administered 24 hours after the last chemotherapy dose, although same-day administration is currently under investigation. Its prolonged half-life is the consequence of pegylation of the filgrastim molecule.

(continued)

▼ BOX 22-2   Cell Line Stimulating Factors (*Continued*)

Nursing Implications
Hypersensitivity reactions may occur. Administer slowly, observing for
    signs/symptoms of respiratory distress.
Check insurance coverage guidelines for each patient; reimbursement criteria
    differ among providers.
Monitor WBC and differential.
Prepare patient for possible side effects: fever, bone pain, pain and redness at
    injection site.

Granulocyte macrophage colony stimulating factor (GMCSF, sargramostim, IL-3)

Dose
Single daily IV or SQ dose of 250 μg/m^2 per protocol. Administer over 2 hours IV.
Should not be used 24 hours before to 24 hours after the administration of
    antineoplastic chemotherapy.

Nursing Implications
Local skin reaction is common; rotate sites daily.
Prepare patient for side effects of fever, bone pain, myalgias, facial flushing,
    and redness at injection site.
Mild capillary leak syndrome is rare side effect.
The following electrolyte imbalances may occur: increased glucose, BUN, cho-
    lesterol, bilirubin, creatinine, ALT, and alkaline phosphatase; and decreased
    albumin and calcium.
Therapy should be continued until WBC count reaches 20,000 cells/mm^3.

Thrombopoietin growth factor (oprelvelkin, Neumega)

Dose
Single dose of 50 μg/kg SQ every day.

Nursing Implications
Mild to moderate fluid retention without weight gain and blurred vision.
Rare transient dysrhythmias (eg, atrial fibrillation).
Therapy should be continued until postnadir platelet count is greater than
    50,000 cells/mL.

Epoetin alfa (erythropoietin alfa, darbepoetin alfa)

Dose
Single dose of 50–150 units/kg every week SQ or a single dose of 40,000 units
    SQ every week.
IV doses must be 40% to 50% higher than SQ doses.
Darbepoetin has a prolonged half-life due to the addition of sailic acids to the
    molecule and is administered as an IV or SQ injection of 1–4.5 mcg/kg
    every 1 to 3 weeks. A common alternative dosing regimen is 200 mcg IV or
    SQ every 2 weeks

Nursing Implications
Do not shake vial.
Prepare patient for side effects of fever, headache, and fatigue.
Therapy should be continued until HCT reaches 34% to 36%.
Thrombotic events and hypertension may be indications for discontinuation of
    this agent.

▼ BOX 22-3 | **Intravenous Administration of Immune Globulin Infusions**

Agent
IVIGm Gammagard, Gammar-IV, Iveegam, Sandoglobulin, Venoglobuline-S

Administration Guidelines
Single IV dose of 100–200 mg/kg and retest IgG levels (level should be >300 mg/dL after infusion therapy.
Dilute in large volume of fluid (approximately 1 L) and administer over at least 2 hours.

Nursing Implications
Hypersensitivity may occur. Administer slowly, observing frequent vital signs (every 15 minutes) and signs/symptoms of respiratory distress for the first 30–60 minutes of infusion.
High-volume infusion may precipitate congestive heart failure in susceptible patients. Monitor to detect signs and symptoms early.
Administer through central venous access only; produces severe phlebitis.
Dose may be repeated monthly if levels decrease or clinical improvement is not evident.

1. Potential for infection
   a. *Problem:* Patients with reduced numbers or activity of WBCs are at risk for the development of life-threatening infections. The type of infecting organism will depend on which WBC activities are altered and other host risk factors. The signs and symptoms of infection in the immunocompromised host are subdued because there is insufficient WBC activity to produce the usual inflammatory symptoms.
   b. *Interventions*
      (1) Assess for signs and symptoms of infection (see Table 22–3) or sepsis/septic shock (Box 22–5).
         (a) Monitor temperature every 2 to 4 hours (inpatient). Rectal temperatures are not advised due to the possibility of breaking the mucosal integrity.
         (b) Observe all dressings daily for signs and symptoms of infection.
         (c) Inspect all orifices (oral cavity, rectal area, urethra) every shift for evidence of localized infection.
         (d) Inspect all excrement every shift for cloudiness, altered color, or odors that may signify infection.
         (e) Assess for any localized pain; inspect painful area for erythema, swelling, exudate, or rebound tenderness of abdomen that may signal pocketed infection.
         (f) Auscultate breath sounds at least every shift and report new adventitious sounds or diminished breath sounds that may herald pulmonary infection.
         (g) Monitor WBC elevations for evidence of infections and response to interventions. If the WBC count is low, assess WBC total count and ANC daily.
      (2) Control environmental risks of infection.

▼ **BOX 22-4** | **Intravenous Administration of Granulocytes**

Administration Guidelines

Granulocytes must be gamma irradiated before administration.

Administer premedications 15–30 minutes before transfusion of WBC, diphenhydramine 25–50 mg, and acetaminophen 650 mg. Some patients require Solucortef 100 mg.

Obtain baseline vital signs, oxygen saturation, and breath sounds. Notify physician of abnormalities. Ongoing vital signs and breath sounds assessment are performed frequently during the infusion.

Administer via standard blood tubing, primed with normal saline only, without additional filters. Product must be transfused by gravity. Some infusion pumps are thought to damage the cells.

Transfusion must begin within 30 minutes of arrival on unit and infused at a rate of 1×10^{10}.

Cells per 30 minutes, not to exceed 500 mL/h.

Gently agitate bottom of bag every 15 minutes to ensure mixing of cells in solution and to prevent settling of WBC in bottom of bag, resulting in bolus effect.

Nursing Implications

Reactions are common, ranging from rash and hives to anaphylaxis and severe respiratory distress.

WBCs should migrate to the site of infection, and the patient may demonstrate rapid onset of symptoms reflecting this WBC infiltration (eg, dyspnea and crackles in the presence of pneumonia).

Have emergency equipment, oxygen delivery system, and suction available.

For rigors during transfusion, administer Demerol 10 mg. IVP every 5 minutes up to 50 mg.

Avoid infusion of amphotericin within 6 hours of WBC transfusion.

(a) Strict handwashing between patients and all procedures to reduce nosocomial infection.

(b) Follow universal precautions.

(c) Cohort neutropenic patients and do not assign with patients who are infected.

(d) Monitor visitors for any recent history of communicable disease and institute precautions as indicated.

(e) Clean all multipurpose equipment (eg, oximeter probes, noninvasive blood pressure (BP) cuffs, bedscale slings, infusion pumps, electronic thermometers) between patient use.

(f) Do not permit live flowers or standing water (eg, in vases) in the patient's room because these may harbor bacteria.

(3) Implement patient care routines to prevent infections and to enhance immune system functioning.

(a) Bathe patient and change linen daily; perform oral care three to four times daily and perineal care twice daily.

▼ BOX 22-5 | **Phases of Sepsis**

Hyperdynamic (Warm Shock)	**Hypodynamic (Cold Shock)**
SBP (systolic blood pressure) <90 mm Hg, or >40 mm below baseline, low diastolic pressure	Profound hypotension, relatively high diastolic pressure
High cardiac output	Low cardiac output
UO < 0.5 mL/kg/h	Anuria
Warm, flushed, dry skin	Cold, pale, clammy skin
Increased heart rate	Tachycardia, dysrhythmias
Bounding pulses	Weak, thready pulse
Fever	Decreased core body temperature
Decreased level of consciousness	Decreased LOC
Increased respiratory rate	Shortness of breath
Decreased respiratory depth	Decreased respiratory depth
Crackles	Crackles, wheezes
Increased WBC count	Increased or decreased WBC count
Hyperglycemia, amylase increased	Hypoglycemia, increased serum and lipase
Metabolic acidosis/respiratory alkalosis	Metabolic/respiratory acidosis
Thrombocytopenia increased	Decreased clotting factors, liver transaminases
Increased fibrine degradation products (FDPs)	Increased bilirubin, BUN
Increased creatinine	

Minimize use of lotions and deodorants, which enhance bacterial growth.

(b) Ensure that nutritional needs are being met.

(c) Protect the patient from consuming possibly contaminated foods by labeling all foods brought from home to be discarded in 1 to 2 days. Avoid commercial foods with meat, seafood, eggs, or mayonnaise. Clean fresh fruits and vegetables before giving them to the patient. Some institutions require a "cooked food diet," in which only foods previously cooked are permitted—no fresh fruits or vegetables, nuts, or unprocessed herbs are permitted; patients drink only bottled water and processed beverages. This practice has not been validated by research (Shelton, 2003).

(d) Ensure that sleep needs are being met.

(e) Control glucose levels so unintentional hyperglycemia does not occur (hyperglycemia compromises phagocytic activities that fight infection).

(f) Use sterile technique for inserting and dressing IV catheters. Dressings should be changed at least every 24 hours if site is draining, less frequently if site is dry and dressing is occlusive.

(g) Cover all open wounds with a sterile dressing. Skin abrasions may be treated with antimicrobial ointment and dressings—or open air, provided that frequent cleansing is performed.

(h) Encourage incentive spirometry or deep breathing and coughing.

(i) Encourage ambulation if patient is physically able, or turn bedridden patients every 2 to 4 hours to prevent skin breakdown and atelectasis.

(j) If building construction is occurring, consider applying a mask on the patient during intrahospital transport. If hepa-filtration or other airflow protection is provided to patients while in the unit and building air systems are old, masks may be considered for transport of these patients as well.

(k) Avoid stopcocks in hospital IV systems; use closed injection-site systems.

(l) Change IV tubing every 96 hours if a closed system is maintained. More frequent changes are advocated if the line is open, or blood or total parenteral nutrition has been administered through the tubing.

(m) Consider closed endotracheal tube suction systems, provided there is an in-line flush port to clean the catheter after each use.

(n) Change oxygen set-ups that have standing water (eg, nasal cannula) every 24 hours.

(4) Institute rapid treatment measures for suspected infections.

(a) For first fever or new fever, perform routine culture and assessment activities as indicated or ordered before initiation of antimicrobial therapy. New fever is defined as one that exceeds 38.3°C initially or after 72 hours on an antibiotic regimen. A temperature of 38.0°C on two separate occasions at least 4 hours apart may also be considered a new fever (Shelton, 2003). Box 22–6 lists the routine culture and assessment functions that should be performed.

(b) Administer antimicrobial therapy as ordered. These agents should not be missed and should be changed to IV form if the patient is unable to take medication orally.

(c) Perform antimicrobial peak and trough levels as ordered. Be certain that the exact time of the last dose of antimicrobials is listed to calculate levels accurately.

(d) Be alert to superinfection with fungal flora usually 7 to 10 days after initiation of broad-spectrum antibiotics. Prophylaxis (eg, oral nystatin or topical nystatin powder to skin folds) may be started in some individuals.

(e) If prolonged neutropenia exists, discuss with the multidisciplinary team the use of nontraditional support measures such as late administered granulocyte stimulating factor and administration of granulocyte transfusions (see Box 22–4).

(f) Report characteristics of excrement or wound drainage.

(g) Check IgG levels; if low, consider the IV administration of immune globulin infusions (see Box 22–3).

▼ **BOX 22-6** | **Routine Culture and Assessment Activities for First Fever and New Fever**

Blood cultures from all venous/arterial catheters, plus a peripheral blood culture

Urine culture

Stool culture (if diarrhea is present, cultures are performed daily for 3 consecutive days)

Sputum culture

Chest x-ray (recent literature suggests this may be optional in the absence of respiratory symptoms [Shelton, 2003])

Orifices cultured—nose, mouth, rectum (some institutions advocate culture of skin where moistness is a problem, such as skinfolds, axilla, groin, buttocks)

Assess breath sounds and report adventitious or diminished sounds

    c. *Desired outcomes*
      (1) Patient will have no fever.
      (2) Patient will have no clinical signs or symptoms of sepsis.
      (3) Patient will have no growth on blood, excrement, or skin surface cultures.
  2. Decreased cardiac output related to infection or sepsis-induced myocardial dysfunction
    a. *Problem:* Leukopenia predisposes patients to great risk of infection. Infection and sepsis cause hyperdynamic cardiovascular function to compensate for vasodilation, reduced blood volume due to increased capillary permeability, and increased energy requirements. This is manifested as the hyperdynamic phase of sepsis. The cardiovascular system initially responds with increased work but will become exhausted and demonstrate decreased cardiac function and potential shock, presenting as hypodynamic sepsis.
    b. *Interventions*
      (1) Monitor vital signs frequently for fever and for hypotension. Diastolic BP will decrease initially due to vasodilation, then the systolic BP will decrease due to capillary permeability or reduced cardiac performance.
      (2) Monitor symptoms of sepsis/septic shock (see Box 22–5).
        (a) Systolic BP < 90 mm Hg
        (b) Urine output <0.5 mL/kg/hr
        (c) Altered mental status
      (3) Evaluate spectrum of antimicrobial therapy, broaden as needed; consider antifungal therapy.
      (4) Administer IV fluids as ordered to replete the vascular space and reduce risk of hypotension.
    c. *Desired outcomes*
      (1) Patient will have a normal blood pressure.
      (2) Patient will exhibit signs of adequate tissue perfusion (ie, normal mental status, adequate urinary output)

3. Altered comfort related to fevers, chills, headaches, myalgias, and arthralgias associated with leukopenia and infection

    a. *Problem:* Leukopenia is often accompanied by infections that cause a multitude of uncomfortable symptoms, which are amenable to nursing intervention. Infections that commonly occur in the immunocompromised patient produce an elevated body temperature that increases metabolic demands and causes discomfort and physical decompensation.

    b. *Interventions*

       (1) Administer acetaminophen as ordered for fever or mild discomfort. Acetaminophen is given with caution for people with compromised liver function, or before broad-spectrum antimicrobial therapy has been implemented.

       (2) Encourage restful environment (controlled temperature, absence of noise, relaxation activities) and limit visitors.

       (3) Apply warmth to aching muscles or joints or cool compress to head as needed. Apply warmed blankets as needed for chills.

       (4) Administer meperidine 12 to 25 mg IV or other opiate or benzodiazepine as ordered for chills.

       (5) Bathe patient or change linen after fever subsides.

       (6) Monitor platelet count because it may decrease due to the hypermetabolism of hyperthermia.

       (7) Avoid enteral feeding when the patient is febrile because nausea and vomiting are common associated symptoms and intestinal motility may be altered.

       (8) Avoid additional causes of fever while trying to resolve condition (eg, try not to give blood products until fever is resolved).

       (9) Monitor respiratory status during hyperthermia; oxygenation often goes down, but the effects of increased temperature may make oxygen saturation remain the same.

    c. *Desired outcomes*

       (1) Patient will not experience chills.

       (2) Patient will verbalize a pain rating of "0" with treatment plan.

       (3) Patient is able to perform activities of daily living without discomfort.

       (4) Patient's body temperature remains less than 38.3°C.

E. Discharge Planning and Patient Education

    1. Teach the patient to take his or her temperature and call the doctor if it is >38.3°C.

    2. Teach the patient and significant other the signs and symptoms of infection.

    3. Advise the patient to avoid exposure to communicable diseases. This may include screening visitors, avoiding crowds, or wearing a mask in transport.

    4. Instruct the patient on clean technique principles to be used at home or with venous access device (VAD) care. Observe return demonstration by patient or significant other.

    5. Provide infection prevention instructions to the patient and significant other.

    6. Assess home circumstances for risk of infection, and refer to public health or home care nursing for assistance in modifications of this environment as needed (eg, well water may need to be replaced with

bottled drinking water and patient and family may need to be taught other methods of purifying water for use by the patient at home).
7. Instruct the patient or significant other on administration of growth factors. Observe return demonstration.

ANEMIA

I. Definition
   A. Most often defined by the serum levels of circulating red blood cells (RBC; hematocrit) or their oxygen-carrying capacity (hemoglobin)
      1. A reduction of hemoglobin or hematocrit by one third or more of normal (hemoglobin less than 10 g/dL or a hematocrit less than 30 mg/dL).
      2. Actual values and patient tolerance vary, and many cancer patients with slowly developing or chronic anemia tolerate much lower values without cardiopulmonary compromise.
      3. More accurate definition: Lowered hemoglobin or hematocrit value that results in altered tissue perfusion as determined by alterations in mental status, oxygenation, blood pressure, urine output, or combinations of these clinical indicators.

II. Etiology: Anemia in the cancer patient categorized by physiologic mechanism (Box 22–7)
   A. Inadequate Production
      1. Bone marrow suppression
      2. Inadequate amounts of necessary elements for red cell formation
      3. Tumor infiltration of the bone marrow (more often presenting with thrombocytopenia and leukopenia earlier in the disease process, and anemia as a late symptom)
      4. Renal disease–induced erythropoietin deficiency
   B. Abnormal Hemolysis and Sequestration
      1. The RBCs of the body are normally sensitized and removed by the spleen when they are senescent, deformed, or dysfunctional.
      2. The spleen can become oversensitized by the development of RBC autoantibodies that detect normal RBCs as foreign tissue and signal splenic macrophages to remove and destroy them.
      3. In addition, the RBC autoantibodies may be circulating in the serum and may initiate extrasplenic hemolysis.
      4. Abnormal sequestration in the spleen or intravascular hemolysis result in hemolytic anemia. It is commonly a secondary disorder, arising as a complication of liver and splenic disease, autoimmune disorders, malignancy, bone marrow transplantation, or drug toxicity.
      5. Transfusion reactions may also cause hemolysis, although a persistent hemolytic anemia is unusual in these situations.
   C. Blood Loss: Blood loss anemia is common in bleeding disorders associated with cancer and cancer treatment. The pathophysiology of bleeding due to mucosal, vascular, and tissue injury is physiologically the same as bleeding in noncancer situations. The management of this problem may be slightly different due to concomitant coagulopathies.

III. Patient Management
   A. Assessment
      1. Nutrition history: The required amount of specific nutrients necessary for RBC development will vary with clinical complications, such

▼ **BOX 22-7** | **Etiologies of Anemia in the Cancer Patient**

Abnormal Production
Bone metastases
Radiation to long bones
Chemotherapy agents
Antiretroviral therapy—reverse transcriptase inhibitors

Abnormal Sequestration
Autoimmune hemolytic syndrome—malignant lymphomas

Hemolysis
Hemolytic transfusion reaction
Autoimmune hemolytic syndrome—bone marrow transplantation

Blood Loss
Mucositis
GI erosion
Stress ulcer
Colon tumors
GI tract radiation exposure (esophageal, colon)

as malabsorption or blood loss. The most important nutrients for production of RBCs are iron, folate, vitamin B_{12}, and protein.

2. History of surgeries is important to ascertain because lower gastric or duodenal surgeries remove the cells that make hydrochloric acid and intrinsic factor, which aid in absorption of vitamin B_{12}. Inadequate B_{12} absorption leads to pernicious anemia.

3. History of recent infectious disease will reveal viral infectious etiologies (eg, Epstein-Barr virus, cytomegalovirus) that may precipitate hemolytic anemia.

4. Medication history reveals the potential etiology of marrow suppression, nutritional deficits, or hemolysis.
   a. Most antimetabolite, alkylating, and antibiotic antineoplastic agents given for more than one monthly cycle will induce anemia.
   b. Histamine blockers are important to note because they abrogate absorption of vitamin B_{12}.
   c. Other medications that may induce anemia include allopurinol, reverse transcriptase inhibitor antiretrovirals, antidysrhythmics, and anticonvulsants.

5. History of bleeding is important to evaluate the patient's potential risk for anemia.
   a. Large blood losses or chronic blood loss induces clinical anemia, requiring intervention.
   b. The most common sites of bleeding in these patients are oral mucous membranes, gastrointestinal (GI) tract, genitourinary tract, and the vagina.

6. Body muscle mass will determine the baseline normal RBC volume.
   a. Greater muscle mass translates to higher RBC counts.

    b. Decreased RBC production occurs with muscle atrophy.
    c. Hypermetabolism breaks down muscle proteins for energy.
  7. Hormones serve to regulate RBC production. When androgen or estrogen levels are manipulated in reproductive organ malignancies (eg, ovarian, uterine, breast, testicular, or prostate cancer), RBC abnormalities may occur. Anemia is most often associated with increased estrogen or decreased androgen.
  8. Body temperature is decreased in anemia. The loss of insulation from the RBC mass causes hypothermia.
  9. Heart rate is elevated in anemic conditions as the body attempts to compensate for diminished oxygen delivery.
    a. Orthostatic tachycardia, where the heart rate increases at least 20 beats per minute when the patient moves from a lying to sitting position or sitting to standing, signals the gravitational changes associated with RBC loss.
    b. Orthostatic tachycardia is a more sensitive indicator of blood loss than orthostatic hypotension.
  10. Blood pressure, after RBC loss
    a. At first, blood pressure is normal or elevated as a sympathetic response to reduced circulating volume.
    b. With continued loss, the blood pressure will decrease and/or the patient may become orthostatic.
    c. Blood loss usually results in systolic hypotension with a normal to elevated diastolic pressure.
  11. Respiratory rate increases in an attempt to compensate for decreased oxygen-carrying capacity of hemoglobin with resultant decrease in tissue oxygenation.
  12. Respiratory distress, angina, and other symptoms of reduced oxygen-carrying capacity reflect the severity of the oxygen deficit. These symptoms are usually demonstrated in patients with significant RBC loss without replacement.
  13. Noninvasive assessment of oxygen-carrying capacity by way of pulse oximetry will be lower than 90% in severe anemia, particularly when respiratory or cardiac compensation mechanisms fail.
  14. Oliguria is the result of reduced renal perfusion and oxygenation and/or occlusion from hemolyzed cells.
  15. When red cells are hemolyzed and inefficiently removed by the spleen, unconjugated bilirubin accumulates in the serum, resulting in jaundice.
  16. Splenic and liver enlargement and tenderness are consequences of abnormal sequestration of senescent or damaged RBC. Sequestration by the liver or spleen may occur due to truly abnormal cell structure or as the result of autoantibody action against the RBC.
B. Diagnostic Parameters
  1. Serum tests (Table 22–4)
  2. Urine tests: Urine urobilinogen levels may be elevated in hemolytic anemia due to increased hemolysis byproduct excretion by the kidneys.
  3. Other tests
    a. Bone marrow aspiration and biopsy involves needle aspiration of red bone marrow from the axial skeleton (sternum, iliac crest) to detect normal RBC precursors and early differentiation. This test

(Text continues on page 330)

TABLE 22–4 Laboratory Tests in Anemia

Test	Normal Value	Clinical Implications of Abnormal Result
Hemoglobin (HgB)	12–15 mg/dL	Levels decreased with reduced RBC production, blood loss, and hemolysis. Levels may appear decreased when hemoglobin is abnormal (eg, sickle cell anemia). The hemoglobin level is usually one third of the hematocrit; variations in this ratio may indicate intervening variables affecting the accuracy of one test or the other.
Hematocrit (Hct)	35%–45%	Decreased with reduced RBC production, blood loss, and hemolysis. Levels are easily influenced by fluid volume status. Hypervolemia leads to lower hematocrit without actual decreased RBC, and hypovolemia and hemoconcentration reflect a higher hematocrit than actually exists. Immature RBCs (eg, reticulocytes) that have a large mass will make the hematocrit appear higher.
Erythrocyte count	3.5–$5.0 \times 10^6/mm^3$	Levels decreased with reduced RBC production, blood loss, and hemolysis. Abnormally shaped RBCs (eg, sickle cells, schistocytes, helmet cells, target cells) will not be counted in the RBC level.
RBC smear	Normocytic, normochromic cells	Evidence of schistocytes (fragmented RBCs) on smear are evidence of sheared and damaged RBCs, which occur during the hemolysis process. Other abnormalities occur with liver disease, renal failure, hypertension, and artificial heart valves.
Reticulocyte count	0.5%–2% total RBC count	Increased reticulocyte (immature RBCs) count occurs in response to blood loss. As the RBC mass decreases, the body's compensatory response is to release reticulocytes to replace RBCs until stabilization occurs. Small elevations (2%–4%) of reticulocytes occur with recent blood loss, but levels exceeding 4% of the total RBC mass indicate hemolysis.
Mean corpuscular volume (MCV)	80–96 μm^3	This test of the average size of each RBC reflects the maturity level and degree of hemoglobin content. Large immature cells, such as reticulocytes, increase the MCV, and inadequate hemoglobin content causes microcytosis and decreases MCV.
Mean corpuscular hemoglobin (MCH)	26–34 pg/cell	This test of the average amount of hemoglobin in each RBC reflects the amount of active and functional hemoglobin. Disorders of hemoglobin production (eg, iron deficiency, sickle cell anemia) cause decreased MCH.

(continued)

TABLE 22-4 Laboratory Tests in Anemia (Continued)

Test	Normal Value	Clinical Implications of Abnormal Result
Mean corpuscular hemoglobin concentration (MCHC)	31–37 g/dL	This test of the average saturation of oxygen to hemoglobin in each RBC reflects the amount of functional hemoglobin. The MCHC is reduced when oxygen saturation is inadequate due to abnormal hemoglobin (eg, sickle cell anemia), or when another gas has replaced oxygen in the hemoglobin molecule (eg, carbon monoxide poisoning).
Platelet count	150,000–400,000/mm^3	Platelet production by the bone marrow is reduced when the marrow is exposed to radiation, toxic chemicals, or certain medications. Decreased platelets also occur as platelets are trapped in small clots of hemolyzed RBCs, and due to excessive sensitivity of the spleen to remove cells. When a large foreign body is in the bloodstream (eg, intravenous catheters, heart valves, pacemakers), platelets will adhere to the foreign object and cause decreased platelet counts at least temporarily. Inflammatory processes stimulate platelet aggregation and may cause initial decreases in platelet count, but the body usually compensates by accelerating production.
WBC count	5.0–10.0 × 10^6/mm^3	Inflammatory processes result in leukocytosis, occurring secondary to the other disorders.
BUN	2–20 mg/dL	Increased creatinine and BUN occur when the level of hemolysis is so significant that intravascular heme, globin, iron, and waste products cause toxic damage to the kidneys and induce renal dysfunction.
Creatinine	0.2–1.0 mg/dL	See above.
Bilirubin (total)	0.2–1.2 mg/dL	When the demand for conjugation of RBC breakdown products exceeds the body's ability to maintain a constant removal, hyperbilirubinemia is the result. More rapid onset of hemolysis is likely to produce higher levels of bilirubin. The bilirubin level correlates to the degree of jaundice; higher levels produce more jaundice.
Erythrocyte sedimentation rate (ESR)	0–20 mm/h	RBCs quickly settle (stack in a straight column within a capillary tube) when they are the usual tiny biconcave disks. With inflammation, this process of settling requires more time. The ESR is prolonged with inflammatory disorders such as autoimmune disease. ESR may be used to monitor response to treatment, but it is not diagnostic of any disorder.

Serum folate	1.5–10 ng/mL	The serum folate reflects the amount of available vitamin building blocks for creation of normal RBCs. Folate is low in folic acid deficiency.
Serum iron level	75–175 µg/dL	Iron stores in the body are usually constant through means of normal intake and recirculation from hemolyzed RBCs, but levels are decreased in iron deficient anemia, pregnancy, or certain GI diseases. Peptic acid of the stomach aids absorption of iron, so iron deficient anemia can occur when the stomach is diseased or resected.
Total iron binding capacity (TIBC)	20%–55%	Iron is bound to hemoglobin approximately one third of the time but may be decreased if iron stores are inadequate. Iron deficient anemia usually requires low serum iron levels and poor binding capacity.
Ferritin level	20–200 ng/mL	Ferritin is a precursor to iron and is reflective of the body's ability to create new iron stores. Ferritin may be low in iron deficient anemia, related to nutritional deficit, and it must be present for the body to accelerate RBC production in times of blood loss.
Transferrin level	200–400 mg/dL	Transferrin is used to bind and recirculate iron from hemolyzed cells. Transferrin may be low when hemolysis has occurred or when large amounts of iron are bound to transferrin.
Haptoglobin level	60–270 mg/dL (fasting)	Haptoglobin normally binds with heme to facilitate removal from the circulation, so free levels of haptoglobin decrease when extrasplenic hemolysis is occurring, because more heme needs to be transported back to the liver before removal or recirculation.
Hemoglobin electrophoresis	Normal A and S	The proteins involved in hemoglobin demonstrate a specific pattern when separate, but abnormal hemoglobin S is present with sickle cell anemia.
Coombs' test (direct/indirect)	Negative	The presence of minor RBC antigens (not the usual A or B antigens) can be detected through this agglutination test. Some minor antigens detected through this means are Kell, E, and cold agglutinins.
LDH	25–75 mg/dL	Increased LDH is indicative of RBC breakdown. LDH is an enzyme released in RBC destruction.

is used when RBC production is thought to be impaired and removal of the suspected precipitator does not improve the RBC
count.

b. RBC survival is tested by administration of indium-tagged RBCs.
Serial nuclear scans are performed to observe the location of the
RBCs (eg, abnormal spleen uptake) or their life span. This may
be used in hemolytic syndromes, or when splenic sequestration
is suspected, but not confirmable, by splenomegaly alone.

C. Treatment (Box 22–8 and Tables 22–5 and 22–6)

D. Nursing Diagnoses

(Text continues on page 334)

▼ **BOX 22-8** | **Treatment of Anemia**

Ferrous sulfate 325 mg PO TID
Folic acid 0.25–1.0 mg PO QD
B_{12} 30 μg IM or deep SQ × 5–10 days, then 100–200 μg IM q month
Erythropoietin alfa:
    Renal failure: 50–100 U/kg SQ 3×/week
    Antiretroviral induced: 100 U/kg IV 3×/week
    Chemotherapy induced: 100–150 U/kg 3×/week or 40,000 U 1/week
    Anemia of chronic illness (darbepoetin only): see above dosing
    Key dosing guidelines:
        Evaluate HCT 2×/week until within 3% of HCT of 36%, or for 2–8
            weeks after every dose change.
        Change dose in increments of 25%
        Hold for 1 week if >4-point rise in HCT within any 2-week period.
Androgens (nandrolone deconate or fluoxymesterone)
Blood transfusions
Hemoglobin substitute
    Fluosol 10–20 mg/kg IV, repeated as needed (half-life 8–12 h)
Staphylococcal protein A is a component of the cell wall of staphylococci
    and is capable of trapping IgG complexes, which are thought to cause
    RBC autoantibodies in hemolytic anemia.
    Administration guidelines:
        Begin plasma reinfusion at a rate of 25 mL/h for 15 min, then increase
            to 100 mL/h.
    Nursing care:
        Assess for hypersensitivity reactions.
        Assess for fluid shifts into the interstitial spaces during infusion, or
            within 6–12 h after infusion (eg, crackles in lungs, edema).
Administer antiplatelet medications (eg, salicylate acid or indomethacin) as
    ordered to reduce ischemia damage of hemolytic anemia.
If autoantibodies or abnormal splenic sequestration is implicated in ane-
    mia, then immunosuppressive agents, such as steroids, azathioprine or
    cyclophosphamide, are given as ordered.

TABLE 22-5 Blood Transfusions

Blood Product	Description	Indications	Administration	Special Considerations
Whole blood	One 500-mL unit contains approximately 200 mL RBC and 300 mL plasma.	Massive blood loss, exchange transfusion	Large-gauge needle for administration; use 0.9% normal saline for starter fluid and flush; use blood administration set with filter pore size of 170 microns.	Be certain blood is ABO and Rh compatible; monitor patient for fluid volume overload; infuse over 2–4 h.
Packed RBCs	One 250-mL unit contains 200 mL RBC and 50 mL plasma.	Low Hct, inadequate oxygen-carrying capacity	Same as with whole blood, but surface area filter may be arger to increase infusion rate.	Be certain blood is ABO and Rh compatible; administer within 30 min of receipt.
Washed RBCs, buffy cells, leukocyte-poor cells	One 200-mL unit contains 50 mL of normal saline solution and has few WBCs and platelets	History of febrile or allergic transfusion reactions	Same as with whole blood, but microaggregate filter is not necessary.	Blood comes in special bag and connections are not as tight; premedication with acetaminophen and/or diphenhydramine may be recommended.
Frozen, deglycerized RBCs	One 200-mL unit contains 50 mL of normal saline; washed free of most WBCs and platelets.	Rare blood types; special needs for oxygen-rich blood, because nonci-trate preservative conserves 2,3-DPG better	Same as with packed washed RBCs.	Thawing process takes approximately 1 h; blood reactions should be decreased, but consult physician about premedication.
Plasma (fresh, fresh-frozen, single-donor)	One 200–300-mL unit of fresh-frozen plasma contains all coagulation factors plus 400 mg fibrinogen; single-donor plasma contains less of factors V and VII.	Coagulation deficiencies; dysfibrinogenemia; liver disease	Allow 45 min for plasma to thaw; may infuse rapidly; smaller needle size may be used; microaggregate filter is not necessary.	ABO compatibility is necessary, but Rh compatibility is not; administer within 6 h of thawing; febrile and allergic reactions are possible.
Platelets	35–50-mL unit contains 7×10^7 platelets.	Thrombocytopenia and thrombocytopathies; bone marrow aplasia	Use special platelet filter (not microaggregate); administer 100 mL over approximately 15 min.	ABO and Rh compatibility not necessary; febrile and allergic reactions are common; obtain postplatelet count to monitor effectiveness.

TABLE 22-6 **Blood Transfusion Reactions**

Type of Reaction	Cause	Signs and Symptoms
IMMEDIATE		
Hemolytic reactions	ABO or Rh incompatibility; intradonor incompatibility; improper storage	Shaking, chills, fever, nausea, vomiting, chest pain, dyspnea, hypotension, oliguria, hemoglobinuria, flank pain, abnormal bleeding; may progress to shock and renal failure
Febrile	Presence of bacterial lipopolysaccharides	Fever, chills, rigors, flank pain, headache
Allergic	Recipient reacts to allergen in donor's blood	Pruritus, urticaria, fever, chills, nausea, vomiting, facial swelling, wheezing, laryngeal edema; reaction may progress to anaphylactic reaction
Plasma protein incompatibility	IgA incompatibility	Flushing, abdominal pain, diarrhea, chills, fever, dyspnea, hypotension
Reaction to bacterial contamination	Presence of gram-negative organisms, which can survive cold (eg, certain species of *Pseudomonas*)	Chills, fever, vomiting, abdominal cramping, diarrhea, shock, renal failure
Circulatory overload	Too rapid or too large an infusion	Dyspnea, chest tightness, dry cough, distended neck veins, crackles, pulmonary edema on chest x-ray
Air embolism	Air in bloodstream by way of blood tubing	Sudden shortness of breath, sharp chest pain, anxiety, coughing, hypotension
REACTIONS TO MULTIPLE TRANSFUSIONS		
Hemosiderosis	Increased hemosiderin	Iron plasma level > 200 mg/dL
Bleeding tendencies	Low platelet count in stored blood, causing dilutional thrombocytopenia	Abnormal bleeding and oozing from breaks in skin surface

Treatment	Prevention
Stop transfusion; maintain IV access; monitor BP; treat shock using IV fluids, oxygen, epinephrine, diuretics, and vasopressors, as indicated by patient condition; obtain posttransfusion blood and urine samples for evaluation; observe patient for signs of hemorrhage resulting from DIC.	Proper identification of donor and recipient blood types to make sure blood is compatible; confirm accurate patient identification before transfusion; transfuse blood slowly for first 10–15 min; observe patient closely for first 20–30 min of transfusion.
Stop transfusion; provide symptomatic relief with antipyretic, antihistamine, or meperidine.	Premedicate patient before blood transfusion with antipyretic, antihistamine, and possibly steroids; use leukocyte-poor or washed blood products or leukocyte filter.
Stop transfusion; administer antihistamines; monitor patients for anaphylactic reaction; administer epinephrine and steroids as indicated.	Give antihistamines as premedication to patients with a history of allergic reactions; observe patient closely for first 20 min of transfusion.
Treat patient for shock by administering oxygen, fluids, epinephrine, and possibly steroids as ordered.	Transfuse only IgA-deficient blood or well-washed RBCs.
Stop transfusion; treat patient with broad-spectrum antibiotics and steroids.	Observe blood before transfusion for gas, clots, and dark purple color; use air-free, touch-free method to draw and deliver blood; maintain strict storage control; change blood tubing and filter every 4 h; infuse each unit of blood over 2–4 h, but terminate after 4 h; maintain sterile technique when administering blood.
Stop transfusion; place patient in semi-Fowler's position; possibly administer oxygen or diuretics.	Transfuse blood slowly; avoid use of whole blood; administer diuretics before giving transfusions to patients at risk for circulatory overload.
Turn patient on left side; administer 100% oxygen by face mask; treat patient for shock.	Expel air from tubing before starting the transfusion; do not allow blood bag to run dry; observe for air in tubing when infusing under pressure.
Perform phlebotomy to remove excess iron.	Administer blood only when absolutely necessary.
Administer platelets; monitor platelet count.	Use only fresh blood that is less than 7 days old when possible.

(continued)

TABLE 22-6 Blood Transfusion Reactions (Continued)

Type of Reaction	Cause	Signs and Symptoms
REACTIONS TO MULTIPLE TRANSFUSIONS		
Increased oxygen affinity for hemoglobin	Decreased level of 2,3-DPG in stored blood causing an increase in the oxygen's affinity for hemoglobin; oxygen stays in the patient's bloodstream and is not released to the tissues	Depressed respiratory rate, especially in patients with chronic lung disease who depend on low oxygen level to breathe
Elevated blood ammonia level	Increased level of ammonia in stored blood	Forgetfulness, confusion
Hypothermia	Rapid infusion of large amounts of cold blood, which decreases myocardial temperature	Shaking, chills, hypotension, ventricular fibrillation, cardiac arrest if core temperature falls below 30°C
Hypocalcemia	Citrate toxicity occurs when citrate-treated blood is infused rapidly, when citrate binds with calcium causing a calcium deficiency, or when normal citrate metabolism is hindered by hepatic disease	Tingling in fingers, muscle cramps, nausea, vomiting, hypotension, cardiac arrhythmias, convulsions, hypokalemia
Potassium intoxication	Abnormally high level of potassium is in stored plasma, caused by red cell lysis	ECG changes with tall, peaked T waves; bradycardia proceeding to cardiac standstill; intestinal colic; diarrhea, muscle twitching, oliguria, renal failure
Renal failure	Heme from hemolyzed RBCs causing renal tubular damage	Oliguria; increased urobilinogen

1. Decreased tissue perfusion related to decreased oxygen-carrying capacity
   a. *Problem:* Reduced numbers or abnormal function of RBCs cause reduced tissue oxygenation. In hemolytic anemia, poor tissue oxygenation from RBC fragment-related thrombosis is an additional problem. Symptoms of compensatory mechanisms or decreased circulating RBCs usually indicate the need for intervention.
   b. *Interventions*
      (1) Assess for sensitive indicators of altered tissue perfusion: mental status, urine output, pulse oximetry, bowel sounds.

Treatment	Prevention
Monitor arterial blood gas results; give respiratory support as needed.	Use only RBCs or fresh blood if possible.
Monitor patient's ammonia level; decrease the amount of protein in diet; if indicated, give neomycin sulfate.	Use only blood products that have been stored less than 7 days, especially if patient has hepatic disease.
Stop transfusion; warm the patient with blankets; obtain electrocardiogram (ECG).	Warm blood to 35°C–37°C with blood warmer, especially before massive transfusions.
Slow or stop transfusion depending on reaction; slowly administer calcium gluconate IV; note that reaction may be worse in hypothermic patients with elevated potassium levels.	Infuse blood slowly; monitor potassium and calcium levels; use blood less than 2 weeks old if multiple units are to be given.
Obtain ECG; administer Kayexalate orally or by enema.	Use fresh blood, less than 1 week old, when massive amounts are to be given.
Administer alkalinized fluids.	Maintain high IV flow rate during high-risk time.

(2) Assess cardiovascular system compensation for reduced oxygen-carrying capacity with every office visit (or shift if hospitalized): check for capillary refill within 3 seconds, full and bounding equal pulses, absence of heart murmur.

(3) Check for orthostasis with every set of vital signs.

(4) Assess eyelids, lips, and ears for central cyanosis, indicative of compromised oxygen-carrying capacity.

(5) Reduce oxygen consumption of patient by providing frequent rest periods.

(6) Periodically assess and maintain adequate vascular volume.

(7) Administer oxygen therapy as ordered if the oxygen level is <60 mmHg or oxygen saturation is <90%.

(8) Avoid hypothermia, which can worsen vasoconstriction and peripheral tissue perfusion.

(9) Position patient to optimize ventilation (high Fowler's or reverse Trendelenburg).

(10) Provide sedation or pain medication if anxiety and pain are contributing to increased oxygen demands.

(11) Administer RBC growth factor or transfuse blood products as ordered (see Box 22–2).

  c. *Desired outcomes*

(1) Patient will maintain a normal RBC count, hematocrit, and hemoglobin.

(2) Patient will have Pao_2 >60 mmHg and oxygen saturation >90%.

(3) Patient will not experience central cyanosis.

(4) Patient's peripheral pulses will be equal and of normal strength, SBP >90, pulse < 100

(5) Patient's urine output will exceed 750 mL/24 h period or 30 mL/h.

2. Altered breathing pattern related to compensation for decreased oxygen-carrying capacity

  a. *Problem:* Tachypnea occurs as a compensatory effort to deliver more oxygen to the tissues. Prolonged tachypnea and oxygen deficit may also result in orthopnea, dyspnea, or frank air hunger.

  b. *Interventions*

(1) Place patient in a position of comfort for improved breathing: reverse Trendelenburg's, semi-Fowler's, extra pillows under head and shoulders.

(2) Provide supplemental oxygen as needed to maintain oxygen saturation >90%.

(3) Provide emotional reassurance and instruction in relaxation techniques to diminish feelings of air hunger.

(4) Monitor work of breathing. Report accessory muscle use or nasal flaring that may indicate need for RBC transfusions.

  c. *Desired outcomes*

(1) Patient will maintain a respiratory rate <20

(2) Patient will maintain oxygen saturation >90%.

(3) Patient verbalizes comfort with breathing pattern.

3. Altered thermoregulation due to decreased RBC mass

  a. *Problem:* Loss of RBC mass leads to reduced body insulation, heat loss, and the clinical manifestation of hypothermia.

  b. *Interventions*

(1) Monitor body temperature with each clinic visit or every 4 hours with vital signs.

(2) Observe for other signs and symptoms of infection because body temperature may not rise with anemic patients.

(3) Provide additional warm clothing or covering as needed by the patient.

(4) Teach the patient to avoid excess exposure to cold because intrinsic insulating protection is altered.

(5) Interpret pulse oximetry with the understanding that readings may be falsely high due to hypothermia and decreased uptake of oxygen by the tissues.

c. *Desired outcomes*

(1) Patient's body temperature will remain above 37.8°C (98.8°F).

(2) Patient does not verbalize cold intolerance.

4. Potential for injury due to altered mobility or thought processes

a. *Problem:* Decreased RBC mass leads to orthostatic cardiovascular changes due to decreased viscosity of the blood and its tendency to pool in the lower extremities. Orthostatic changes may cause dizziness, blurred vision, confusion, and gait disturbances.

b. *Interventions*

(1) Check orthostatic status with each clinic visit or daily in hospitalized patients.

(2) Question the patient about the presence of visual, hearing, or perceptual deficits.

(3) Advise patients to move slowly from lying to standing position and to assess their tolerance.

(4) Provide a safe environment; institute fall precautions.

(5) Provide assistance when patient is out of bed.

c. *Desired outcomes*

(1) Patient will not experience neurologic symptoms.

(2) Patient will maintain normal sensory perceptions.

5. Alteration in comfort related to splenic or hepatic enlargement or dry, itching skin from jaundice

a. *Problem:* Hemolysis of RBCs causes fragmented circulating cells that are sequestered and removed by normal mechanisms in the liver and spleen. Engorgement of the liver and spleen with these damaged cells leads to enlargement of the organ and somatic pain. Excess RBC hemolysis leads to hyperbilirubinemia, jaundice, and associated pruritus.

b. *Interventions*

(1) Assess patient's perception of comfort at least every shift.

(2) Palpate the abdomen every shift to determine the splenic and hepatic enlargement, which may contribute to abdominal discomfort.

(3) If abdominal distention is present, obtain abdominal girths at least daily.

(4) Examine the sclera and skin for evidence of jaundice.

(5) Apply lotion or mentholated creams to relieve itching as needed.

(6) Administer antipruritic medications as ordered.

c. *Desired outcomes*

(1) Patient will deny the presence of abdominal discomfort.

(2) Patient will have a nonpalpable spleen and liver.

(3) Patient will maintain normal skin color, without yellowish tint.

(4) Patient will deny itching skin.

6. Alteration in urinary elimination related to renal dysfunction from heme destruction of nephrons

    a. *Problem:* Decreased circulating RBCs lead to reduced renal oxygenation and to slowed glomerular filtration with reduced urine output. RBC hemolysis and immune complexes can also cause obstruction in the microvasculature of the kidneys. Ischemic damage leads to slowed glomerular filtration and acute renal failure.

    b. *Interventions*

        (1) Insert Foley catheter as ordered.

        (2) Monitor urine output frequently, and report intake and output according to ordered parameters.

        (3) Monitor free hemoglobin levels of the urine, urobilinogen, and urine specific gravity.

        (4) Monitor renal function through BUN and creatinine levels.

        (5) Monitor electrolytes (especially potassium, calcium, phosphorus) and fluid balance as renal dysfunction progresses.

        (6) Monitor intake and output totals every shift to evaluate fluid balance. Limit fluid intake by concentrating medications and blood products.

        (7) Weigh daily to assess fluid balance.

        (8) Monitor peak and trough drug levels, which may reflect effective renal clearance of medications.

        (9) Administer antihypertensive medications as ordered.

    c. *Desired outcomes*

        (1) Patient will have normal BUN, creatinine, and electrolyte levels.

        (2) Patient will have a urine output that exceeds intake.

        (3) Patient will have a stable weight.

        (4) Blood pressure is within normal limits for the patient's preillness blood pressure.

  7. Fatigue related to decreased RBC and WBC counts and reduced energy reserve. Follow recommendations in Chapter 25.

E. Discharge Planning and Patient Education

  1. Assess the patient's neurologic and cardiovascular tolerance of the anemia, and implement safety measures as indicated.

  2. Initiate a home health nurse consultation for assessing the safety of the home and presence of support systems if the patient becomes more symptomatic.

  3. Administer RBC stimulants, such as erythropoietin, or blood transfusions in the home, if appropriate. This may require specially trained home care nurses.

  4. Perform a serum complete blood count at least weekly for patients with chronic anemia related to the malignancy or treatment. This will provide trending information and may be used to determine the success of specific treatment modalities.

  5. Teach the patient subtle symptoms of bleeding: coffee ground emesis; black, tarry stools; minor gum bleeding. Teach the patient to move from lying to sitting to standing positions slowly to avoid potential injury.

THROMBOCYTOPENIA AND BLEEDING DISORDERS

I. Definition

A. Disorders of Quantity of Coagulation Components
    1. Thrombocytopenia
    2. Hypofibrinogenemia
    3. Reduced clotting factors
B. Disorders of Quality of Coagulation Components
C. These deficiencies can result in life-threatening hemorrhage.

II. Etiology

A. The etiologies of coagulation disorders are classified by the step of the coagulation process that is affected. The four phases and associated coagulation disorders are shown in Figure 22–1.
B. The three most common etiologies are noted in Table 22–7.
C. Thrombocytopenia is a low platelet count that may occur due to decreased production, consumption, or abnormal splenic removal.
    1. Thrombocytopenia is the most common cause of bleeding in cancer patients.
    2. The prevalent etiologic factors are noted in Box 22–9.
D. Platelet dysfunction can occur due to medications (eg, salicylates or nonsteroidal antiinflammatory agents), uremia, or GI disease (see Box 22–9).
E. Coagulation Protein Deficiency
    1. Can occur when important precursors (ie, vitamin K) are not available. Production of vitamin K-dependent factors is compromised with
        a. Gastric surgery—interferes with intrinsic factor production that aids absorption
        b. Large bowel disease
        c. Certain antibiotics
        d. Other medications
    2. Liver failure—hepatitis, cirrhosis
F. Dysfunction of coagulation proteins occurs with liver failure.
G. The major disorder of clot lysis is disseminated intravascular coagulation (DIC; see Chapter 33).

III. Patient Management

A. Assessment
    1. Petechiae (tiny purplish red dots) and ecchymoses (bruises) indicate capillary/microvascular bleeding in the soft tissue. They may occur with minor injury, dependent pressure (eg, from lying on one area), or gravitational pressure (eg, limbs hanging) in fragile vessels with inadequate coagulation factors.
    2. Overt bleeding from wounds, body orifices, or around existing tubes occurs immediately if platelets are inadequate, because the platelet plug is the first step of the clotting cascade. Bleeding that is delayed 20 minutes to 2 hours indicates coagulation protein deficit. In many severe disorders, spontaneous and continuous bleeding occurs from open vessels.
    3. Enlarged and tender liver or spleen
        a. An indication that abnormal or fragmented cells are being captured by these organs.

Process		Coagulation abnormalities
Vasoconstriction reduces the loss of blood	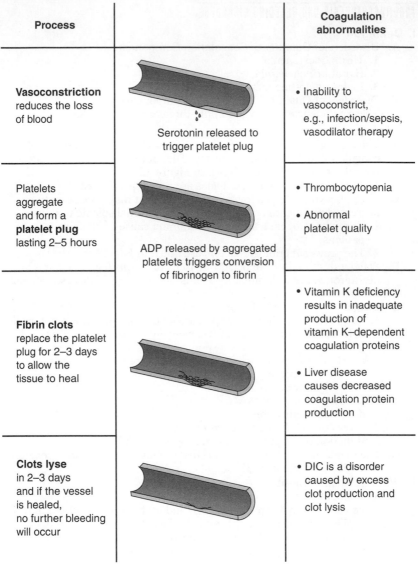 Serotonin released to trigger platelet plug	• Inability to vasoconstrict, e.g., infection/sepsis, vasodilator therapy
Platelets aggregate and form a **platelet plug** lasting 2–5 hours	ADP released by aggregated platelets triggers conversion of fibrinogen to fibrin	• Thrombocytopenia • Abnormal platelet quality
Fibrin clots replace the platelet plug for 2–3 days to allow the tissue to heal		• Vitamin K deficiency results in inadequate production of vitamin K–dependent coagulation proteins • Liver disease causes decreased coagulation protein production
Clots lyse in 2–3 days and if the vessel is healed, no further bleeding will occur		• DIC is a disorder caused by excess clot production and clot lysis

Figure 22–1. The clotting process.

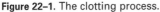

    b. Excessive removal can be a normal compensatory mechanism when there are cell fragments, such as with massive thromboses.
    4. Oliguria occurs when the microvasculature of the kidneys is thrombosed (or ruptured) and the compromised blood flow to the kidneys causes slowed glomerular filtration.

(Text continues on page 345)

TABLE 22-7 Coagulopathies

	Platelet Disorder	Hepatic Coagulation Protein Disorder	Disseminated Intravascular Coagulation
Definition	Thrombocytopenia—A reduced number of circulating and functional platelets for use in the body's clotting mechanism	The liver is the production site of all coagulation proteins except Factor VIII. When significant liver disease or malabsorption of vitamin K (necessary for some protein production) occurs, there is a failure to produce an adequate supply of functional coagulation proteins. Without coagulation proteins, a fibrin clot is not formed and bleeding will go unchecked. Patients with hepatic-induced coagulopathies may have an intact platelet plug, but, after the platelet plug dissolves, bleeding from the injured site will occur.	In normal circumstances, the clotting system is triggered by tissue injury, vessel injury, or a foreign body in the bloodstream. Hemostasis and fibrinolysis balance each other to produce a state of equilibrium between clot formation and dissolution. In severe disease, the stimulus to clot is overwhelming and does not remit, which leads to excess stimulation of clotting. This massive microvasculature clotting is the predominant feature; however, the clotting depletes coagulation factors, shears RBC, and leads to fibrin clot breakdown products (fibrin degradation products [FDP]), which all serve to increase the bleeding tendency. Thrombosed vessels also have a tendency to rupture, and depleted coagulation factors are unable to stave the flow of blood from the site.
Etiology	See Box 22-9.	Most common—Liver disease. Central lobar damage, such as seen with hepatitis, late cirrhosis, and end-stage hepatic disease, must occur before coagulopathies are evident. Anticoagulant medications (eg, heparin, warfarin) achieve their therapeutic action through interference with these coagulation proteins; therefore, over-treatment with these medications may induce bleeding symptoms.	Sepsis Trauma Burns Surgery, especially abdominal or prostate surgery Cancer Obstetric emergencies—Amniotic fluid embolism, postpartum hemorrhage, eclampsia, HELLP syndrome *(continued)*

341

TABLE 22-7 Coagulopathies *(Continued)*

	Platelet Disorder	Hepatic Coagulation Protein Disorder	Disseminated Intravascular Coagulation
		Gastrointestinal (GI) malabsorption syndromes or limited oral intake diminish the amount of vitamin K absorbed from the GI tract, resulting in insufficient production of the vitamin K-dependent coagulation factors and a bleeding tendency. Certain broad-spectrum antibiotics (eg, beta-lactam antibiotics) destroy the normal GI flora, which aid in vitamin K absorption, leading to coagulopathies.	Foreign bodies in the bloodstream—Fat embolism, sickle cell crisis
Pathophysiology	Platelets may not be adequately or normally made, signaling a bone marrow disease such as aplastic anemia, leukemia, or radiation injury to the marrow. Platelets may also be abnormally destroyed or rendered dysfunctional after leaving the marrow. Platelet problems are evident in capillary injury and early after any injury, because the platelet plug is the first line of coagulation after injury to the vessel has occurred.	Lack of production of coagulation proteins results in the body's inability to form a stable fibrin clot after the platelet plug has dissolved. Initial platelet response may be adequate, but rebleeding will occur after the platelet plug dissolves in 20 min to 2 h.	See Chapter 33.

Signs/symptoms	Petechiae Ecchymosis Occult blood in excrement Micro-organ hemorrhages (eg, kidneys [renal failure], brain [intracranial bleeds]) Mucous membrane bleeding (eg, oral cavity, urine) Spontaneous infiltrative hemorrhage, especially dependent areas—retroperitoneal alveolar, intracerebral	Initial hemostasis with rebleeding from site of injury Occult blood in excrement Discrete bleeding from sites of injury (eg, a vessel punctured from prior blood draw, small ulcerations in GI tract) May be symptomatic in rare cases where no potential bleeding sites exist	Thrombotic presentation is usually earliest symptomatology (eg, oliguria, cyanosis, hypoxia, cardiac ischemia, DVT, altered level of consciousness). Bleeding symptoms occur later in the process, once clots have been made and are dissolving (eg, hematuria, GI bleeding, alveolar hemorrhage, intracranial bleeding, bleeding from every orifice and injured skin surface). Symptoms of cell turnover, such as jaundice or increased BUN, vary among patients.
Diagnostic tests	Decreased platelet count Decreased platelet survival Prolonged bleeding time Positive platelet autoantibody if immune mediated	Prolonged prothrombin time (PT) Prolonged partial thromboplastin time (PTT) Prolonged thrombin time (TT) Decreased fibrinogen level	Decreased platelet count Prolonged PT Prolonged PTT Prolonged TT Decreased fibrinogen level Elevated fibrin degradation products Elevated D-dimer fibrin degradation product Decreased antithrombin III levels

(continued)

TABLE 22-7 Coagulopathies *(Continued)*

	Platelet Disorder	Hepatic Coagulation Protein Disorder	Disseminated Intravascular Coagulation
Comments	Thrombocytopenia is the most common coagulation defect in the oncology patient. Platelets are fragile cells easily damaged by a variety of problems experienced by ICU patients (eg, fever, dialysis filters, large-bore catheters, prosthetic heart valves).	Coagulation protein deficiencies are a late manifestation of most hepatic diseases. Some anticoagulant medications that cause abnormalities in the coagulation cascade may be reversed by specific reversal agents, vitamin K, or administration of fresh frozen plasma. Bleeding that persists despite replenishment of platelets and normalization of PT may require Factor VIII replacement (cryoprecipitate) because this factor is not made by the liver.	The most common causes of this syndrome are (1) sepsis, (2) trauma, (3) burns. Mortality rate exceeds 50%. Frequently occurs concomitantly with ARDS (it is uncertain which syndrome triggers which). May be acute or chronic symptomatology—Slow tissue injury such as with malignancy more frequently presents with chronic symptoms. Treatment of underlying etiology is essential for recovery. Replacement of lost blood components is essential while awaiting the patient's improvement.

Shelton, B. K. (1996a). Hematologic disorders. In J. Hebra & M. M. Kuhn (Eds.), *Manual of critical care nursing* (pp. 192–194). Boston, MA: Little, Brown.

▼ **BOX 22-9   Etiologies of Platelet Disorders**

Bone Marrow Suppression

Aplastic anemia

Burns

Cancer chemotherapy

Exposure to inonizing radiation

Nutritional deficiency (vitamin B_{12}, folate)

Platelet Destruction Outside Bone Marrow

Heat stroke

Heart valves

Heparin

Infections, severe or sepsis

Large-bore intravenous line (eg, pheresis or dialysis catheters)

Splenic sequestration of platelets

Sulfonamides

Transfusions

Trimethoprim sulfamethoxazole

Immune Response Against Platelets

Idiopathic thrombocytopenia purpura

Mononucleosis

Thrombotic thrombocytopenic purpura

Vaccinations

Viral illness

Interference with Platelet Production (other than nonspecific marrow suppression)

Alcohol

Histamine-2 blocking agents

Histoplasmosis

Hormones

Thiazide diuretics

Interference with Platelet Function

Aminoglycosides

Catecholamines (eg, epinephrine, dopamine)

Cirrhosis of the liver

Dextran

Diabetes mellitus

Hypothermia

Loop diuretics (eg, furosemide)

Malignant lymphomas

Nonsteroidal antiinflammatory agents

Phenothiazines

Salicylate derivatives

Sarcoidosis

Scleroderma

Systemic lupus erythematosus

Thyrotoxicosis

Tricyclic antidepressants

Uremia

Vitamin E

5. Occult or overt bleeding in excrement (urine, feces, emesis)
   a. The mucous membranes of the body have capillaries close to the surface and are, hence, the earliest to bleed when coagulation mechanisms are inadequate.
   b. Bleeding may be occult and only detected by laboratory examination, or visible from body orifices or in body secretions.
   c. The mucous membranes of the body that tend to bleed include the nasopharynx, oral mucosa, GI tract, urinary tract, and upper airways.

6. Bloody sputum is an unusual but possible manifestation of diffuse pulmonary bleeding that occurs with inflammation or traumatic injury of the airway (eg, after endotracheal suctioning).
   a. Sputum may be pink-tinged if lower airway injury has occurred, or frankly bloody in upper airway injury.
   b. The risk of bloody sputum is increased when coagulation deficits occur in conjunction with other airway disorders (eg, pneumonia or intubation of the airway).

B. Diagnostic Parameters: These depend on the specific disorder of coagulation. Generalized abnormalities are described below. Table 22–7 outlines distinctive diagnostic parameters that are unique to each disorder.
   1. Serum tests: Decreased HCT and HgB will occur with all coagulation disorders when a sufficient amount of blood is lost to demonstrate a functional anemia.
   2. Urine tests: Guaiac-positive test of urine signifies occult blood in the urine, which occurs in most coagulation disorders because the mucous membranes are the most sensitive to bleeding when there is a coagulation deficit.
   3. Other tests: Guaiac-positive test of stool or emesis signifies blood in the stool and emesis, which occurs in many coagulation disorders because the mucous membranes are the most sensitive to bleeding when there is a coagulation deficit.

C. Treatment: Bleeding disorders are treated in multiple ways.
   1. The first priority in treatment of a bleeding disorder is to correct the underlying cause.
      a. This may involve administration of an important nutrient or precursor (eg, AquaMEPHYTON administration when vitamin K-dependent proteins are inadequate; see Table 22–7).
      b. It may also involve blood component transfusions, such as RBCs or platelets in coagulopathies related to blood loss (see Tables 22–5 and 22–6).
   2. When correction of the underlying problem is unsuccessful or not possible, other supportive strategies are employed.
      a. Bleeding may be treated symptomatically by applying ice or pressure to the site of bleeding. This causes vasoconstriction and reduces blood loss, but does not prevent bleeding from recurring.
      b. Other supportive, local measures to decrease bleeding from a specific site include topical agents, such as Gelfoam, topical thrombin, or Avitene.
   3. Systemic treatments for coagulation disorders involve stimulation of the body's normal processes to produce factors or agents known to decrease the bleeding tendency.
      a. One bone marrow growth factor is licensed by the U. S. Food and Drug Administration (FDA) to stimulate bone marrow production of platelets (oprelvelkin, interleukin-11).
      b. Amicar (aminocaproic acid) blocks plasminogen breakdown of plasmin.
      c. Somatostatin (octreotide) enhances activity of a normally occurring GI enzyme with a procoagulant effect. It has been used for management of GI bleeding.

    d. High-dose estrogen has also been used to enhance normal clotting mechanisms, but its efficacy for use in the bleeding patient has not been established.

D. Nursing Diagnoses

  1. Potential for bleeding related to low platelet count, decreased platelet quality, hepatic coagulation defects, or DIC

    a. *Problem:* Coagulopathies increase the risk of spontaneous bleeding, as well as bleeding related to injury. The nature of the bleeding may be predicted based on the etiology, but severity depends more on extent of the coagulation deficit and type of injury.

    b. *Interventions*

      (1) Implement bleeding prevention strategies, such as keeping the head of bed elevated, avoiding medications that induce coagulopathies (eg, aspirin), limiting invasive procedures, padding bed rails, allowing patients out of bed only with assistance and padding, avoiding rectal procedures, maintaining oral hygiene, and keeping nares and lips softened.

      (2) Ensure that there is a stable blood-drawing access to avoid unnecessary venipunctures.

      (3) Use automatic BP cuff and clip on oximeter probes cautiously to prevent injury.

      (4) Monitor all excrement for occult blood.

      (5) Examine body (including cavities) every shift for bleeding, bruising, or petechiae.

      (6) Administer topical hemostatic agents (eg, Gelfoam, topical thrombin) when procedures must be performed.

      (7) Use paper tape and skin barrier on skin to prevent skin tears and bleeding. Duoderm or other skin covering may be used to apply tape that must be changed frequently.

      (8) Administer blood components as ordered (see Table 22–2), and monitor for transfusion reactions (see Table 22–3).

      (9) Monitor HCT, HgB, RBC, platelets, PT, PTT, fibrinogen, FDP, D-dimer, thrombin time as ordered.

    (10) Estimate blood losses through excrement or exsanguination. If blood loss looks significant, run a hematocrit on drainage.

    (11) Monitor volume status (intake and output, central venous pressure) and blood pressure when patient is actively bleeding to detect symptoms of hypovolemic shock.

    c. *Desired outcomes*

      (1) Patient will have absence of bleeding.

      (2) Patient will have stable HCT and Hgb.

      (3) Patient will have normal coagulation studies.

  2. Altered body image due to bleeding, bruising, or hematoma formation

    a. *Problem:* Vascular occlusion and tendencies to bleed can cause cyanosis, extensive subcutaneous tissue bleeding, or overt bleeding resulting in purplish bruising in all body areas, edema with purplish discoloration, petechiae, bleeding from every orifice or puncture site, bloody urine, bloody stool, and bloody tears. Patients or their families may be very distressed regarding these changes in body image.

    b. *Interventions*

      (1) Provide patient and family with an idea of expected changes that may occur with these disorders.

      (2) Be sensitive to nursing interventions that may worsen these symptoms. The nurse should avoid the following when treating a patient with a bleeding disorder.

        (a) Automatic BP cuff

        (b) Trendelenburg positioning

        (c) Use of nonelectric razors

        (d) Intramuscular (IM) or subcutaneous (SQ) injections

        (e) Rectal procedures (eg, temperatures) and medications

        (f) Patient getting constipated or straining during defecation

        (g) Patient getting dry mucous membranes of the nose or mouth

      (3) Reassure patient and family that the blood in the subcutaneous tissue will be reabsorbed as the patient gets better.

      (4) Encourage family to participate in providing comfort measures.

    c. *Desired outcomes*

      (1) Patient and family will be prepared for the body image changes that may occur with bleeding disorders.

      (2) Patient and family will see resolution of ecchymoses.

3. Potential fluid volume deficit due to hemorrhage

    a. *Problem:* Blood lost through micro- and macrovascular bleeding will deplete blood volume, as well as produce a deficit of coagulation components.

    b. *Interventions*

      (1) Monitor fluid status through intake and output measurements.

      (2) Monitor vascular volume through central venous pressures, orthostatic vital signs, and jugular venous pulsations.

      (3) Obtain daily weights to compare to intake and output records.

      (4) Administer isotonic IV fluids (eg, Ringer's, normal saline) or blood products to replenish lost vascular volume.

    c. *Desired outcome:* Patient will have normal blood pressure, central venous pressure, and stable weights.

4. Potential alteration in oxygenation related to intrapulmonary bleeding

    a. *Problem:* When intrapulmonary bleeding occurs, the upper airways are occluded with blood or clots, or the alveoli are filled with blood, hindering the normal exchange of gases. This leads to hypoxemia and hypercarbia.

    b. *Interventions*

      (1) Administer supplemental oxygen as ordered.

      (2) Maintain humidification of airways by way of humidified air, humidified oxygen, nasal sprays, or nebulizer treatments.

      (3) Perform nasotracheal suctioning only with a physician's order. Avoid unnecessary suctioning for platelet counts $\leq 20,000/mm^3$.

(4) Use nasopharyngeal airway when needed to reduce trauma while suctioning.

(5) Administer coagulation factors (platelets, FFP) as needed before nasopharyngeal airway insertion or suctioning.

(6) Administer positive pressure ventilation assistance (eg, CPAP mask, BiPAP) for intrapulmonary bleeding as ordered.

(7) Monitor arterial blood gases periodically, and monitor oxygen saturation continuously.

(8) Report to physician any acute onset of dyspnea, cough, desaturation, or bloody sputum.

(9) Maintain position of optimal ventilation—Trendelenburg's or Fowler's.

(10) Obtain chest x-rays as ordered to monitor bleeding and degree of congestion.

   c. *Desired outcomes*

(1) Patient's Pao_2 will remain $\geq$ 80 mmHg by arterial blood gas.

(2) Patient's Pco_2 will remain $\leq$ 45 mmHg by arterial blood gas.

(3) Patient's pulse oximetry oxygen saturation will remain >90%.

(4) Patient will not have bloody sputum, dyspnea, or cough.

(5) Patient will have a normal chest x-ray.

5. Decreased urinary output related to hemorrhagic cystitis

   a. *Problem:* When coagulopathy is present, and particularly in the presence of preexisting bladder injury (eg, caused by cyclophosphamide), hemorrhagic cystitis may occur.

   b. *Interventions*

(1) Provide adequate hydration (ie, 150 to 500 mL/h) throughout administration and clearance of cyclophosphamide. Hydration adequacy can be determined by adequacy of urine output and presence of occult blood in the urine.

(2) Use other measures to assess fluid status in addition to urine output, because urine output is altered by amount of blood in the urine.

(3) Assess for distended bladder, which could increase risk of hemorrhagic cystitis occurrence.

(4) Assess for bladder spasms, especially in the context of blood in the urine. Spasms often indicate retained clots and require evacuation bladder irrigations.

   (a) Administer prescribed irrigation solution by way of three-way Foley catheter, allowing continuous inflow and outflow simultaneously.

   (b) Increase inflow rate if bloody urine is noted—returning irrigant should only be pink, or clots are likely to occur.

   (c) Add hemostatic agents (eg, alum, prostaglandin E_2) to irrigant as prescribed.

   (d) Check for irrigation fluid overfill and add into output so accurate output is registered (eg, some 2-L containers contain 2,070 mL). Accurate fluid values can be obtained by weighing the irrigating solutions.

   c. *Desired outcome:* Patient will not have occult or frank blood in the urine.

6. Altered sensory perception (vision) due to bleeding
   a. *Problem:* Thrombosis (in DIC) and bleeding occur in the microvasculature of the retina, particularly if accompanied by hypertension. These hemorrhages alter visual acuity and may cause temporary or permanent visual deficits.
   b. *Interventions*
      (1) Assess visual sensation every shift in awake patients.
      (2) Presume visual deficits in the disoriented patient, and provide verbal descriptions of all nursing care behavior and all personnel who enter the room.
      (3) Note ophthalmic findings and communicate with peers regarding the patient's status.
      (4) Explain to family why the patient may be unable to focus vision on them when spoken to.
   c. *Desired outcome:* Patient will have normal visual acuity or will compensate for visual deficits by way of other senses.
7. Altered cognition due to bleeding
   a. *Problem:* Patients with coagulation defects are at significant risk for spontaneous or injury-induced intracranial bleeding.
   b. *Interventions*
      (1) Maintain target platelet count, or coagulation test results through transfusion of blood components.
      (2) Implement measures to prevent risk of intracranial hemorrhage. Assist patients when out of bed, establish a safe environment free of obstructions, maintain head of bed elevation 30 degrees at all times, do *not* use Trendelenburg positioning for management of hypotension or insertion of a central venous access line.
      (3) Perform a thorough bilateral motor and sensory neurologic assessment when any cognition, sensory, or musculoskeletal symptoms occur.
      (4) Immediately report to the physician the presence of any high-risk symptoms such as severe headache, unequal motor strength, visual disturbances, pupillary changes, hypertension.
   c. *Desired outcomes*
      (1) Absence of mental status changes
      (2) Absence of focal neurologic deficits
E. Discharge Planning and Patient Education
   1. Teach the patient and family the nature of the disorder, when it is likely to occur, clinical manifestations, and reportable symptoms.
   2. Teach patient the chronicity of the disorder. In patients receiving chemotherapy, the disorder may be short-lived; in patients receiving radiotherapy, it may be late in onset; and when bone metastases are the etiology, effects are permanent.
   3. Explain to the patient that chemotherapy decreases the platelet count and outline the predictable nadir (deepest amount of decrease). The patient should be particularly careful to avoid injury and be alert to excess bleeding in the time just before to just after the nadir. Discourage strenuous physical activity, activities placing patient at risk for injury, and sexual intercourse during this time period.

4. Monitor blood counts near the point of nadir to detect how low the platelet counts actually become. Patients with coagulopathies related to liver disease will require more frequent blood count monitoring because they have less predictable clotting deficit.

REFERENCES

Baldwin, P. D. (2002). Febrile nonhemolytic transfusion reactions. *Clinical Journal of Oncology Nursing, 6*(3), 171–172, 174.

Baltic, T., Schlosser, E., & Bedell, M. K. (2002). Neutropenic fever: One institution's quality improvement project to decrease time from patient arrival to initiation of antibiotic therapy. *Clinical Journal of Oncology Nursing, 6*(6), 337–340.

Barber, F. D. (2001). Management of fever in neutropenic patients with cancer. *Nursing Clinics of North America, 36*(4), 631–644, v.

Bedell, C. (2003). Pegfilgrastim for chemotherapy-induced neutropenia. *Clinical Journal of Oncology Nursing, 7*(1), 55–57.

Bron, D., Meuleman, N., & Mascaux, C. (2001). Biological basis of anemia. *Seminars in Oncology, 28*, 1–6.

Brown, M., & Whalen, P. K. (2000). Red blood cell transfusion in critically ill patients. Emerging risks and alternatives. *Critical Care Nurse* (Suppl), 1–14, quiz 15–6.

Buchsel, P. C., Forgey, A., Grape, F. B., & Hamann, S. S. (2002). Granulocyte macrophage colony-stimulating factor: Current practice and novel approaches. *Clinical Journal of Oncology Nursing, 6*(4), 198–204.

Buchsel, P. C., Murphy, B. J., & Newton, S. A. (2002). Epoetin alfa: Current and future indications and nursing implications. *Clinical Journal of Oncology Nursing, 6*(5), 261–266.

Byars, L. (2002). Neutropenia risk assessment and management in the ambulatory care setting. *Oncology Supportive Care, 1*(1), 27–39.

Compston, J. E. (2002). Bone marrow and bone: A functional unit. *Journal of Endocrinology, 173*, 387–394.

Fitzpatrick, L. (2002). When to administer modified blood products. *Nursing. 32*(5), 36–41, quiz 42.

Freedman, M.L. (1999). Aging in the blood. In W.B. Abrams & R. Berkow (Eds.), *The Merck manual of geriatrics* (4th ed.). Rahway, NJ: Merck, Sharp & Dohme Research Laboratories.

Fritsma, M.G. (2003). Use of blood products and factor concentrates for coagulation therapy. *Clinical Laboratory Science, 16*(2), 115–119.

Fung, Y. L., Goodison, K. A., Wong, J. K., & Minchinton, R. M. (2003). Investigating transfusion-related acute lung injury (TRALI). *Internal Medicine Journal, 33*(7), 286–290.

Gillespie, T. W. (2003). Anemia in cancer: Therapeutic implications and interventions. *Cancer Nursing, 26*(2), 119–28, quiz 129–30.

Hellstrom-Lindberg, E., Willman, C., Barrett, A. J., & Saunthararajah, Y. (2002). Achievements in understanding and treatment of myelodysplastic syndromes. *Hematology* (American Society of Hematology Educational Program), pp. 110–132.

Higgins, C. (2000–2001). The risks associated with blood and blood product transfusion. *British Journal of Nursing, 9–10*(22), 2281–2290.

Kullavanuaya, P., Manotayam S., Thong-Ngamm, D., Mahachai, V., & Kladchareon, N. (2001). Efficacy of octreotide in the control of acute upper gastrointestinal bleeding. *Journal of the Medical Association of Taiwan, 84*(12), 1714–1720.

Mank, A., & van der Lelie, H. (2003). Is there still an indication for nursing patients with prolonged neutropenia in protective isolation? An evidence-based nursing and medical study of 4 years experience for nursing patients with neutropenia without isolation. *European Journal of Oncology Nursing, 7*(1), 17–23.

Miller, R. L. (2001). Blood component therapy. *Orthopedic Nursing, 20*(5), 57–65, quiz 66–68.

Milligan, P., & Pirie, L. (2000). Enhancing care for transfusion patients. *Professional Nurse, 15*(11), 700–703.

Pantanowitz, L., Kruskall, M. S., & Uhl, L. (2003). Cryoprecipitate. Patterns of use. *American Journal of Clinical Pathology, 119*(6), 874–881.

Perry, M. C. (Ed.). (2001). *The chemotherapy source book* (p. 562). Baltimore, MD: Williams & Wilkins.

Price, T. H. (2002). Granulocyte transfusion in the G-CSF era. *International Journal of Hematology, 76*(Suppl 2), 77–80.

Reigle, B. S., & Dienger, M. J. (2003). Sepsis and treatment-induced immunosuppression in the patient with cancer. *Critical Care Nursing Clinics of North America, 15*(1), 109–118.

Rogers, B. (2002). Management of anemia in the ambulatory patient with cancer. *Oncology Supportive Care, 2,* 9–25.

Rowe, R., & Doughty, H. (2000). Observation and documentation of bedside blood transfusion. *British Journal of Nursing, 9*(16), 1054–1058.

Rust, D. M., Simpson, J. K., & Lister, J. (2000). Nutritional issues in patients with severe neutropenia. *Seminars in Oncology Nursing, 16*(2), 152–162.

Shelton, B. K. (2003). Evidence-based care for the neutropenic patient with leukemia. *Seminars in Oncology Nursing, 19*(2), 133–141.

_____. (2001). Hematological and immune disorders. In M. L. Sole, M. L. Lamborn & J. C. Hartshorn (Eds.), *Introduction to critical care nursing* (3rd ed., pp. 405–457). Philadelphia, PA: W. B. Saunders.

_____. (1999a). Sepsis. *Seminars in Oncology Nursing, 15*(3), 209–221.

_____. (1996b). Hematologic disorders. In J. Hebra & M. M. Kuhn (Eds.), *Manual of critical care nursing* (pp.192–194). Boston, MA: Little, Brown.

_____. (1996). Immunologic disorders. In J. Hebra & M. M. Kuhn (Eds.), *Manual of critical care nursing* (pp. 221–225). Boston, MA: Little, Brown.

Shelton, B. K., Ashenbrenner, D. A., Shane, K. (2002). Biological therapy. In D. Ashenbrenner (Ed.), *Pharmacologic therapy* (pp. 583–610). Philadelphia: Lippincott Williams & Wilkins.

Simmons, P. (2003). A primer for nurses who administer blood products. *Medical-Surgical Nursing, 12*(3), 84–90, quiz 191–2.

Smith, L. H., & Besser, S. G. (2000). Dietary restrictions for patients with neutropenia: A survey of institutional practices. *Oncology Nursing Forum, 27*(3), 515–520.

Trewitt, K. G. (2001). Bone marrow aspiration and biopsy: Collection and interpretation. *Oncology Nursing Forum, 28*(9), 1409–1415, quiz 1416–1417.

Walker, J., & Criddle, L. M. (2002). Massive transfusion: Don't stop. *Journal of Emergency Nursing, 28*(2), 176–178.

Walter-Coleman, S. (1996). Transfusion therapy for patients critically ill with cancer. *AACN Clinical Issues in Critical Care, 7*(1), 37–45.

Wilson, B. J. (2002). Dietary recommendations for neutropenic patients. *Seminars in Oncology Nursing, 18*(1), 44–49.

Wright-Kanuth, M. S., & Smith, L. A. (2002). Developments in component therapy: Novel components and new uses for familiar preparations. *Clinical Laboratory Science, 15*(2), 116–124, quiz 125–7.

23 Constipation and Diarrhea

Katherina Violette

I. Overview of Disorders of Intestinal Motility

A. Abnormalities of intestinal motility can involve the processes of absorption, secretion, or peristalsis.

1. Normal bowel absorption is primarily affected by the functional capacity of the villi.
2. Normal bowel secretion is regulated by cells in the crypts.
3. Normal bowel peristalsis is stimulated by the presence of substances in the gastrointestinal (GI) tract and affected by neuromuscular disorders.
4. Normal transit time for food in the GI tract is 24 to 48 hours.
5. Elder patients may have baseline alterations in motility that influence their risk of developing complications.
   a. Slowed and less effective absorption
   b. Reduced lymphocyte activity of the gut decreases inflammatory response and decreases antibody responses
   c. Decreased peristalsis

B. Definitions

1. *Constipation*—Less stool output and dryer, harder consistency than normal
2. *Diarrhea*—More stool output and more liquid consistency than normal

C. Prevalence

1. GI complaints are present in >50% of adults and children with advanced cancer (Campbell, Draper, Reid & Robinson, 2001; Komurcu, Nelson, Walsh, Ford & Rybicki, 2002).
2. Nearly all patients having radiation that includes the pelvis or GI tract experience alterations in motility.
3. More than 50% of patients with cancer experience alterations in motility caused by chemotherapeutic agents (Brown et al., 2001; Gossel, 2002).
4. Gastrointestinal dysfunction is a common toxicity of antineoplastic therapy that causes therapy delays.
5. Studies reflect that family caregivers are unable to accurately assess the intensity of these symptoms (Potter, Hami, Bryan & Quigley, 2003)

CONSTIPATION

I. Definition

A. Decrease in the usual frequency of bowel movements, resulting in difficult passage of hard, dry stool

B. Defining Features

    1. Failure to have a bowel movement for 3 days despite normal intake

    2. Hard, dry stool

    3. Straining at stool

    4. Feeling of incomplete evacuation

  C. Ranked in top three distressing symptoms by patients with advanced cancer (Campbell et al., 2001)

II. Etiology

  A. Pathophysiologic mechanisms may include one or several of these mechanisms:

    1. Increased absorption.

    2. Decreased secretion.

    3. Decreased peristalsis.

  B. Decreased oral intake of both fluids and fiber with resultant dehydration.

  C. Decreased physical activity related to hospitalization, generalized weakness, fatigue, or lethargy can reduce neurologic stimulus to pass stool.

  D. Depression and anxiety can result in decreased oral intake or decreased physical activity. Antidepressant medications may also enhance the risk of constipation.

  E. Carcinomas of the bowel may alter normal bowel function or cause lumen obstruction.

  F. Surgical Procedures

    1. Any operative manipulation of the bowel will slow peristalsis.

    2. Anesthetic agents used for surgery slow peristalsis.

    3. Surgical procedures involving the GI tract may affect any component of normal absorption, secretion, or peristalsis.

  G. Chemotherapeutic Agents

    1. Vinca alkaloids (eg, vincristine, vinblastine) cause autonomic neuropathy in about 30% of patients that can result in constipation or paralytic ileus that peaks in incidence 3 to 7 days after chemotherapy administration (Brown et al., 2001).

    2. Thalidomide

  H. Opiates (Pappagallo, 2001)

    1. Incidence is 45% to 98% of patients receiving regular regimen of opioids.

    2. Dose related.

  I. Medical Disorders

    1. Addison's disease.

    2. Cushing's disease.

    3. Diabetes mellitus causes autonomic neuropathy.

    4. Hypothyroidism.

    5. Spinal cord compression between T8 and L3 can cause relaxation of the anal sphincter and fecal retention.

  J. Other Medications

    1. Aluminum-containing antacids

    2. Antiemetics

    3. Anticholinergics (eg, loperamide, medications to treat bladder spasms)

    4. Antihypertensives—Calcium channel blockers, centrally acting agents (eg, clonidine)

     5. Calcium or iron supplements
     6. Diuretics
     7. Phenothiazines
     8. Sympathetic stimulation—Antidepressants, antiparkinson agents
     9. Sleep medications
    10. Tricyclic antidepressants
K. Electrolyte Disturbances
     1. Hypokalemia causes decreased intestinal motility and paralytic ileus due to neuromuscular irritability.
     2. Hypercalcemia impedes the transmission of stimuli causing atony of the GI tract and constipation.
L. Increased Sympathetic Tone
     1. Chronic pain or stress
     2. Use of sympathetic stimulating agents: Dopamine, antidepressants
M. Older age may be the most important adjunctive risk factor in patients receiving medications known to cause constipation.
N. Changes in routine that disrupt normal bowel toileting
     1. Travel.
     2. Lack of time—When bowel evacuation is delayed from initial urges, the stimulation and sensation of having to defecate weaken.
     3. Lack of privacy.

III. Patient Management

A. Assessment
     1. Patient history
         a. Risk factors
         b. Normal bowel habits
         c. Diet history—Fluid, fiber, caffeine
         d. Medication history for risk factors
         e. Use of laxatives
         f. Activity level
     2. Patient complaints
         a. Frequency of stool.
         b. Consistency of stool.
         c. Associated symptoms—Lower back discomfort, feeling of fullness, rectal pressure, abdominal pain, abdominal cramping or gas, abdominal distention, anorexia, nausea, headache.
         d. The constipation assessment scale (CAS) is a common valid and reliable assessment scale that addresses constipation and its related symptoms as well as the distress experienced by the patient (McMillan & Williams, 1989; Quanta Healthcare Solutions, 2003).
     3. Physical findings
         a. Performance status and ability to increase activity level
         b. Bowel sounds
         c. Abdomen firmness, tenderness to palpation
         d. Manual detection of stool in rectum
B. Diagnostic Parameters: There are no definitive diagnostic tests for constipation; it is a diagnosis made by clinical evidence.
C. Treatment
     1. Lifestyle alterations
         a. Diet—Increase fluid, increase fiber
         b. Exercise—Increase aerobic exercise

2. Complementary therapies
   a. Herb teas—1 tsp of substance in boiling water; dried dandelion blooms, licorice root, mullein, slippery elm, raspberry leaves, rhubarb root tincture, guelder rose bark tincture (Brown, 2001)
   b. Aloe vera juice several times a day
   c. Flax or linseed seeds crushed into a porridge or chewed
3. Surgical therapy
   a. Lower endoscopy for diagnosis or management of refractory constipation (Pepin & Ladabaum, 2002)
   b. Laparoscopy-assisted bowel resection
   c. Percutaneous cecostomy (Wills, Trowbridge, Disario & Fang, 2003)
4. Medications (Table 23–1)
D. Nursing Diagnoses
1. Constipation related to cancer, cancer treatment, or adverse effects
   a. *Problem:* Constipation can be caused by multiple factors and is often the result of several interacting risk factors. Constipation can result in bowel obstruction, reabsorption of metabolic toxins, and discomfort.
   b. *Interventions*—Will vary based on causative factors and the patient's ability to comply with some interventions, and should, therefore, be individualized. The following interventions are listed in the order they are usually initiated, from least invasive to most comprehensive.
      (1) Increase fluid intake (2 to 3 L daily). Warm fluids may act as a peristaltic stimulant and assist with evacuation.
      (2) Increase fiber intake. High-fiber foods include whole grains, bran, fresh raw fruits and vegetables, nuts, coconuts, corn, popcorn, raisins, dates, and prunes.
      (3) Avoid caffeine because it can act as a diuretic, decreasing water volume.
      (4) Avoid cheese products and refined grains.
      (5) Increase physical activity, which will increase gut motility. If confined to bed, contract and relax abdominal muscles and move lower extremities.
      (6) Provide for regular toilet habits, including:
         (a) Consistent daily toilet time (after breakfast is a time when gut motility is naturally high)
         (b) Privacy
         (c) A bedside commode rather than a bedpan when possible
      (7) Anticipate treatment regimens likely to cause constipation and implement preventive stool softeners or bulk producers. Regimens to reduce opioid-induced constipation include both a stool softener and a peristaltic stimulant.
         (a) Senna 1 to 2 tablets daily at bedtime.
         (b) Docusate 1 to 2 tablets daily in the morning.
         (c) If patients do not move their bowels at least once per day, each can be increased by 1 tablet daily until a maximum of 4 tablets three times a day is reached, or 3 to 4 days without a bowel movement.
      (8) Add bulk producers and stool softeners as needed (see Table 23–1).

(9) Additional pharmacologic interventions (see Table 23–1).

(10) Participate in referral for surgical management of bowel obstruction when indicated.

  (a) Possible candidates: Tumor-associated constipation and luminal obstruction, or severe high fecal impaction.

  (b) Diagnostic tests defining location and extent of fecal obstruction include abdominal flat plate and lateral x-rays, abdominal computed tomography (CT) scan, or abdominal ultrasound.

  (c) Serum ammonia levels may aid in determining severity of toxic metabolic waste absorption.

(11) Teach the patient pelvic Kegel exercises to enhance rectal muscle tone.

  c. *Desired outcomes*

  (1) Patient will maintain regular, comfortable passage of soft, formed stool.

  (2) Patient will have fewer complaints of discomfort or constipation.

  (3) Patient will have decreased need for laxatives or other interventions.

2. Potential for infection due to bowel obstruction or rupture.

  a. *Problem:* Severe and intractable constipation can lead to bowel obstruction and possible rupture. If the large bowel ruptures, peritoneal sepsis will ensue.

  b. *Interventions*

  (1) Frequent abdominal assessment when the patient has known constipation.

    (a) Bowel sounds.

    (b) Abdominal pain—Report rebound tenderness immediately.

    (c) Abdominal distention.

  (2) Vital sign monitoring every shift or ambulatory visit. Investigate possible abdominal sepsis if the patient is febrile.

  (3) Serial abdominal circumferences if distention is present.

  (4) If acute obstruction or rupture is suspected, prepare for:

    (a) Stat abdominal flat plate x-ray.

    (b) Wide open infusion of intravenous (IV) fluids and possible transfer to an intensive care unit for vasopressors.

    (c) Stat IV antibiotics that usually include metronidazole or a fluoroquinolone.

    (d) NPO until it is determined whether the patient is a candidate for surgery.

    (e) Frequent vital signs and intake and output measurement.

    (f) Laboratory specimens for serum chemistry, amylase, and lactate.

  c. *Desired outcome:* Constipation is resolved before abdominal crisis occurs.

IV. Discharge Planning and Patient Education

  A. Educate patients who are at high risk for constipation, especially if they are receiving opiates or plant alkaloid antineoplastic agents.

  B. Teach patients the importance of constipation prevention by increasing fluids, fiber, physical activity and maintaining any prescribed prophylactic medication regimen.

TABLE 23-1 Treatment of Constipation

Category	Examples	Action	Onset (hours)	Side Effects	Comments
Aminoguanidine indole partial 5HT$_4$ antagonist	Tegaserod	Prokinetic properties	May not see any effects for days, and maximal efficacy about 1 month	Dizziness, headache, nausea, vomiting, abdominal pain, flatulence	Has only been approved for use by women having constipation as predominant irritable bowel syndrome, but used investigationally for constipation of other etiologies.
Naltrexone derivatives	Methylnaltrexone	Opioid antagonists	2–8	Hypertension, tachycardia, pupillary constriction, tremors, insomnia, dizziness, nervousness, anxiety	Newer agents do not cross the blood–brain barrier and cause the same degree of withdrawal symptoms as pure antagonists such as naloxone.
Bulk laxatives	Bran Metamucil (psyllium) Citrucel (methylcellulose)	Increases size and weight of stool by absorbing water from the gut Softens stool	12–24 (could be up to 72)	May cause bloating, flatulence, or abdominal cramping Possible intestinal obstruction if not taken with sufficient water	Requires high fluid intake Avoid administering psyllium products with salicylates or digitalis—it may decrease action of these drugs
Saline laxatives	Milk of magnesia Magnesium citrate Sodium phosphate	Draws water into intestinal lumen and distends bowel, thus stimulating peristalsis	0.5–3	Causes abdominal cramping, flatulence, liquid stools	Most useful as preparative agents for diagnostic tests Avoid magnesium laxatives in patients with renal dysfunction Avoid sodium laxatives in patients with CHF or hypertension
Osmotic laxatives	Lactulose Sorbital	Promotes water retention Increases volume in colon	24–48	Unpalatably sweet	Produces an osmotic catharsis Often effective in treatment of vincristine- or narcotic-induced constipation

Category	Drug	Action	Onset (h)	Side effects	Comments
Softener	Docusate (Colace)	Promotes water retention / Softens stool	24–72		Helps prevent straining due to hard stool
Lubricant	Mineral oil	Lubricates and softens the stool	6–8	Possible lipid pneumonia from aspiration / May cause anal leakage	
Stimulant laxatives	Bisacodyl (Dulcolax) / Anthraquinones (Senokot, Cascara)	Stimulates peristalsis in the colon	6–10	May produce excessive catharsis / Possible electrolyte disturbances / May be habit forming	Effective in the treatment of opiate-induced constipation
	Castor oil	Same as above	2–6		
Suppositories	Glycerine	Stimulates sensory receptors in the rectum / Draws fluid into rectum	0.5–1	May cause irritation or burning sensation in the rectum	Onset is more rapid
	Bisacodyl	Also contains stimulant laxative	0.25–1		
Enemas	Tap water	Adds water to stool		Only evacuates distal colon	Useful for constipation related to diagnostic procedures or the management of fecal impaction
	Soap suds	Adds water and irritant effect			
	Fleets (sodium phosphate/biphosphate)	Exerts osmotic effect		Chance of bowel perforation	Reserve for when other methods have been ineffective
	Oil retention	Softens and lubricates			

DIARRHEA

I. Definition
   A. Frequent passage of soft or liquid stools.
   B. May or may not be associated with discomfort.
   C. Stool may contain abnormal constituents such as blood, pus, or mucus.

II. Etiology
   A. Major Pathophysiologic Mechanisms
      1. Osmotic diarrhea—Abnormal absorption function causes pulling of water into the bowel lumen, increasing the water content of the GI contents.
         a. Ingestion of poorly absorbable hyperosmolar substances (eg, high sugar)
         b. Absorption defect (eg, deficient lactase, gluten sensitivity [celiac disease], pancreatic insufficiency)
      2. Secretory diarrhea—Overstimulation of the intestinal tract's secretory capacity
         a. Characterized by:
            (1) Large stool volume (can exceed 1 L/h in well-hydrated adults)
            (2) Absence of red or white blood cells in the stool
            (3) Absence of fever or other systemic symptoms (except those due to dehydration)
            (4) Persistence of diarrhea with fasting (volume may diminish, however)
            (5) Lack of excess osmotic gap in stool electrolytes. The stool usually has low Na^+ and Cl^- and high K^+, but with secretory diarrhea levels are nearly the same as serum levels (Field, 2003).
         b. Common causes
            (1) Bacterial enterotoxins
               (a) *Campylobacter*
               (b) *Clostridium difficile*
               (c) *Cryptosporidium*
               (d) *Escherichia coli*
               (e) *Giardia lamblia*
               (f) *Listeria*
               (g) *Salmonella*
               (h) *Shigella*
               (i) *Yersinia*
            (2) Endocrine hormone-secreting neoplasm
               (a) Gastrinoma
               (b) Pheochromocytomas
               (c) Ganglioneuromas (childhood)
               (d) Medullary thyroid cancer
               (e) Carcinoid
               (f) Mastocytosis
            (3) Dihydroxy bile acids with poor absorption—Crohn's disease, distal small bowel resection (>100 cm resected; Wildt, Norby Rasmussen, Lysgard Madsen & Rumessen, 2003)

(4) Hydroxylated fatty acids that reach the large colon are poorly absorbed and attract water and secretions, worsening diarrhea.
    (a) High-fat diet
    (b) Gallbladder or pancreatic insufficiency
    (c) Abnormal lymphatic function within the GI tract (lymph nodes assist in fat absorption)
(5) Inflammatory mediators (most common etiology of diarrhea with biologic therapies)

3. Exudative diarrhea—Loss of the epithelial layer of the intestinal tract
  a. Pathophysiology—Hydrostatic pressure in the blood vessels and lymphatics will cause water and electrolytes, mucus, protein, and cells to accumulate luminally.
  b. Most common cause of diarrhea with most chemotherapeutic agents.
    (1) Alkylating agents
    (2) Antitumor antibiotics—Dactinomycin, idarubicin, mithramycin, mitoxandrone
    (3) Antimetabolite fluoropyrimidines—The degree of diarrhea in these agents has been linked to elevated blood levels of the drug, and may be abrogated by a schedule change (DiPaolo, 2002)
    (4) Camptothecins
    (5) Platinol derivatives
    (6) Topoisomerase inhibitors—Highest risk
    (7) Arsenic
  c. Local radiation therapy injury to the pelvis, abdomen, lower thorax, and lumbar spine.
  d. Chronic health conditions can lead to protein loss with hypoalbuminemia and hypoglobulinemia.

4. Diarrhea from motility disturbances
  a. Increased peristalsis.
    (1) Hyperkalemia (Taylor, Zwillich, Kaehny, Levi & Popovtzer, 2003)
    (2) Hypermagnesemia
  b. Transient diarrhea is seen after celiac plexus block for pain management. With normal bowel function, adjustment is usually rapid (Chambers, 2003; Okayama et al., 2002).

5. Acute T-cell activation with release of inflammatory mediators (especially tumor necrosis factor; eg, graft-versus-host disease).

III. Patient Management
  A. Assessment
    1. Patient history for risk factors
      a. Normal bowel habits
      b. Diet history—Fluid, fat, caffeine
      c. Familial diseases—Crohn's disease, celiac disease, cystic fibrosis, hyperthyroidism, diabetes mellitus
      d. Medication history
        (1) Antacids
        (2) Antiarrhythmics
        (3) Antihypertensives

        (4) Antimicrobials—Macrolides; tetracycline; second-, third-, and fourth-generation cephalosporins; sulfa drugs

        (5) Theophylline

    e. Use of antidiarrheals and their effectiveness

    f. Activity level—Heavy exercise may induce diarrhea, but light to moderate exercise should not (Simren, 2002)

  2. Patient complaints

    a. Frequency of stool

        (1) More than three to six stools a day, but based on an increase from baseline

        (2) Timing—Early morning bowel is most active, after eating, not in relation to intake

    b. Consistency of stool

        (1) Formed or liquid.

        (2) Color—Light color may indicate lack of bile salts.

        (3) Odor—Possible indication of infection, or inadequate fat metabolism.

        (4) Presence or absence of other constituents (eg, blood [increases gut transit time], pus [indicates infection or inflammation])

    c. Associated symptoms that may help identify the etiology or interventions likely to be effective

        (1) Nausea

        (2) Flushing, feeling hot

        (3) Diaphoresis

        (4) Sense of incontinence

        (5) Abdominal cramping, bloating, or gaseous feeling

    d. The assessment scale—Graded by severity (see Table 23–2 for NCI toxicity grading scale [Cancer Therapeutics Evaluation Program, 1999])

  3. Physical findings

    a. Signs of dehydration if fluid loss has been significant.

    b. Stool characteristics.

    c. Presence of related symptoms.

    d. Presence of fecal impaction—Diarrhea may occur as absorption at the site of obstruction is impaired and only fluid passes the obstructed area. This is especially suspected if acute and severe cramping occurs before small amounts of diarrhea that is unrelated to other risk factors, or in patients at risk for obstruction.

B. Diagnostic Parameters—No specific diagnostic tests validate diarrhea, but several tests may elucidate the etiology.

  1. Stool test for bacteria, fungus, ova, parasites, specific bacterial toxins (eg, *Clostridium difficile*)

  2. Stool test for pus, blood, fat

  3. Stool test for celiac disease that may have been undiagnosed before oncologic diagnosis and therapy— antiendomysial antibody testing, antitransglutaminase (Thomson et al., 2001).

C. Treatment varies and is driven by the etiology and pathophysiologic mechanism as well as provider preference. An overview of guidelines

TABLE 23-2 NCI-CTC Criteria for Grading Severity of Diarrhea

	Grade 0	Grade 1	Grade 2	Grade 3	Grade 4
Diarrhea					
Patients without colostomy	None	Increase of <4 stools/day over pretreatment	Increase of 4–6 stools/day, or nocturnal stools	Increase of ≥7 stools/day or incontinence; or need for parenteral support for dehydration	Physiologic consequences requiring intensive care; or hemodynamic collapse
Patients with a colostomy	None	Mild increase in loose, watery colostomy output compared with pretreatment	Moderate increase in loose, watery colostomy output compared with pretreatment, but not interfering with normal activity	Severe increase in loose, watery colostomy output compared with pretreatment, interfering with normal activity	Physiologic consequences, requiring intensive care; or hemodynamic collapse

Cancer Therapeutics Evaluation Program, 1999.

developed for chemotherapy-induced diarrhea is included in
Figure 23–1.
1. Oral rehydration with fluids is effective in secretory diarrhea where
   absorptive capacity is not impaired. Fluids derived from rice or
   other grains have proven helpful (Field, 2003).
2. Emergency management of diarrhea-associated complications such
   as hypotension or acidosis may be an initial priority.
3. Lifestyle alterations.
   a. Diet
      (1) Increase fiber.
      (2) Avoid caffeine, spicy foods, or other peristaltic stimulants.
      (3) Limit warm fluids that enhance bowel content transit time.
      (4) Some suggest that increasing intake of calcium may assist in
          management of diarrhea for some people (Ukleja, Scolapio
          & Buchman, 2002).
      (5) Nutritional supplements glutamine and growth hormone may
          alleviate some symptoms (Ukleja, Scolapio & Buchman, 2002).
   b. Exercise—Maintain consistent exercise regimen without exten-
      sive heavy exercise.
4. Complementary therapies
   a. Juice of black currant berries
   b. Tea using 1 to 2 tsp leaves in boiling water—Agrimony, bilberry,
      carob, cloves, lady's mantle, meadowsweet, nutmeg, ribwort,
      plantain, purple loosestrife
5. Treat specific etiologies
   a. Replace pancreatic enzymes as needed.
   b. Adjust fat intake if fat intolerant.
   c. Eliminate gluten if congenital or acquired celiac disease is pre-
      sent (Stewart & Southcott, 2002).
   d. Eliminate milk products if lactose intolerance is the problem.
6. Medications (Table 23–3)
7. Probiotics (replacement of normal GI flora) has been helpful in a
   number of patient populations with persistent or chronic diarrhea.
   These must be considered carefully in the patient who may be experiencing neutropenia (Cremonini et al., 2002; Delia et al., 2002; Periti & Tonelli, 2002; Sullivan & Nord, 2002; Wullt, Hagslatt, & Odenholt, 2003).
8. If the patient is receiving supplemental enteral feedings and experiencing persistent diarrhea, specific feeding-related measures may be
   indicated.
   a. If hypoalbuminemia is a potential cause, use an isotonic for-
      mula, initiate at a low rate (20 mL/h), and advance slowly (10
      mL every 12 hours).
   b. If short bowel syndrome is present, use an elemental formula.
   c. If stools are loose but volume is not significant, try a fiber-con-
      taining formula that will absorb excess fluid.
   d. If diarrhea occurs with bolus enteral feeding, administer as con-
      tinuous infusion and advance slowly.
   e. Hyperosmolar formula may need to be diluted with water and
      gradually increased in strength as tolerated or changed to an iso-
      tonic formula.

First Report of Diarrhea to Clinician

Evaluate condition of patient

1. Obtain history of onset and duration of diarrhea.
2. Description of number of stools and stool composition (eg, watery, blood in stool)
3. Assess patient for fever, dizziness, abdominal pain, weakness (ie, rule out risk for sepsis, bowel obstruction, dehydration).
4. Medications profile (ie, to identify any diarrheogenic agents).
5. Dietary profile (ie, to identify diarrhea-enhancing foods).

Management

1. Stop all lactose-containing products, alcohol, and supplements.
2. Drink 8 to 10 large glasses of clear liquids a day (water, Gatorade, broth).
3. Eat frequent small meals (bananas, rice, applesauce, toast, plain pasta).

Treatment

Administer standard dose of loperamide: initial dose 4 mg followed by 2 mg every 4 hours or after every unformed stool.

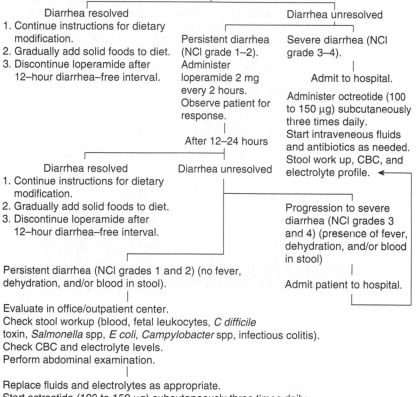

12–24 hours later

Diarrhea resolved
1. Continue instructions for dietary modification.
2. Gradually add solid foods to diet.
3. Discontinue loperamide after 12–hour diarrhea–free interval.

Persistent diarrhea (NCI grade 1–2). Administer loperamide 2 mg every 2 hours. Observe patient for response.

Diarrhea unresolved

Severe diarrhea (NCI grade 3–4).

Admit to hospital.

Administer octreotide (100 to 150 µg) subcutaneously three times daily. Start intravenous fluids and antibiotics as needed. Stool work up, CBC, and electrolyte profile.

After 12–24 hours

Diarrhea resolved
1. Continue instructions for dietary modification.
2. Gradually add solid foods to diet.
3. Discontinue loperamide after 12–hour diarrhea–free interval.

Diarrhea unresolved

Progression to severe diarrhea (NCI grades 3 and 4) (presence of fever, dehydration, and/or blood in stool)

Admit patient to hospital.

Persistent diarrhea (NCI grades 1 and 2) (no fever, dehydration, and/or blood in stool).

Evaluate in office/outpatient center.
Check stool workup (blood, fetal leukocytes, *C difficile* toxin, *Salmonella* spp, *E coli*, *Campylobacter* spp, infectious colitis).
Check CBC and electrolyte levels.
Perform abdominal examination.

Replace fluids and electrolytes as appropriate.
Start octreotide (100 to 150 µg) subcutaneously three times daily.

Figure 23–1. Expert panel's recommended guidelines for the treatment of chemotherapy-induced diarrhea. (Wadler, S., et al. [1998]. Recommended guidelines for the treatment of chemotherapy-induced diarrhea. *Journal of Clinical Oncology, 16*[9], 3169–3178.)

      f. Cold enteral feeding is more likely to produce diarrhea, so administer at room temperature.

D. Nursing Diagnoses

  1. Diarrhea related to medical conditions, cancer or cancer treatment

    a. *Problem:* Diarrhea is caused by multiple cancer and non-cancer-related factors. Diarrhea is uncomfortable, disrupts activities of daily living, and can lead to serious health problems.

    b. *Interventions* will vary with etiologic factor and must, therefore, be individualized.

      (1) Plan small frequent meals that can be more easily digested and produce less dumping syndrome.

      (2) Increase fluid intake to provide fluids necessary to support diarrhea and rehydrate the patient.

      (3) Initially implement a low-residue diet that is high in protein and calories. Proteins are easily digested, causing less irritation than fats or carbohydrates. Calories are needed to replace lost nutrition.

      (4) Administer multivitamin as needed, recognizing that both water-soluble and fat-soluble vitamins are less absorbed with diarrhea. Studies also suggest that additional zinc may be helpful in reducing diarrhea (Meier, Burri & Steuerwald, 2003).

      (5) Limit foods that may be stimulating or irritating, including whole grains, fried or fatty foods, spicy foods, fresh fruits and vegetables, caffeine, carbonated beverages.

      (6) Serve foods at room temperature. Extremely warm or cold foods may stimulate peristalsis.

      (7) Encourage nonpharmacologic/herbal methods of managing diarrhea.

      (8) Probiotics (replacement of normal GI flora; see Treatment section).

      (9) Use medications as prescribed (see Table 23–3).

        (a) For mild diarrhea, give medications prn.

        (b) For severe or uncontrolled diarrhea, give medications at regular intervals around the clock until diarrhea is controlled.

    c. *Desired outcomes*

      (1) Patient reestablishes normal bowel function.

      (2) Patient is able to maintain adequate nutrition.

      (3) Patient is able to maintain or maximize quality of life and activities of daily living.

  2. Fluid volume and electrolyte deficit due to diarrhea

    a. *Problem:* Extremely large volumes of fluid can be lost when a patient has diarrhea. Diarrhea can also cause severe electrolyte disturbances such as hypokalemia and hypocalcemia.

    b. *Interventions*

      (1) Monitor intake, output, and weight that will provide information about fluid losses.

      (2) Monitor orthostatic vital signs and central venous pressure as available to estimate body fluid balance.

      (3) Replenish fluids as needed.

TABLE 23-3 Treatment of Diarrhea

Category	Medications	Action	Comments
Antibiotics	Metronidazole Vancomycin HCl	Treatment of bacterial infections, specifically *Clostridium difficile*	Vancomycin must be given po to treat this type of infection
Anticholinergics/ Antispasmodics	Atropine sulfate Scopolamine Belladonna Donnatal	Reduce gastric secretions and decrease intestinal peristalsis	Use when a patient is having painful cramping
Natural products	Aluminum carbonate (Basogel) Donnagel aluminum hydroxide gel (Amphojel)	Absorbent plus anticholinergic activity	Useful in diarrhea with abdominal cramping
	Bismuth subsalicylate (Pepto-Bismol)	Antisecretory	Relieves abdominal cramping May turn stools black Contains salicylates
	Kaolin and pectin (Kaopectate)	An attapulgite (clay-containing material), which acts as an absorbent	Does not decrease gastric motility
	Psyllium hydrophilic mucilloid (Metamucil)	Absorbent Bulk-forming agent	Encourage additional fluids
Serotonin antagonist	Octreotide acetate (Sandostatin)	Acts like the naturally occurring hormone somatostatin to inhibit growth hormone, insulin, serotonin, and gastrin. Inhibits gallbladder contractility.	Given as a subcutaneous injection Available as a one to three times daily injection or sustained-release monthly injection Injection site pain may be reduced with ice at site before injection

   (a) Oral rehydration with water, rice- or grain-derived fluids, or isotonically balanced and electrolyte-enriched fluids used for diarrhea in children (eg, Pedialyte).

   (b) Avoid high-sugar, caffeinated, or carbonated fluids, or high-fiber fruit juices.

  (4) Monitor serum electrolytes as warranted, depending on the severity of the fluid loss.

   (a) Replace electrolytes orally or intravenously as needed (especially potassium, calcium) if problem is in small bowel, and phosphorus if problem is in large bowel.

   (b) To ascertain type of diarrhea, assess stool osmolarity and electrolytes.

   (c) Assess for neuromuscular and cardiovascular abnormalities indicative of electrolyte disturbances, such as tetany, twitching, cramps, palpitations, irregular pulse.

  (5) Assess albumin levels that will reflect nutrition and, if low, worsen diarrhea.

  (6) If oral rehydration is unsuccessful, consider parenteral hydration and nutrition until the diarrhea has resolved.

  (7) If an etiology has not been determined and diarrhea is persistent, antimicrobial therapy may be considered.

 c. *Desired outcome:* Patient will maintain fluid and electrolyte balance.

 3. High risk for infection related to impaired skin integrity secondary to diarrhea

  a. *Problem:* Frequent and watery stools can cause excoriation of the skin in the perianal area.

  b. *Interventions*

   (1) Clean perianal area with warm soap and water or baby wipes and pat dry after each bowel movement.

   (2) Use ointments (eg, A & D ointment, Desitin, petroleum jelly) as a protective barrier on the skin surrounding the anus.

   (3) Use local anesthetics (Tucks, Nupercainal) as necessary.

   (4) Encourage warm sitz baths after bowel movements and as desired.

   (5) Keep perianal area dry. Encourage wearing absorbent cotton clothing, drying well after toileting, and leaving area exposed to air when possible.

  c. *Desired outcome:* Patient will be free of pain and excoriation in the perianal area.

IV. Discharge Planning and Patient Education

 A. Teach high-risk patients the signs and symptoms of diarrhea requiring medical attention. Some patients may be provided antidiarrheal medications for prn use, and only need report excessive or refractory diarrhea.

 B. Teach patients and significant others to recognize signs and symptoms of dehydration—thirst, poor skin turgor, headache, nausea, dizziness, infrequent urination.

 C. Refer for nutrition counseling if patient's normal diet patterns may contribute to risk of diarrhea.

 D. Plan for follow-up laboratory assessment for electrolyte disturbances in patients with persistent diarrhea.

REFERENCES

Bennett, V., & Engelking, C. (2002). *Current perspectives on cancer treatment-induced diarrhea (CTID)*. Tampa, FL: Moffitt Cancer Center.

Berg, D. T. (2001). Diarrhea. In J. M. Yasko (Ed.), *Nursing management of symptoms associated with chemotherapy* (5th ed., pp. 109–130). West Conshohocken, PA: Meniscus.

Boushey, R. P., & Dackiw, A. P. (2002, August). Carcinoid tumors. *Current Treatment Options in Oncology, 3*(4), 319–326.

Bovee-Oudenhoven, I. M., Lettink-Wissink, M. L., Van Doesburg, W., Witteman, B. J., & Van Der Meer, R. (2003). Diarrhea caused by enterotoxigenic *Escherichia coli* infection of humans is inhibited by dietary calcium. *Gastroenterology, 125*(2), 469–476.

Brown, D. (2001). *New encyclopedia of herbs and their uses*. New York: DK Publishing.

Brown, K. A., Esper, P., Kelleher, L. O., Brace O'Neill, J. E., Polovich, M., & White, J. M. (Eds.). (2001). *Chemotherapy and biotherapy guidelines and recommendations for practice*. Pittsburgh, PA: Oncology Nursing Society.

Campbell, T., Draper, S., Reid, J., & Robinson, L. (2001). The management of constipation in people with advanced cancer. *International Journal of Palliative Nursing, 7*(3), 110–119.

Cancer Therapeutics Evaluation Program. (1999). *Common toxicity criteria* (Version 2.0). Bethesda, MD.

Cardenas, A., & Kelly, C. P. (2002). Celiac sprue. *Seminars in Gastrointestinal Disease, 13*(4), 232–244.

Carroccio, A., Volta, U., Di Prima, L., Petrolini, N., Florena, A. M., Averna, M. R., Montalto, G., & Notarbartolo, A. (2003). Autoimmune enteropathy and colitis in an adult patient. *Digestive Diseases and Sciences, 48*(8), 1600–1606.

Chambers, P. C. (2003). Coeliac plexus block for upper abdominal cancer pain. *British Journal of Nursing, 12*(14), 838–844.

Chey, W. D. (2003). Tegaserod and other serotonergic agents: What is the evidence? *Review of Gastroenterology Disorders, 3*(Suppl. 2), S35-S40.

Cremonini, F., Di Caro, S,, Nista, E. C., Bartolozzi, F., Capelli, G., Gasbarrini, G., & Gasbarrini, A. (2002). Meta-analysis: The effect of probiotic administration on antibiotic-associated diarrhoea. *Alimentary Pharmacology and Therapeutics, 16*(8), 1461–1467.

Curtiss, C. P. (1999). Constipation. In C. H. Yarbro, M. H. Frogge & M. Goodman (Eds.), *Cancer symptom management* (2nd ed., pp. 508–520). Sudbury, MA: Jones & Bartlett.

De Bruyn, G. (2003). Diarrhoea in adults. *Clinical Evidence, 9*, 767–775.

Delia, P., Sansotta, G., Donato, V., Messina, G., Frosina, P., Pergolizzi, S., & De Renzis, C. (2002). Prophylaxis of diarrhoea in patients submitted to radiotherapeutic treatment on pelvic district: Personal experience. *Digestive and Liver Diseases, 34*(Suppl. 2), S84-S86.

Di Carlo, G., & Izzo, A. A. (2003). Cannabinoids for gastrointestinal diseases: Potential therapeutic applications. *Expert Opinion Investigational Drugs, 12*(1), 39–49.

Dickey, W. (2002). Colon neoplasia co-existing with coeliac disease in older patients: Coincidental, probably; important, certainly. *Scandinavian Journal of Gastroenterology, 37*(9), 1054–1056.

DiPaolo, A., Ibrahim, T., Danesi, R., Maltoni, M., Vannozzi, F., Flamini, E., Zoli, W., Amadori, D., & Del Tacca, M. (2002). Relationship between plasma concentrations of 5-fluorouracil and 5-fluoro-5,6-dihydrouracil and toxicity of 5-fluorouracil infusions in cancer patients. *Therapeutic Drug Monitoring, 24*(5), 588–593.

Engelking, C., Stuckey-Marshall, L., & Viele, C. (2002). *Nurse's pocket guide. Assessment and management of cancer-related diarrhea*. New York: Cancer Care.

Field, M. (2003). Intestinal ion transport and the pathophysiology of diarrhea. *Journal of Clinical Investigation, 111*(7), 931–943.

Gossel, T. A. (2002). *Management of constipation in institutionalized, immobilized, and elderly patients*. New York: Power-Pak C.E.

Hawkins, R. A. (2000). Constipation. In D. Camp-Sorrell & R. A. Hawkins (Eds.), *Clinical manual for the oncology advanced practice nurse* (pp. 339–342). Pittsburgh, PA: Oncology Nursing Press.

Held-Warmkessel, J. (2000). Diarrhea. In D. Camp-Sorrell & R. A. Hawkins (Eds.), *Clinical manual for the oncology advanced practice nurse* (pp. 343–350). Pittsburgh, PA: Oncology Nursing Press.

Johnston, S. D., McMillan, S. A., Collins, J. S., Tham, T. C., McDougall, N. I., & Murphy, P. (2003). A comparison of antibodies to tissue transglutaminase with conventional serological tests in the diagnosis of coeliac disease. *European Journal of Gastroenterology and Hepatology, 15*(9), 1001–1004.

Komurcu, S., Nelson, K. A., Walsh, D., Ford, R. B., & Rybicki, L. A. (2002). Gastrointestinal symptoms among inpatients with cancer. *American Journal of Hospice and Palliative Care, 19*(5), 351–355.

Kurz, A., & Sessler, D. I. (2003). Opioid-induced bowel dysfunction: Pathophysiology and potential new therapies. *Drugs, 63*(7), 649–671.

Layer, P., Keller, J., & Lankisch, P. G. (2001). Pancreatic enzyme replacement therapy. *Current Gastroenterology Reports, 3*(2), 101–108.

Lin, E. M., (2001). Constipation. In J. M. Yasko (Ed.), *Nursing management of symptoms associated with chemotherapy* (5th ed., pp. 95–108). West Conshohocken, PA: Meniscus.

Marteau, P., Seksik, P., & Jian, R. (2002). Probiotics and intestinal health effects: A clinical perspective. *British Journal of Nutrition, 88*(Suppl. 1), S51-S57.

Martz, C. M. (1999). Diarrhea. In C. H. Yarbro, M. H. Frogge & M. Goodman (Eds.), *Cancer symptom management* (2nd ed., pp. 522–544). Sudbury, MA: Jones & Bartlett.

McCormick, D. (2002). Carcinoid tumors and syndrome. *Gastroenterology Nursing, 25*(3), 105–111.

McMillan, S. C., & Moody, L. E. (2003). Hospice patient and caregiver congruence in reporting patients' symptom intensity. *Cancer Nursing, 26*(2), 113–118.

McMillan, S. C., & Williams, F. A. (1989). Validity and reliability of the Constipation Assessment Scale. *Cancer Nursing, 12,* 183–188.

Meier, R., Burri, E., & Steuerwald, M. (2003). The role of nutrition in diarrhoea syndromes. *Current Opinions in Clinical Nutrition and Metabolic Care, 6*(5), 563–567.

Nelsen, D. A., Jr. (2002). Gluten-sensitive enteropathy (celiac disease): More common than you think. *American Family Physician, 66*(12), 2259–2266.

Okuyama, M., Shibata, T., Morita, T., Kitada, M., Tukahara, Y., Fukushima, Y., Ikeda, K., Fuzita, J., & Shimano, T. (2002). A comparison of intraoperative celiac plexus block with pharmacological therapy as a treatment for pain of unresectable pancreatic cancer. *Journal of Hepatobiliary and Pancreatic Surgery, 9*(3), 372–375.

Pappagallo, M. (2001). Incidence, prevalence, and management of opioid bowel dysfunction. *American Journal of Surgery, 182*(5A Suppl), 11S-18S.

Pepin, C., & Ladabaum, U. (2002). The yield of lower endoscopy in patients with constipation: Survey of a university hospital, a public county hospital, and a Veterans Administration medical center. *Gastrointestinal Endoscopy, 56*(3), 325–332.

Periti, P., & Tonelli, F. (2002). Biotherapeutics and biotherapy of surgical enteropathies. *Digestive and Liver Disease, 34*(Suppl. 2), S87-S97.

Potter, J. Hami, F., Bryan, T., & Quigley, C. (2003). Symptoms in 400 patients referred to palliative care services: Prevalence and patterns. *Palliative Medicine, 17*(4), 310–314.

Quanta Healthcare Solutions. (2003, June). Chapter 10: Gastroenterology. In *The Medical Algorithms Project,* (Release 11.1). Available: www.medal.org/index/html.

Rivkin, A. (2003). Tegaserod maleate in the treatment of irritable bowel syndrome: A clinical review. *Clinical Therapeutics, 25*(7), 1952–1974.

Robinson, C. B., Fritch, M., Hullett, L., Petersen, M. A., Sikkema, S., Theuninck, L., & Timmer, K. (2000). Development of a protocol to prevent opioid-induced constipation in patients with cancer: A research utilization project. *Clinical Journal of Oncology Nursing, 4*(2), 79–84.

Schumann, C. (2002). Medical, nutritional, and technological properties of lactulose. An update. *European Journal of Nutrition, 41*(Suppl. 1), 117–125.

Simren, M. (2002). Physical activity and the gastrointestinal tract. *European Journal of Gastroenterology and Hepatology, 14*(10), 1053–1056.

Stewart, A. J., & Southcott, B. M. (2002). Coeliac disease following high-dose chemotherapy. *Clinical Oncology (Royal College of Radiologists), 14*(6), 494–496.

Sullivan, A., & Nord, C. E. (2002). The place of probiotics in human intestinal infections. *International Journal of Antimicrobial Agents, 20*(5), 313–319.

Taylor, J. G., Zwillich, C. W., Kaehny, W. D., Levi, M., & Popovtzer, M. M. (2003). Hyperkalemia with concomitant watery diarrhea: An unusual association. *American Journal of Kidney Disease, 42*(2), E9-E12.

Thomson, A. B., Keelan, M., Thiesen, A., Clandinin, M. T., Ropeleski, M., & Wild, G. E. (2001). Small bowel review: Disease of the small intestine. *Digestive Diseases and Sciences, 46*(12), 2555–2566.

Tsavaris, N., Kosmas, C., Vadiaka, M., Zonios, D., Papalambros, E., Papantoniou, N., Margaris, H., Zografos, G., Rokana, S., Retalis, G., & Koufos, C. (2003). Amifostine, in a reduced dose, protects against severe diarrhea associated with weekly fluorouracil and folinic acid chemotherapy in advanced colorectal cancer: A pilot study. *Journal of Pain and Symptom Management, 26*(3), 849–854.

Ukleja, A., Scolapio, J. S., & Buchman, A. L. (2002). Nutritional management of short bowel syndrome. *Seminars in Gastrointestinal Disease, 13*(3), 161–168.

Wadler, S., Benson III, A. B., Engelking, C., Catalano, R., Field, M., Kornblau, S. M., Mitchell, E., Rubin, J., Trotta, P., & Vokes, E. (1998). Recommended guidelines for treatment of chemotherapy-induced diarrhea. *Journal of Clinical Oncology, 16*(9), 3169–3178.

Wanitschke, R., Goerg, K. J., & Loew, D. (2003). Differential therapy of constipation—A review. *International Journal of Clinical Pharmacology and Therapeutics, 41*(1), 14–21.

Wildt, S., Norby Rasmussen, S., Lysgard Madsen, J., & Rumessen, J. J. (2003). Bile acid malabsorption in patients with chronic diarrhoea: Clinical value of SeHCAT test. *Scandinavian Journal of Gastroenterology, 38*(8), 826–830.

Wills, J. C., Trowbridge, B., Disario, J. A., & Fang, J. C. (2003). Percutaneous endoscopic ceostomy for management of refractory constipation in the adult patient. *Gastrointestinal Endoscopy, 57*(3), 423–426.

Wullt, M., Hagslatt, H. L., & Odenholt, I. (2003). Lactobacillus plantarum 299v for the treatment of recurrent *Clostridium difficile*-associated diarrhoea: A double-blind, placebo-controlled trial. *Scandinavian Journal of Infectious Disease, 35*(6–7), 365–367.

Yavuz, M. N., Yavuz, A. A., Aydin, F., Can, G., & Kavgaci, H. (2002). The efficacy of octreotide in the therapy of acute radiation-induced diarrhea: A randomized controlled study. *International Journal of Radiation Oncology, Biology, and Physics, 54*(1), 195–202.

24 Delirium

Karin Taylor
Laura Herald Hoofring

I. Definition: A clinical syndrome that affects the functioning of the brain in which there are disturbances of consciousness with reduced ability to focus, sustain or shift attention; changes in cognition; and the development of a perceptual disturbance not accounted for by a preexisting or developing dementia. Also known as encephalopathy, intensive care unit (ICU) psychosis, sundowning (American Psychiatric Association, 1994).

II. Etiology

    A. Medications and especially polypharmacy (eg, opiates, benzodiazepines, anticholinergics, steroids, antifungals, chemotherapy agents)

    B. Metabolic encephalopathies (eg, hypoxia; electrolyte imbalances; renal, hepatic, pancreatic, pulmonary insufficiencies)

    C. Infections (eg, urinary tract infection [UTI], pneumonia)

    D. Head trauma

    E. Epilepsy

    F. Neoplasms: especially intracranial or central nervous system (CNS) lesions

    G. Vascular disorders

    H. Hematologic disorders

    I. Allergic responses

    J. Withdrawal syndromes

III. Prevalence

    A. Frequently missed or misdiagnosed by doctors and nurses

        1. Lack of knowledge.

        2. Symptoms may be mild and not noticed, especially in hypoalert–hypoactive delirium.

        3. The fluctuation of symptoms and limited time spent with a patient contribute to missing diagnosis.

        4. Many of the symptoms of delirium appear to be symptoms of other disorders such as major depression, mania, and psychosis, and lead to incorrect diagnosis.

    B. Widely reported to frequently occur in the medically ill elderly, cancer patients, patients entering palliative care, the terminally ill, and patients in the ICU.

        1. 25% to 40% of patients with cancer at some point during the illness.

        2. Increases to 85% of cancer patients when terminal (Anderson & Holmes, 1993).

3. Over 80% of ICU patients experience delirium (Ely, Siegel & Inouye, 2001).

C. Patients with delirium have increased medical complications, higher morbidity and mortality rates, and longer lengths of stay.
   1. 17.5 million in-patient days and over $4 billion in Medicare expenditures for elderly patients in the United States (U.S. Bureau of the Census, 1996).

D. It is important that delirium is recognized early in patients.
   1. Protected from the effects of inactivity, fearfulness, and agitation.
   2. Causes are detected and, if possible, eliminated or minimized.

IV. Course
A. May last a few hours, days, weeks, or months.
B. Develops acutely over hours to days and resolves if causes are removed unlike dementia, which evolves slowly over time and there is no disturbance of consciousness.
C. Sleep–wake cycle is disturbed.
D. Often begins and is worse at night.
E. Symptoms tend to wax and wane but become sustained as delirium worsens.

V. Signs and Symptoms
A. Hypoalert–Hypoactive (depending on the severity)
   1. Is often drowsy, has difficulty staying awake, falls asleep during interactions.
   2. Can become stuporous or comatose.
   3. Quiet and withdrawn.
   4. Apathetic.
   5. Lacks spontaneous speech and conversation and, as delirium worsens, may become incoherent or mute.
   6. Becomes disoriented to time → place → person.
   7. Has difficulty finding words or naming objects.
   8. Has poor concentration.
   9. Has difficulty shifting or sustaining attention. May perseverate.
   10. Has impaired memory (especially short term) and recall.
   11. Lacks ability to think abstractly or understand multiple directions.
   12. Impaired written language.

B. Hyperalert–Hyperactive (depending on the severity)
   1. Exhibits same difficulties of sustaining and focusing attention, poor concentration, language disturbances, disorientation, and memory difficulties as seen in hypoalert–hypoactive.
   2. Restless and agitated.
   3. May become aggressive and violent.
   4. Uncooperative, argumentative, and unable to be reasoned with.
   5. Is talkative, but speech is often rapid and disorganized.
   6. Easily distracted.

C. Mixed
   1. Patient fluctuates between periods of being hypoalert–hypoactive to being hyperalert–hyperactive.

D. Perceptual Disturbances and Delusions
   1. More common in hyperalert–hyperactive and mixed delirium.
   2. More likely to occur at night.

3. Illusions—Perception in which actual external stimuli are misinterpreted or misperceived (eg, intravenous [IV] pole appears to be a person standing by the bed).
4. Hallucinations—Perceptions without an actual stimulus (eg, sees/hears dead relative in the room).
   a. Visual most common/auditory second.
   b. Tactile, gustatory, or olfactory also possible.
5. Delusions—Fixed, false, idiosyncratic belief
   a. Tends to be of a persecutory nature (eg, patient believes his nurse is trying to harm him despite reassurance).

E. **Mood**
1. Patients with delirium will often exhibit a wide variety of moods (eg, demoralization, irritability, euphoria, fear, anxiety).
2. They are often scared or frightened because they have difficulty understanding what is happening and may become aggressive.

VI. Assessment

A. Assess and evaluate patient's mental status and clinical presentation carefully on admission and daily or with each outpatient visit looking for signs and symptoms of delirium.
1. Family members are particularly helpful in gathering information about the patient's mental status both recent and past. Especially helpful in elderly and identifying a possible underlying dementia.
2. Must ask questions related to hallucinations, illusions, delusions because patients will often not share information or only tell family members.

B. Screens and Tests
1. Wide variety of tools to screen/assess delirium (eg, Confusion Assessment Scale (CAM), Memorial Delirium Rating Scale, Intensive Care Delirium Rating Scale)
   a. Vary by length and skill level needed to use
2. Mini-Mental Status Exam (MMSE; Box 24–1)
   a. Most widely used screening tool for assessing cognitive impairment
   b. Well-established reliability and validity
   c. Takes only 5 to 10 minutes to administer
   d. Generally scores below 24 show impairment but may be impacted by a person's age, educational level, and language barriers (Folstein, Folstein & McHugh, 1975)

VII. Interventions

A. Once delirium is diagnosed, treatment and interventions should focus on correcting the cause(s), protecting the patient, optimizing the environment, and managing agitation and perceptual disturbances (Slavney, 1998).

B. Correct the Cause(s)
1. Communicate to all team members the presence of the delirium.
2. Assess patient for all possible obvious causes (see II).
3. If patient is agitated, assess for possible causes of agitation (eg, bladder retention, uncontrolled pain, anticholinergic medications).
4. Take steps to alleviate causes.

▼ **BOX 24-1** | **The Mini-Mental Status Examination**

When giving the examination, it is best to minimize all distractions, make sure there is adequate lighting, and make sure patients have corrective devices in place.

Orientation
• What is the date? (year)(season)(date)(day)(month)—5 points
• Where are we? (state)(county)(town)(hospital)(floor)—5 points

Registration
• Name three objects: one second to say each. Ask the patient all three after you have said them. Give one point for each correct answer. Then repeat them until he/she learns all three. Count trials and record. The first repetition determines the score, but, if the patient cannot learn the words after six trials, then recall cannot be meaningfully tested. Maximum score—3 points.

Attention and calculation
• Serial 7s, beginning with 100 and counting backward. One point for each correct; stop after five answers. Alternatively, spell WORLD backward (one point for each letter that is in correct order). Maximum score—5 points.
• Ask for the three objects repeated above. One point for each correct. Maximum score—3 points.
• Show and ask patient to name a pencil and wrist watch—2 points
• Repeat the following, "No ifs, ands, or buts." Allow only one trial—1 point
• Follow a three-stage command, "Take a paper in your right hand, fold it in half, and put it on the floor." Score one point for each task executed. Maximum score—3 points.
• On a blank piece of paper, write "close your eyes" and ask the patient to read and do what it says—1 point
• Give the patient a blank piece of paper and ask him or her to write a sentence. The sentence must contain a noun and verb and be sensible—1 point
• Ask the patient to copy a design (eg, intersecting pentagons). All ten angles must be present, and two must intersect—1 point

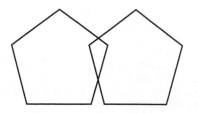

C. Protect the Patient
1. Frequent checks by nursing staff or family if at home.
2. Constant supervision if delirium is causing issues of patient safety (eg, at higher risk for falls, dislodging lines or tubes).
3. Do not leave medications at patient's bedside.
4. Restraints
   a. Only if constant supervision and direction fail to adequately protect the patient or others in their environment.
   b. Use temporarily if unable to protect patient in any other manner.
   c. Use least restrictive device (eg, mitts on hands instead of wrist restraints).
   d. Remove as quickly as able because restraints are frequently agitating.
D. Optimize the Environment
1. Quiet, stable environment.
2. Clock, calendar, name/location of hospital within patient's eyesight.
3. Lighting: Full illumination during day/partial at night.
4. Do not wake at night unless necessary.
5. Use simple concepts and short sentences.
6. Make sure patients understand what has been said.
7. Give explanation before touching the patient.
8. Consistent, familiar caregivers when possible.
9. Encourage caregivers to visit: Bring familiar objects in to have at the bedside.
10. Family education to decrease their anxiety and assist with reporting unusual behavior for the patient.
11. Minimize the number of procedures.
12. Make sure the patient has corrective devices (eg, hearing aids, glasses) in place.
13. Assist patient with activities of daily living (ADL) and have daily routine.
E. Managing Symptoms (agitation and perceptual disturbances/delusions)
1. Haloperidol: Drug of choice in controlling agitation, perceptual disturbances, and delusions
   a. May be given by mouth (PO), intramuscularly (IM), or IV.
   b. Generally, it is best to start with smaller doses if symptoms are mild or the patient is elderly (eg, 0.5 mg to 1 mg).
   c. Larger doses can be given if symptoms more severe.
   d. May respond better to scheduled doses (bid) with prn as necessary.
   e. Dosage and frequency can be decreased as patient improves.
   f. Best to decrease and discontinue daytime doses before nighttime ones because symptoms tend to occur and continue more frequently at night.
   g. Change to oral form if using IM or IV when patient is able to take oral medications.
   h. Side effects may actually be less frequently seen when using IV form of administration.
      (1) Dystonia: Muscle rigidity most often noted in the muscles in the jaw, neck, shoulders, legs.

        (a) Can be treated with Benadryl or Cogentin.

        (b) Both medicines are anticholinergic and may worsen the delirium.

    (2) Akathesia: Restlessness and the inability to sit or lie still. Restlessness temporarily relieved if patient is able to get up and walk.

        (a) Relieved if medicine stopped or dose decreased.

    (3) Parkinsonian: Drooling, tremor, pin rolling, shuffling gait.

2. Other neuroleptics

  a. Risperidone and olanzapine have also been used for the treatment of symptoms.

    (1) Have decreased likelihood of extra-pyramidal symptoms (EPS)

    (2) Can only be given PO, although olanzapine does come in oral disintegrating tablet (ODT) for those patients who have difficulty swallowing

3. Benzodiazepines

  a. Uses

    (1) Treat agitation

    (2) Drug of choice for treating alcohol withdrawal

    (3) Medical contraindications for use of neuroleptics

  b. May actually worsen delirium, especially in the elderly.

  c. Important to carefully assess patient's response after receiving dose to make sure mental status and agitation are not worsened.

  d. Short-acting benzodiazepines (eg, lorazepam, midazolam) are usually better choices than longer-acting ones (eg, diazepam or clonazepam) because they are metabolized and excreted faster than their counterparts.

  d. Doses can be given on scheduled or prn basis.

  e. Benzodiazepines will not treat perceptual disturbances and/or delusions so a neuroleptic should also be used unless contraindicated.

  f. Give small doses and slowly increase as indicated.

REFERENCES

American Psychiatric Association. (1994). *Diagnostic and statistical manual of mental disorders* (4th ed.). Washington, DC: Author.

Anderson, B., & Holmes, W. (1993). Altered mental status: An algorithm for assessment of the delirium in the cancer patient. *Current Issues in Cancer Nursing Practice Updates, 2*(5), 1–10.

Bergeron, N., Dubois, M., Dumont, M., Dial, S., & Skrobik, Y. (2001, April 20). Intensive care delirium screening checklist: Evaluation of a new screening tool. *Intensive Care Medicine*. Available: www.springer-ny.com.

Breitbart, W., Rosenfeld, B., Roth, A., Smith, M. J., Cohen, K., & Passik, S. (1998, February). The Memorial Delirium Assessment Scale. *Journal of Pain and Symptom Management, 15*(2), 73–75.

Ely, E. W., Siegel, M. D., & Inouye, S. (2001). Delirium in the intensive care unit: An under-recognized syndrome of organ dysfunction. *Seminars in Respiratory Critical Care Medicine, 22*(2), 115–126.

Folstein, M. F., Folstein, S. E., & McHugh, P. R. (1975). Mini-Mental State: A practical method for grading the cognitive state of patients for the clinician. *Journal of Psychiatric Research, 12,* 189.

Inouye, S. K., van Dyck, C. H., Alessi, C. A., Balkins, S., Siegal, A. P., & Horwitz, R. I. (1990). Clarifying confusion: The confusion assessment method: A new method for detecting delirium. *Annals of Internal Medicine, 113,* 941–948.

Slavney, P. (1998). *Psychiatric dimensions of medical practice.* Baltimore, MD: The Johns Hopkins University Press.

U. S. Bureau of the Census. (1996). *Statistical abstract of the United States.* Washington, DC: Author.

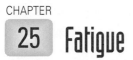

25 Fatigue

Victoria Mock

I. Definition: Cancer-related fatigue is a persistent, subjective sense of tiredness related to cancer or cancer treatment that interferes with usual functioning (Mock et al., 2003).

- **A.** Fatigue is the most commonly reported distressful symptom experienced by cancer patients and may be a side effect of the cancer diagnosis, the treatments, or the pathologic disease process (Ahlberg, Ekman, Gaston-Johansson & Mock, 2003).
- **B.** Fatigue is a subjective experience that is best described by the person experiencing it.

II. Etiology: Multiple interacting physiologic, psychological, and situational factors affect the fatigue experience of cancer patients. Some factors known to contribute to fatigue in patients with cancer are listed below.

- **A.** Malnutrition: Hypermetabolism may result from tumor growth and from competition of normal tissue with tumors for nutrients. Hypermetabolism increases nutrient requirements, whereas malabsorption, anorexia, nausea, or vomiting may lead to inadequate intake of nutrients.
- **B.** Lack of Adequate Sleep and Rest: This may be a consequence of pain, anxiety, depression, or cancer treatments.
- **C.** Altered Body Chemistry: An accumulation of toxic byproducts of cellular destruction may result from radiotherapy, chemotherapy, biotherapy, and tumor growth.
- **D.** Emotional Distress: Emotional responses to the uncertain future that accompanies a cancer diagnosis include anxiety and depression, both of which are characterized by fatigue.
- **E.** Oxygen Deficit: Anemia or alterations in oxygen/carbon dioxide exchange (such as those caused by lobectomy or lung disease) may cause hypoxia and fatigue.
- **F.** Deconditioning: Prolonged inactivity related to pain, nausea, or other symptoms may result in a decrease in functional capacity and tolerance for physical activity.
- **G.** Physiologic Alterations: Infection, pain, hypercalcemia, hypoglycemia, and other side effects of treatment or disease alter energy and stamina.

III. Patient Management
- **A.** Assessment
  1. The following are defining characteristics that may indicate fatigue.
     - **a.** Verbalization of an unremitting and overwhelming lack of energy or need for rest
     - **b.** Inability to maintain usual routines

    c. Perceived need for additional energy to accomplish routine tasks; weakness

    d. Increase in physical complaints

    e. Emotional lability or irritability

    f. Impaired ability to concentrate; lethargy or listlessness

    g. Decreased ability to perform physical and mental work or feeling accident prone

    h. Disinterest in surroundings or introspection

    i. Muscle weakness

2. If fatigue is suspected, a comprehensive physical and emotional assessment of the patient should be performed.

    a. Note pattern of fatigue: intensity, duration, time of occurrence (AM versus PM), degree of distress, and any other factors that seem to precipitate, increase, or alleviate fatigue.

    b. Observe ability to engage in usual activities. Decreases in tolerance for physical activities and impaired ability to concentrate are common characteristics of fatigue.

    c. Assess signs and symptoms of concurrent health problems. Disease-related anemia, dyspnea, pain, or tachycardia may contribute to fatigue.

    d. Evaluate patterns of rest and sleep. Insomnia, lethargy, and irritability may indicate inadequate sleep. Excessive resting may reflect a decreased tolerance for activity.

    e. Observe coping ability. Anxiety, depression, worry, and stress are commonly seen in conjunction with fatigue.

    f. Assess alterations in lifestyle and quality of life, as they have been reported to contribute to fatigue.

B. Diagnostic Parameters

    1. The clinical diagnosis of fatigue is based on the presence of the defining characteristics listed in the Assessment section of this chapter. There are no accepted serum or laboratory tests for fatigue.

    2. A visual analogue scale, similar to that commonly used for clinical assessment of pain, with anchors of "0—No fatigue" to "10—Worst fatigue imaginable," may be used for a quick clinical assessment of fatigue or to monitor fatigue levels. The rating also suggests how debilitating the symptoms are considered by the patient. Consistent ratings of 4 and above should prompt the care provider to perform a comprehensive assessment and plan appropriate interventions (Mock et al., 2003).

C. Treatment: There are no specific medical treatments for fatigue. However, other medical conditions that contribute to fatigue (eg, anemia, depression) should be treated appropriately. Complaints of fatigue may be indicative of problems listed in section II. See nursing interventions below to help manage fatigue.

D. Nursing Diagnosis and Related Interventions and Outcomes (Clark & Lacasse, 1998; Nail, 2002; Ream & Richardson, 1999)

    1. Activity intolerance related to cancer treatment and decreased activity levels

        a. *Problem:* Decrease in tolerance for usual activities occurs as the result of biochemical alterations from tumor pathology and cancer treatments. Symptoms should be assessed for physical and emotional causes that can be corrected or treated. (See section II.) In addition, prolonged periods of decreased activity from fatigue or other symptoms eventually reduce functional capacity and tolerance for physical activity.

  b. *Interventions*

    (1) Regularly assess for fatigue and monitor fatigue levels, especially in response to new cancer treatments or nursing interventions.

    (2) Assist the patient to conserve energy by:

      (a) Identifying energy-depleting factors.

      (b) Developing an activity/rest plan for carrying out priority activities.

      (c) Delegating more fatiguing or less-valued activities.

    (3) Assist the patient to use energy effectively by:

      (a) Scheduling more strenuous or high-priority activities during peak energy periods.

      (b) Pacing activities to prevent overexertion and loss of energy reserves.

      (c) Maintaining activity levels to prevent progressive loss of function.

    (4) Assist the patient to plan and carry out energy restorative activities, such as:

      (a) Eating a well-balanced, nutritious diet.

      (b) Enhancing restful sleep.

      (c) Engaging in stress management/coping activities.

      (d) Participating in a regular exercise program, developed in consultation with a physiatrist or physical therapist, to maintain or improve functional capacity (Mock et al., 2001).

    (5) Administer medications or treatments to relieve discomforts (such as pain or nausea) that exacerbate fatigue or decrease tolerance for activity.

    (6) Evaluate effectiveness of nursing interventions for fatigue by reviewing the patient's self-report and observing for a decrease in defining characteristics.

  c. *Desired outcomes*

    (1) The patient will verbalize a decrease in fatigue.

    (2) The patient will pace activities, balancing rest and exertion.

    (3) The patient will request assistance as needed and delegate tasks as indicated.

    (4) The patient will use energy conservation and restoration techniques.

    (5) The patient will participate in a regular exercise program.

2. Altered nutrition, less than body requirements, related to anorexia, nausea/vomiting, and hypermetabolism

  a. *Problem:* Malnutrition contributes to loss of weight and muscle mass, weakness, delayed wound healing, and insufficient energy for activities of daily living (ADLs; Brown, 2002).

  b. *Interventions:* Follow recommendations in Chapter 28.

  c. *Desired outcomes:* See Chapter 28.

3. Sleep pattern disturbance related to emotional distress and cancer treatment

  a. *Problem:* The anxiety and depression that accompany a cancer diagnosis and treatment may interfere with normal sleep patterns. In addition, some cancer treatments such as steroids, as well as unmanaged symptoms such as pain or nausea, may interrupt sleep.

  b. *Interventions*

  (1) Encourage a regular sleep schedule.

  (2) Provide a quiet environment.

  (3) Plan a warm bath at bedtime.

  (4) Administer mild sedatives, as indicated.

  (5) Administer pain medications or antiemetics, as indicated.

  c. *Desired outcomes*

  (1) The patient will maintain a normal sleep pattern.

  (2) The patient will verbalize adequate rest and sleep.

4. Knowledge deficit related to lack of information about fatigue as a side effect of treatment.

  a. *Problem:* Fatigue is a common side effect of cancer treatments and cancer pathology. Lack of knowledge about fatigue can cause anxiety about the meaning of fatigue and distress related to unmanaged fatigue.

  b. *Interventions*

  (1) Teach patient to expect fatigue.

  (2) Explain fatigue mechanisms.

  (3) Teach patient interventions that may decrease fatigue-related symptoms.

  c. *Desired outcomes*

  (1) The patient will verbalize awareness of fatigue as a possible side effect of treatment.

  (2) The patient will verbalize understanding of fatigue mechanisms.

  (3) The patient will verbalize understanding of interventions that may decrease fatigue-related symptoms.

5. Anxiety related to ineffective individual coping

  a. *Problem:* The situational crisis of a cancer diagnosis, treatment decisions, and the cancer treatments themselves are commonly accompanied by moderate to high anxiety levels. Anxiety is an energy-depleting response and is characterized by acute and chronic fatigue.

  b. *Interventions:* Follow recommendations in Chapter 31.

  c. *Desired outcomes:* See Chapter 31.

E. Discharge Planning and Patient Education

  1. Teach patients who are scheduled to receive surgery, chemotherapy, radiotherapy, or biotherapy about the potential for fatigue before they begin treatment.

  2. Plan for prevention and treatment of fatigue. The success of a plan to manage fatigue depends on the education, understanding, and partnership of both patient and family.

REFERENCES

Ahlberg, K. M., Ekman, T., Gaston-Johansson, F., & Mock, V. (2003). Evaluation and management of cancer-related fatigue: A review. *Lancet, 362,* 640–650.

Brown, J. K. (2002). A systematic review of the evidence on symptom management of cancer-related anorexia and cachexia. *Oncology Nursing Forum, 29*(3), 517–532.

Clark, P. M., & Lacasse, C. (1998). Cancer-related fatigue: Clinical practice issues. *Clinical Journal of Oncology Nursing, 2*(2), 45–53.

Mock, V., Atkinson, A., Barsevick, A., Piper, B., et al. (2003). Cancer-related fatigue: Clinical practice guidelines in oncology. *JNCCN—Journal of the National Comprehensive Cancer Network, 1*(3), 308-331 (see *www.nccn.org*).

Mock, V., Pickett, M., Ropka, M., Lin, E., Stewart, K., Rhodes, V., McDaniel, R., Grimm, P., Krumm, S., & McCorkle, R. (2001). Fatigue and quality of life outcomes of exercise during cancer treatment. *Cancer Practice, 9*(3), 119–127.

Nail, L. (2002). Fatigue in patients with cancer. *Oncology Nursing Forum, 29*(3), 537–544.

Ream, E., & Richardson, A. (1999). From theory to practice: Designing interventions to reduce fatigue in patients with cancer. *Oncology Nursing Forum, 26*(8), 1295–1303.

26 Neuropathies

Susan E. Sartorius-Mergenthaler

I. Definition: Neuropathy is a direct or indirect interruption in the nerve pathway resulting in a disruption or disturbance of the specific nerve function. The loss of function (neuropathy) can occur at any location in the nervous system, and the severity of loss can be either temporary or permanent (Table 26–1).

  A. The nervous system is a complex and intricate matrix of nerve cells, responsible for sensory perception, motor coordination, and autonomic function.

  B. The two subsystems of the nervous system are the central nervous system (CNS) and peripheral nervous system.

  1. The CNS includes the brain and spinal cord. Deficits may include confusion, alteration in gait, and diminished reflexes.

  2. The peripheral nervous system includes the autonomic, parasympathetic, and sympathetic systems. Deficits occur outside the CNS and may include myalgias, paresthesias, motor weakness, and paralytic ileus.

  C. Types of Neuropathy

  1. Mononeuropathy—caused by lesions of the nerve root or peripheral nerve fiber and asymmetric

  2. Polyneuropathy—affecting many nerves and usually bilaterally symmetric

II. Etiology: Cancer patients are particularly vulnerable to neuropathies for a variety of treatment- and disease-related reasons.

  A. Pathophysiologic Mechanisms

  1. Direct injury

  a. Associated with direct destruction or cumulative dose or blood level of neurotoxic substances. In these cases are usually irreversible (eg, cisplatin).

  b. May be further divided into metabolic and toxic

  c. Certain cases are reversible for unexplained reasons (eg, oxaliplatin) (Grothey, 2003)

  d. Reports of neuropathy occurring at lower drug levels may occur when pre-existing neuropathy or high-risk conditions (eg, diabetes mellitus) exist (Chaudhry et al., 2003; Sommer, 2003; Verstappen et al., 2003)

  e. May involve specific nerve fibers (small sensory, large motor) that predict whether symptoms will be sensory, motor, autonomic, or combinations of these

  f. May be related to the solubilizer rather than the medication; for example, paclitaxel is combined with cremophor for solubility

TABLE 26–1 National Cancer Institute Common Toxicity Criteria for Neurotoxicity

Toxicity	Grade 0	Grade 1	Grade 2	Grade 3	Grade 4
Neuropathy, cranial	Absent	—	Present, not interfering with activities of daily living (ADL)	Present, interfering with ADL	Life-threatening, disabling
Neuropathy, motor	Normal	Subjective weakness, but no objective findings	Mild objective weakness, interfering with function, but not interfering with ADL	Objective weakness interfering with ADL	Paralysis
Neuropathy, sensory	Normal	Loss of deep tendon reflexes or paresthesias (including tingling) but not interfering with function	Objective sensory loss or paresthesia (including tingling), interfering with function, but not with ADL	Sensory loss or paresthesia interfering with ADL	Permanent sensory loss that interferes with function

Cancer Therapy Evaluation Program (2003, March 31). Common terminology criteria for adverse events (Version 3.0, DTCD, NCI, NIH, DHHS). Available: http://ctep.cancer.gov.

reasons, and the cremophor is actually thought to be the neurotoxic agent (ten Tije et al., 2003)
   2. Inflammatory- or immune-mediated
      a. Further classified as autoimmune (antibody-induced) or infective
      b. Proposed mechanism for neuropathies from infection, autoimmune, post-transplant, and multiple myeloma or monoclonal gammopathy
      c. More acute pain is experienced in this type of neuropathy
      d. Motor fibers are more affected in this type of neuropathy
      e. This type of neuropathy may be more responsive to plasmapheresis or immunoglobulin (Donofire, 2003; Kiprov & Hoffman, 2003)
   B. Part of nerve involved may lend clues to etiology, predict signs and symptoms, or guide treatment (Bishop, 2000)
      1. Anatomic pattern—nerve root, plexus, nerve or combinations
      2. Fibers involved—motor, or large sensory
      3. Part of nerve involved—neuronal, axonal
      4. Specific pathologic alteration—axonal degeneration, demyelination, conduction block
   C. Treatment Related
      1. Surgery
      2. Chemotherapy and biologic response modifiers (Box 26-1)
      3. Radiation therapy
      4. Blood and marrow transplant (Rabinstein et al., 2003)
   D. Combination Treatment/Disease Related
      1. Tumor impingement on nerves or other structures
      2. Decreased renal function

▼ **BOX 26-1** | **Chemotherapy and Biologic Response Modifiers Associated With Neuropathies**

Peripheral Nervous System	Central Nervous System
Carboplatin	Asparaginase
Cisplatin	Carboplatin
Cytarabine (bolus, high dose)	Cisplatin
Docetaxel	Cytarabine
Etoposide	5-FU
Gemcitabine	Ifosfamide
Interferon alfa	Methotrexate
Paclitaxel	Oxaliplatin
Purine analogues (fludarabine, pentostatin)	Procarbazine
Suramin	Tumor necrosis factor
Velcade	Vinblastine
Vinblastine	Vincristine
Vincristine	Vinorelbine
Vinorelbine	

  3. Decreased hepatic function
  4. Infection or bleeding
  5. Electrolyte abnormalities—hypercalcemia, hypocalcemia, hypokalemia
E. Comorbidity
  1. Diabetes mellitus
  2. Chronic use of alcohol
  3. Atherosclerotic heart disease
  4. Charcot-Marie-Tooth disease (a hereditary neuropathy)
  5. Herpes zoster
  6. Human immunodeficiency virus (HIV) infection—may include multiple viral, inflammatory, and medication mechanisms
  7. Sarcoidosis
  8. Thyroid disorder
D. Concurrent Medications
  1. Steroids
  2. Diuretics
  3. Antiemetics
  4. Antiretrovirals
  5. Aminoglycoside antibiotics
  6. Pain medications
  7. Thalidomide
  8. Antidepressants

III. Patient Management

A. Assessment: All patients receiving neurotoxic agents need to have a baseline neurologic assessment.
  1. *Sensory dysfunction* is characterized as a gradual loss of sensation in the extremities. Patients may also experience pain or hyperesthesia (increased sensitivity). The feet are typically affected more than the hands because longer nerve fibers are usually affected first. Assessment of sensory dysfunction may include evaluation of patient's ability to sense pain, temperature, touch, and vibration. Position sense and fine discrimination may also be tested.
  2. *Motor dysfunction* is evidenced as a decrease in muscle strength and reflexes particularly of the feet, which can interfere with the ability to walk, stand, and maintain balance. Assessment of motor dysfunction may involve evaluation of muscle tone, strength, flexion, and extension as well as overall coordination. Pupil size, shape, equality, and light reflex may also be tested.
  3. *Cerebellar dysfunction* can affect posture, walking, and speech. Cerebellar change is gradual and can be reversible. Indications of cerebellar dysfunction may include nystagmus, changes in speech patterns, alterations in posture or gait, ataxia, decreased mobility, and tremors.
  4. *Cerebral dysfunction* may be manifested as changes in mental status or level of consciousness, loss of memory and ability to concentrate, or change in behavior. Seizures may also occur, especially in the presence of brain tumors or metastasis. Patients should be assessed for any changes in mental status, including disorientation, memory loss, poor abstract thinking, loss of arithmetic ability, changes in emotional affect, and inability to follow commands.

5. *Autonomic nervous system (parasympathetic and sympathetic) dysfunction* may be manifested as a loss of involuntary body functions. Patients should be assessed for loss of bladder and bowel function including adynamic ileus and neurogenic bladder. Changes in vital signs may also be evident.

B. Diagnostic Parameters
   1. Nerve conduction studies may be done to evaluate the etiologic mechanism (eg, inflammatory, demyelinating), degree of nerve loss in the extremities. This may include evaluation for deep tendon reflexes, paresthesia, and sensory perception (Krarup, 2003).
   2. Electromyelogram (EMG) may be performed to further assess the specific pathophysiologic mechanism of nerve injury.
   3. A sequential neurologic examination may be done to monitor for changes in sensation, strength, reflexes, facial palsy, or muscle atrophy.
   4. Mental status evaluations (eg, mini-mental state examination) may be performed to assess for subtle or progressive changes.
   5. Nerve biopsies can detect nerve density and specific injury associated with unique etiologies (eg, HIV infection, herpes zoster infection) (Luciano, Pardo, & McArthur, 2003).
   6. Serum or cerebrospinal fluid antibody levels can detect immunoglobulin M or immunoglobulin G antibodies that may be the cause of some polyneuropathies (eg, myeloma-related) (Kornberger & Pestronk, 2003).

C. Treatment
   1. The prevention and treatment of neuropathies are largely experimental. The level of severity, discomfort, and the patient's pain rating are evaluated. Some groups of patients may receive prophylactic analgesics such as ibuprofen for myalgias and arthralgias, whereas other patients may need short-term opiate support for pain relief.
   2. Once neuropathies have been identified, the only way to prevent further progression or damage is to remove the cause. Most often, the cause is treatment related. A patient receiving potentially neurotoxic treatment will be closely monitored for any changes in neurologic status. If the neuropathy is not life threatening, is not permanently life-altering, is tolerable, and the treatment is effective, often the patient will maintain the treatment plan or therapy dose adjustments will be considered.
   3. The use of amifostine as prophylaxis against peripheral neuropathy associated with cisplatin, paclitaxel, and carboplatin therapy. This agent is not yet licensed by the Food and Drug Administration for this purpose, but ongoing trials have yielded mixed results (Moore et al., 2003; Schucter et al., 2003).
      a. Dose—740 mg/m² IV over 15 minutes
      b. Adverse effects—infusion-related hypotension, nausea, vomiting
      c. Prevention/management of adverse effects—prehydration, antiemetics, rapid infusion, vital sign monitoring
   4. Evidence-based practice standards for treatment of peripheral neuropathy (Smith, Whedon & Bookbinder, 2002)
      a. Level 1—Over-the-counter pain relievers such as acetaminophen 1,300 mg tid or nonsteroidal antiinflammatory agents (eg, ibuprofen 800 mg tid).

b. Level 2—Burning pain is treated with neuroleptics and tricyclic antidepressants, such as amitriptyline, imipramine, nortriptyline 25 to 75 mg at bedtime. Anticonvulsants, such as gabapentin, phenytoin, or carbamazepine, are used for sharp or shooting pain.

c. Level 3—Involves the use of opioid medications for treatment of refractory severe pain.

5. Investigational pharmacologic and nutrient therapies
   a. Nerve growth factors have been used investigationally in treatment of diabetic neuropathy. Quantitative nerve improvement was not demonstrated, but subjective improvement was noted in 45% of 1,019 patients treated (Apfel et al., 2000).
   b. Glutamine 10 mg tid for 4 days starting 24 hours after administration of paclitaxel showed potential benefit in a single small sample size study (Vahdat et al., 2001)
   c. Gabapentin/Neotrofin (AIT-082) is currently in trials (U. S. National Library of Medicine, 2002)

6. Nonpharmacologic therapies
   a. Transcutaneous electrical nerve stimulation (TENS) can block the conduction of pain nerve signals to the brain
   b. Relaxation techniques can facilitate relief of muscle tension associated with pain, and hence reduce pain perceptions.
   c. Exercise may be helpful in reducing pain, maintaining muscular tone, and improving balance in patients with peripheral neuropathy (Richardson, Sandman & Vela, 2001).
   d. Capsaicin cream, created from chili peppers, is thought to decrease levels of substance P (Huebscher, 2000).

D. Nursing Diagnosis and Related Interventions and Outcomes: Close monitoring and careful assessment can assist in early detection of neurologic changes. Interventions can then be implemented to maximize function and comfort.

1. Alterations in comfort related to neuropathic changes
   a. *Problem:* Patients with neuropathies may develop increased sensitivity (hyperesthesia); burning, numbness, and tingling in their fingers and toes; or muscle and joint achiness. Pain is most common in patients who experience sensory complications of neuropathy.
   b. *Interventions:* Follow recommendations in Chapter 30.
   c. *Desired outcome:* The patient's symptoms will be controlled. (Follow recommendations in Chapter 30.)

2. Potential for self-care deficit related to neuropathies
   a. *Problem:* Patients with neuropathies can experience a wide variety of problems that can interfere with their ability to perform normal, self-care activities. They can develop weakness, loss of feeling in their extremities, difficulty walking or standing, and inability to perform fine motor functions, such as buttoning and writing. These and other symptoms can inhibit their ability to care for themselves and perform normal work.
   b. *Interventions*
      (1) Assess the patient's ability to perform normal self-care and work activities. Identify specific areas where assistance may be needed.

(2) Assess the patient's social support network for potential resources.

(3) Encourage the patient to discuss worries and concerns about changes in ability to perform self-care.

(4) Collaborate with other care professionals (eg, physical and occupational therapists) to aid the patient in adaptive techniques for performing activities of daily living (ADL).

c. *Desired outcome:* The patient's ability to perform ADL will be maximized.

3. High risk of injury related to neuropathic changes

a. *Problem:* Sensory and motor dysfunction increases the risk of complications such as falls, burns, cuts, skin breakdown, and loss of muscle strength and joint mobility. Patients experiencing CNS dysfunction are at an increased risk of injury related to falls, seizures, and confusion.

b. *Interventions*

(1) Thoroughly assess the type, degree, and level of neuropathy experienced by the patient.

(2) For patients with sensory deficits, instruct them to use caution when using sharp objects and avoid extremes in temperature. Encourage them to wear shoes, particularly soft-soled shoes that tie.

(3) For patients with muscle weakness or cerebellar dysfunction, evaluate the need for aids to assist with ambulation. Evaluate their environment for safety risks that may increase the chance of falling.

(4) For patients with CNS dysfunction, monitor for mental status changes and seizures. Instruct the caregiver about what to watch for and how to increase the safety of the environment.

(5) For patients who are immobile, provide passive range of motion and perform interventions to decrease the risk of skin breakdown.

c. *Desired outcome:* The patient will avoid safety risks and not be injured.

E. Discharge Planning and Patient Education

1. Educate and provide information to the patient and family about the treatment and potential side effects.

2. Teach patient and family to look for signs and symptoms related to neuropathy and report any changes to the health care provider.

3. A quick screening assessment for symptoms in patients who may not recognize or report specific symptoms includes asking the following questions (Aventis Pharmaceuticals, 2002):

a. Do you have difficulty walking or problems of balance?

b. Do you tend to hug the wall when you walk?

c. Do you drop things?

d. Do you have difficulty buttoning a shirt or blouse?

e. Do you have difficulty closing a zipper?

f. Do you have numbness in your fingers and toes?

g. Do you have a feeling of "pins and needles" or tingling in your fingers and toes?

4. Teach patient and family the self-injury/risk factors associated with neuropathy and the importance of a safe home environment.
5. Refer patient to specialized supportive health care services.
   a. Occupational therapy
   b. Physical therapy
   c. Psychosocial support

REFERENCES

Apfel, S. C., Schwartz, S., Adornato, B. T., et al. (2000). Efficacy and safety of recombinant human nerve growth factor in patients with diabetic polyneuropathy: A randomized trial. *Journal of the American Medical Association, 284,* 2215–2221.

Aventis Pharmaceuticals, Inc. (2002). How do I know if I have peripheral neuropathy? A common side effect of some anticancer treatments. *Patient Information and Weekly Diary.* Bridgewater, NJ: Aventis Pharmaceuticals.

Bishop, R. A. (2002). Approach to the patient with polyneuropathy. *Lippincott's Primary Care Practice, 4*(6), 563–579.

Brown, K. A., Esper, P., Kelleher, L. O., Brace O'Neill, J. E., Polovich, M., & White, J. M. (Eds.). (2001). *Chemotherapy and biotherapy guidelines and recommendations for practice* (pp. 145–148). Pittsburgh, PA: Oncology Nursing Society.

Chaudhry, V., Chaudhry, M., Crawford, T. O., Simmons-O'Brien, E., & Griffin, J. W. (2003). Toxic neuropathy in patients with pre-existing neuropathy. *Neurology, 60*(2), 337–340.

Chaudhry, V., Rowinsky, E. K., Sartorius, S. E., et al. (1994). Peripheral neuropathy from taxol and cisplatin combination chemotherapy: Clinical and electrophysiological studies. *Annals of Neurology, 35,* 304–311.

Decker, G. M. (2002). Glutamine indicated in cancer care? *Clinical Journal of Oncology Nursing, 5.* 112–115.

Donofrio, P. D., (2003). Immunotherapy of idiopathic inflammatory neuropathies. *Muscle and Nerve, 28*(3), 273–292.

Furlong, T. G. (1993). Neurologic complications of immunosuppressive cancer therapy. *Oncology Nursing Forum, 20,* 1337–1352.

Grothey, A. (2003). Oxaliplatin-safety profile: Neurotoxicity. *Seminars in Oncology, 30*(4 Suppl. 15), 5–13.

Huebscher, R. (2000). Peripheral neuropathy: Alternative and complementary options. *Nurse Practitioner Forum, 11,* 73–77.

Kiprov, D. D., Hofmann, J. C. (2003). Plasmapheresis in immunologically mediated polyneuropathies. *Therapeutic Apheresis and Dialysis, 7*(2), 189–196.

Kornberg, A. J., & Pestronk, A. (2003). Antibody-associated polyneuropathy syndromes: Principles and treatment. *Seminars in Neurology, 23*(2), 181–190.

Krarup, C. (2003). An update on electrophysiological studies in neuropathy. *Current Opinion in Neurology, 16*(5), 603–612.

Lubejko, B. J., & Sartorius, S. E. (1993). Nursing considerations in paclitaxel (Taxol) administration. *Seminars in Oncology, 20* (4 Suppl 3), 26–30.

Luciano, C. A., Pardo, C. A., & McArthur, J.C. (2003). Recent developments in the HIV neuropathies. *Current Opinions in Neurology, 16*(3), 403–409.

Marrs, J., & Newton, S. (2003). Updating your peripheral neuropathy "know-how." *Clinical Journal of Oncology Nursing, 7*(3), 299–305.

Moore, D. H., Donnelly, J., McGuide, W. P., et al. (2003). Limited access trial using amifostine for protection against cisplatin- and three-hour paclitaxel-induced neurotoxicity: A phase II study of the Gynecologic Group. *Journal of Clinical Oncology, 21*(22), 4207–4213.

Rabinstein, A. A., Dispenzieri, A., Micallef, I. N., et al. (2003). Acute neuropathies after peripheral blood stem cell and bone marrow transplantation. *Muscle and Nerve, 28*(6), 733–736.

Ricardson, J. K, Sandman, D., & Vela, S. (2001). A focused exercise regimen improves clinical measures of balance in patients with peripheral neuropathy. *Archives of Physical Medicine and Rehabilitation, 82,* 205–209.

Schucter, L. M., Hensley, M. L., Meropol, N. J., et al. (2002). 2002 update of recommendations for the use of chemotherapy and radiotherapy protectants: Clinical practice guidelines of the American Society of Clinical Oncology. *Journal of Clinical Oncology, 20*(12), 2895–2903.

Smith, E. L., Whedon, M. B., & Bookbinder, M. (2002). Quality improvement of painful peripheral neuropathy. *Seminars in Oncology Nursing, 18,* 36–43.

Sommer, C., (2003). Painful neuropathies. *Current Opinion in Neurology, 16,* 623–628.

ten Tije, A. J., Verweij, J., Loos, W. J., & Sparreboom, A. (2003). Pharmacologic effects of formulation vehicles: Implications for cancer chemotherapy. *Clinical Pharmacokinetics, 42*(7), 665–685.

U. S. National Library of Medicine. (2002). Current clinical trials. Available: http://clinicaltrials.gov/ct/gui/action.

Vahdat, J.M., Papadopoulos, K., Lange, D., et al. (2001). Reduction of paclitaxel-induced peripheral neuropathy with glutamine. *Clinical Cancer Research, 7,* 1192–1197.

Verstappen, C. C., Heimans, J. J., Hockman, K., & Postma, T. J. (2003). Neurotoxic complications of chemotherapy in patients with cancer: Clinical signs and optimal management. *Drugs, 64*(15), 1549–1563.

Vital, A. (2001). Paraproteinemic neuropathies. *Brain Pathology, 11*(4), 399–407.

Wilkes, G. M. (1996). Neurological disturbance. In S. L. Groenwald, M. H. Frogge, M. Goodman, & C. H. Yarbro (Eds.), *Cancer symptom management* (pp. 324–355). Boston: Jones & Bartlett.

27 Nausea and Vomiting

Katherina M. Violette

I. Definition: Nausea and vomiting are two of the most common side effects of chemotherapy. They are also among the top concerns and fears for any patient who is about to receive chemotherapy.

    A. Nausea is an uncomfortable wavelike feeling of distress in the epigastrium, abdomen, or in the back of the throat. It results in diminished gastric tone and reduced peristalsis. It is often associated with parasympathetic symptoms such as sweating or hypersalivation. It can be experienced alone or in combination with vomiting.

    B. Vomiting is the forceful expulsion of the contents of the stomach, duodenum, or proximal jejunum through the mouth and nose.

    C. Patterns of Nausea and Vomiting

        1. *Anticipatory nausea or vomiting* is a conditioned or learned response to the previous emetogenic effects of therapy and their associated environmental stimuli. It is characterized by the onset of nausea or vomiting triggered by a sensory stimulus that reminds the person of circumstances in which they experienced nausea or vomiting from true physiologic causes. Anticipatory nausea and vomiting have been associated with all types of cancer therapy. This type of nausea can be significantly reduced if acute and delayed nausea and vomiting are minimized from the onset of therapy.

        2. *Acute nausea or vomiting* occurs within the first 24 hours after therapy. The most common treatment-related cause is chemotherapy.

        3. *Delayed nausea or vomiting* develops at least 24 hours after the administration of therapy. This is most common in patients receiving cisplatin, carboplatin, cyclophosphamide, anthracyclines, high doses of chemotherapy, and radiation therapy. The pathophysiology of delayed nausea and vomiting is poorly understood and research is ongoing.

II. Etiology: Vomiting is a complex process that must involve coordination of input from both the brain and the gastrointestinal (GI) tract. The vomiting center (VC) is located in the lateral reticular formation of the medulla. The VC is stimulated by one of five different afferent pathways or by stimulation from the chemoreceptor trigger zone (CTZ), which is located anterior to the medulla in the fourth ventricle. Several factors may contribute to nausea and vomiting in the cancer patient.

    A. Afferent pathway stimulation from any mechanism causes stimulation of the vomiting center.

        1. *Vagal visceral afferents* are associated with irritation of the GI tract.

        2. *Sympathetic visceral afferents* are stimulated when organs of the chest and abdomen are irritated, obstructed, or ischemic.

   3. *Vestibulocerebellar afferents* involve the labyrinth of the inner ear. This is generally not of concern in chemotherapy-related nausea and vomiting.
   4. *Midbrain afferents* respond during increased intracranial pressure.
   5. *Cerebral cortex and limbic system afferents* respond to stimulation of the senses, including sights, tastes, and odors. This is where classical conditioning is manifested as anticipatory nausea and vomiting.
B. CTZ Stimulation
   1. It is believed that chemotherapy-related vomiting is primarily the result of stimulation of the CTZ. It is thought that metabolites of chemotherapy irritate the CTZ by way of direct blood supply or the exposure to cerebrospinal fluid. Vomiting results when the CTZ stimulates the VC.
   2. Several neurotransmitters have been identified as being present or affecting this area. They include dopamine, serotonin (5-HT), gamma-aminobutyric acid (GABA), histamine, acetylcholine, norepinephrine, prostaglandin, glutamate, corticosteroid, cannabinoid, opiate, and neurokinin-1 (NK1).
   3. Chemotherapy stimulates enterocromaffin cells in the GI tract to release serotonin.
C. Other Factors
   1. Radiation therapy involving the brain, chest, abdomen, or back will cause stimulation of sympathetic visceral afferents and possibly vagal visceral afferents. Total body irradiation often causes nausea and vomiting.
   2. Constipation, GI obstruction, renal dysfunction, or biliary obstruction can all cause nausea and vomiting because of sympathetic and vagal visceral afferents.
   3. Brain metastases can directly or indirectly stimulate midbrain afferents.
   4. Severe anxiety or pain causes stimulation of cerebral cortex afferents that result in nausea or vomiting.
   5. Electrolyte abnormalities, especially hypercalcemia and hyponatremia, can cause nausea and vomiting. The suspected mechanisms are stimulation of vagal visceral afferents or direct effects on the CTZ.
   6. Other medications (eg, opioids, nonsteroidal antiinflammatory agents, salicylate-containing medications).

III. Patient Management
A. Assessment
   1. Nausea
      a. Dizziness is thought to occur in conjunction with nausea because of vagally induced bradycardia and hypotension.
      b. Pallor usually occurs in conjunction with hypotension.
      c. Diaphoresis, abdominal cramping, and hypersalivation coincide with parasympathetic afferent vagal stimulation.
      d. Tachycardia occurs due to the sympathetic stimulation of the stress response when a person is nauseated.
   2. Vomiting
      a. Excessive salivation occurs with vagal visceral afferent stimulation. This often precedes actual vomiting.

  b. Increased heart rate before vomiting and decreased heart rate during vomiting. The stressor of impending vomiting causes tachycardia, but, as vagal stimulation occurs with vomiting, the heart rate decreases.
  c. Decreased blood pressure occurs with bradycardia.
  d. Increased rate and depth of respiration.
  e. Generalized feeling of weakness.
 3. Nausea and vomiting assessment scales and standards
  a. Nausea is a subjective symptom; vomiting is objective.
  b. There are variable and subjective degrees of distress associated with these symptoms.
  c. Self-report is the most important and reliable method of collecting information about nausea and vomiting because it is the amount of distress it induces that may dictate interventions for persistent symptoms.
  d. Nausea and vomiting should be assessed for about 3 days after acute emetogenic therapy and indefinitely in therapies known to cause delayed nausea and vomiting.
  e. The Nausea and Vomiting Symptom Distress Adaptation Scale originally developed by Rhodes, Watson and Johnson is one of the most common instruments used to assess nausea and vomiting (Rhodes, Watson & Johnson, 1984).
  f. Other multisymptom assessment tools may include questions addressing the presence or severity of nausea and vomiting.
 4. Assessment of nausea and vomiting should include evaluation for potential complications.
  a. Electrolyte abnormalities
  b. Dehydration
  c. Anorexia/cachexia
  d. Mallory-Weis tear (esophagus-stomach junction tears with forceful vomiting and causes sudden and severe upper GI bleeding)
  e. Aspiration pneumonia
  f. Pathologic fractures
  g. Dental carries
B. Diagnostic Parameters
 1. There are no specific tests used to diagnose nausea and vomiting.
 2. A general assessment and history of the patient may indicate the occurrence of nausea and vomiting.
  a. Patient's response to nausea or vomiting in other situations, such as pregnancy, flu, car-sickness, or nervousness, may give an indication as to the response to nausea and vomiting during the cancer experience. The presence of four or more of the following specific characteristics with the first chemotherapy treatment has been found to significantly predict subsequent anticipatory nausea development. This anticipatory nausea typically will occur by the fourth cycle of chemotherapy (Morrow, Lindke & Black, 1991).
   (1) Actual presence of nausea or vomiting with first cycle
   (2) Patient report that nausea/vomiting was "moderate, severe, or intolerable"
   (3) <50 years old

      (4) Susceptibility to motion sickness

      (5) Feeling warm or hot all over and/or sweating with first treatment

      (6) Feelings of generalized weakness after first treatment

  b. History of chronic or high alcohol intake has been associated with a lesser occurrence of nausea or vomiting (Markman, 2002).

  c. Females are more likely to experience nausea or vomiting than males (Markman, 2002).

  d. Elderly patients are less likely to experience nausea and vomiting than younger patients (Markman, 2002).

  e. Previous strategies or medications used to treat nausea or vomiting and their success are important to note and incorporate into the patient's treatment plan.

  f. Patient's expectations or anxiety regarding treatment may be related to previous personal and anecdotal experiences, and may include misconceptions regarding the symptom or its management.

  g. The emetogenic potential of the chemotherapeutic agent, at least in part, predicts the risk of its occurrence (Table 27–1). Some chemotherapeutic agents have a higher incidence of nausea and vomiting as a side effect, which would make them more emetogenic.

  h. Concomitant radiation therapy also increases the risk of nausea and vomiting in patients.

C. Treatment: General Guidelines

  1. Nonpharmacologic interventions

    a. Provide a calm, reassuring environment.

    b. Minimize distinctive odors or sights, including perfumes, room deodorizers, and disinfectants. Strong smells can trigger nausea. Smells can also produce a conditional response.

    c. Provide adequate ventilation in the room.

    d. Use distractions, including music or television.

    e. Use relaxation techniques, such as progressive muscle relaxation and guided imagery.

    f. Use hypnosis and systematic desensitization.

    g. Consider aromatherapies thought to help alleviate nausea and vomiting, such as peppermint.

    h. Consider ginger, which has been reported by patients as helpful.

    i. Acupuncture and acupressure may be tried. Mild pressure applied to the inner aspect of the wrist (P-6 acupressure point) can be applied by using acupressure bands.

    j. Encourage light aerobic exercise, as patient tolerates.

    k. Have an emesis basin close at hand, but not in sight.

    l. Offer frequent mouth care.

    m. Plan dietary interventions (see Chapter 28).

      (1) Offer mints or sour candy during chemotherapy administration to help decrease metallic or drug taste.

      (2) Serve foods that are room temperature or colder to minimize the odors that can often make a patient nauseous.

      (3) Avoid fatty or spicy foods.

TABLE 27–1 Emetogenic Potential of Chemotherapeutic Drugs

Level 5(>90%)
  Carmustine >250 mg/m^2
  Cisplatin >50 mg/m^2
  Cyclophosphamide >1,500 mg/m^2
  Dacarbazine
  Mechlorethamine
  Streptozocin

Level 4 (60% to 90%)
  Busulfan >4 mg/d
  Carboplatin
  Carmustine <250 mg/m^2
  Cisplatin <50 mg/m^2
  Cyclophosphamide >750 mg/m^2
    <1,500 mg/m^2
  Cytarabine >1 g/m^2
  Dactinomycin
  Doxorubicin >60 mg/m^2
  Melphalan >50 mg/m^2
  Methotrexate >1,000 mg/m^2
  Procarbazine

Level 3 (30% to 60%)
  Amifostine >500 mg/m^2
  Cyclophosphamide <750 mg/m^2
  Doxorubicin 20 to 59 mg/m^2
  Epirubicin <90 mg/m^2
  Ifosfamide
  Interleukin-2 >12 to 15 million units/m^2
  Irinotecan
  Lomustine
  Methotrexate 250 to 1,000 mg/m^2
  Mitoxantrone <15 mg/m^2
  Topotecan

Level 2 (10 to 30%)
  Capecitabine
  Cytarabine (low dose)
  Docetaxel
  Doxorubicin (liposomal)
  Etoposide
  5-FU <1,000 mg/m^2
  Gemcitabine
  Methotrexate >50 mg/m^2 <250 mg/m^2
  Mitomycin
  Paclitaxel
  Temozolomide

Level 1 (<10%)
  alfa Interferon
  Asparaginase
  Bleomycin
  Chlorambucil (oral)
  Fludarabine
  Hydroxyurea
  Melphalan
  Methotrexate <50 mg/m^2
  Pentostatin
  Rituximab
  Vinblastine
  Vincristine
  Vinorelbine

Adapted from Ettinger, D. E., and The NCCN Antiemesis Panel Members. (2003). Antiemesis Clinical Practice Guideline Version 2. Retrieved on 4/12/03 from www.nccn.org/physician_gls/f_guidelines.html.

(4) Avoid strong-tasting and favorite foods so that these foods will not be associated with nausea or vomiting should either develop.
(5) Encourage clear liquids or broths.
(6) Encourage carbonated beverages.
(7) Avoid caffeinated beverages.
(8) Remove food covers outside of the patient's room.
(9) Try peppermint oil, one or two drops, either in a glass of water or on a gauze pad (when inhaled, it may decrease nausea).
  2. Pharmacologic interventions (Table 27–2 and Figure 27–1)

(*text continues on page 401*)

TABLE 27–2 Pharmacologic Management of Nausea and Vomiting

Category	Action	Medication and Dose	Comments
Antihistamines	Histamine H1 receptor antagonist	Antihistamines	Generally not used alone to treat nausea and vomiting but as an adjunct; may cause sedation, hypotension; prevents or treats extrapyramidal symptoms (EPS) or dystonic reactions; use with caution in patients with hepatic dysfunction.
Benzodiazepines	CNS depressant; sedative—interferes with afferent nerves from cerebral cortex	Lorazepam (Ativan) PO or SL: 0.5–2 mg q4h IV: 0.5–2.0 mg q4h Diazepam (Valium) PO: 2–4 mg q4–6h IV: 2–10 mg q4–6h	May cause sedation, amnesia; use with caution in patients with hepatic or renal dysfunction.
Butrophenones	Dopamine antagonist in the CTZ	Haloperidol (Haldol) PO: 1–2 mg q4h IM/IV: 1–3 mg q4–6h Droperidol (Inapsine) IM: 2–10 mg IV: 0.5–2.0 mg q3–4h	May cause sedation, hypotension, tachycardia, EPS (especially in young patients); prevent or treat EPS with diphenhydramine 25–50 mg PO or IV.
Cannabinoids	Suppresses pathways to VC	Dronabinol (Marinol) PO: 5–10 mg q4h	May cause sedation, dysphoria or disorientation, dry mouth, orthostasis, tachycardia.

Phenothiazines	Dopamine antagonist in CTZ inhibits VC by blocking autonomic afferent impulses by way of vagus nerve	Prochlorperazine (Compazine) PO: 10 mg q4–6h IM/IV: 10 mg q4–6h PR: 25 mg q12h Promethazine (Phenergan) PO: 12.5–25 mg q4–6h IM/IV: 10–25 mg q4–6h PR: 25 mg q4–6h Chlorpromazine (Thorazine) PO: 10–50 mg q4–6h IM/IV: 25–50 mg q4–6h PR: 25–100 mg q4–6h	May cause sedation, orthostasis, dizziness, EPS (more common in young patients); dystonia can occur with chlorpromazine or prochlorperazine; prevent or treat EPS with diphenhydramine 25–50 mg PO or IV.
Serotonin antagonists	5–HT$_3$ antagonist	Ondansetron (Zofran) PO: 8 mg q12h or 16–24 mg qd IV: 8–32 mg Granisetron (Kytril) PO: 2 mg qd, or 1 mg q12h IV: 1.0 mg Dolasetron (Anzemet) PO: 100 mg qd IV: 100 mg	May cause hypotension, headache, constipation; not recommended for delayed nausea/vomiting; use with caution on patients with hepatic dysfunction; efficacy improved when combined with a steroid; prolongation of cardiac conduction intervals has been reported.

(continued)

399

TABLE 27-2 Pharmacologic Management of Nausea and Vomiting (Continued)

Category	Action	Medication and Dose	Comments
Steroids	Unknown; has central and peripheral effect. Synergistic effect when given with serotonin antagonists.	Dexamethasone (Decadron) PO: 10–20 mg q4–6h IV: 4–20 mg q4–6h	May cause insomnia, euphoria/anxiety, hypertension; rapid IV infusion may cause perineal, rectal, or vaginal itching or burning.
Substituted benzamide	Dopamine antagonist in the CTZ; increases GI motility and gastric emptying; high concentrations found to block 5-HT$_3$ receptors.	Metoclopramide (Reglan) PO: 20–40 mg q4–6h IV: 10 mg—up to 2 mg/kg q3–4h	May cause sedation, diarrhea, anxiety or EPS, headache, hypotension; prevent or treat EPS with diphenhydramine 25–50 mg PO or IV.
Neurokinin-1 (NK-1) receptor antagonists	Antagonist of human substance P (neurokinin 1) (NK$_1$) receptors	Aprepitant (Emend) PO: 125 mg PO 60 min before chemotherapy on day 1 then 80 mg PO on days 2 and 3.	New class of agents, which may be effective for acute and/or delayed nausea or vomiting. Initial and repeated courses of highly emetogenic chemotherapy may affect warfarin levels and oral contraceptive efficacy. Use cautiously in patients receiving concomitant medicinal products metabolized by way of the Cyp3A4 pathway, as blood levels of the agents may become elevated or prolonged. (eg, Docetaxel, paclitaxel, vinblastine, ifosfamide, midazolam).

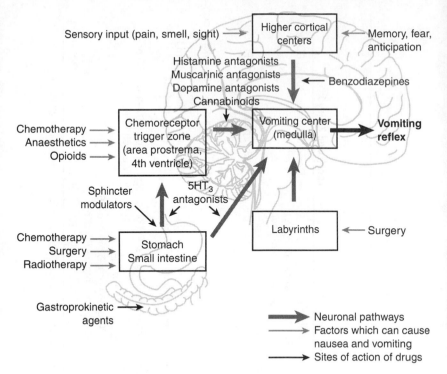

Figure 27–1. Nausea and vomiting pathophysiology. (Reproduced with permisson by CeNeS. Copyright 2002 CeNeS.)

    a. Administer antiemetic therapy to prevent and treat nausea and vomiting.

        (1) Prevention is the primary objective of therapy, but antiemetic agents may also be used to treat breakthrough or refractory nausea and vomiting.

        (2) Use for moderate or highly emetogenic chemotherapy around-the-clock for 24 to 36 hours after conclusion of therapy, instead of on an as-needed basis.

    b. Administer antiemetics 30 minutes before chemotherapy.

    c. Monitor the patient for signs of extrapyramidal side effects (EPS) caused by the antiemetics (Table 27–3). EPS is characterized by a feeling of restlessness or agitation, muscle twitches or tremors, and possible torticollis, which involves spasms and contractions of the muscles of the neck and lower jaw. EPS has a higher incidence of prevalence in the younger patient population (<30 years old; McEvoy, Litvok, Welsh, et al., 2000).

    d. Administer sedatives or anxiolytics to help decrease the patient's anxiety and allow the patient to sleep through the most severe periods of nausea. These agents may also provide an amnesic

TABLE 27-3   Antiemetic Schema

Start before chemotherapy.
Repeat daily for fractionated doses of chemotherapy.

High (Level 3–5) Day 1	Then Day 2–4	N/V Continues	Low (Level 2) Day 1
• Granisetron 2 mg po qd or 1 mg PO bid or I mg IV or • Ondansetron 8 mg PO bid or 16–24 mg PO qd or 8–32 mg IV or • Dolasetron 100 mg PO or IV qd +Dexamethasone 20 mg PO or IV ±Lorazepam 0.5–2 mg PO or IV q4–6h	• Granisetron 2 mg PO qd or 1 mg PO bid/× 3 days or • Ondansetron 8 mg PO bid or 16 mg PO qd/× 3 days or • Dolasetron 100 mg PO qd × 3 days +Dexamethasone 8 mg PO bid × 3 days ±Lorazepam 0.5–2 mg PO q6h	PRN options: Prochlorperazine 10 mg PO or IV q4–6h or 25 mg supp pr q12h Metoclopramide 10–20 mg PO q4–6h ± diphenhydramine 25–50 mg PO q4–6h or 1–2 mg/kg IV q3–4h + diphenhydramine 25–50 mg IV q4h Lorazepam 0.5–2 mg PO or IV q4–6h Haloperidol 1–2 mg PO q4–6h or 1–3 mg IV q4–6h Dronabinol 5 mg/m^2 PO q4h or 1–5 mg IV q4–6h	• Dexamethasone 20 mg PO or IV qd or • Prochlorperazine 10 mg PO or IV q4–6h or • Metoclopramide 1–2 mg/kg IV or 10–20 mg PO q4h +Diphenhydramine 25–50 mg PO or IV q4–6h PRN ±Lorazepam 0.5–1 mg PO or IV q4–6h PRN

Adapted from Ettinger, D. E., and The NCCN Antiemesis Panel Members. (2003). Antiemesis Clinical Practice Guideline Version 2. Retrieved on 4/12/03 from www.nccn.org/physician_gls/f_guidelines.html.

effect that will help the patient to cope with nausea and vomiting during future treatment.

D. Nursing Diagnosis and Related Interventions and Outcomes: The problem of nausea and vomiting in the cancer patient population creates many patient care issues and nursing diagnoses. Most of the nursing diagnoses are closely related, and, therefore, interventions will provide positive outcomes for several diagnoses at the same time. Because of this, a general overview of nursing interventions is provided in the treatment section of this chapter. Specific nursing diagnoses and interventions are listed below.

1. Anxiety, ineffective individual coping, and impaired social interaction related to nausea or vomiting
   a. *Problem:* Nausea or vomiting, whether perceived or actual, produces a tremendous amount of anxiety. This anxiety may interfere with a person's ability to cope. Fear of becoming nauseous or fear of vomiting may cause a person to restrict activities and social interactions, possibly cutting off much needed support and encouragement.
   b. *Interventions*
   (1) See Treatment section (III.C) for general guidelines.
   (2) Obtain a referral to a mental health professional as needed (see Chapter 31).
   (3) Administer sedatives or amnesics as ordered. Patients may need to cope with nausea and vomiting by sleeping.
   (4) Provide take-home antiemetics for delayed or persistent nausea and vomiting.
   (5) Follow up with patients sent home to ensure that they are coping adequately with nausea and vomiting.
   (6) Encourage support of family and friends for patients anxious and fearful about nausea and vomiting.
   c. *Desired outcome:* Patient verbalizes ability to positively cope with unresolved nausea and vomiting.

2. Noncompliance and altered health maintenance related to side effects of treatment
   a. *Problem:* Difficulty with nausea or vomiting may result in missed appointments or refusal of further courses of chemotherapy. Severe nausea or vomiting may cause treatment delays or dose reductions that may adversely affect patient survival.
   b. *Interventions*
   (1) See Treatment section (III.C) for general guidelines.
   (2) Provide personal follow-up for scheduled appointments.
   (3) Refer to mental health professional to assess ability and appropriateness of continuing therapy when concerned that it will affect the patient's willingness to continue therapy.
   c. *Desired outcome:* Treatment continues as planned.

3. Fluid volume deficit related to decreased fluid intake or vomiting
   a. *Problem:* The loss of fluid and electrolytes through vomiting can be significant and can lead to dehydration and electrolyte imbalances. Dehydration can increase the toxicity of nephrotoxic drugs.

    b. *Interventions*
      (1) See Treatment section (III.C) for general guidelines.
      (2) Monitor for metabolic alkalosis (because hydrogen ions and chloride are lost), hypokalemia, hypercalcemia, and hypomagnesemia.
      (3) Record intake and output or have outpatients who are vomiting keep a daily record.
      (4) Record daily weight; note any decrease from patient's baseline normal.
      (5) Record urine specific gravity. When a patient becomes dehydrated, the specific gravity will rise.
      (6) Assess skin turgor and moistness of mucous membranes for signs of dehydration.
      (7) Encourage electrolyte replacement fluids (eg, Pedialyte, sport drinks) if tolerated.
      (8) Provide intravenous (IV) fluids to prevent severe dehydration. The condition of dehydration causes the symptom of nausea independent of other etiologies.
      (9) Replace electrolytes as necessary to maintain normal metabolic balance. Hypokalemia and hypomagnesemia are associated with nausea and vomiting independent of other etiologies.
     (10) Have patients wait 2 hours after vomiting before trying to drink again. Instruct patients to begin with ice or sips of water and work toward other clear liquids, and saving milk products until certain that more nausea and vomiting has ceased.
     (11) Assess orthostatic vital signs if dehydration is suspected.
     (12) Assess central venous pressures if a central line is in place.
    c. *Desired outcomes*
      (1) Normal skin turgor, mucous membrane integrity.
      (2) Adequate urine output and weight maintenance.
      (3) Normal vital signs.
      (4) Verbalization of symptom relief.
  4. Alteration in nutrition, less than body requirements, related to nausea or vomiting
    a. *Problem:* Nutrition is not retained when a patient vomits before complete nutrient digestion. Vomiting also decreases the desire to eat or drink due to a fear of more vomiting. Anticipated nausea or vomiting may result in decreased intake of foods or fluids.
    b. *Interventions*
      (1) See Treatment section (III.C) for general guidelines.
      (2) Encourage patient to take antiemetics 30 minutes before meals.
      (3) Encourage small frequent meals.
      (4) Place patient on calorie count if nutrition is compromised for more than 7 days.
      (5) Weigh patient at least weekly.
      (6) Assess serum protein values for hypoalbuminemia, indicating altered nutrition.

      c. *Desired outcomes*
        (1) Weight maintenance.
        (2) Ability to consume meals without vomiting.
        (3) Normal serum albumin.
  5. Activity intolerance related to inadequate nutrition
      a. *Problem:* Vomiting expends a large amount of energy. Nourishment is not retained, and the desire to eat or drink is diminished for fear of vomiting. Fluid deficits, electrolyte imbalances, and malnutrition related to nausea and vomiting also reduce energy.
      b. *Interventions*
        (1) See Treatment section (III.C) for general guidelines.
        (2) Encourage rest periods as needed.
        (3) Encourage light exercise as tolerated. Has been proven to reduce reported nausea and vomiting in some people (Durak, Harris, & Ceriale, 2001).
        (4) Supplement depleted electrolytes.
        (5) Maintain adequate hydration.
      c. *Desired outcome:* The patient will be able to maintain normal activities of daily living.
E. Discharge Planning and Patient Education
  1. Instruct the patient that nausea and vomiting can be controlled with current medications and interventions.
  2. Explore the patient's view of using complementary therapies to reduce nausea and vomiting, and refer to wellness experts for advice.
  3. Assess the patient's previous experiences and anticipated distress with nausea and vomiting.
  4. Instruct the patient on use and dosage of antiemetics and reportable side effects (see Table 27–2).
  5. Reinforce importance of prophylactic antiemetics.
  6. Refer patients to home care services for fluids, electrolyte replacement, home nutrition, or laboratory test monitoring as needed.

REFERENCES

Bender, C. M., McDaniel, R. W., Murphy-Ende, K., Pickett, M., Rittenberg, C. N., Rogers, M. P., Schneider, S. M., & Schwartz, R. N. (2002). Chemotherapy-induced nausea and vomiting. *Clinical Journal of Oncology Nursing, 6*(2), 94–102.

Brown, K. A., Esper, P., Kelleher, L. O., Brace O'Neill, J. E., Polovich, M., & White, J. M. (Eds.). (2001). *Chemotherapy and biotherapy guidelines and recommendations for practice.* Pittsburgh, PA: Oncology Nursing Society.

Durak, E. P., Harris, J., & Ceriale, S. M. (2001). The effects of exercise on quality of life improvements in cancer survivors: The results of a national survey. *Journal of Exercise Physiology* [on-line journal], *4*(4).

Ettinger, D. E., and The NCCN Antiemesis Panel Members. (2003). Antiemesis Clinical Practice Guideline Version 2. Retrieved on 4/12/03 from www.nccn.org/physician_gls/f_guidelines.html.

Goodman, M. (1997). Risk factors and antiemetic management of chemotherapy-induced nausea and vomiting. *Oncology Nursing Forum, 24*(7), 20–32.

Hogan, C. M., & Grant, M. (1997). Physiologic mechanisms of nausea and vomiting in patients with cancer. *Oncology Nursing Forum, 24*(7), 8–12.

King, C. R. (1997). Nonpharmacologic management of chemotherapy-induced nausea and vomiting. *Oncology Nursing Forum, 24*(7), 41–48.

Markman, M. (2002). Progress in preventing chemotherapy-induced nausea and vomiting. *Cleveland Clinic Journal of Medicine. 69*(8), 609–617.

McEvoy, G., Litvok, K., & Welsh, O. (Eds.). (2000). *American hospital formulary service drug manual* (p. 2677). Bethesda, MD: American Hospital Formulary Service.

Morrow, G. R., Lindke, J., & Black, P. M. (1991). Predicting development of anticipatory nausea in cancer patients: Prospective examination of eight clinical characteristics. *Journal of Consulting Clinical Psychologists, 53*(4), 447–454.

Pisters, K. M. W., & Kris, M. G. (1999). Chemotherapy-induced nausea and vomiting. In R. Pazdur, L. R. Coia, W. J. Moskins & L. D. Wagman (Eds.), *Cancer management. A multidisciplinary approach medical to surgical and radiation oncology* (3rd ed.). Melvill, NY: PRR.

Rittenberg, C. N. (2002). A new class of antiemetic agents on the horizon. *Clinical Journal of Oncology Nursing, 6*(2), 103–104.

Rhodes, V. A. (1997). Criteria for assessment of nausea, vomiting, and retching. *Oncology Nursing Forum, 24*(7), 13–19.

Rhodes V. A., Watson P. M., & Johnson M. H. (1984). Development of reliable and valid measures of nausea and vomiting. *Cancer Nursing, 7*, 33–41.

Wickham, R. (1999). Nausea and vomiting. In C. H. Yorbro, M. H. Frogge & M. Goodman, M. (Eds.), *Cancer symptom management* (pp. 228–263). Sudbury, MA: Jones & Bartlett.

Wickham, R. S. (2001). Nausea and vomiting. In J. M. Yasko (Ed.), *Nursing management of symptoms associated with chemotherapy* (5th ed.). West Conshohocken, PA: Meniscus.

28 Nutritional Problems

Tara Kellner

I. Definition
   A. Nutritional problems in the cancer patient can result from complications of the disease itself or from its treatment.
   B. Problems can be mechanical or biochemical in nature.
   C. If severe, the result is a compromised nutritional state characterized by loss of skeletal muscle protein and fat stores and micronutrient (vitamin, mineral, and trace element) deficiencies.
   D. Up to 50% of patients present at the initial cancer diagnosis with some degree of weight loss.

II. Etiology: The etiology of nutritional problems in the patient with cancer is usually multifactorial.
   A. Systemic and localized effects of the tumor (Box 28–1)
   B. Adverse effects of antineoplastic treatment (Box 28–2)

III. Patient Management
   A. Assessment: The following factors should be considered in the nutritional assessment of the cancer patient to develop an appropriate plan for intervention.
      1. Percentage of weight loss from usual weight evaluated when the patient is euvolemic, with significant loss being 10% or more over 3 months or 5% over 1 month
      2. Factors that impact the patient's ability to eat or absorb nutrients
         a. Dysgeusia—Altered taste sensation.
         b. Mucositis—Inflammation and breakdown of the gastrointestinal (GI) mucosa (see Chapter 29).
         c. Xerostomia—Oral mucosal dryness.
         d. Dysphagia/odynophagia—Difficulty swallowing or pain with swallowing.
         e. Anorexia—Lack of desire to eat.
         f. Nausea/vomiting (see Chapter 27).
         g. Early satiety—Sensation of fullness after ingesting only a small portion of food or fluid
         h. Constipation—Can contribute to fullness and anorexia (see Chapter 23).
         i. Diarrhea—If persistent or painful, can result in decreased intake; if severe, can indicate malabsorption (see Chapter 23).
         j. Extent and location of disease (localized versus metastasized), with GI tract involvement impacting greatest on intake and absorption.

Nutritional Problems Associated with the Presence of Neoplastic Disease

Anorexia with progressive weight loss and undernutrition
Taste changes causing depressed or altered food intake
Alterations in protein, carbohydrate, and fat metabolism
Hypermetabolism
Impaired food intake and malnutrition secondary to bowel obstruction at any level

Malabsorption associated with:
- Deficiency or inactivation of pancreatic enzymes.
- Deficiency or inactivation of bile salts. Failure of food to mix with digestive enzymes (eg, enzymes dilution; pancreaticobilial asynchrony).
- Fistulous bypass of small bowel.
- Infiltration of small bowel or lymphatics and mesentery by malignant cells.
- Blind loop syndrome occurring with depressed gastric secretion or partial upper–small bowel obstruction leading to bacterial overgrowth.
- Malnutrition-induced villous hypoplasia.
- Protein-losing enteropathy with various malignancies

Hormonal abnormalities induced by tumors
- Hypercalcemia induced by increased serum calcitriol and other hormones or by osteoclastic processes.
- Osteomalacia with hypophosphatemia, often associated with depressed serum calcitriol.
- Hypoglycemia of insulin-secreting tumors.
- Hyperglycemia (eg, with islet glucagonoma or somastostatinoma)
- Anemia from chronic blood loss

Electrolyte and fluid problems with:
- Persistent vomiting due to intestinal obstruction or intracranial tumors
- Intestinal fluid losses through fistulas or diarrhea
- Intestinal secretory abnormalities due to hormone-secreting tumors (eg, carcinoid syndrome, Zollinger-Ellison syndrome [gastrinoma], Verner-Morrison syndrome, increased calcitonin of villous adenoma)
- Inappropriate antidiuretic hormone secretion associated with certain tumors (eg, lung carcinomas)
- Hyperadrenalism due to tumor-producing corticotropin or corticosteroid

Miscellaneous organ dysfunction with nutritional implications (eg, intractable gastric ulcers with gastrinomas, Fanconi's syndrome with light chain disease, coma with brain tumors).

Shils, M. E. (1999). Nutrition and diet in cancer. In M. E. Shils, J. A. Olson, M. Shike, & A. C. Ross, *Modern nutrition in health and disease.* Philadelphia: Lippincott Williams & Wilkins.

Nutritional Problems Associated with Anti-Cancer Therapies

Radiation Therapy
- Brain: effects on chemoreceptor zone causes nausea, vomiting
- Oropharyngeal area: destruction of sense of taste, xerostomia, odynophagia, loss of teeth
- Lower neck and mediastinum: esophagitis with dysphagia, fibrosis with esophageal stricture, nausea
- Abdomen and pelvis: acute and chronic bowel damage, diarrhea, malabsorption, stenosis and obstruction, fistulization

Surgical Treatment
- Radical resection of oropharyngeal area: Chewing and swallowing difficulties
- Esophagectomy: Gastric stasis and hypochlorhydria secondary to vagotomy, steatorrhea secondary to vagotomy, diarrhea secondary to vagotomy, early satiety, regurgitation
- Gastrectomy (high subtotal or total): dumping syndrome, malabsorption, achlorhydria and lack of intrinsic factor and R protein, hypoglycemia, early satiety
- Intestinal resection—jejunum: Decreased efficiency of absorption of many nutrients
- Intestinal resection—ileum: vitamin B12 deficiency, bile salt losses with diarrhea or steatorrhea, hyperoxaluria and renal stones, calcium and magnesium depletion, fat and fat-soluble vitamin malabsorption
- Massive bowel resection: life-threatening malabsorption, malnutrition, metabolic acidosis, dehydration
- Ileostomy and colostomy: complications of salt and water balance
- Blind loop syndrome: vitamin B12 malabsorption
- Pancreatectomy: malabsorption (especially fats, fat-soluble vitamins), diabetes mellitus

Drug Treatment
- Corticosteroids: fluid and electrolyte problems, nitrogen and calcium losses, hyperglycemia
- Antimicrobials—dysgeusia, anorexia, nausea, vomiting, diarrhea
- Sex hormone analogues: fluid retention, nausea, anorexia, Megesterol acetate glucocorticoid effects
- Cytotoxic chemotherapy: dysgeusia, mucositis, dysphagia/odynophagia, anorexia, nausea/vomiting, early satiety, constipation, diarrhea

Biologic Therapies
- Tumor necrosis factor (TNF): anorexia, nausea, vomiting, diarrhea, disorders of metabolism
- Interleukin-2: anorexia, dysgeusia, nausea, vomiting, diarrhea, mucositis, azotemia, disorders of metabolism
- Interferon: anorexia, nausea, vomiting, diarrhea, azotemia

Shils, M. E. (1999). Nutrition and diet in cancer. In M. E. Shils, J. A. Olson, M. Shike, & A. C. Ross, *Modern nutrition in health and disease*. Philadelphia: Lippincott Williams & Wilkins.

   k. Type and duration of future antineoplastic therapy and expected severity of GI side effects will determine the type (oral, tube feeding, or intravenous [IV]) of nutritional support required.

   l. Other medical complications the patient may be experiencing and their impact on the GI tract and intake or absorption (eg, history of inflammatory bowel disease, hiatal hernia, steroid-induced ulcer disease, diabetes, hepatic or renal dysfunction).

   m. Psychosocial issues.

     (1) Depression can exacerbate anorexia and result in decreased motivation to adhere to nutritional recommendations.

     (2) Inadequate physical and emotional support at home can impact on a patient's ability to adhere to nutritional recommendations.

     (3) Financial resources can affect the patient's ability to purchase food items and nutritional supplements required.

3. Prognosis must be considered in formulating any nutritional care plan.

   a. If a patient is being actively treated, full nutritional support is indicated.

   b. If prognosis is poor and further antineoplastic treatment is not planned, aggressive nutritional support may not be indicated.

   c. If a patient has a functional GI tract, quality of life may be maintained or improved by enteral tube feeding.

   d. The decision to use parenteral nutrition (PN) in a patient with end-stage disease who does not have a functioning GI tract is a very controversial and emotional issue. PN may not make the patient feel stronger and is not without complications. The pros and cons of this therapy need to be reviewed with the patient and family.

B. Diagnostic Parameters: Many traditional nutritional assessment parameters cannot be used, or must be used cautiously in assessment of this patient population. Abnormalities of traditional nutritional parameters can reflect side effects of the neoplastic treatment or other medical factors.

1. Serum tests

   a. Serum proteins (albumin, transferrin, and prealbumin) are all affected by blood volume and other clinical conditions.

     (1) Dehydration causes overestimation of transferrin and albumin levels, and overhydration gives a false low value.

     (2) Infection and stress decrease albumin levels even in the setting of adequate nutrient intake.

     (3) Hepatic disease may affect protein production.

     (4) Both albumin and transferrin will be lowered with nephrotic syndrome and protein-losing enteropathy.

     (5) The prealbumin level is lowered with infection, stress, and hepatic dysfunction.

   b. Total lymphocyte count is suppressed when antineoplastic therapy causes immunosuppression.

   c. Hemoglobin/hematocrit values can be low from the hematopoietic toxicity of antineoplastic therapy.

2. Other tests

   a. Anthropometrics: Weight and skinfold measurements will both be affected by fluid status. These measurements will not provide pertinent information in the patient with edema or ascites. Skin-fold measurements also reflect activity level and can decrease with inactivity despite adequate nutritional support.

   b. Skin antigen panel will be anergic when the patient is immuno-suppressed from antineoplastic therapy.

   c. Nitrogen balance requires 24-hour urine collection for assessment. Accuracy of results is affected if the specimen is contaminated by feces, or if hepatic or renal dysfunction is present.

C. Patient Management

  1. See Table 28–1 for summary of therapeutic treatment options for nutritional problems.

  2. Nursing diagnoses

    a. Gustatory sensory alteration

      (1) *Problem:* Chemotherapy and radiation therapies damage cells that have rapid turnover rates. This includes the taste buds, resulting in altered taste sensation. The central nervous system (CNS) is also involved in taste sensation, and, therefore, tumor involvement of the cranial nerves can result in dysgeusia. Other contributing factors include certain antibiotics or analgesics, oral infections (eg, thrush), and xerostomia.

      (2) *Interventions*

        (a) Determine type of dysgeusia and provide suggestions to minimize effects.

- If metallic taste, offer hard candy to mask the taste.
- If sweet aversion exists, avoid traditional liquid supplements that are likely to taste sweet, and offer tart flavors (eg, lemon, cranberry).
- If overall sense of taste is decreased (hypogeusia), try salty or spicy foods as tolerated; use herbs to increase flavor; use tart flavors.
- If red meat is unappealing, try alternate protein sources (eg, poultry, fish, eggs, beans, dairy products).
- If nausea or vomiting occurs, avoid spicy foods.
- If mucositis occurs, avoid tart flavors.

        (b) Emphasize good oral hygiene to minimize the bad taste from decaying material and bacterial buildup.

      (3) *Desired outcomes*

        (a) Patient can identify one strategy to help cope with dysgeusia.

        (b) Patient will maintain adequate nutrient intake and weight through diet modification and use of nutritional supplements.

    b. Mucositis and impaired swallowing due to treatment-related mucosal injury

      (1) *Problem:* Because the GI mucosa consists of cells with a rapid turnover rate, chemotherapy and radiation treatment destroy these cells along with the neoplastic cells, causing mucositis. Oral infection can exacerbate the injury and its associated symptoms.

      (2) *Interventions* (see Chapter 29 for specific guidelines)

(Text continues on page 419)

TABLE 28–1 Nutritional Support Options

	Enteral Nutrition	Parenteral Nutrition (Central Access)	Parenteral Nutrition (Peripheral Access)
Indications	• Functional GI tract • Moderate–severe nutrient deficiency	• Nutritional support required >2 weeks or when attempts at enteral feeding have failed • Moderate to severe nutrient deficiency • Complete intestinal obstruction • Short bowel syndrome • High-output intestinal fistulas • Severe intractable diarrhea or emesis • Severe malabsorption • Edematous or friable bowel • After extensive GI surgery or bleed • Severely malnourished or catabolic patient (required to be NPO for 5 days)	• For short-term use (3–5 days) in patients who have limited oral intake because of frequent tests requiring NPO status or during an evaluation of possible obstruction • Short-term bowel dysfunction • Mild–moderate nutrient deficiency
Total caloric	1,800–2,800 calories daily Polymeric formula: Standard: 1 calorie/mL; 80% to 85% water. Concentrated: 1.5–2.0 calorie/mL; 70% to 75% water. (Use for fluid-restricted patients.) Partially hydrolyzed: One or more micronutrients are partially or completely broken down into smaller components. Use is limited; may be required in some	2,000–4,000 calories daily Dextrose 20% to 50% (provides 3.4 calorie/g): Use to meet 50% to 60% of calorie requirements. Maximum recommended infusion rate in adults is 5 mg/kg/min. Lipids (10% solution provides 1.1 calorie/mL; 20% solution provides 2 calorie/mL): Use to meet 30% of calorie requirements. Provides essential fatty acids to prevent deficiency. Use of lipids has been shown	1,400–2,000 calories daily Dextrose 5% to 10% solution is maximum concentration that can be administered peripherally (3–4 L/day). Lipids: Use of lipids is required to reduce overall osmolarity. The maximum concentration that may be administered peripherally is 10% to 20% (500 mL/day) Protein: Protein solutions suitable for peripheral administration are 3% to 4.5% (1–2 L/day) Vitamins: Use standard parenteral multi-

cases of malabsorption

Disease specific: These products are expensive and their efficacy is controversial (ie, hepatic, renal, pulmonary).

Considerations in choosing a formula:

1. Calorie and protein requirements
2. Fluid requirements and restrictions
3. Known patient intolerances (eg, fat)

to decrease elevated hepatic function tests and hepatic steatosis compared to dextrose-only based regimens.

Protein (provides 4 calorie/g): Use standard 4.5% or 8% concentration to meet 10% to 20% calorie requirements. Standard formulas contain essential and nonessential amino acids. Restriction is indicated occasionally (eg, in hepatic encephalopathy or in renal failure if dialysis is not being used).

Vitamins: Use standard parenteral multivitamin preparation; add vitamin K (1 mg/day) separately.

Trace elements: Use standard parenteral preparation, which includes zinc, copper, manganese, chromium, and selenium.

Electrolytes: Average daily recommendations for TPN electrolytes for adults:
Sodium—100 mEq
Potassium—60–120 mEq
Phosphorus—10–22 mmol
Magnesium—8–20 mEq
Calcium—10–15 mEq
Chloride—100 mEq

vitamin preparation; vitamin K (1 mg/day) is usually administered separately or as an intramuscular injection.

Trace minerals: Use standard parenteral preparation, which includes zinc, copper, manganese, chromium, and selenium.

Electrolytes: Concentrations for peripheral administration are different than parenteral. Maximum peripheral infusion rate for potassium—20 mEq/h.

(continued)

TABLE 28–1 Nutritional Support Options *(Continued)*

	Enteral Nutrition	Parenteral Nutrition (Central Access)	Parenteral Nutrition (Peripheral Access)
Site of delivery	Enteral via gastric tube, gastrostomy tube, or jejunal tube	Intravenous via central venous catheter	Intravenous by way of peripheral venous access. At least 20-gauge needle, although 18-gauge or higher is preferred.
Method of delivery	Continuous: Used for any patient and any site of delivery, especially those who have been NPO for more than 1 week. With gastric feedings, once tolerance to continuous infusion has been established, conversion to cyclic or bolus infusion can be attempted if desired. Cyclic: Used for a 12-hour nocturnal infusion, allowing mobility during the day. If administered via gastric or duodenal sites, implement aspiration precautions. Bolus: For patients who wish to take feedings that mimic meals. This is an acceptable method for gastric feedings. The feeding may be administered via a syringe or gravity drip. Prevent potential complications.	Continuous: Parenteral nutrition is generally initiated at a continuous 24-hour infusion rate. Cyclic: Once tolerance to goal rate is established, conversion to a nocturnal, cyclic schedule may be possible. This permits unrestricted ambulation during the day.	Continuous: This method does not provide for nutritional repletion or, in most patients, even nutritional maintenance. Rapid progression to centrally administered PN or oral/tube feeding is recommended.

Special assessment

1. Assess for nausea and vomiting, bloating, and increased abdominal girth, indicating delayed motility and may require decreasing infusion rate or discontinuation of feeding.
2. Assess volume status for dehydration. The estimated daily fluid requirement is 30 mL/kg. Include water used for tube flushing. Overhydration can be monitored via input/output records and rapid weight gain.
3. Assess for diarrhea.
4. Assess for constipation. Adequate fluid intake is essential to aid in prevention. A fiber-containing formula may be beneficial as well.

1. Assess line access site for signs or symptoms of infection at least daily.
2. Use a dedicated line, not breaking integrity. Fluids and tubing should be changed daily due to infection.
3. If the new bag of solution is unavailable, hang dextrose 10%.
4. Monitor for electrolyte imbalances and notify responsible health care professionals (physicians, pharmacists, nutritionists) to alter TPN formulation as needed.
5. Ensure vitamin and mineral replacement.
6. In prolonged therapy, assess for acalculous cholecystitis (elevated bilirubin, RUQ discomfort, jaundice).

1. Assess line access for signs and symptoms of phlebitis or infection.
2. Monitor glucose and electrolytes periodically.
3. After 3–5 days of therapy, consider whether extended support will necessitate another method of nutritional supplementation.

(continued)

415

TABLE 28–1 Nutritional Support Options *(Continued)*

	Enteral Nutrition	Parenteral Nutrition (Central Access)	Parenteral Nutrition (Peripheral Access)
Unique nursing management	1. Minimize risk of aspiration by checking residuals. With continuous feedings, check q4h until tolerance to goal infusion rate is established. New literature suggests that assessing residual volumes may not be reflective of the aspiration risk or intolerance, and the need to hold feeding based upon residual volume alone is not appropriate (McClave & Snider, 2002). This remains a controversial stance, and many still consider the following guidelines as standard of care (McClave et al, 2002). Residuals of 100 mL or less are acceptable and should be reinfused so the patient is not missing needed nutrients. If residuals are high, the infusion rate may be lowered.	1. Prevention of metabolic complications: *Hyperglycemia:* Most common with infection or on corticosteroids. Dextrose content of PN should be decreased. Maximal use of lipids can replace the dextrose calories. Addition of insulin therapy is commonly needed. Electrolyte abnormalities: May be affected by other medications or clinical conditions, and alleviated or exacerbated by parenteral nutrition. *Hypertriglyceridemia:* Reduce lipid calories if level is 400 mg/dL. 2. Avoid overfeeding total calories. 3. Hepatic abnormalities: Avoid overfeeding. Mild, transient elevations can occur in any hepatic function, which peaks within 10–15 days of PN initiation.	1. Use a 20-gauge or larger IV catheter. 2. Maintain a dedicated line for peripheral nutrition. 3. Change IV tubing and fluid daily.

With bolus feedings, check before each feeding and hold for 150 mL or greater. In patients taking oral feeding in addition to tube feeding, evaluation of residuals is not possible.

2. Minimize the risk of aspiration for gastric or duodenal feedings by elevating the head of the bed by at least a 45-degree angle. Stop feedings for 2 hours prior to and during any procedure requiring prolonged supine positioning.

3. Avoid tube clogging by flushing with 30–60 mL water after any medication administration and before and after each bolus or cyclic feeding.

4. Medications should be in liquid form, or pills finely crushed. Time-released pills cannot be crushed and should not be administered via a tube. Check with the pharmacist regarding medication administration via a jejunostomy, because some medications may have special mixing instructions to ensure bioavailability, and the osmolality may be too high for jejunal administration.

4. Cholestasis/cholecystitis: Lack of GI stimulation during the prolonged fasting frequently associated with PN can contribute to gall bladder abnormalities. Some form of oral or tube feeding is encouraged as soon as the patient can tolerate

5. Hypercapnia: Can result from excess dextrose calories. Avoid overfeeding, and replace a portion of the dextrose calories with lipid calories to help decrease carbon dioxide production.

(continued)

TABLE 28–1 Nutritional Support Options (Continued)

	Enteral Nutrition	Parenteral Nutrition (Central Access)	Parenteral Nutrition (Peripheral Access)
	5. Minimize risk of infection and diarrhea by careful handling of formula. For continuous feedings: hang no more than 4 hours worth of formula; do not add new formula to that already hanging; insert feeding administration container with water before adding new formula; refrigerate unused portion of canned formula in a covered container. Discard formula after 24 hours and change feeding administration container and tubing daily.		
Laboratory monitoring	• Daily, progressing to weekly in chronic use: Serum/plasma glucose Metabolic panel: sodium, potassium, chloride, carbon dioxide, blood urea nitrogen, creatinine, phosphate, calcium, magnesium • Several times a week, progressing to every 2–4 weeks in chronic use: Serum nutritional tests—albumin, prealbumin, transferrin Liver function tests Triglycerides	• Twice daily, progressing to weekly in chronic use: Serum/plasma glucose Metabolic panel: sodium, potassium, chloride, carbon dioxide, blood urea nitrogen, creatinine, phosphate, calcium, magnesium • Several times a week, progressing to every 2–4 weeks in chronic use: Serum nutritional tests—albumin, prealbumin, transferrin Liver function tests Triglycerides	• Once to twice daily: Serum/plasma glucose Electrolytes • Baseline only or weekly if continued that long: Metabolic panel: Sodium, potassium, chloride, carbon dioxide, blood urea nitrogen, creatinine, phosphate, calcium, magnesium Serum nutritional tests—albumin, prealbumin, transferrin Liver function tests Triglycerides

(a) Encourage drinking cold or frozen fluids that may be soothing to a sore mouth.

(b) Mechanical soft diet.

(c) Assess presence of the gag reflex prior to allowing to eat in patients with severe enough mucositis to alter their ability to swallow.

(d) Maintain intake diary to encourage the patient to achieve specific fluid and food intake goals, and identify the need to consider supplemental nutrition methods.

(3) *Desired outcomes*

(a) Patient will identify foods easiest to tolerate during mucositis.

(b) Patient will maintain adequate nutrient intake and weight through diet.

c. Xerostomia due to altered mucous membranes

(1) *Problem:* Xerostomia results from altered saliva production, leaving the oral mucosa more susceptible to damage from mechanical and thermal irritants. Without the antimicrobial effect of saliva, the risk of infection is greater. The patient's ability to chew/swallow food and take medications is compromised. Although radiation is the main cause, narcotics and some antiemetics can contribute to oral dryness.

(2) *Interventions* (see Chapter 29 for specific guidelines)

(a) Encourage casseroles and foods topped with sauces and gravies to increase moistness.

(b) Include a beverage with meals to assist swallowing.

(c) Suggest tart foods and beverages to help saliva production, but discourage if mucositis is present.

(d) Offer hard candy and popsicles between meals to provide some relief of dry mouth.

(e) Encourage the patient to avoid plain meat and chicken or dry bread products because they are generally not tolerated.

(f) Offer artificial saliva solutions; however, patient acceptance is variable.

(g) Encourage frequent oral hygiene to promote oral moistness.

(h) Administer amifostine as indicated to prevent xerostomia (see Chapter 29).

(3) *Desired outcomes*

(a) Patient will identify one strategy to relieve oral dryness.

(b) Patient maintains adequate nutrient intake and weight through diet modification and use of nutritional supplements.

d. Altered nutrition, less than body requirements, due to impaired swallowing

(1) *Problem:* Dysphagia/odynophagia can result from radiation damage, infection, or a tumor impinging on the throat or esophagus.

(2) *Interventions* (see Chapter 29)

(a) In severe cases, use a gastrostomy or jejunostomy feeding tube, if indicated. If use of these routes is unsuccessful, PN may be required.

(b) Assess integrity of gag reflex. If compromised, implement aspiration precautions.

(3) *Desired outcomes*

(a) Patient can identify one strategy to cope with dysphagia.

(b) Patient will remain free of aspiration pneumonia.

(c) Patient maintains adequate nutrient intake and weight through diet modification and use of nutritional supplements.

e. Altered nutrition, less than body requirements, due to anorexia

(1) *Problem:* Neoplasms can produce substances that cause loss of appetite (anorexia). Tumor-induced aberrations in glucose and lipid metabolism; all antineoplastic therapies; and many antibiotics, antifungal agents, and narcotics can contribute to anorexia. Other factors involved include impaired organ function (eg, hepatic, renal), pain, fatigue, and depression. Cancer-related anorexia-cachexia affects two thirds of all patients with cancer (Finley, 2000).

(2) *Interventions*

(a) Plan small, frequent meals. It is important not to overwhelm the patient with large portions of food. Because these patients prefer not to eat, it is necessary to present very small quantities of food at one sitting.

(b) Redefine meals. A bowl of cereal or an ounce of cheese with several crackers can be a meal.

(c) Use liquid nutritional supplements to maximize calorie and protein intake. Many patients find them easiest to take by drinking 1 to 2 ounces per hour.

(d) Help the patient to make every bite count. Excess use of water and other calorie-free beverages should be avoided. Discourage reduced calorie or diet products.

(e) Help the patient to plan meals. Some patients find it helpful to set up a time schedule for meals and use an alarm clock to remind them when to eat.

(f) Encourage the patient to always have snacks available, especially when traveling, so no meals are missed.

(g) Consider including an alcoholic beverage with a meal to act as an appetite stimulant. Consult the physician for approval.

(h) Use an appetite stimulant to help in some cases.

(i) Megestrol acetate (Megace): Administered 400 mg bid. Adverse effects: Hypertension, thrombotic disorders, diarrhea, impotence, hyperglycemia, fluid retention, rash.

(ii) Dronabinol (Marinol): Administered beginning with 2.5 mg before lunch and dinner, or, if intolerant, a single 2.5-mg dose may be taken at bedtime. Adverse effects: CNS symptoms (dizziness, feeling high, somnolence, confusion). Dose can be reduced to qd before bed to relieve these symptoms. Dronabinol is contraindicated in patients who are sensitive to sesame oil or any cannabinoid (Jatoi et al., 2002).

    (i) Agents under investigation: Dexamethasone (Decadron), infliximab (Remicade), thalidomide (Thalomid), adenosine triphosphate (Agteresch et al, 2002; Jatoi & Loprinzi, 2001a; Wilkes, Ingwersen & Barton-Burke, 2002).

(3) *Desired outcome:* Patient maintains adequate nutrient intake and weight through diet modification and use of nutritional supplements.

f. Altered nutrition, less than body requirements, due to nausea and vomiting

    (1) *Problem:* The mechanisms of chemotherapy- and radiation-induced nausea or vomiting involve the vomiting center and chemoreceptor trigger zones of the brain, but other factors may also contribute to the problem (see Chapter 27).

    (2) *Interventions*

        (a) Administer antiemetics. Use of regularly scheduled antiemetics is essential for persistent nausea. Additional medications should be available on a prn basis for breakthrough symptoms.

        (b) If there is an anticipatory or anxiety component to the nausea or vomiting, teach relaxation techniques that may be helpful.

        (c) Discourage intake until nausea is well controlled. This will prevent patients from forming strong food aversions.

        (d) Initiate intake with a clear liquid diet and advance, as tolerated, to bland, solid foods.

        (e) Offer small food portions frequently. In many cases, it is not what has been eaten that causes vomiting, but that too much has been eaten at one sitting.

        (f) Explain to the patient that fried, greasy, and spicy foods are not generally tolerated.

        (g) Encourage cold food items because they are better tolerated than hot foods; the aroma of hot foods can exacerbate nausea.

        (h) Encourage the patient to sip beverages slowly between meals to avoid bloating with meals, which can contribute to nausea and vomiting. Discourage the patient from reclining for at least 1 hour after a meal.

        (i) Use enteral tube (jejunostomy) or parenteral feeding if the patient is unable to maintain adequate oral intake or experiences weight loss.

    (3) *Desired outcomes*

        (a) Nausea and vomiting will be controlled with pharmacologic and nonpharmacologic interventions.

        (b) Patient will maintain adequate nutrient intake and weight through diet modification.

g. Altered nutrition, less than requirements, due to early satiety

    (1) *Problem:* The feeling of premature satiety can occur with delayed gastric emptying. An esophagectomy or partial gastrectomy can cause early satiety because the new gastric pouch is smaller. If the vagus nerve is severed, gastric atony with delayed emptying results. In some patients, atrophic changes have been noted in the small intestine mucosa and may result in increased transit time and delayed digestion. Delayed digestion may provide subsequent continuous stimuli to the satiety center.

(2) *Interventions*

(a) Use Reglan (metoclopramide 10 to 20 mg) three times daily to increase gastric motility so food doesn't remain in the stomach for an extended time.

(b) Plan small, frequent meals.

(c) Help the patient to make every bite count. Discourage reduced-calorie or diet products.

(d) Discourage large beverages with meals because this will hasten early satiety.

(3) *Desired outcome:* Patient will maintain adequate nutrient intake and diet through modification and use of nutritional supplements.

h. Constipation

(1) *Problem:* Constipation can result from narcotics and certain chemotherapeutic agents (eg, vincristine). Inadequate fluid intake and inactivity can compound this problem. Constipation, when accompanied by abdominal pain and distention, can significantly limit intake (see Chapter 23).

(2) *Interventions*

(a) Recommend increased fiber intake. Gradual increase is advised to avoid flatulence and cramping, which can be associated with high-fiber intake. High-fiber suggestions include whole grain breads and cereals, beans, legumes, nuts, and fresh fruits and vegetables.

(b) Maintain adequate fluid intake. Most adults require approximately 2 L daily. Some people find use of hot beverages most effective.

(c) Use Metamucil, Citrucel, or other bulk fiber agents.

(3) *Desired outcomes*

(a) Patient will maintain adequate nutrient intake and diet through diet modification.

(b) Patient will resume a normal bowel pattern.

i. Diarrhea

(1) *Problem:* Diarrhea can result from GI mucosal damage that occurs with chemotherapy and radiation. Other potential contributing factors include antibiotics, biotherapy, intestinal infection, and any neoplasm or surgery that causes malabsorption. Diarrhea, when accompanied by abdominal pain and cramping, can significantly impact intake (see Chapter 23).

(2) *Interventions*

(a) Discourage fresh fruits and vegetables, beans, legumes, and nuts. Fruit juice intake should be limited. Use of fruit drinks or punch is acceptable.

(b) In some cases, restrict foods high in fat because they may exacerbate symptoms.

(c) If the patient is lactose intolerant, use lactose-reduced dairy products.

(d) Maintain adequate fluid intake to avoid dehydration. Most adults require approximately 2 L daily. Limit caffeinated beverages because these tend to dehydrate and, in some cases, increase GI motility.

(e) If severe, restrict patient to a clear liquid diet for 24 hours. In some cases, NPO with use of IV fluids and PN may be required.

(f) For specific interventions (including those related to enteral feedings), consult Chapter 23.

(3) *Desired outcomes*

(a) Patient will modify diet to minimize contribution of oral intake to diarrhea while maintaining weight.

(b) Patient will resume a normal bowel pattern.

j. Weight loss due to altered nutrition, less than body requirements

(1) *Problem:* Weight loss can result from multiple tumor- and treatment-related side effects.

(2) *Interventions*

(a) If a patient continues to lose weight, encourage consultation with a dietitian for individual counseling. Many patients require individualized diet instruction to adjust their diet to meet nutritional requirements. A summary comparison of nutritional supplementation method is included in Table 28–1.

• Determine estimated requirements (Box 28–3).

  i. Energy (calorie) requirements

  ii. Protein requirements

  iii. If a patient is unable to meet estimated requirements by way of meals and liquid nutritional sup-

---

▼ **BOX 28-3 | Estimated Nutrient Requirement Equations**

Harris-Benedict Equation (estimates basal energy expenditure [BEE])

Male: 66.5 + (13.75 × weight in kg) + (5.00 × height in cm) −
(6.775 × age in years)

Female: 655.1 + (9.563 × weight in kg) + (1.850 × height in cm) −
(4.676 × age in years)

Total Energy Requirements

Weight maintenance: BEE × 1.2–1.3

Weight gain (if persistently febrile or on steroids): BEE × 1.5

Protein Requirements

Maintenance: kg × 1

Anabolic/Repletion: kg × 1.5

Harris, J., & Benedict, F. (1919). A biometric study of basal metabolism in man. Washington, DC; Carnegie Institute of Washington.
www-users.med.cornell.edu/~spon/picu/calc/beecalc.htm, accessed 1/28/04.

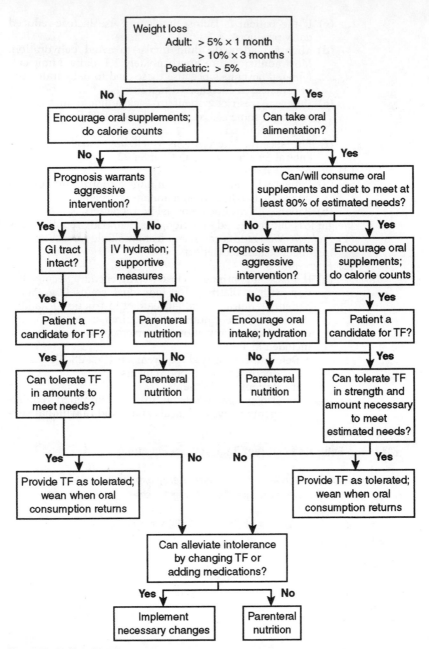

Figure 28–1. Algorithm for nutritional support of the oncology patient. (Adapted from Alexander, H. R. & Norton, J. A. [2001]. Nutritional supportive care. In P. A. Pizzo & D. G. Poplack [Eds.], *Principles and practice of pediatric oncology* [4th ed.]. Philadelphia: Lippincott Williams & Wilkins.

plements, evaluate alternative means of nutritional support. As noted in the algorithm in Figure 28-1, prognosis must be considered when planning nutritional support. Aggressive nutritional support in the absence of aggressive treatment of the neoplasm is not routinely recommended.

• Consider nutritional additives or special formulations—arginine, glutamine, omega-3 fatty acids, nucleotides (Kelly & Wischmeyer, 2003; Sargent, Murphy & Shelton, 2002; Gershwin, German, & Keen, 2000).

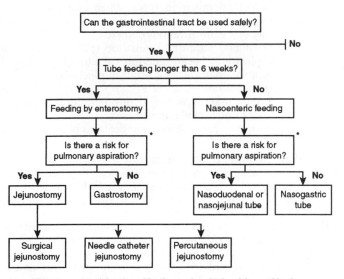

* In addition to expected duration of feeding and aspiration risk, consider the following factors to determine feeding site: (1) Presence of intractable emesis, or future therapy anticipated to be highly emetogenic, would preclude feeding into the stomach (use of jejunostomy feeding would likely be preferable). (2) Impaired gastric motility may preclude feeding into the stomach. (3) Location of any obstructions (e.g., esophageal obstruction would require use of gastrostomy or jejunostomy; gastric or upper intestinal obstruction would require use of jejunostomy). (4) Whether the patient is a surgical candidate (if not, patient would require percutaneous or fluoroscopic placement).

Figure 28–2. Decision-making algorithm for selection of enteral feeding sites. (Adapted from Ideno, K. [1993]. Enteral nutrition. In Gottschlich, M. M., et al. [Eds.]. *Nutritional support dietetics: Core curriculum* [2nd ed.]. Silver Spring, MD: American Society for Parenteral and Enteral Nutrition. Includes information from Schattner, M. [2003]. Enteral nutrition support of the patient with cancer: Route and role. *Journal of Clinical Gastroenterology, 36*[4], 297–302; Shils, M.E. [1999]. Nutrition and diet in cancer. In M.E. Shils, et al., *Modern nutrition in health and disease*. Philadelphia: Lippincott Williams & Wilkins: Shike, M., & Bloch, A. S. [1998]. Enteral nutrition. *Gastrointestinal Endoscopy Clinics of North America, 8*[3]; Guenter, P. [2001]. *Tube feeding: practical guidelines and nursing protocols*. Gaithersburg, MD: Aspen; Haddad, R. Y., & Thomas, D. R. [2002]. Enteral nutrition and enteral tube feeding: Review of the evidence. *Clinics in Geriatric Medicine, 18*[14], 867–881.)

- Growth hormone supplementation in the face of severe malnutrition has been proposed as beneficial. Research studies have been inconclusive. Due to its expense and uncertain benefit, its use should be reserved for people with unresolvable complications related to malnutrition (Sargent, Murphy & Shelton, 2002; Takala et al., 1999; Trujillo, Robinson & Jacobs, 2001).

(b) Enteral tube feedings: If the GI tract is functional, use enteral tube feedings as the route of nutritional support (see algorithm for selection of enteral feeding sites in Figure 28–2; Haddad & Thomas, 2002; Schattner, 2003).

(c) Parenteral nutrition (PN): When attempts with enteral feedings fail or if the GI tract is not functional, use PN by way of a central venous catheter.

(d) Peripheral parenteral nutrition (PPN): PPN has limited applications because peripheral administration of hyperosmolar solutions can result in phlebitis.

(3) *Desired outcomes*

(a) Patient maintains weight through diet modification and use of nutritional supplements.

(b) Patient does not have complications of enteral/parenteral support.

IV. Discharge Planning and Patient Education

A. Counsel the patient regarding diet modifications required for coping with the multiple side effects of malignancy and therapy to attain and maintain adequate oral intake. Arrange for postdischarge nutrition follow-up with a dietitian, if available.

B. Counsel the patient on proper use of medications (ie, antiemetics, analgesics) to minimize treatment side effects affecting intake.

C. If the patient is receiving an enteral tube or parenteral tube, contact a home care company to provide feeding solutions, supplies, and feeding administration instruction. The patient's insurance coverage needs to be investigated because policies differ widely in their coverage and often stipulate use of specific home care companies. If these feedings are for supplemental or temporary use, the patient should understand the goal of oral intake required to discontinue the feedings.

D. Educate the patient regarding the need to contact the doctor if oral intake is insufficient or weight loss occurs.

REFERENCES

Agteresch, H. J., Rietveld, T., Kerkhofs, L. G. M., et al. (2002). Beneficial effects of adenosine triphosphate on nutritional status in advanced lung cancer patients: A randomized clinical trial. *Journal of Clinical Oncology, 20,* 371–378.

Alexander, H. R. (2001). Nutritional support. In P. A. Pizzo & D. G. Poplack (Eds.). *Principles and practice of pediatric oncology* (4th ed.). Philadelphia: Lippincott Williams & Wilkins

Alpers, D. H. (2002). *Manual of nutritional therapeutics* (4th ed.). Philadelphia: Lippincott Williams & Wilkins.

DeWitt, R. C., & Kudsk, K. A. (1998). Enteral nutrition. *Gastroenterology Clinics of North America, 27*(2), 371–386.

Finley, J. P. (2000). Management of cancer cachexia. *AACN Clinical Issues, 11*(4), 590–603.

Gershwin, J., German J. B., & Keen, C. L. (2000). *Nutrition and immunology: Principles and practice.* Totowa, NJ: Humana Press.

Gottschlich, M. M., Matarese, L. E., & Shronts, E. P. (Eds.). (1993). *Nutrition support dietetics: Core curriculum.* Silver Spring, MD: American Society for Parenteral & Enteral Nutrition.

Guenter, P. (2001). *Tube feeding: Practical guidelines and nursing protocols.* Gaithersburg, MD: Aspen.

Haddad, R. Y., & Thomas, D. R. (2002). Enteral nutrition and enteral tube feeding. Review of the evidence. *Clinical Geriatric Medicine, 18*(4), 867–881.

Harris, J., & Benedict, F. (1919). *A biometric study of basal metabolism in man.* Washington, DC; Carnegie Institute of Washington.

Heber, D., Blackburn, G. L., & Go, V. L. W. (1999). *Nutritional oncology.* San Diego, CA: Academic Press.

Ideno, K. (1993). Enteral nutrition. In M. M. Gottschlich et al. (Eds.), *Nutritional support dietetics: Core curriculum* (2nd ed.). Silver Spring, MD: American Society for Parenteral and Enteral Nutrition.

Jatoi, A., & Loprinzi, C. L. (2001a). An update: Cancer-associated anorexia as a treatment target. *Current Opinion in Clinical Nutrition and Metabolic Care, 4*(3), 179–182.

_____. (2001b). Current management of cancer-associated anorexia and weight loss. *Oncology, 15*(4), 497–502, 508, discussion 508–510.

Jatoi, A., Windschitl, H. E., Loprinzi, C. L., et al. (2002). Dronabinol versus megestrol acetate versus combination therapy for cancer-associated anorexia: A north central cancer treatment group study. *Journal of Clinical Oncology, 20*(2), 567–573.

Katz, D. L. (2000). *Nutrition in clinical practice.* Philadelphia: Lippincott Williams & Wilkins.

Kelly, D., & Wischmeyer, P. E. (2003). Role of L-glutamine in critical illness: New insights. *Current Opinion in Clinical Nutrition and Metabolic Care, 6*(2), 217–222.

McClave, S.A., DeMeo, M.T., DeLegge, M.H., et al. (2002). North American Summit on Aspiration in the Critically Ill Patient: Consensus statement. *Journal of Parenteral and Enteral Nutrition, 26*(6 Suppl.), S80–S85.

McClave, S.A., & Snider, H.L. (2002). Clinical use of gastric residual volumes as a monitor for patients on enteral tube feeding. *Journal of Parenteral and Enteral Nutrition, 26*(6 Suppl.), S43–S48; discussion S49–S50.

Morrison, G., & Hark, L. (1999). *Medical nutrition and disease* (2nd ed.). Malden, MA: Blackwell Science.

National Cancer Institute. (1998). *Eating hints for cancer patients.* Bethesda, MD: Author.

Sargent, C., Murphy, D., & Shelton, B. K. (2002). Clinical update: Nutrition in critical care. *Clinical Journal of Oncology Nursing, 6*(5), 287–289.

Sauberlich, H. E. (1999). *Laboratory tests for the assessment of nutritional status* (2nd ed.). Boca Raton, FL: CRC Press.

Schattner, M. (2003). Enteral nutrition support of the patient with cancer: Route and role. *Journal of Clinical Gastroenterology, 36*(4), 297–302.

Shils, M. E. (1999). Nutrition and diet in cancer. In M. E. Shils, J. A. Olson, M. Shike, & A. C. Ross. *Modern nutrition in health and disease.* Philadelphia: Lippincott Williams & Wilkins.

Shils, M. E., Olson, J. A., Shike, M., & Ross, A. C. (1999). *Modern nutrition in health and disease* (3rd ed.). Philadelphia: Lippincott Williams & Wilkins.

Takala, J., Ruokonen, E., Webster, N. R., et al. (1999). Increased mortality associated with growth hormone treatment in critically ill adults. *New England Journal of Medicine, 341,* 785–792.

Trujillo, E. B., Robinson, M. K., & Jacobs, D. O. (2001). Feeding critically ill patients: Current concepts. *Critical Care Nursing, 21*(4), 60–71.

Whitney, E. N. (2002). *Understanding normal and clinical nutrition* (6th ed.). Belmont, CA: Wadsworth.

_____. (1999). *Understanding nutrition* (8th ed.). Belmont, CA: West/Wadsworth.

Wilkes, G. M., Ingwersen, K., & Barton-Burke, M. (2002). *2002 Oncology nursing handbook.* Sudbury, MA: Jones & Bartlett.

29 Oral Complications

Tracy T. Douglas
Brenda K. Shelton

I. Definition
  A. Mucositis is also known as stomatitis.
   1. A broad term that encompasses functional and degenerative changes in the gastrointestinal (GI) system, resulting in inflammation, epithelial tissue sloughing, and ulceration.
   2. The GI tract is affected in its entirety, but the term *mucositis* is most often used to describe oral mucosal injury.
   3. The severity of mucositis can affect the course of treatment and the patient's quality of life.
   4. Incidence ranges from 10% of patients receiving adjuvant chemotherapy to 89% of blood and marrow transplantation patients. Average of approximately 35% to 40% incidence of mucositis with antineoplastic therapy
   5. Toxicity may be severe enough to require a chemotherapy or radiotherapy dose reduction or delay in the next treatment cycle.

II. Etiology
  A. Pathophysiology
   1. The oral mucosa is an injury-sensitive but rapidly regenerating tissue that can be damaged by multiple stressors in cancer patients.
      a. The outer epithelial layer is replaced every 7 to 14 days.
      b. The short life cycle of these cells is primarily responsible for their increased sensitivity to the stresses of cancer therapy.
   2. Saliva contains enzymes that protect the oral mucosa from dryness and infection. Decreased production of saliva enhances the risk of mucositis.
   3. Indirect toxic effects in the mouth by the release of inflammatory mediators
   4. The mouth has diverse and complex microflora that cause infection of damaged tissues. Recent studies have not shown a decrease in mucositis in patients using antimicrobial lozenges.
   5. Altered nutritional status impedes the body's ability to regenerate healthy tissue.
   6. Mucositis is more prevalent in younger people, thought to be related to a more rapid epithelial cell turnover rate
  B. The most common etiologic factors for mucositis are listed in Table 29–1.

(Text continues on page 432)

TABLE 29–1 Etiologies and Physiologic Mechanisms of Mucositis

Disorder/Agent	Examples	Clinical Features of Mucositis
Alkylating agents	Busulfan Cisplatin Carboplatin Cyclophosphamide Hepsulfan Ifosfamide Mechlorethamine Melphalan Procarbazine Thiotepa	Chemotherapy prevents immediate regeneration of mucosal membranes, resulting in a peak incidence of mucositis occurring 2–14 days after initiation of cancer therapy. Type of chemotherapy with highest association to mucositis.
Antimetabolites	Cyclocytidine Cytosine arabinoside 5-Fluorouracil Floxuridine Gemcitabine Hydroxyurea (high doses) Mechlorethamine 6-Mercaptopurine Methotrexate 6-Thioguanine	Chemotherapy prevents immediate regeneration of mucosal membranes, resulting in a peak incidence of mucositis occurring 2–14 days after initiation of cancer therapy. Direct injury from chemotherapy secreted in saliva (eg, methotrexate) may also induce epithelial damage.
Antimicrobials	Erythromycin	Broad-spectrum antimicrobials destroy the normal protective flora of the mouth, increasing the risk of fungal superinfection (esp. *Candida*).
Antitumor antibiotics	Actinomycin D Bleomycin sulfate Dactinomycin Daunorubicin Doxorubicin Epirubicin Idarubicin Mithramycin Mitomycin C Mitoxantrone	Chemotherapy prevents immediate regeneration of mucosal membranes, resulting in a peak incidence of mucositis occurring 2–14 days after initiation of cancer therapy.
Biologic response modifiers— cytokines	Interferon Interleukin-2 Tumor necrosis factor	Biologic therapy produces mucositis beginning 2–5 days after initiation of therapy and lasting 7–10 days after the treatment is complete. Forty percent of patients receiving cytokines develop mucositis.

(continued)

TABLE 29-1 Etiologies and Physiologic Mechanisms of Mucositis *(Continued)*

Disorder/Agent	Examples	Clinical Features of Mucositis
Biologic response modifiers—antibodies	Gemtuzumab	Poorly defined specific features
Graft-versus-host disease (GVHD)	Acute GVHD Chronic GVHD	Severe mucositis occurs in 80% of blood and marrow transplant patients 2 or more weeks after transplantation. The mechanism of injury is thought to be T-lymphocytic infiltration of normal epithelial tissue. Mucositis presents in a significant number of individuals. Chronic GVHD after allogeneic bone marrow transplant causes fibrotic changes in skin and mucous membranes that result in hyposalivation and a risk of oral infection that may also cause mucositis.
Hepatic disease	Hyperammonemia increases bleeding risk, mucosal changes, and taste alterations. High urea levels increase bleeding risk, alter mucosal integrity, and cause taste alterations.	Leads to an excessive amount of ammonia in saliva, causing spontaneous bleeding of gums, gray exudate, and complaints of a salty metal taste. Dry mouth with taste changes precede mucosal breakdown.
Mechanical irritation	Endotracheal tubes Ethanol Frequent oral suction Orogastric tubes Smoking and other tobacco products	Oral irritation in the location of the tube or suction can cause injury ranging from mild to hemorrhagic. Reducing the strength of suction can decrease the severity of oral injury.
Miscellaneous anti-neoplastic agents	L-asparaginase Trimetrexate	Chemotherapy prevents immediate regeneration of mucosal membranes, resulting in a peak incidence of mucositis occurring 4–10 days after initiation of therapy.
Miscellaneous nonchemotherapeutic agents	Menogaril	
Neutropenia	Depth of aplasia increases risk of mucositis.	Preexisting WBC abnormalities and prolonged neutropenia associated with hematologic malignancies and HIV disease lead to three to seven times higher incidence of mucositis than in other patient groups

▐ TABLE 29–1 **Etiologies and Physiologic Mechanisms of Mucositis** *(Continued)*

Disorder/Agent	Examples	Clinical Features of Mucositis
	Prolonged neutropenia (>10 days) increases risk of mucositis. Other disorders interfering with WBC function (eg, diabetes mellitus, renal dysfunction, hepatic dysfunction, autoimmune disease)	.
Nutritional deficiencies	Intake of high-calorie, high-sugar foods to maintain body weight, but also enhance oral bacterial growth. Insufficient fluid uptake leads to dry and vulnerable oral mucosa.	
Plant alkaloids	Etoposide (high doses) Vinblastine Vinorelbine	Chemotherapy prevents immediate regeneration of mucosal membranes, resulting in a peak incidence of mucositis occurring 7–14 days after initiation of therapy.
Periodontal disease (preexisting)	Caries and caries-associated periapical pathology increase the risk of infection-related mucositis. Abnormal oral bites, oral bridges, and dentures. Phenytoin causes gingival hyperplasia, along with gum tenderness and a greater risk of injury.	The preexisting bacterial load of the oral cavity causes oral infection when the patient becomes neutropenic or immunocompromised. Poor oral hygiene enhances proliferation of oral microbes. *Candida albicans* infection is the most common infection, and herpes simplex virus is second in prevalence. Ulcerative mucositis places the patient at risk for streptococcal bacteremia.
Radiation therapy	One hundred percent of patients receiving radiation to the neck area have mucositis.	Peak incidence within second week of therapy, or after 2,000 cGy has been administered.

(continued)

TABLE 29-1 **Etiologies and Physiologic Mechanisms of Mucositis** *(Continued)*

Disorder/Agent	Examples	Clinical Features of Mucositis
Taxanes	Paclitaxel Docetaxel	Chemotherapy prevents immediate regeneration of mucosal membranes, resulting in a peak incidence of mucositis occurring 7–14 days after initiation of therapy.
Xerostomia	Radiation therapy to the head and neck region is a common etiology. Medications that reduce saliva production: anticholinergics, antiemetics, antidepressants, antihistamines, diuretics, opiates, phenothiazines. Other etiologies: NPO status, oxygen therapy, tachypnea, mouth breathing, and oral or nasal gastric suction.	May be irreversible when caused by radiation.

Brown et al., 2001; Peterson & Schubert, 1997.

III. Patient Management
    A. Assessment
        1. Key points to guide assessment
            a. The onset of mucositis begins right after chemotherapy; however, the symptoms peak 7 to 10 days after therapy.
            b. The period of greatest mucosal damage correlates with the white cell nadir.
            c. The areas of the mouth that are most susceptible to mucosal damage are the soft tissues of the soft palate, floor of the mouth, tongue, and buccal mucosa.
        2. Signs and symptoms of mucositis
            a. Oral pain often precedes mucositis development. The pain is often a burning sensation.
            b. Dry mouth (xerostomia) and thick, ropy saliva are often associated with the early stages of mucositis.
            c. Oral erythema is the result of epidermal cell sloughing and the capillaries being closer to the skin surface.
            d. Oral edema occurs at the edges of the tongue and along the left and right buccal mucosa.
            e. Pseudomembranes are whitish coverings over the oral mucosa, with tender erosive tissue beneath the surface. Pseudomembranes may or may not be painless but often reflect the location where ulcerations will occur.

f. Ulcerations are shallow abrasions involving the entire epithelial tissue layer. They are common along the teeth line, the buccal mucosa, the lip mucosa, the floor of the mouth, and the ventral surface of the mouth. When severe ulceration occurs, hypersalivation is a more common presentation.

B. Diagnostic Parameters

  1. There are no serum or urine tests used to diagnose or indicate the presence of mucositis; however, the presence of neutropenia or thrombocytopenia may exacerbate the clinical manifestations of mucositis.

  2. Oral assessment is the only way to diagnose the presence of mucositis.

  a. Although many assessment tools are available, none has shown a clear advantage over another.

  b. The main objective of assessment is to perform consistent and ongoing observation of the oral cavity.

  c. Mucositis is rated as mild, moderate, or severe based on numeric scores compiled from findings in all areas of the mouth.

  d. Assessment scales

  (1) A simple and easy-to-use oral assessment scale derived from the World Health Organization (WHO) scale is used in the National Cancer Institute's (NCI) Common Toxicity Index version 3.0 (Fig. 29–1).

  (2) Oral Mucositis Assessment Scale (OMAS) was created by a multidisciplinary work group of experts for research on mucositis (Sonis et al., 1999). This tool was determined valid and reliable in a multicenter study, and highly correlated with the NCI scoring system.

  (3) Oral Mucositis Index (OMI) is a 34-question index for dental professionals; however, it has been recently converted to OMI-20 for nondental health professionals. The OMI-20 is a valid and reliable tool for rating mucositis (McGuire et al., 2002).

  (4) Oral Assessment Guide (OAG) is an "oral cavity assessment tool," not just a mucositis tool. The user evaluates eight parameters, grading them as normal, somewhat abnormal, and severely abnormal. The parameter totals are calculated to create a numeric score and grading of mucositis as absent or mild, moderate, and severe (Eilers, 2003).

  e. The components of the oral examination are universal regardless of whether a research-based assessment instrument is used. (A sample assessment procedure can be found in Table 29–2.)

  f. Common features of abnormal assessment findings are noted in Table 29–3.

C. Treatment

  1. There are no specific therapies to prevent mucositis.

  2. Mucositis is treated primarily symptomatically with oral cleansing, rinsing, topical agents, and pain medication.

  3. Therapy breaks or dose restrictions of antineoplastic therapy can prevent mucositis recurrence or reduce severity in future treatment cycles.

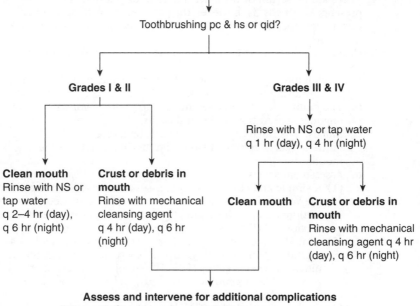

Mucositis Quick–Guide

Grade I: Erythema of the mucosa.
Grade II: Patchy ulcerations or pseudomembranes.
Grade III: Confluent ulcerations or pseudomembranes; bleeding with minor trauma.
Grade IV: Tissue necrosis; significant spontaneous bleeding; life-threatening consequences

Toothbrushing pc & hs or qid?

Grades I & II

Grades III & IV

Rinse with NS or tap water
q 1 hr (day), q 4 hr (night)

Clean mouth
Rinse with NS or
tap water
q 2–4 hr (day),
q 6 hr (night)

Crust or debris in mouth
Rinse with mechanical
cleansing agent
q 4 hr (day), q 6 hr
(night)

Clean mouth

Crust or debris in mouth
Rinse with mechanical
cleansing agent q 4 hr
(day), q 6 hr (night)

Assess and intervene for additional complications
Dry mouth: Consider saliva substitute
Pain: Ulcerease 10 cc q 2 hr prn; swish and expectorate
Lip dryness: Lip lubricant prn
Pain > 3: Implement "Management of Patient with Pain" protocol

Figure 29–1. Oral care algorithm. (Johns Hopkins Oncology Center)

    4. There is a plethora of studies in the literature using common and
unusual treatments to prevent and reduce severity of mucositis.
      a. An overview of some of these agents is included in Table 29–4.
      b. The U. S. Food and Drug Administration (FDA) has approved
two drugs for prevention or treatment of xerostomia: pilocarpine
and amifostine.
  D. Nursing Diagnoses
    1. Altered mucous membranes related to radiation therapy,
chemotherapy, graft-versus-host disease, infection, trauma, medications, altered nutrition, and altered health maintenance
      a. *Problem:* Damage to rapidly dividing epithelial tissues leads to
altered tissue integrity, discomfort, and increased risk of infection. Oral mucosal injury occurs approximately 7 to 14 days
after antineoplastic chemotherapy, and at other times when
related to other etiologic factors.

TABLE 29–2 **Oral Assessment Procedure**

Steps of the Oral Assessment Procedure	Implications of Clinical Findings
Explain to the patient that the oral cavity will be inspected for overall hygiene and mucositis.	Patient cooperation can be maximized when they are well informed.
Turn on overhead lights and don gloves.	Promotes visualization
Gather supplies: Tongue blade Light source Gauze	Implements assist in optimal visualization
Ask the patient to rate oral cavity pain at the time of assessment. If the oral examination is normal but pain is present, this must be noted.	If oral pain is greater than 3 on a 10-point scale, protocol for pain management is initiated, and more detail about the oral discomfort should be described. The patient often at first describes a mucosal "burning" sensation. The pain is usually continuous and exacerbated by mouth care, swallowing, and sleeping (due to mouth breathing). Other common descriptors patients use to describe mucositis pain are: tender, aching, and sharp. Mouth pain is particularly difficult to control because it is difficult for patients to swallow pain medication. Hospital admissions can be attributed to mucositis pain and dehydration.
Inspect the lips. Note the following: All lip edges (inner and outer) intact? Are lips smooth? Are there moles or birthmarks?	Note any moles, birthmarks, cracking or peeling, ulcerations, red marks, or edema. The lips are a relatively transparent layer of cells, not keratinized (horny) where evaporation occurs. Healthy lips are smooth with clear edges. Observe for presence of cheilitis or fissures and or white plaques at the corners of the mouth.
Have patient open his or her mouth.	Facilitates visualization
Turn on the light source and look into the mouth.	Facilitates visualization
Observe dentition: Are all teeth present? If there are dentures, remove before performing oral examination. Are any teeth fractured? Are any teeth decayed? Where are fillings and bridges? Do they appear intact? Are teeth shiny and white? Note any debris on or between teeth.	Note any broken or missing teeth, the fit of dentures, any decayed teeth, fractured teeth, or missing fillings. The crown portion of the tooth is above the gum line and covered with enamel dentin to create a shiny white appearance of a calcified substance. Pulp contains blood vessels and nerves; if there is decay reaching the pulp, it causes pain.

(continued)

TABLE 29–2 Oral Assessment Procedure *(Continued)*

Steps of the Oral Assessment Procedure	Implications of Clinical Findings
Observe the gingivae.	Note if the gums are receded or hyperplastic. Redness along the line of dentition may indicate infection below the gum surface. Gums that bleed easily may indicate gingival infection, hormonal disturbance, or thrombocytopenia.
Observe if saliva is present (visually, or detected on the tongue blade used throughout the examination): Is it clear? Is it thin and watery or thick and ropey?	If the tongue blade sticks to the tongue's surface, there is inadequate saliva. Thick and ropey saliva is also an indication of inadequate production. Both the absence of saliva and copious thick saliva can occur in the presence of mucositis.
Place the tongue blade on the buccal mucosa. Take tongue blade and place it between the gum line and buccal mucosal wall. Starting on the right side, and using the light to illuminate the oral cavity, look for erythema, swelling, lesions, or bleeding of the buccal mucosa. Repeat this procedure on the left side of the mouth.	Assess the rest of the mouth and the inside of the lips for erythema, pseudomembranes (whitish overcoating), edema, lesions, and bleeding. Use a tongue blade to assess the buccal mucosa for lesions caused by the trauma of mastication. The mouth and the inside of the lips are lined with mucous membrane of stratified squamous nonkeratinized cells. The stratified layer protects the mouth from abrasive food.
Gently pull out the labial mucosa (lip mucosa) and observe.	The lips are very moisture dependent and are good indicators of oral health.
Shine the light into the center of the mouth and inspect the tongue.	Look for erythema, dry appearance, prominent papillae, or smooth papillae, signaling disease. Any discolorations or lesions should also be noted.
Have the patient lift the tongue, move it to the right, then to the left.	
Use a light to inspect the floor of the mouth, the underside of the tongue, and the sides of the tongue.	The ventral side of the tongue and the floor of the mouth is an area often affected by mucositis.
If the patient is unable to lift the tongue, use a gauze on the tongue and a tongue blade against the buccal mucosa to lift the tongue, separate tissues, and visualize the area.	
Using the light source, inspect the hard and soft palate. Press on the center of the tongue, and ask the patient to say "ah" while the tongue surface is held down with a tongue blade to assist in visualizing the soft palate and uvula.	

TABLE 29-2 Oral Assessment Procedure (Continued)

Steps of the Oral Assessment Procedure	Implications of Clinical Findings
Assess dysphagia by determining the patient's ability to swallow liquids and solid foods.	Dysphagia indicates mucositis in the posterior oropharynx. One study demonstrated an alarming incidence of "silent" aspiration in head and neck cancer patients with radiation induced mucositis (Eisbruch et al., 2002).
Assess voice.	Interpret loss of voice as a possible indication of the severity of mucositis in the esophagus. Loss of voice indicates severe edema around the vocal cords and should alert the health care provider to prepare to artificially maintain the airway.

b. *Interventions*
   (1) Perform oral assessment every shift or daily during the time periods when mucositis is at greatest risk. The NCI toxicity assessment scale (Box 29–1) can be used to target interventions.
   (2) Instruct the patient to brush with a soft, narrow-headed toothbrush at a 45-degree angle at the gum line. Encourage the

TABLE 29-3 Appearance of Specific Oral Lesions

Suspected Disorder	Assessment Findings
Candida albicans	White pseudomembranous lesion that does not scrape off, bleeds easily, often painful, presence of cheilitis
Herpes simplex	Shallow, round or oval ulceration (vesicles are often not observed); regular shape border to lesion; raised (often whitish colored) border along edge of ulcer, often along gum line or on buccal mucosa; often very painful
Kaposi's sarcoma	Reddish, purplish, or blackish raised lesion, ranging from a few millimeters to several centimeters in size; irregular shape border to lesion, although usually circular or oval
Oral hairy leukoplakia	Hard, keratinized, white lesion, usually on the tongue or along gum line; lesion has prominent papillae-like projections that give it a hairy appearance
Pseudomonas	Small, punctuated, often brown-colored lesions found anywhere in the mouth
Staphylococcus	Small- to moderate-sized, round lesions; may have pustule appearance; tender to touch
Streptococcus	Erythematous, irregular-shaped lesions, with clear to whitish exudate; usually extremely painful

Beck, 1992; Beck & Yasko, 1993; Shelton & Weikel, 1990.

TABLE 29-4 **Management of Mucositis**

Agent	Indications	How Administered
Amifostine	High risk for xerostomia, eg, head and neck radiation therapy	200 mg/m^2 over 3 min before every treatment of standard fractionated radiation therapy
Bicarbonate solution	Oxidizing agent	1 tsp baking soda to 8 oz water or saline. Cleanses debris from normal saline. Swish the solution, then spit. Rinse mouth with water afterward.
Cetacaine spray	Oral anesthetic	2% solution sprayed over irritated area for 2 s or less; monitor dose to not suppress gag reflex.
Chlorhexidine	Antibacterial and antifungal	Rinse for 1–2 min and expectorate; 15 mL bid.
Glyoxide	Oral rinse with anesthetic properties	Rinse with approximately 10 gtt for 1 min, then expectorate. Specific lesions may have a few drops placed directly on site and expectorated after 1–3 min.
Hydrogen peroxide solution	Oxidizing agent, cleansing solution	Create 1/4 strength peroxide, rinse then spit, qid. Rinse with water afterward.
Listerine antiseptic	Antibacterial oral rinse	15 mL rinse and expectorate bid.
Moisture swabs, spray	Saliva substitute and oral rinsing agent	Spray or swab mouth as needed for dry mouth or to clean mouth.
Normal saline	Rinsing solution	Rinse with room temperature or cool solution as desired. Increased rinsing frequency decreases oral bacterial load, helps remove debris, and moistens mouth.
Nystatin swish, troches, pastilles	Antifungal prophylaxis and treatment for oral or esophageal candidiasis	15–30 mL swish, then swallow. When used prophylactically, solution may be spit rather than swallowed. Nystatin troches and pastilles are used as a lozenge, allowing the medication to melt and be swallowed.
Pilocarpine	Saliva stimulant	Oral 5 mg three times/day
Salivart	Saliva stimulant	Spray oral cavity as needed for dry mouth.

(continued)

TABLE 29–4 Management of Mucositis (Continued)

Agent	Indications	How administered
Sucralfate slurry	Oral anesthetic	15–30 mL liquidated sucralfate swished, then swallowed if used for esophagitis or gastric ulceration, or spit if used as prophylactic agent.
Tessalon perles	Topical anesthetic	100 mg/perle. Bite to express liquid, to relieve pain, then swish and expectorate. Maximum of 6 per 24 h.
Ulcerease	Topical anesthetic	15 mL qid, swish and spit.
Viadent (sanguinaria) mouthwash	Antibacterial mouth rinse	15 mL rinse and expectorate bid.
Viscous xylocaine	Topical anesthetic	15 mL qid; swish, gargle, and expectorate to relieve pain. Not to exceed 120 mL in 24 h.
Xerolube	Saliva substitute	Spray or squeeze bottle. Use as needed for dry mouth.

Beck, 1992; Johns Hopkins Oncology Center Nursing, 1996; Shelton & Weikel, 1990.

patient to exert gentle pressure on the brush at the gum line, on biting surfaces, and on the tongue. This method of tooth-brushing helps prevent formation of plaque and massages the gums and tongue. Massaging these tissues stimulates circulation, removes debris, restores tissue tone, stimulates salivation, and promotes the keratinization of the epithelial mucosa.

(3) Instruct or assist the patient to floss with waxed or unwaxed dental floss after toothbrushing, then to gargle with water to remove debris.

(4) Keep the lips lubricated to prevent injury and infection.

▼ **BOX 29-1**   **National Cancer Institute Toxicity Grading Criteria for Mucositis**

The mouth changes are grouped into four categories according to the NCI Common Toxicity Criteria v3.0:

Grade 0   Oral mucosa without erythema, plaques, ulcers, discolorations, bleeding or oral pain
Grade 1   Erythema of the mucosa
Grade 2   Patchy ulcerations or pseudomembranes
Grade 3   Confluent ulcerations or pseudomembranes; bleeding with minor trauma
Grade 4   Tissue necrosis; significant spontaneous bleeding; life-threatening consequences
Grade 5   Death

(5) If the mouth contains debris, or if periodontal disease exists, encourage the use of an oxidizing (cleansing) agent three times daily. Two common oxidizing agents are hydrogen peroxide (one-fourth strength) and sodium bicarbonate (1 teaspoon in 1 quart of solution; see Fig. 29–1 and Table 29–4). The patient should then recleanse with a water solution of the patient's choosing (tap, sterile, saline).

(6) Assist the patient to perform mouth care at least four times a day. This should be performed after meals and at bedtime or spaced throughout the day (see Fig. 29–1).

(7) Oral rinsing may be performed more frequently than brushing, flossing, and oxidized cleansing. To remove bacteria and debris, the rinsing frequency is increased to about six times daily if oral mucosa is ulcerated or has lesions.

(8) Antimicrobial mouthwashes (eg, chlorhexidine) may be used if preexisting periodontal disease or extensive debris is present.

(9) Document patient responses to mucositis interventions. Alter cleansing and rinsing regimen as mucositis characteristics change (see Fig. 29–1 and Table 29–4).

  c. *Desired outcomes*

    (1) Patient will have pink, intact, and moist mucosa.

    (2) Patient's teeth will be clean, shiny, and without debris.

2. Alteration in comfort or acute pain related to impaired oral mucosal integrity

  a. *Problem:* Mucositis causes tissue necrosis and sloughing of the epithelial tissue layer in the mouth. The loss of this superficial tissue exposes nerves, causing pain of the mouth.

  b. *Interventions*

    (1) Assess oral pain every shift during peak mucositis incidence periods and while erythema, edema, lesions, or ulcerations are present.

    (2) Implement pain protocols as indicated by institutional policy.

    (3) Provide oral topical anesthetics as desired by the patient. Common agents and their proposed mechanism of action are included in Table 29–4.

    (4) If soothing to the patient, offer ice chips to moisten the oral mucosa and reduce discomfort.

    (5) Maintain mouth moistness with frequent rinsing or saliva substitutes because a dry mouth is more uncomfortable.

    (6) Provide alternative methods of communication because mouth pain may deter speaking.

    (7) Avoid commercial mouthwashes that contain high percentages of alcohol, which exacerbates oral dryness and pain.

    (8) Make mouth care solutions and implements readily available at the patient's bedside. Compliance may depend on availability.

  c. *Desired outcomes*

    (1) Patient will be free of oral pain.

    (2) Patient will be satisfied with the ability to communicate needs to health care personnel.

3. Potential for infection related to altered oral tissue integrity

    a. *Problem:* Mucositis produces breaks in the integrity of the oral mucosa, which predisposes the exposed underlying tissue to invasion by normal oral organisms or to pathogens entering by food, drink, or contaminated devices.

    b. *Interventions*

        (1) Avoid use of dentures that do not fit. Dentures should be removed nightly and soaked in a disinfectant denture-soaking solution. The solution should be changed daily. Rinse dentures, brush with denture cleaner, and then rinse again before returning to the mouth.

        (2) Rinse toothbrush with very hot water before use. This helps destroy bacteria and softens the toothbrush. Change toothbrushes weekly to reduce the risk of infection transmission by toothbrush.

        (3) Antimicrobial mouthwashes (eg, chlorhexidine) may be used if preexisting periodontal disease or excessive debris is present.

        (4) Monitor oral lesions every shift, noting increases in size or changes in character. Report new or infectious-looking lesions. Oral infections are not always painful. When ordered, obtain bacterial, fungal, or viral cultures of the lesions.

        (5) Note and report difficulty swallowing, which may indicate oral infection further back in the oropharynx that cannot be assessed by visualization.

        (6) Administer prophylactic oral antimicrobials as ordered (eg, nystatin swish for oral *Candida*).

        (7) Always check the entire oral cavity for infectious lesions when the patient exhibits a new fever.

    c. *Desired outcomes*

        (1) Patient will be free of oral lesions indicative of infection.

        (2) Oral cultures are negative for pathogenic organisms.

4. Altered nutrition, less than body requirements, related to inability to eat due to severe mucositis (see Chapter 28)

    a. *Problem:* Mouth pain and edema deter the patient from obtaining adequate nutrition and necessary fluid intake, and may necessitate nutritional supplementation from other, nonoral sources.

    b. *Interventions*

        (1) Assess oral intake before and during mucositis.

        (2) Assess caloric needs and whether they are being met during mucositis.

        (3) Assess intake and output measurements and possible insensible losses through hypersalivation. Determine if fluid volume deficit from inadequate intake or excess loss is possible.

        (4) Assess skin and mucous membranes for signs and symptoms of dehydration.

        (5) Provide a small amount of water to assess gag and swallow reflex. This will determine the patient's ability to safely continue oral intake during mucositis.

      (6) Encourage cool fluids and foods to reduce trauma and discomfort of eating.

      (7) Encourage mechanical soft diet if mucositis causes oral discomfort.

    c. *Desired outcome:* Patient will be able to eat and drink adequate amounts of fluids and food to maintain proper nutrition.

5. Impaired swallowing related to oral edema from mucositis (see Chapter 28)

    a. *Problem:* Oral mucositis or infectious complications may involve the oropharynx, causing edema and difficulty swallowing or talking. This impaired swallowing may alter nutrient intake or affect airway clearance.

    b. *Interventions*

      (1) Provide a small amount of water to assess gag and swallow reflex. This will determine the patient's ability to safely continue oral intake during mucositis.

      (2) Encourage cool fluids and foods to reduce oropharyngeal trauma and the discomfort of eating.

      (3) Encourage mechanical soft diet if mucositis causes difficulty swallowing.

      (4) Encourage head-of-bed elevation when severe mucositis impairs swallowing in order to reduce the risk of inadvertent aspiration.

      (5) Provide the patient with easy access to oral suction, which assists in removal of excess secretions and reduces aspiration risk.

    c. *Desired outcome:* Patient will be able to eat and drink without swallowing difficulties.

6. Ineffective airway clearance related to oral edema from mucositis

    a. *Problem:* Oral mucositis or infectious complications may involve the oropharynx, causing edema. This edema and impaired swallowing may affect airway clearance.

    b. *Interventions*

      (1) In the presence of mucositis, assess upper airways (trachea and bronchi) for stridor (indicative of bronchospasm) and gurgles (indicative of retained secretions).

      (2) Assess patient for dyspnea, tachypnea, air hunger, mental status changes, or other symptoms of poor gas exchange in relation to oropharyngeal edema.

      (3) Assess pulse oximetry for oxygen saturation, and arterial blood gases for hypoxemia and hypercarbia, if severe airway edema is present and causing a risk for impaired gas exchange.

      (4) Provide a small amount of water to assess gag and swallow reflex. This will determine the patient's ability to safely continue oral intake during mucositis.

      (5) Encourage head-of-bed elevation when severe mucositis impairs swallowing in order to reduce the risk of inadvertent aspiration.

(6) Provide the patient with easy access to oral suction, which assists in removal of excess secretions and reduces aspiration risk.

(7) Administer corticosteroids systemically or topically, or racemic epinephrine (local oropharyngeal spray) as ordered, if severe airway stridor places the patient at risk for impaired gas exchange.

  c. *Desired outcomes*

    (1) Patient will not have stridor and gurgles on breath sound assessment.

    (2) Patient will present with no signs or symptoms of respiratory distress, hypoxemia, or hypercarbia.

7. Potential for bleeding related to oral mucosal injury

  a. *Problem:* Mucositis causes erosion of the outer epithelial layer of the oral mucosa, resulting in multiple mucosal capillaries being exposed and having the potential to bleed with minimal injury. Oral bleeding may be exacerbated by coagulopathies also suffered by the patient.

  b. *Interventions*

    (1) Note and report the degree and location of oral bleeding to the physician.

    (2) Monitor platelet count and coagulation tests for abnormalities that increase the risk of oral bleeding.

    (3) Administer ice chips or cold fluids to stop minimal oral bleeding.

    (4) Modify the toothbrushing regimen if oral bleeding occurs with toothbrushing. A softer toothbrush, less vigorous brushing, or use of Toothettes may be substituted.

    (5) Apply gauze and pressure or topical hemostatics (eg, Gelfoam, topical thrombin, Avitene) as needed for bleeding oral lesions.

    (6) Provide readily available oral suction to prevent aspiration of blood from the oral cavity.

    (7) Encourage frequent oral rinsing to remove the bloody taste from the patient's mouth, and to reduce the amount of blood swallowed that may induce nausea or vomiting.

  c. *Desired outcome:* Patient will be free of oral bleeding.

E. Discharge Planning and Patient Education

  1. Teach the patient and family about ways to detect and manage mucositis. Patients should be aware of when mucositis is likely to occur, how long it should last, and what it may look like.

  2. Give the patient specific instructions on mucositis prevention, interventions, and common complications addressed in the Patient Management section of this chapter. Instructions must include the necessity for fluid, nutrition, and pain control to prevent unnecessary readmission to the hospital.

  3. Instruct the patient to look for signs of infectious complications (eg, thrush).

REFERENCES

Awidi, A., Homsi, U., Kakail, R., Mubarak, A., Hassan, A., Kelta, M., Martinez, P., Sulaiti, S., Al Qady, A., Jamhoury, A., Daniel, M., Charles, C., Ambrose, A., & El-Aloosy, A. (2001). Double-blind, placebo-controlled cross-over study of oral pilocarpine for the prevention of chemotherapy-induced oral mucositis in adult patients with cancer. *European Journal of Cancer, 37*(16), 1971–1975.

Beck, S. L. (1992). Prevention and management of oral complication in the cancer patient. In S. Hubbard, P. Greens, & M. T. Knobf (Eds.), *Current issues in cancer nursing practice updates* (pp. 1–12). Philadelphia: Lippincott-Raven.

Beck, S. L., & Yasko, J. M. (1993). *Guidelines for oral care* (2nd ed.). Crystal Lake, IL: Sage.

Brown, K., Esper, P., Kelleher, L., O'Neill, J., Polovich, M., & White, J., (2001). *Chemotherapy and biotherapy. Guidelines and recommendations for practice.* Pittsburgh, PA: Oncology Nursing Society.

Cancer Therapy Evaluation Program. (2003, March 31). Common terminology criteria for adverse events (Version 3.0, DTCD, NCI, NIH, DHHS). Available: http://ctep.cancer.gov.

Cerchietti, L., Navigante, A., Bonomi, M., Zaderajko, M., Menendez, P., Pogany, C., & Roth, B. (2002). Effect of topical morphine for mucositis-associated pain following concomitant chemoradiotherapy for head and neck carcinoma. *Cancer, 95*(10), 2230–2236.

Culy, C., & Spencer, C. (2001). Amifostine: An update on its clinical status as a cytoprotectant in patients with cancer receiving chemotherapy or radiotherapy and its potential therapeutic application in myelodysplastic syndrome. *Drugs, 61*(5), 641–684.

Eilers, J. (2003). When the mouth tells us more than it says—The impact of mucositis on quality of life. *Oncology Supportive Care, 1*(4), 31–43.

Eisbruch, A., Lyden, T., Bradford, C., Dawson, L., Haxer, M., Miller, A., Teknos, T., Chepeha, D., Hogikyan, N., Terrell, J., & Wolf, G. (2002). Objective assessment of swallowing dysfunction and aspiration after radiation concurrent with chemotherapy for head-and-neck cancer. *International Journal of Radiation Oncology, Biology, Physics, 53*(1), 4–5.

Etiz, D., Orhan, E., Demirustu, C., Ozdamar, K., & Cakmak, A. (2002). Comparison of radiation-induced oral mucositis scoring systems. *Tumori, 88*(5), 379–384.

Johns Hopkins Oncology Center Nursing. (1996). *Mucositis standards of care.* Baltimore, MD: The Johns Hopkins Oncology Center.

Kolbinson, D. A., Schubert, M. M., Flournoy, N., et al. (1991). Early oral changes following bone marrow transplantation. *Oral Surgery, Oral Medicine, and Oral Pathology, 66*, 130–138.

McGuire, D., Peterson, D., Muller, S., Owne, D., Slemmons, M., & Schubert, M. (2002). The 20 item oral mucositis index: Reliability and validity in bone marrow and stem cell transplant patients. *Cancer Investigation, 20*(7–8), 893–903.

Peterson, D., & Schubert, M., (1997). Oral toxicity. In M. Perry (Ed.), *The chemotherapy source book* (2nd ed.). Baltimore, MD: Williams & Wilkins.

Poland, J. (1991). Prevention and treatment of oral complications in the cancer patient. *Oncology, 5*(7), 45–50.

Regnard, C., & Fitton, S. (1989). Mouth care: A flow diagram. *Palliative Medicine, 3*, 67–69.

Rocke, L., Loprinzi, C., Lee, J., et al. (1993). A randomized clinical trial of two different durations of oral cryotherapy for prevention of 5-fluorouracil-related stomatitis. *Cancer, 72*, 2234.

Rothenberger, S. (1993). Assessment of the oral cavity. In M. Frank-Stromberg (Ed.), *Instruments for clinical research* (pp. 391–400). Boston, MA: Jones & Bartlett.

Shelton, B. K., & Weikel, D. (1990). Alterations in the oral mucosa: Assessment to intervention. In *American Association of Critical Care Nurses [AACN] National Teaching Institute Proceedings* (pp. 233–237). Laguna, Niguel, CA: AACN.

Sonis, S., Eilers, J., Epstein, J., LeVeque, F., Liggett, W., Mulagha, M., Peterson, D., Rose, A., Schudert, M., Spiijkervet, F., & Wittes, J. (1999). Validation of a new scoring system for the assessment of clinical trial research of oral mucositis induced by radiation or chemotherapy. *Cancer, 85*(10), 2103–2113.

Sprinzl, G., Galvan, O., de Vries, A., Ulmer, H., Gunkel, A., Lukas, P., & Thumfart, W. (2001). Local application of granulocyte-macrophage colony stimulating factor (GM-CSF) for the treatment of oral mucositis. *European Journal of Cancer, 37*(16), 2003–2009.

Stiff, P. (2001). Mucositis associated with stem cell transplantation: Current status and innovative approaches to management. *Bone Marrow Transplantation* (Suppl. 2), S3-S11.

Stokman, M., Spijkervet, F., Burlage, F., Dijkstra, P., Manson, W., de Vries, E., & Roodenburg, J. (2003). Oral mucositis and selective elimination of oral flora in head and neck cancer patients receiving radiotherapy: A double-blind randomized clinical trial. *British Journal of Cancer, 88*(7), 1012–1016.

U. S. Department of Health and Human Services, Public Health Services, National Institutes of Health, & Office of Medical Applications of Research. (1989). *Oral complications of cancer therapies: Diagnosis, prevention, and treatment* [National Institutes of Health Consensus Development Conference Statement]. Bethesda, MD: Author.

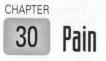

30 Pain

Suzanne Amato Nesbit

I. Definition: Pain is a multidimensional experience characterized by physiologic and psychological components. It is a complex phenomenon that involves both perception of a stimulus and response to it. One third of cancer patients in active therapy and 60% to 90% of patients with advanced disease have pain. One critically important aspect related to the definition of pain is to understand that it is subjective. Cancer pain is unique in many ways. Patients can have pain in more than one site, it can have more than one cause, and patients can have more than one syndrome. In addition, they can have acute and chronic pain simultaneously, and the pain can vary in its pattern, intensity, and duration. As a result of its multiple causes and presentation, cancer pain often requires more than one treatment. The patient's perception of pain and the subsequent self-report are the most reliable measures that health care providers should use to assess and control pain successfully.

  A. Types of Pain
   1. *Nociceptive pain* occurs when nociceptors are activated by noxious stimulus (eg, injury, disease).
     a. *Somatic pain* is the most common type of pain and can occur in cutaneous or deep tissues (eg, with bone metastases).
     b. *Visceral pain* is another type of nociceptive pain (eg, distention of the liver capsule and the intestinal viscera).
   2. *Neuropathic pain* occurs as a result of injury to nerves (eg, tumor infiltrating the brachial plexus, chemotherapy-induced peripheral neuropathies).

  B. Classification of Pain
   1. *Acute pain* is characterized as a "complex, unpleasant experience with emotional and cognitive, as well as, sensory features that occur in response to tissue trauma." It is usually nociceptive and associated with subjective and objective physical signs and activation of the autonomic nervous system. The cause of the pain is usually known (Chapman & Nakamura, 1999).
   2. *Chronic pain* continues after an injury is healed. It may be nociceptive, neuropathic, or both. Hyperactivity of the autonomic nervous system is less common. Patients may not "appear" to be in pain.
   3. *Cancer pain* can be caused by the disease (eg, tumor invasion, compression of nerves) or by treatment or procedures (eg, biopsy, chemotherapy, surgery). It can have features of nociceptive pain, neuropathic pain, or both. It can be acute or chronic in nature.

  C. Goals of Cancer Pain Treatment (Table 30–1)
   1. Control pain.
   2. Prevent or minimize side effects.

TABLE 30-1 Preferred Treatment

I. Preliminary pain assessment data are obtained. This includes a brief history, physical examination, laboratory data, and pain intensity information.

II. Patient comfort is maximized with prompt administration of analgesics. This facilitates the evaluation process.
   a. Mild pain is usually treated with nonopioids, whereas the opioid analgesics are used for moderate to severe pain.
   b. The oral route of administration is preferred for virtually all patients.
   c. Analgesics with short half-lives are used to facilitate rapid dose escalation and prompt relief of pain.
   d. Analgesics are given "around the clock" rather than "as needed."
   e. Once baseline opioid requirements are determined, sustained-release opioid preparations can be used to reduce the number of pills taken each day.
   f. PRN medications are available for breakthrough pain.
   g. A prophylactic bowel regimen is initiated with all opioid therapy. Nausea and vomiting are treated with aggressive antiemetic therapy. These may become less prominent after the first several days of opioid therapy.
   h. The dose of each analgesic is maximized before considering changes in drugs or routes of administration.
   i. Changes in analgesics or routes of administration are generally based on the development of significant toxicities that are not responsive to usual measures rather than the total administered dose.
   j. Equi-analgesic tables are used to approximate opioid dose conversions.
   k. Serial pain intensity ratings are obtained and documented in the medical record.

III. A comprehensive pain assessment is completed as outlined in the text.

IV. The treatment approach and diagnoses are reassessed based on the results of the pain assessment and relief scores.

V. The potential benefits and risks of the following approaches to pain management are assessed.
   a. Antineoplastic therapies
   b. Adjuvant analgesics
   c. Neurostimulatory techniques
   d. Nonpharmacologic approaches
   e. Regional anesthesia
   f. Neuroablative procedures

VI. Consider referral to an experienced multidisciplinary pain team if attempts to control pain in patients with the following difficult-to-manage problems are not successful.
   a. Patients with neuropathic pain
   b. Patients with episodic or incident pain
   c. Patients with impaired cognitive or communicative function
   d. Patients with a history of substance abuse

Grossman, S. A., & Nesbit, S. A. (2004). Cancer pain. In M. D. Abeloff et al. (Eds.), *Clinical oncology* (3rd ed.). Philadelphia: W. B. Saunders.

3. Enhance patient's quality of life.
   D. Barriers to Pain Relief
      1. Problems related to health care professionals (eg, inadequate knowledge of pain management, incomplete assessment, fear of addiction)

2. Problems related to patients (eg, reluctance to report pain, fear that pain means disease is worse, reluctance to take pain medicines because of fear of addiction and side effects)
3. Problems related to the health care system (eg, pain a low priority, access to pain treatments, costs of treatment, and restrictive regulations of controlled substances)

II. **Etiology:** Table 30–2 lists common cancer pain syndromes from all causes.
   A. Disease-related causes (ie, tumor that has infiltrated bones, nerves, and viscera) are the most common reason for cancer pain. Tumor-related causes can be both acute and chronic in nature.

TABLE 30–2 Common Cancer Pain Syndromes*

Associated With Tumor Infiltration	Associated With Cancer Therapy
Base of skull	Postsurgical pain syndromes
Orbital	Postmastectomy
Middle fossa	Post-thoracotomy
Clivius metastases	Post–radical neck dissection
Odontoid fracture	Phantom limb and stump pain
Parasagittal	Postradiation pain syndromes
Jugular foramen	Fibrosis or brachial or lumbosacral plexus
Sphenoid sinus metastases	Acute radiation dermatitis or mucositis
Cranial nerve	Radiation-induced peripheral nerve tumors
Glossopharyngeal neuralgia	Radiation myelopathy
Trigeminal neuralgia	Postchemotherapy pain syndromes
Peripheral nerve	Peripheral neuropathy
Intercostal neuropathy	Steroid pseudorheumatism
Peripheral neuropathy	Mucositis
Plexus	Acute herpetic and posttherpetic neuralgia
Cervical plexopathy	
Brachial plexopathy	
Lumbosacral plexopathy	
Epidural space	
Epidural cord compression	
Epidural metastases	
Subarachnoid space	
Neoplastic meningitis	
Intraparenchymal CNS	
Brain metastases	
Spinal cord metastases	
Visceral involvement	
Obstruction of hollow viscus or ducts	
Rapid growth in solid organs	
Other	
Vascular compromise	
Necrosis or ulceration of mucous membrane	
Pleural and pericardial involvement	

*Examples of common pain syndromes unrelated to cancer: Lumbar or cervical disk disease, migraine.

Adapted from Grossman, S., & Gregory, R. (1996). Pain. In J. Kirkwood, M. Lotze, & J. Yasko (Eds.), *Current cancer therapeutics* (2nd ed., p. 374). Philadelphia: Current Medicine.

B. Treatment-related causes include those brought on by procedure, diagnostic methods, surgery, chemotherapy, and radiation. These causes can also be either acute or chronic in nature.
C. Causes unrelated to cancer or its treatment account for the smallest percentage of pain in cancer patients. However, it is important for the clinician to differentiate between cancer- and non-cancer-related causes, because the treatments may be very different.

III. Patient Management
A. Assessment: The following are physical indications of pain:
   1. Facial grimacing
   2. Moaning
   3. Guarding
   4. Increased heart and respiratory rates
   5. Increased blood pressure
B. Diagnostic Parameters: A comprehensive assessment is conducted for a new pain or a significant change in an existing pain. A simpler assessment, such as asking a patient about current pain intensity and degree of relief, is warranted before and after administering an analgesic. Pain assessment is of particular importance in patients who have communication difficulties (eg, non-English speaking, children, and the elderly). The frequency of assessment is directly related to the success of adequate pain control. The following are essential pain assessment parameters:
   1. Assessment of pain intensity and character
      a. Onset and temporal character: When did it start? How often does it occur?
      b. Location: Where is it?
      c. Quality: What does it feel like? (stabbing, shooting, cramping, dull, aching)
      d. Intensity: What is the intensity of current pain?
         (1) Numerical rating scale: On a scale of 0 to 10, with 0 being no pain and 10 being the worst pain imaginable, ask the patient to select a number between 0 and 10 that best describes the pain.
         (2) Verbal descriptor scale: Ask the patient to indicate if he or she is in pain. If so, ask if the pain is mild, moderate, or severe.
         (3) Hopkins Pain Rating Instrument (a plastic, portable, 10-cm, double-sided instrument): Show the patient the side that contains no numbers but has "no pain" on one end and "worst pain imaginable" on the other. Ask the patient to slide the plastic tab to the place that represents the pain. Look at the reverse side of the instrument to see the numerical rating of the pain (Fig. 30–1).
   2. Aggravating and relieving factors: What makes the pain better or worse?
      a. Previous treatment: What treatments were used in the past and how successful were they?
      b. Relief from current treatment: Is relief of pain complete, almost complete, partial, very little, or none?
      c. Side effects of current treatment: Are you experiencing any side effects to current treatment?

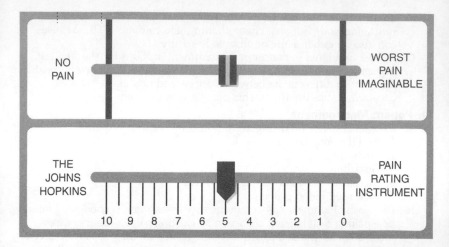

Figure 30–1. The Johns Hopkins Pain Rating Instrument. The upper panel shows the front side of the instrument; the lower panel shows the back. Thus, when the tab is at "the worst pain imaginable" rating (front), the score reads "10" (back).

3. Assess psychosocial factors.
   a. Effect of pain on patient and family members
   b. Meaning of pain to patient and family
   c. Usual coping strategies for pain and other stressors
   d. Mood states
   e. Effect of pain on sleep and fatigue
   f. Concern about addiction and side effects of medication
   g. Concern about costs of treatment
4. Diagnostic tests are performed to determine the causes of pain and aid in selection of the most appropriate intervention. Performing physical and neurologic examinations and ordering and reviewing diagnostic tests are the responsibility of the physician or primary provider. Tests should be appropriate to the body area and function, and to the possible etiology of the pain.
C. Treatment: The administration of analgesics is one of the most common nursing activities to help control pain. The nurse must possess adequate knowledge about analgesic pharmacology.
   1. Categories of analgesics
      a. Nonopioids (for mild/moderate pain): Have a peripheral mechanism of action; have a ceiling effect; are used alone or in combination with opioids. They include acetaminophen, aspirin, non-steroidal antiinflammatory drugs (NSAIDs), and COX-2 inhibitors (Tables 30–3, 30–4, 30–5, 30–6, 30–7)
      b. Opioids (for moderate/severe pain): Have a central mechanism of action; do not have a ceiling effect; are given on a scheduled basis with prn for breakthrough pain. Most patients have successful management with the oral route. (See Tables 30–4, 30–5, 30–6, 30–7, 30–8 and Box 30–1 for general comments, side effects, and routes of administration.)

TABLE 30-3 Adult Dosing Data for Nonopioids

Acetaminophen	650 mg q4h 975 mg q6h	APAP lacks the peripheral antiinflammatory and antiplatelet activities of the other NSAIDs.
Aspirin	650 mg q4h 975 mg q6h	The standard against which other NSAIDs are compared. May inhibit platelet aggregation for >1 week and may cause bleeding. Aspirin is contraindicated in children with fever or other viral disease because of its association with Reye's syndrome.
Carprofen	100 mg tid	
Choline magnesium trisalicylate	1000–1500 mg tid	May have minimal antiplatelet activity.
Choline salicylate	870 mg q3–4h	May have minimal antiplatelet activity.
Diclofenac	50–75 mg q12–24h	
Diflunisal	500 mg q12h	
Etodolac	200–400 mg q6–8h	
Fenoprofen	300–600 mg q6h	
Flubiprofen	50–100 mg q12h	
Ibuprofen	400–600 mg q6h	
Indomethacin	25–50 mg q6–8h	
Ketoprofen	25–60 mg q6–8h	
Ketorolac tromethamine	PO 10 mg q4–6h (maximum dose 40 mg/day) IM: 60 mg initially, then 30 mg q6h IV: 30 mg initially, then 15 mg q6h	Duration of use not to exceed 5 days
Magnesium salicylate	650 mg q4h	
Meclofenamate sodium	50–100 mg q6h	Coombs'-positive autoimmune hemolytic anemia has been associated with prolonged use.
Mefenamic acid	250 mg q6h	
Meloxicam	7.5–15 mg q24h	
Nabumetone	500 mg q24h	
Naproxen	250–275 mg q6–8h	
Naproxen sodium	275 mg q6–8h	
Phenylbutazone	100 mg q8h	
Piroxicam	10–20 mg q24h	
Sodium salicylate	325–650 mg q3–4h	
Sulindac	150–200 mg q12–24g	
Tolmetin	400–800 mg q8h	
COX-2 Inhibitors		
Celecoxib	100–200 mg q12h	
Rofecoxib	12.5–25 mg q24h	
Valdecoxib	10 mg q24h	

Grossman, S. A. (1999). Management of cancer pain: National comprehensive cancer network guidelines. *Oncology, 13,* 33–44; American Pain Society. (1999). *Principles of analgesic use in the treatment of acute pain and chronic cancer pain: A concise guide to medical practice* (4th ed.) Glenview, IL: Author; Jacox, S., Carr, D., Payne, R., et al. (1994). *Management of cancer pain: Clinical practice guideline No. 9* (AHCPR Publication No. 94-0592; p. 48). Rockville, MD: Agency for Health Care Policy and Research, U.S. Dept. of Health and Human Services.

TABLE 30-4 Routes of Administration

Route	Definition and Notes	Drug Types	Comments
Oral	By mouth (per os) Requires functioning GI tract, intact swallowing mechanism, sufficient GI tract for absorption to occur	Nonopioids, opioids, adjuvant analgesics	Advantages: convenient, noninvasive, cost-effective, flexible, less discomfort than injections with comparable efficacy Disadvantages: requires functional GI system; slow onset of action and relatively delayed peak effects; requires patient compliance
Rectal	Insertion of suppository into rectum	Nonopioids, opioids	Useful in patients who cannot take medications by mouth Any opioid may be compounded for rectal administration
Intramuscular	Injection into large muscle (e.g., gluteus or vastus lateralis)	Some nonopioids, opioids	IM administration should not be used, especially for chronic treatment, due to multiple disadvantages: • Painful injections • Wide fluctuations in drug absorption make it difficult to maintain consistent blood levels • Rapid fall-off of action compared with PO administration • Chronic injections may damage tissue (fibrosis, abscesses); IV and SC injections are appropriate alternatives
Intravenous	Injection into vein; may be single or repetitive bolus or continuous infusion with or without PCA	Some nonopioids, opioids, adjuvant analgesics	IV is most efficient ROA for immediate analgesia and permits rapid titration IV bolus produces rapid onset of effect, but shorter duration of action than IM; not recommended for drugs with long half-lives Continuous IV infusion provides steadier drug blood levels, which maximize pain relief while minimizing side effects
Subcutaneous	Placement of drug just under skin with small needle Continuous SC infusion can be obtained with a small needle	Some opioids	Advantages: produces steady blood levels; time until onset of effect is comparable to IM administration and effects are longer lasting, with less painful administration; cheaper than IV administration; obviates need for GI function Disadvantages: slower onset and offset and lower peak effects than IV administration, time consuming, often disliked by patients

Route	Description	Drugs	Comments
Topical	Applied directly to the skin, where the drug penetrates	NSAIDs, local anesthetics (eg, lidocaine patch and gel, EMLA), capsaicin	Advantages: local effect (ie, no significant serum levels) limits side effects to local reactions, no drug–drug interactions; easy to use, no titration needed Disadvantages: may cause local skin reactions
Transdermal	Absorbed through skin with gradual release into the systemic circulation	Some opioids, adjuvant analgesics	Advantages: convenient, noninvasive, provides prolonged, relatively stable analgesia Disadvantages: delayed onset of action with first dose, drug absorption influenced by internal or external heat
Oral transmucosal	Delivery of drug to mouth, including sublingual (under tongue) and buccal/gingival administration	Some opioids	Advantages: easy, requires little staff supervision; avoids significant liver metabolism associated with oral opioids Disadvantages: variable absorption, bitter taste, dose is limited
OTFC	Fentanyl incorporated into a sweetened matrix on a stick for consumption	Fentanyl	Some absorption by way of oral mucosa, but most by way of GI tract; yields higher drug levels and better bioavailability than oral fentanyl
Intranasal	Small aerosol device placed inside nostril that delivers a calibrated dose of a drug	Butorphanol, sumatriptan	Takes advantage of rich blood supply to nose and also avoids significant liver metabolism associated with some drugs
Intraspinal	Epidural and intrathecal administration		
Other (sublingual, vaginal)	Placement of drug under the tongue (sublingual) or in the vagina	Opioids	Most opioids can be absorbed sublingually or vaginally in patients who have problems such as impaired swallowing, short gut syndrome, or poor IV access

EMLA: Eutectic Mixture of Local Anesthetics (lidocaine and prilocaine); GI: gastrointestinal; IM: intramuscular; IV: intravenous; NSAIDs: nonsteroidal antiinflammatory drugs; OTFC: oral transmucosal fentanyl citrate; PCA: patient-controlled analgesia; PO: per os (orally); ROA: route of administration; SC: subcutaneous.

Berry P. H., Chapman C. R., Covington E. C., et al, (2001). *Pain: Current understanding of assessment, management, and treatments.* Reston VA: National Pharmaceutical Council and the Joint Commission for Accreditation of Healthcare Organizations.

TABLE 30–5 PCA and Regional Anesthesia

Route	Definition	Example Drug Types	Comments
PCA	Use of infusion pump that allows patient to self-administer small doses of analgesics via one of several routes (eg, IV, SC, epidural)	Opioids (eg, morphine, hydromorphone, fentanyl, meperidine), some NSAIDs	Used for numerous surgeries (eg, C-section, abdominal, orthopedic) and medical conditions (cancer pain, sickle cell crisis, burn pain, HIV pain, pancreatitis, kidney stones, fractures) Advantages: less delay in onset of analgesia than PRN dosing Compared with IM, improved analgesia with smaller doses of opioids and fewer side effects Disadvantages: Patient must understand technique, so less useful in some clinical populations
Single or repetitive epidural bolus	Injection or infusion of agent into the epidural space via insertion of a needle (single bolus) or catheter (repetitive bolus)	Opioids (eg, morphine, fentanyl hydromorphone), local anesthetics (eg, bupivacaine, ropivacaine), corticosteroids, clonidine, baclofen	Used for diagnostic and therapeutic nerve blocks; the latter include surgeries (eg, C-section, gynecologic, urological surgeries) Advantages: simple, no need for infusion device, delivery to site close to site of action (spinal cord) permits more intense analgesia (greater analgesia for given drug) Disadvantages: limited number of suitable agents, higher incidence of side effects, requires personnel to reinject catheter, higher risk of catheter contamination, does not permit PCA
Continuous epidural	Continuous infusion of agent(s) into the epidural space via a catheter. A long-term catheter can be tunneled under the skin or surgically implanted for long-term pain management (eg, cancer pain, CNCP)	Opioids, local anesthetics	Used for acute pain (eg, postoperative, obstetrical, posttraumatic pain) and chronic pain (eg, cancer pain, neuropathic pain) Advantages: permits concomitant use of local anesthetic and shorter-acting opioids, eliminates need for catheter reinjection, reduces rostral spread of analgesia, less risk of catheter contamination, greater potency than systemic administration Disadvantages: Potential for catheter migration and side effects (eg, of skin and subcutaneous tissue around catheter site; rarely, hematoma, abscess, or meningitis)

PCEA	Continuous infusion of drugs into epidural space, controlled by a patient-operated infusion pump	Opioids	Allows patient to manage dynamic changes in pain related to activity
Bolus or continuous intrathecal (spinal)	Injection or infusion of agent into the subarachnoid space by way of insertion of a needle (single bolus) or catheter (repetitive bolus); an indwelling intrathecal catheter can be placed for long-term analgesia to reduce the risk of infection	Opioids (eg, morphine, hydromorphone, fentanyl), local anesthetics (eg, lidocaine, bupivacaine, mepivacaine)	Uses include cancer pain (regionalized pain below T1), neuropathic pain Single bolus more commonly used for acute pain due to difficulty in maintaining indwelling intrathecal catheters. May be cost-effective for patients with cancer or CNCP Advantages: provides intense analgesia at lower doses than systemic administration Disadvantages: can be difficult to titrate drug effect, risk of infection and other side effects Onset and duration of effect reflect lipid solubility of agent; greater effects of drug at given dose than with systemic administration
Local infiltration	Infiltration of various body structures with local anesthetics and/or corticosteroids	Local anesthetics (eg, bupivacaine), corticosteroids	Used for acute pain (eg, postoperative pain, postoperative joint pain, acute bursitis, tendonitis, muscle spasm) and chronic pain (eg, painful scars, neuromata, trigger points for myofascial syndromes, arthritis, facet syndrome)
Spinal nerve block	Blockade of spinal neurons outside the spinal canal in the paravertebral region or anywhere along its course	Local anesthetics	Includes cervical spinal blocks, occipital blocks, thoracic spinal blocks, lumbar and sacral spinal nerve blocks, sympathetic blockade Used for severe acute or chronic pain (eg, postoperative, posttraumatic, postamputation, PVD, cancer pain, visceral pain, CRPS, neuralgias)
Topical application	Application of local anesthetics to skin (eg, patch, gel, cream, paste)	Topical local anesthetics (eg, lidocaine, EMLA); other local anesthetics (eg, cocaine, benzocaine)	Oral agents used for pain in mucous membranes of mouth Topical anesthetics used for procedural pain (EMLA) and some chronic pain (eg, lidocaine patch or gel for postherpetic neuralgia)

C-section: Cesarean section; CNCP: chronic noncancer pain; CRPS: chronic regional pain syndrome; EMLA: Eutectic Mixture of Local Anesthetics (lidocaine and prilocaine); HIV: human immunodeficiency virus; IM: intramuscular; IV: intravenous; NSAIDs: nonsteroidal antiinflammatory drugs; PCA: patient-controlled analgesia; PCEA: patient-controlled epidural analgesia; PRN: as needed; PVD: peripheral vascular disease; SC: subcutaneous.

Berry P. H., Chapman C. R., Covington E. C., et al, (2001). *Pain: Current understanding of assessment, management, and treatments.* Reston VA: National Pharmaceutical Council and the Joint Commission for Accreditation of Healthcare Organizations.

TABLE 30–6 Examples of Psychological Methods Used to Manage Pain

Intervention	Definition	Purpose/Goals	Uses
Patient education	Provision of detailed information about disease or interventions and methods of assessing and managing pain (eg, preoperative instruction about importance of deep breathing, coughing, and ambulating postoperatively; teaching patients with chronic pain about what may aggravate and relieve pain)	Can reduce pain, analgesic use, and length of hospital stay	Postoperative pain, chronic pain
Contingency management[a]	CM involves the manipulation of environmental consequences of pain behavior in a way that helps patients to modify their behavior; it involves use of social reinforcers to increase "well behavior" (eg, exercise, nonmedical conversation) and decrease "sick role" behavior	Refers to methods not for treating the pain per se but rather helping patients to change behaviors. Studies suggest that CM effectively reduces pain	Chronic pain
CBT	CBT combines cognitive therapy techniques (eg, attention diversion) with behavioral techniques (eg, relaxation, assertiveness training); there are two major CBT subtypes: cognitive restructuring and coping skills training	Helps patients alter their perceptions or labeling of pain (ie, decrease negative thoughts, emotions, and beliefs), increase sense of control, and decrease maladaptive behaviors	Chronic pain especially, but also useful for acute pain
Cognitive restructuring	Type of CBT in which patients are taught to monitor and evaluate negative thoughts	The goal is to generate more accurate and adaptive thoughts	Chronic pain
Coping skills training	Type of CBT that helps patients develop coping skills, which includes relaxation and imagery techniques, adaptive coping self-statements, and group psychotherapy	Directed at helping patients to develop skills to manage pain and stress	Multiple types of pain (see below)

Therapy	Description	Types of pain
Relaxation with imagery	Includes progressive muscle relaxation, imagery, visualization, and meditation One of most widely used nonpharmacologic treatments for pain that can increase focus on feelings of well-being as well as diminish tension, anxiety, depression, and pain-related inactivity.[b]	Postoperative pain, chronic headache, chronic LBP, cancer pain, arthritis pain, labor pain, TMD
Hypnosis	Technique in which a patient's susceptibility to suggestion is heightened, facilitating modification of memory and perception; hypnosis can be used alone or as a means of enhancing the effectiveness of another clinical intervention[b]	Postoperative, burn, dental, labor, cancer, procedural, neuropathic, and musculoskeletal pain; headache
Distraction	Includes repeating reaffirming phrases, singing, talking, etc., to distract attention from unpleasant awareness of pain; in patients with CNCP, it also may include social and recreational activities	Multiple acute and chronic types of pain
	Hypnosis may provide comfort and reduce anxiety and suffering associated with acute, recurrent, and chronic types of pain; it reduces cortical activation associated with painful stimuli The goal is for the patient to actively occupy his or her attention with an activity or topic other than pain	
Biofeedback	Patient learns to take voluntary control over physiological body activities by receiving input (eg, visual or auditory cues) about these activities (eg, heart beat, muscle tension, skin temperature) Directed at teaching a patient how to take control of body responses by way of mental activity	Most support for use with vascular HA; also used for chronic LBP and other HA, myofascial pain, rectal pain
Psychotherapy	Treatment for a mental illness or maladaptive behaviors that involves a therapist establishing a relationship with a patient to achieve certain goals; includes individual (supportive and dynamic), group, and family psychotherapy Goals of psychotherapy include modifying symptoms, changing maladaptive behaviors, and promoting growth and development	Chronic pain, cancer pain, pain associated with HIV infection

[a]The terms "contingency management" and "operant conditioning" are used interchangeably. Overlap exists between CM and CBT, but CM focuses more on modifying behavior and CBT helps more with altering patient perceptions or labeling of sensations. (Fordyce, W. E. [2001]. Operant or contingency therapies. In J. S. Loeser, et al. [Eds.], *Bonica's management of pain* [3rd ed.] Baltimore, MD: Lippincott Williams & Wilkins.)

[b]These methods can be taught quickly but patients do best with encouragement from health care professionals and family members. Audiotapes and printed materials also can be helpful.[24]

CBT: cognitive-behavioral therapy; CM: contingency management; CNCP: chronic noncancer pain; HA: headache; HIV: human immunodeficiency virus; LBP: low back pain; TMD: temporomandibular disorder.

Berry P. H., Chapman C. R., Covington E. C., et al (2001). *Pain: Current understanding of assessment, management, and treatments.* Reston VA: National Pharmaceutical Council and the Joint Commission for Accreditation of Healthcare Organizations.

TABLE 30–7 Examples of Physical Methods Used to Manage Pain

Intervention	Definition	Purpose/Goals	Examples of Uses
Stretching	Gentle exercise to improve flexibility	Improve ROM, function, comfort	Arthritis, LBP, fibromyalgia, myofascial pain syndrome
Exercise/ reconditioning	Reconditioning exercises can improve strength and endurance as well as combat stiffness and weakness associated with pain-related inactivity	Useful in regaining muscle and tendon strength, as well as improving ROM, endurance, comfort, and function. Transforms painful activities into more easily tolerated ones. Minimizes atrophy, demineralization, and deconditioning	Arthritis, LBP, fibromyalgia, CRPS
Gait and posture training	Appropriate attention to gait and posture, including preventive and therapeutic ergonomics	Relieve pain and restore function; prophylaxis against further pain	LBP, neck pain, tension HA
Applied heat or cold	Application of cold (cryotherapy) to decrease pain and swelling and improve function; later application of heat (thermotherapy) to augment performance and diminish pain	Application of cold produces local analgesia, slows nerve conduction, and promotes tendon flexibility. Application of heat produces local analgesia, dilates (widens) blood vessels, and promotes flexibility	Acute trauma (eg, injury, surgery); repetitive trauma, arthritis, muscle pain or spasm, acute LBP
Immobilization	Reduction of activity and avoidance of strain for certain duration; may involve brace to assist, restrict, or limit function of joint	May be needed to maintain proper alignment during post-injury repair but is generally harmful for patients with CNCP	Some postoperative, injury (eg, fracture)

TENS	Selective stimulation of cutaneous receptors sensitive to mechanical stimuli (mechanoreceptors) by applying low-intensity current via skin electrodes[a]	TENS can reduce pain and analgesic use and improve physical mobility, presumably by interfering with transmission of nociceptive impulses in nerve fibers	Trauma, postoperative, labor, abdominal pain; neuralgias, other neuropathic pain, PVD, angina, musculoskeletal pain
PNS SCS IC	Electrical stimulation of selected regions of the nervous system via implantable devices[b]	The goal of electrical stimulation is to disrupt nociceptive signaling	Chronic pain of the trunk and limbs (eg, PVD), neuropathic pain (deafferentation, poststroke pain), cancer pain
Massage	Rubbing of painful or nonpainful adjacent area	Facilitates relaxation and decreases muscle tension and pain	Postoperative pain, arthritis, fibromyalgia
Acupuncture	Old Chinese healing technique involves insertion of fine needles into the skin at varying depths; application of pressure at acupuncture sites is called acupressure	Acupuncture may cause the secretion of endorphins and interfere with transmission of nociceptive information to relieve pain	Postoperative, radiculopathy, chronic LBP, fibromyalgia

[a]TENS appears to work best when applied to skin close to the pain's site of origin and when sense of touch and pressure are preserved.

[b]The implanted portion of the device consists of a pulse generator and leads connected to electrodes located in fascia in close proximity to a peripheral nerve (PNS), the spinal canal (SCS), or brain (IC). The patient or clinician controls stimulation using nonimplanted system components.

CNCP: chronic noncancer pain; CRPS: chronic regional pain syndrome types I and II; HA: headache; IC: intracerebral stimulation; LBP: lower back pain; PNS: peripheral nerve stimulation; PVD: peripheral vascular disease; ROM: range of motion; SCS: spinal cord stimulation; TENS: transcutaneous electrical nerve stimulation.

Berry P. H., Chapman C. R., Covington E. C., et al, (2001). *Pain: Current understanding of assessment, management, and treatments.* Reston VA: National Pharmaceutical Council and the Joint Commission for Accreditation of Healthcare Organizations.

TABLE 30–8 Common Opioids for Cancer Pain

Drug	Route	Equi-Analgesic Dose (mg)[a]	Peak Effect (h)	Duration of Effect (h)	Comments
Oxycodone	PO	30	0.5	3–6	No ceiling dose if given without fixed combinations; parenteral formulation not available.
	PO SR			12	
Morphine	PO	30–60	1.5–2.0	4–6	Many oral formulations for individual patient needs.
	PO SR	30–60	2.0–3.0	8–12	
	IV/IM	10	0.5–1.0	3–5	
Hydromorphone	PO	7.5	1.0–2.0	3–4	Good choice for subcutaneous route due to potency.
	PR	Unknown	Unknown	Unknown	
	IV/IM	1.5	0.5–1.0	3–4	
Meperidine	PO	300	1.0–2.0	3–6	Not preferred due to CNS toxic metabolite that accumulates in renal failure.
	IV/IM	75	0.5–1.0	2–3	
Levorphanol	PO	4.0	1.0–2.0	6–8	Long T2 (11 hours) necessitates slow dose titration. Drug accumulation may occur.
	IV/IM	2.0	1.0–1.5	6–8	
Fentanyl	TD	Unknown	72	12 or >0.5–1.0	Short T2 (<1 hour). TD dose titration difficult with depot in subcutaneous adipose tissue. Transdermal fentanyl 25 µg/h approx = 45 mg/day oral morphine.
	IV/IM	0.1	<1.0		
Methadone	PO	20	4.0	4–6	Despite long T2 (15–150+ hours), duration of analgesia is not prolonged; however drug accumulation can result in toxicities. Caution is warranted when converting to methadone in patients with high opioid tolerance.
	IV/IM	10	0.5–1.5	4–6	
Butorphanol	IN	2	1.0	3–4	Mixed agonist–antagonist may precipitate withdrawal in patient previously receiving a pure agonist, thus not generally recommended for cancer pain.
	IV/IM	2	0.5–1.0	3–4	

[a]Approximate potency relative to 10 mg of parenteral morphine.

PO = oral; IV = intravenous; SQ = subcutaneous; IN = intranasal; TD = transdermal; (?) = unknown.

Caution: Cross-tolerance between opioids is incomplete. Use caution when performing equianalgesic conversions. Titrate to clinical response.

Drugs of choice for severe cancer-related pain. Opioids do not have an analgesic ceiling effect, and, therefore, dose can be titrated to achieve maximum pain relief.

Constipation is an almost universal complication of opioid use, so all patients should receive prophylactic stimulant laxative therapy unless otherwise contraindicated (eg, by chronic diarrhea).

Sedation is a frequent side effect of initial opioid use; however, tolerance develops soon in most patients.

Respiratory depression rarely occurs except in opioid-naive patients and those with significant pulmonary disease.

True hypersensitivity reactions to opioids are rare. If patients experience such reactions, it is often possible to administer an opioid from another subclass safely.

The subclasses are: phenanthrene derivatives—morphine, codeine, hydromorphone, oxycodone; phenylpiperidine derivatives—merperidine, fentanyl; diphenylheptane derivatives—methadone.

The use of opioid antagonists, such as naloxone, can immediately reverse all opioid effects, including analgesia. Such reversal results in acute withdrawal, which may be complicated by excruciating pain and seizure. Therefore, opioid antagonists are never recommended to reverse non–life-threatening effects, such as confusion or sedation. If used to reverse life-threatening respiratory depression or hypotension, they should be titrated cautiously.

Oral is the preferred route of administration, except for patients who cannot take or tolerate oral medications. When given in appropriate doses, oral opioids are as efficacious as parenteral opioids.

Rectal and transdermal dosage forms are available and are effective noninvasive alternatives when oral medication is not possible.

Rectal suppositories are contraindicated if lesions of the rectum or anus are present.

Repetitive intramuscular (IM) and subcutaneous (SQ) injections should be avoided because they are painful and absorption is inconsistent.

Intravenous (IV) administration may be used when less invasive routes are ineffective or unavailable. IV opioids may be given by bolus or continuous administration (including PCA); however, they require careful monitoring during titration. Inappropriately excessive dosing may carry significant risk of respiratory depression, especially in opioid-naive patients or those with underlying pulmonary pathology.

Low-volume continuous SQ infusion may also be used if venous access is not established.

IV or SQ PCA provides a good steady level of analgesia. It is widely accepted by patients but requires special infusion pumps and staff education. It may not be appropriate for patients with altered mental status or agitation.

Epidural and intrathecal opioids provide good analgesia, when suitable. These routes have significant risk of respiratory depression, which may be delayed, necessitating careful monitoring. Special preservative-free drug formulations are necessary for these routes of administration.

Jacox, S., Carr, D., Payne, R., et al. (1994). Management of cancer pain: Clinical practice guideline No. 9 (AHCPR Publication No. 94-0592; p. 63). Rockville, MD: Agency for Health Care Policy and Research, U.S. Dept of Health and Human Services.

    c. Adjuvant analgesics: Drugs that have analgesic activity that is not their primary indication, or drugs that help with side effects of opioids. They include antidepressants, anticonvulsants, corticosteroids, and psychostimulants (Table 30–9).

  2. Definitions related to analgesic administration

    a. *Tolerance:* Physiologic response in which, after repeated administration, a given opioid begins to lose its effectiveness. Patients report a decrease in duration of pain relief.

    b. *Psychological dependence* ("addiction"): Behavior exhibiting overwhelming involvement with obtaining and using a drug for its psychic effects rather than its intended medical reasons. It is rare in patients who require opioids for legitimate medical reasons.

    c. *Physiologic dependence:* Physiologic response in which withdrawal will occur if opioids are abruptly discontinued.

D. Nursing Diagnoses

  1. Pain related to cancer or cancer treatment

    a. *Problem:* Pain can be caused by many factors and not all of them are known before initiating treatment. Because pain can occur at any time during a patient's illness, ongoing assessment is essential. Unrelieved pain is debilitating and emotionally exhausting, and contributes to worsening of other symptoms. It has a deleterious effect on a patient's and family's quality of life.

    b. *Interventions:* These vary based on the findings from a comprehensive assessment.

      (1) Treat the underlying malignancy with radiation, chemotherapy, or surgery.

      (2) Administer nonopioid and opioid analgesics through a variety of routes.

      (3) Teach behavioral, cognitive, and cutaneous techniques to help relieve pain.

    c. *Desired outcomes*

      (1) Patient will maintain a satisfactory level of relief, as evaluated by the patient and family.

      (2) Patient will be able to tolerate side effects, as evaluated by the patient and family.

      (3) Patient will achieve a maximal quality of life, as evidenced by participation in important activities and family interaction.

  2. Painful constipation

    a. *Problem:* Patient may experience abdominal pain due to constipation resulting from analgesic use.

    b. *Interventions:* Follow recommendations in Chapter 23 and Box 30–1.

    c. *Desired outcome:* Patient will eliminate constipation and be able to continue using analgesics for pain relief.

E. Discharge Planning and Patient Education

  1. Tell the patient about who is responsible for managing pain.

  2. Explain short- and long-term goals, including plans for follow-up.

  3. Teach the patient to report unrelieved or worsening pain, presence of new pain, and unacceptable side effects to pain therapies.

  4. Discuss common side effects of pain treatment and appropriate actions to prevent or relieve symptoms (Table 30–10).

TABLE 30–9 Commonly Used Adjuvant Analgesics for Cancer Pain

Drug Category	Indications	Drugs	Common Toxicities	Comments
Antidepressants	Neuropathic pain	Amitriptyline Nortriptyline Desipramine	Sedation, dry mouth, constipation, postural hypotension, urinary retention	Begin with low doses 10–25 mg, increase dose every few days, expect to see pain relief within several days, mood elevation within several weeks
Anticonvulsants	Neuropathic pain, myoclonic jerks	Phenytoin Carbamazepine Valproic acid Clonazepam Gabapentin	Drowsiness, dizziness, nausea, rash, bone marrow depression	Use loading dose with phenytoin; monitor platelets with carbamazepine
Psychostimulants	Opioid-induced sedation	Dextroamphetamine Methylphenidate Modafinil	Nervousness, irritability, insomnia, dizziness, dry mouth	Give early in the day to avoid insomnia; do not use if patient is already delirious or confused
Corticosteroids	Spinal cord compression, increased intracranial pressure, visceral distention	Decadron Methylprednisolone Prednisone	Gastritis, insomnia, fluid retention, hyperglycemia, proximal myopathy, increased appetite	
Muscle relaxants	Muscle spasm	Diazepam Baclofen Methocarbamol Cyclobenzaprine	Sedation, dizziness, nausea, weakness, confusion	

(continued)

TABLE 30-9 Commonly Used Adjuvant Analgesics for Cancer Pain (Continued)

Drug Category	Indications	Drugs	Common Toxicities	Comments
Benzodiazepines	Muscle spasm, anxiety, insomnia, myoclonus	Diazepam Lorazepam Alprazolam Temazepam Midazolam	Sedation, delirium, hypotension, headache, respiratory depression	Not analgesics, synergistic effect with opioids can cause respiratory depression
Antispasmodics	GI or bladder spasm	Diphenoxylate and atropine Loperamide Scopolamine patch Dicyclomine	Sedation, dry mouth, constipation	
Neuroleptics	Delirium, agitation, nausea and vomiting, hiccoughs	Methotrimeprazine, haloperidol, prochlorperazine, chlorpromazine	Sedation, orthostatic hypotension, confusion, extrapyramidal reactions	Useful for symptoms other than pain; methotrimeprazine has analgesic properties
Bisphosphonates	Bone pain	Pamidrondate Zoledronic acid	Hypocalcemia, fever, GI disturbances, anemia	Delays time to painful skeletal events. Also used with analgesics for bone pain.

Grossman, S. A., & Nesbit, S. A. (2004). Cancer pain. In M. D. Abeloff et al. (Eds.). *Clinical oncology* (3rd ed.). Philadelphia: W. B. Saunders.

▨ TABLE 30–10 Common Side Effcects of Pain Treatment

Side Effect	Management	Specific Agents
Constipation	Begin bowel program when initiating therapy. Combination of agents may be useful.	Stool softeners Irritants Bulk laxatives Lubricants Enemas
Nausea and vomiting	Treat with antiemetics; esp. phenothiazine and anticholinergic agents. Switch to another opiate.	Promethazine Prochlorperazine Scopolamine Hydroxyzine
Sedation	Use of stimulants.	Dextroamphetamine Methylphenidate
Pruritus	Treat with antihistamines. Consider another opiate, avoiding morphine.	Hydroxyzine Diphenhydramine
Myoclonus	Switch to another opiate or lower opiate dose. Avoid meperidine, especially in patients with impaired renal function.	
Withdrawal symptoms	Taper dose by 2 every other day when discontinuing.	Clonidine

Grossman, S. A. & Gregory, E. (1994). Pain. In Kirkwood, M. T., Lotze, M. T.,& Yasko, J. M. (Eds.). In *Current cancer therapeutics.* Philadelphia: Current Medicine.

5. Tell the patient to report to the health care provider if unable to take prescribed medications because of side effects, cost of medicines, or availability at pharmacy.
6. Encourage the patient to keep a pain diary, which would include pain intensity ratings, medications, and presence of side effects.
7. Give the patient age-related and educationally appropriate pain materials. These materials are available from the National Cancer Institute (1–800–4CANCER) and local chapters of the American Cancer Society.

REFERENCES

American Pain Society. (2003). *Principles of analgesic use in the treatment of acute pain and chronic cancer pain: A concise guide to medical practice* (5th ed.). Glenview, IL: Author.

American Pain Society Quality of Care Committee. (1995). Quality improvement guidelines for the treatment of acute pain and cancer pain. *Journal of the American Medical Association, 274,* 1874–1880.

Bosnjak, S., Jelic, S., Susnjar, S., & Luki, V. (2002). Gabapentin for relief of neuropathic pain related to anticancer treatment: A preliminary study. *Journal of Chemotherapy, 14,* 214–219.

Bruera, E., & Neumann, C. M. (1999). Role of methadone in the management of pain in cancer patients. *Oncology, 13,* 1275–1282.

Bruera, E., & Sweeney, C. (2002). Methadone use in cancer patients with pain: A review. *Journal of Palliative Medicine, 5,* 127–138.

Chapman, C. R., et al. (Eds.). (2001). *Bonica's management of pain* (3rd ed., pp. 17–25). Baltimore, MD: Lippincott Williams & Wilkins.

Chapman, C. R., & Foley, K. (Eds.). (1993). Current and emerging issues in cancer pain: Research and practice. Philadelphia: Lippincott-Raven. Available: http://talaria.org/chtoc.html.

Chapman, C. R., & Nakamura, Y. (1999). A passion of the soul: An introduction to pain for consciousness researchers. *Consciousness and Cognition, 8,* 391–422.

Cherny, N. I. (2001). Cancer pain: Principles of assessment and syndromes. In A. M. Berger, R. K. Portenoy & D. E. Weissman (Eds.), *Principles and practice of supportive oncology* (pp. 3–42). Philadelphia: Lippincott-Raven.

Chibnal, J. T. (2001). Pain assessment in cognitively impaired and unimpaired older adults: A comparison of four scales. *Pain, 92,* 173–186.

Coda, B. A., & Bonica, J. J. (2001). General considerations of acute pain. In J. D. Loeser, S. H. Butler, C. R. Chapman, et al. (Eds.), *Bonica's management of pain* (3rd ed., pp. 222–240). Baltimore, MD: Lippincott Williams & Wilkins.

Curtiss, C. P. (2001). JCAHO: Meeting the standards for pain management. *Orthopedic Nursing, 20,* 27–30.

Dunajcik, L. (1999). Chronic nonmalignant pain. In M. McCaffery & C. Pasero (Eds.), *Pain clinical manual* (2nd ed., pp. 467–521). St. Louis, MO: Mosby.

Fordyce, W. E. (2001). Operant or contingency therapies. In J. S. Loeser, et al. (Eds.), *Bonica's management of pain* (3rd ed.). Baltimore, MD: Lippincott Williams & Wilkins.

Grossman, S. A. (1999). Management of cancer pain: National Comprehensive Cancer Network guidelines. *Oncology, 13,* 33–44.

Grossman, S. A., & Gregory, R. E. (1996). Pain. In J. M. Kirkwood, M. T. Lotze & J. M. Yasko (Eds), *Current cancer therapeutics* (2nd ed.). Philadelphia: Current Medicine.

Grossman, S. A., & Nesbit, S. A. (2004). In M. D. Abeloff et al. (Eds.), Clinical oncology (3rd ed.). Philadelphia: W. B. Saunders.

Grossman, S. A., Nesbit, S., & Loscalzo, M. (2002). *Hopkins opioid program—Conversions for the PDA* (Palm OS version). Available: www.hopkinskimmelcancercenter.org/specialtycenters/hop.cfm.

Grossman, S. A., Sheidler, V. R., McGuire, D. B., et al. (1992). A comparison of the Hopkins pain rating instrument with standard visual analogue and verbal descriptor scales in patients with cancer pain. *Journal of Pain and Symptom Management, 7,* 196–203.

Hortobagyi, G. N., Theriault, R. L., Lipton, A., et al. (1998). Long-term prevention of skeletal complications of metastatic breast cancer with pamidronate. *Journal of Clinical Oncology, 16,* 2038–2044.

Loscalzo, M. (2002). Psychological approaches to the management of pain in patients with advanced cancer. *Hematology/Oncology Clinics of North America, 10,* 139–155.

Magrum, L. C., Bentzen, C., & Landmark, S. (1996). Pain management in home care. *Seminars in Oncology Nursing, 12,* 202–218.

McGuire, D. B., & Sheidler, V. R. (1993). Cancer pain. In S. L. Groenwald, M. H. Frogge, M. Goodman & C. H. Yarbro (Eds.), *Cancer nursing: Principles and practice* (3rd ed.). Boston, MA: Jones & Bartlett.

McGuire, D. B., Yarbro, C. H., & Ferrell, B. R. (Eds.). (1995). *Cancer pain management* (2nd ed.). Boston, MA: Jones & Bartlett.

McQuay, H., Carroll, D., Jadad, A. R., et al. (1995). Anticonvulsant drugs for management of pain: A systematic review. *British Medical Journal, 311,* 1047–1052.

Moryl, N., Santiago-Palma, J., Kornick, C., et al. (2002). Pitfalls of opioid rotation: Substituting another opioid for methadone in patients with cancer pain. *Pain, 96,* 325–328.

Pereira, J., Lawlor, P., Vigano, A., et al. (2001). Equianalgesic dose ratios for opioids: A critical review and proposals for long-term dosing. *Journal of Pain and Symptom Management, 22,* 672–687.

Portenoy, R. (1989). Mechanisms of clinical pain. Observations and speculations. *Neurology Clinics of North America, 7,* 205–230.

Rhodes, D. J., Koshy, R., Sheidler, V. R., Waterfield, W., Wu, A., & Grossman, S. A.

(1998). Feasibility of quantitative pain assessment in outpatient oncology practice. *Journal of Clinical Oncology, 19,* 501–508.

Ripamonti, C., Groff, L., Brunelli, C., et al. (1998). Switching from morphine to oral methadone in treating cancer pain: What is the equianalgesic dose ratio? *Journal of Clinical Oncology, 16,* 3216–3221.

Rouff, G., & Lema, M. (2003). Strategies in pain management: New and potential indications for COX-2 specific inhibitors. *Journal of Pain Symptom Management, 25S,* S21-S31.

Seaman, J., & Knight, R. D. (1996). Efficacy of pamidronate in reducing skeletal events in patients with advanced multiple myeloma. *New England Journal of Medicine, 334,* 488–493.

Zech, D. F., Lehmann, K. A., Hertel, D., et al. (1995). Validation of World Health Organization guidelines for cancer pain relief: A 10-year prospective study. *Pain, 63,* 65–76.

31 Psychosocial Issues

Karin Taylor
Laura Herald Hoofring

I. Overview: The emotional responses to a diagnosis of cancer are varied and never static as patients and families make their way through their cancer journey. They often report feeling devastated, shocked, afraid, angry, sad, guilty, demoralized, anxious, depressed, confused, and out of control of their lives. Compounded by the physical problems brought on by their cancer and treatments, coping can be difficult. Fortunately, with assistance and support, many patients and families do well. Nurses can help patients and families. This chapter explores the influence of multiple factors on patients' and caregivers' coping, specific disorders that impede coping, and nurse interventions in caring for patients and families.

COPING WITH LIFE-THREATENING ILLNESS

I. Personality Characteristics

  A. A person's basic personality will affect how he or she responds to the diagnosis and treatment.

  B. These characteristics and responses are on a continuum.

  C. Usually, people respond to illness as they responded to life and stressors in the past.

  D. Stress will make personality characteristics more pronounced.

  E. It is important to find out what they were like before their illness (their premorbid personality [PMP]).

  F. It is important to get feedback from the family or significant others regarding the patient's usual presentation and ways he or she now is different.

  G. Examples:

    1. People who tend to like control will have more anxiety because of their lack of control.

    2. People who withdraw when anxious will do so more now.

    3. People who are optimistic will generally meet their diagnosis and treatment with optimism.

II. Life Story

  A. What people have experienced in their lives that has shaped their view of themselves and the world around them

  B. Assessment

    1. Helpfulness of support systems in the past

    2. Past successes and failures

    3. Past experience with illness and death

    4. How they dealt with past challenges

III. Current Life Role
  A. What their role is now; can be multiple (eg, mother, teacher, daughter, wife, and so forth).
  B. Includes age-specific tasks and determines the demands placed on them.
  C. How have they changed because of their diagnosis or treatment?
  D. What has changed for others in the family because of cancer?
  E. Who depends on them and who will take over their care?
  F. Do they have support systems and how do they use them?

IV. Their life story and personality characteristics along with their current life roles have much to do with their reaction to their diagnoses and treatment.
  A. The interaction of all three can determine the amount and type of emotions they experience (eg, anxiety, optimism, anger).
  B. Concern develops when their emotions and response are different and troublesome from past periods of adversity. This may indicate a greater problem with mood or adjustment, and intervention may be needed.
  C. Include family members' assessment regarding any change.

V. Culture
  A. Lens through which patients and families interpret and understand their experiences.
    1. Practices, beliefs, values
      a. Illness beliefs
      b. Health practices
      c. Death rituals
      d. Family relationships
      e. Symptom management
      f. Activities of daily living
      g. Food practices
    2. Language
  B. Being aware and respectful of the cultural differences of patient, family, and staff is essential to providing good care.
  C. Assessment
    1. Practices, beliefs, values
    2. Impact of the patient's and family's cultural practices, beliefs, and values on their understanding of their illness and treatments
  D. Interventions
    1. Ensure that the plan of care reflects the cultural beliefs, values, and practices of the patient and family.
    2. Seek assistance (eg, experts, literature) to help overcome barriers and increase understanding.

VI. Existential Factors
  A. Meaning of the Illness: Finding meaning or making sense of the illness
    1. Evolves and changes over time.
    2. Reflects each person's interpretation of the disease, treatments and circumstances.
    3. Many variables (eg, culture, past experiences, religion/spirituality, and so forth) influence the meaning that patients and caregivers ascribe to the illness and experiences.
    4. Differences between nurse's own "meanings" of the illness and those of patients and families can be a source of conflict.

     5. Assessment

       a. How have you made sense or what meaning have you found in what is happening to you/your loved one?

B. Suffering

     1. Cancer diagnosis makes people think of pain, suffering, and death.

     2. Has physical, psychological, emotional, and spiritual components for each patient and family member.

     3. Is closely connected to one's sense of the meaning of the illness and circumstances.

     4. Uncontrolled symptoms can increase one's sense of suffering and greatly affect one's sense of hope.

     5. Past experiences with suffering will affect how patients and families respond.

     6. Assessment

       a. Do you have concerns about physical suffering?

       b. What can nurses do to minimize or eliminate any suffering you may experience?

C. Hope

     1. Described as the "activating force of the human spirit" (Fromm).

     2. Patient's and family's sense of hope will be ever-changing and redefined throughout their or their loved ones' illness.

     3. Treatments received, nurses, physicians, and other health care providers are often seen as sources of hope for patients and families.

     4. At times, patients/families may appear to have "unrealistic" hope.

       a. May be needed as a coping mechanism to "protect" their emotional well-being at that time

       b. Becomes concerning if it prevents them from attending to timely concerns (eg, making a will)

     5. Loss of hope can lead to feelings of apathy and meaninglessness and can be a significant indication of major depression (see section below on Major Depression).

     6. Assessment.

       a. What are the things in your life that you are hoping will happen?

       b. If a cure is not possible, what are your hopes for the time you have?

D. Spirituality/Religion

     1. Spirituality speaks to issues of transcendence, interconnectedness, and meaningfulness.

     2. Religion is a specific view with a belief system and is expressed through rituals, practices, and observances.

     3. Is often a sustaining factor in helping patient/family find meaning and hope in the illness and experience.

     4. Studies have repeatedly shown that those with spiritual/religious beliefs have higher sense of well-being.

     5. Assessment.

       a. What role does faith or spirituality play in your life?

       b. What role has it taken in difficult times?

E. Interventions

     1. Honor the importance of your relationship with patients and families.

2. Educate and manage symptoms to increase patient's and family's sense of control and well-being, thus decreasing suffering and increasing hope.
3. Assist in their search for positive meanings and hope by listening, normalizing, validating, and reframing.
4. Assist in setting attainable and realistic goals.
5. Make appropriate referrals (eg, chaplains and clergy, social workers, psychiatric nurses, and psychiatrists) as needed.
6. Assist the patient and family in practicing their religious beliefs (eg, have a Muslim patient's bed face east toward Mecca for prayers, assist an Orthodox Jewish patient in getting kosher foods).

VII. Loss and Grief

A. Definition: A *loss* is an experience in which a person loses connection to a valued object, relationship, situation, or part of self. *Grief* is the natural human response to loss. Grieving is the process of responding to the loss through thoughts, feelings, and behaviors.
B. The losses that patients and families experience are numerous and can be physical, social, occupational, financial, emotional, relational, and spiritual in nature.
C. Many variables affect the response(s) a patient and family have to a loss or losses.
  1. Meaning of the loss
  2. Personality (see section above on Personality Characteristics)
  3. Age and developmental level
  4. Resources and support
  5. Reactions of others
  6. Past experiences with loss and grief
  7. Coping patterns
  8. Cultural values and beliefs
D. There are physical and emotional characteristics in the stages of loss and grief that patients and families experience (Table 31–1).

TABLE 31–1 Physical and Emotional Characteristics of Stages of Loss and Grief

Stage	Characteristics
Shock and disbelief	Emotional and physical denial of loss
Developing awareness	Crying, angry outbursts, shortness of breath, choked feelings, sighing, flashes of anguish, retelling the story, painful dejection, and changes in eating, sleeping, and sexual interest
Bargaining and restitution	Idealizing the loss and contracting for reprieve or deliverance
Accepting the loss	Reliving past experiences, preoccupation with thoughts of loss, painful void in life, crying, somatic symptoms, dreams or nightmares
Resolving the loss	Establishing new relationships, planning for the future, recalling rich memories or past experiences, affirming oneself, and resuming previous roles

  E. Interventions
   1. Encourage patients and families to talk about their losses and grief. Give them permission to grieve.
   2. Provide safe, nonjudgmental environment that allows them to express both positive and negative feelings.
   3. Listen carefully and normalize and validate their feelings and experiences.
   4. Facilitate coping.
      a. Identify effective coping skills.
      b. Make referrals to support groups, bereavement groups, and counseling.
      c. Educate them about expected thoughts, feelings, and behaviors associated with loss and grief and roadblocks to the grief process (eg, social isolation, closed communication).
   5. Encourage use of cultural, religious, and social customs and rituals associated with loss and grief.
   6. Monitor for signs of dysfunctional grieving, which occurs when the grieving process interferes with the usual level of functioning.
      a. Physical changes or decline in physical or psychosocial functioning
      b. Social withdrawal
      c. Critical changes in behavior (eg, oversedation, emotional extremes [guilt, anger, hostility], depression, substance abuse, expression of suicidal intentions) should be reported and appropriate referrals initiated. (See sections below on Major Depression and Suicide, and Substance Abuse/Dependence.)

VIII. Intimacy and Sexuality
  A. Many factors may alter one's sexual health and intimacy with his or her partner.
   1. Changes in physical appearance
   2. Fatigue, pain, and other symptoms associated with cancer and treatment
   3. Surgeries (prostatectomy, hysterectomy, mastectomy, ostomies)
   4. Side effects of medications and treatment that impair libido and sexual gratification
   5. Fear and anxiety
   6. Lack of knowledge
   7. Embarrassment
  B. Alterations can cause a great deal of distress.
   1. Stress and breakdown in relationships
   2. Decrease one's sense of quality of life
   3. Lower one's self-esteem or sense of worth
  C. Often not addressed by nurses and physicians.
   1. Discomfort
      a. Important for nurses to assess their beliefs and comfort related to sexuality and seek education/supervision
   2. Time limitations especially in outpatient settings
   3. Readiness of the patient to discuss sexual health
   4. Lack of knowledge/resources
   5. Seen as an unimportant issue in context of their disease and treatment
  D. Interventions

1. Assess patient's and partner's level of concern and knowledge related to intimacy and sexuality.
   a. Ask open-ended questions: "Many patients with cancer notice changes or problems in their sex lives. Do you have any problems or concerns related to your sexuality?"
   b. Ask about premorbid sexual health to provide basis of understanding of current concerns or problems.
2. Provide safe, open, and nonjudgmental environment when discussing patient's sexual health.
3. If uncomfortable discussing sexual issues, make appropriate referrals to convey a sense of importance and care for the patient's sexual health.
4. Patient/partner education.
   a. Changes secondary to their treatments as related to their sexual health and functioning
   b. Alternative positions for sexual intercourse that may be more comfortable
   c. Use of assistive devices
      (1) Lubricants
      (2) Vaginal dilators
   d. Alternatives to intercourse that provide intimacy: Massage, cuddling, hand holding, manual stimulation, and so forth
   e. Times when sexual activity should be avoided
   f. Medication side effects
   g. Reproductive information
      (1) Egg and sperm banking
      (2) Use of condoms and birth control
5. Informational resources for nurses, patients, and partners.
   a. American Cancer Society—www.cancer.org
   b. National Cancer Institute—www.cancer.gov
   c. Cancer Care—www.cancercare.org

IX. Demoralization
A. Definition: Inability to tolerate the adversity they are experiencing.
B. Often occurs in relationship to physical symptoms, discomfort, or losses.
C. It can be difficult to differentiate from major depression.
D. In demoralization (unlike major depression):
   1. Mood usually improves as their physical state improves.
   2. Patients rarely believe they deserve to suffer.
E. Other causes of mood changes can be medications (steroids, interferon), a delirious state, or anxiety.
F. Presentation.
   1. Mood may be sad, anxious, irritable, depressed, or angry.
   2. They may be withdrawn, demanding, depressed, uncooperative, or suicidal.
   3. This can be a normal reaction to a difficult situation caused by the diagnosis of cancer.
G. Other factors besides their medical condition can cause this response, such as difficulties with family relationships, financial stressors (see sections above on Personality Characteristics, Life Story, and Current Life Role).

H. Interventions.
1. Take physical complaints seriously (pain, nausea, anxiety) and treat.
2. Assess for mood and symptom relief.
3. Increase the choices the patient can make.
4. Encourage the patient to communicate thoughts and feelings and to specify what is difficult.
    a. *Examples:* Diagnosis, physical symptoms, role changes.
    b. Find out what the patient understands about the illness or situation.
    c. Learn about the patient's usual personality characteristics.
5. Normalize the patient's reaction by letting him or her know that many people experience uncomfortable emotions when dealing with cancer.
6. Communicate understanding of the situation. This validates the patient's experience (Slavney, 1998).
7. Let the patient know you understand what he or she is saying, how it makes "sense" in context of adversity.
8. Review coping strategies used in the past.
    a. What worked? What has the patient tried now?
    b. Problem solve which ones to use now.
9. Help the patient make "sense" of his or her response by examining personality characteristics, life story, and role (eg, independent, take-charge person has more difficulty with the dependent role of a patient).
10. Reframe the experience from different perspectives (eg, grandparents caring for children while the patient is too ill gives the grandparents opportunity to bond with their grandchildren rather than it being a burden).
11. Assess the patient's level of knowledge regarding illness and treatment, and teach.
12. Help patient identify resources and support systems including spiritual support if applicable.
13. Use hospital supports of social work and pastoral care.
14. If mood is still low, consider referral to rule out major depression.

DISORDERS THAT IMPEDE COPING

I. Major Depression and Suicide
A. Definition: A state of feeling sad, discouraged, hopeless, helpless, worthless that is present daily for most of the day. Patients experience excessive guilt with disturbances in thinking, concentration, or decision making. They can present as sad, tearful, angry, or irritable.
B. Differential Diagnoses
1. Delirium
2. Demoralization
3. Substance abuse
C. Untreated depression in the medically ill patient results in an increase in hospital days, an increase in medical complications, and a decrease in the quality of life.
D. Prevalence

1. Overall major depression is a common clinical problem with a prevalence of 5% to 9% for women and 2% to 3% for men.
2. Chronic medical illness predisposes patients to depression. Cancer is no exception with rates ranging from 23% to 60% (Newport & Nemeroff, 1998).
3. Certain types of cancer are known to have higher rates of depression.
   a. Pancreatic 50%
   b. Oropharynx 22% to 40%
   c. Breast 10% to 32%
   d. Colon 13% to 25%
   e. GYN 23% (Newport & Nemeroff, 1998)

E. Etiology
1. It is thought that major depression is caused by a chemical imbalance in the brain possibly involving serotonin and/or norepinephrine.
2. Stressful life events may also precipitate neurochemical changes.
3. Risk factors include a personal or family history of depression.
4. Substance abuse can precipitate or mimic the symptoms of a major depression.
5. Some medications or medical conditions can precipitate or mimic a depressive episode: hypothyroidism, Cushing's syndrome, hypercalcemia, steroids, interferon, amphotericin B, tamoxifen, metoclopramide, L-asparaginase, procarbazine, vinblastine, vincristine, cyproterone (Newport & Nemeroff, 1998).

F. Assessment (Box 31–1)
1. Five or more of the symptoms found in Box 31–1.
2. Must include a low/depressed mood or anhedonia, which is the loss of pleasure or interest.
3. Start by asking if the person feels depressed or low for most of the day.
4. Ask if the patient (or family member) has ever experienced a depressive episode before their cancer diagnosis.
   a. Did they take any medication for this?
   b. What was the medication, dose, and did it help?
   c. Who prescribed the medication? How long did they take it and why did they stop?

G. Interventions for Major Depression
1. Spend time with the patient; encourage them to tell you about thoughts/feelings, what this experience has been like (see IX.H.).
2. Monitor for improvement or worsening of symptoms.
3. Inform physician of concerns regarding symptoms.
4. Initiate referrals for psychiatric, spiritual consultation, or social work, if appropriate.
5. A lack of motivation is a symptom of depression.
   a. If a patient does not participate in ADLs and is physically able to, evaluate for major depression or delirium.
6. Give encouragement and teaching about major depression.
7. Assist with ADLs.
8. Encourage patient to be active with PT/OT consult, if appropriate.

▼ **BOX 31-1** | **DSM IV Criteria for Major Depressive Episode**

Five (or more) of the following symptoms have been present during the same 2-week period and represent a change from previous functioning; at least one of the symptoms is either (1) depressed mood or (2) loss of interest or pleasure. **Symptoms cannot be the result of a medical condition or treatment (eg, loss of appetite while receiving chemotherapy).**

- Depressed mood most of the day, nearly every day. *"Rate your mood between one and ten." "Have you ever felt this bad before? When was that?" "Tell me about your mood." "How long have you been feeling this way?" "Does anything make you feel better?" "Do you feel hopeful?"*
- Markedly diminished interest or pleasure in all, or almost all, activities most of the day, nearly every day. *"Is there anything you still enjoy or get enjoyment from?" "Do you derive pleasure from anything (for example, children, grandchildren, friends, hobbies)?"*
- *Significant weight loss when not dieting or weight gain or decrease or increase in appetite nearly every day. *"What are you eating?" "Are you forcing yourself to eat?"*
- *Insomnia or excess sleep nearly every day. "Do you have a hard time getting to sleep or waking up early?" "How many hours a day do you sleep and is this an increase or decrease for you?"
- Psychomotor agitation or retardation nearly every day. *Is the person very slow in verbal responses? Does he or she move slowly or move quickly and appear anxious?*
- *Fatigue or loss of energy nearly every day. *"Do you have the energy to accomplish what you want to do?" Observe what they do each day versus what they are physically able to perform.*
- Feelings of worthlessness or excessive or inappropriate guilt nearly every day (not merely self-reproach or guilt about being sick). *"Do you think you deserve to go through this experience?" "Do you think you are a good person?" "Have you been feeling guilty about anything?"*
- *Diminished ability to think or concentrate, or indecisiveness, nearly every day. *Observe the patient's ability to read, hold conversations, answer questions, and make decisions.*
- Recurrent thoughts of death, recurrent suicidal ideation with a specific plan, or a suicide attempt or a specific plan for committing suicide. *"Do you have any thoughts of harming yourself or killing yourself?" "Do you ever wish you would just not wake up in the morning or you would die from your treatment?"*

---

*Many of oncology patients' depressive symptoms can be accounted for from the illness or treatment.

Adapted from the *Diagnostic and statistical manual of mental disorder,* fourth edition. Copyright American Psychiatric Association, 1994.

H. Passive Death Wish: The wish to die or not wake up but has no plan or intent to harm oneself. This is not uncommon for the demoralized patient as well as the patient with depression.

   1. This thought can become more pronounced when depression or anxiety increases or their physical state declines.

   2. It can decrease as they become healthier or less depressed.

   3. Monitor these thoughts if they become more active (eg, more frequent, intense, or encompass a plan). See section below on Suicide.

I. Suicide

   1. Take statements of wanting to die and harm self seriously.

   2. Always ask! You will not put the thought in their head.

   3. Active suicidal ideation: They have a plan.

      a. What is it?

      b. Are they able to accomplish it (eg, pills, physical ability)?

      c. Do they have access to a gun?

   4. Interventions for suicide (see sections on Depression and Demoralization)

      a. Protect. Do not leave alone and keep environment safe (eg, no knives, glass).

      b. Observe that they take all medications.

      c. Inpatient—Psychiatric consult and follow hospital protocol.

      d. Outpatient—Seen in emergency department for an evaluation.

J. Pharmacologic Treatment for Major Depression

   1. Antidepressants are prescribed because etiology is biochemical (Tables 31–2 and 31–3).

   2. Antidepressants are equally effective and are often chosen by the side-effect profile that will be compatible for the patient.

TABLE 31–2 Selective Serotonin Reuptake Inhibitors (SSRI): Side Effects and Nursing Considerations

Side Effects	Nursing Considerations
Nausea	Administer medications with meals or at bedtime; tolerance can develop
Diarrhea	Bland diet; adequate hydration; lower dose temporarily; antidiarrheal drugs
Insomnia	Dose as early in the day as possible; good sleep regimen; use relaxation techniques; omit caffeine; lower dose
Dry mouth	Encourage adequate hydration; sugar-free lozenges and gum
Nervousness (fluoxetine)	Use relaxation techniques; lower dose; change to a different antidepressant
Headache (fluoxetine)	Medicate with mild analgesics; lower dose; change to a different antidepressant
Sexual dysfunction	Take daily dose after sexual intercourse, not immediately before
Drowsiness (paroxetine)	Dose at bedtime; encourage daytime activity; avoid using machinery
Sweating (paroxetine)	Good hygiene; good hydration; cotton clothing

Laraia, M. & Stuart, G. (1995). *Quick psychopharmacology reference* (2nd ed.) Baltimore, MD: Mosby-Year Book.

TABLE 31–3 Common Antidepressant Medications

Generic Name	Trade Name	Class	Usual Therapeutic Dose (mg/d)	Dose Range (mg/d)	Anticholinergic Side Effects	Cardiac Arrhythmia	Sedation	Orthostatic Hypotension	Insomnia, Agitation	GI Distress
Amitriptyline	Elavil	TCA	100–300	50–300	+4	+3	+4	+4	0	0
Bupropion	Wellbutrin	Atypical	200–450	100–450	0	+1	0	0	+2	+1
Citalopram	Celexa	SSRI	20–40	10–80	0	0	0	0	+2	+3
Fluoxetine	Prozac	SSRI	20–40	20–80	0	0	0	0	+2	+3
Mirtazapine	Remeron	Atypical	15–45	15–45	+1	0	+4	+2	+1	+1
Nefazodone	Serzone	Atypical	50–600	50–600	+1	0	+3	+2	+1	+2
Nortriptyline	Pamelor	TCA	75–150	20–200	+2	+2	+2	+2	0	0
Paroxetine	Paxil	SSRI	20–40	10–50	+1	0	+1	0	2	3
Sertraline	Zoloft	SSRI	50–150	25–250	0	0	0	0	2	3
Venlafaxine	Effexor	Nonselective reuptake	75–225	25–350	0	0	0	0	0	3

From Stuart, G., & Laraia, M. (1998). *Pocket guide to psychiatric nursing* (4th ed.). St. Louis: Mosby; Maxmen J., Ward, N., & Dubrovsky, S. (2002). *Psychotropic drugs fast facts* (3rd ed.). New York: W. W. Norton.

3. Sexual effects.
   a. A decrease in libido is very common for the depressed patient.
   b. Antidepressant medication can also cause a decreased libido, impotence, diminished sexual arousal, and impaired orgasms.
   c. Highest with the selective serotonin reuptake inhibitors (SSRI): fluoxetine, sertraline, paroxetine.
   d. SSRI often delay orgasm.
   e. Impotence seen more with tricyclic antidepressants (TCA): nortriptyline, amitriptyline.
   f. Bupropion has the least amount of sexual side effects and may increase libido.
   g. Educate your patients about the side effects; at first, these may not be an issue because a decreased libido is a common symptom of major depression. As they begin to feel better, noncompliance can result from the sexual side effects.
4. Education for the patient and family.
   a. May take 6 to 8 weeks before the full effect is felt from the medication.
   b. Antidepressants are not addicting, and they do not elevate a person's mood as an "upper" or cocaine would.
   c. Will remain on the medication for a number of months.
   d. Many antidepressants should not be stopped abruptly; they need to be tapered.

II. Anxiety
A. Definition: Diffuse, vague apprehension associated with feelings of uncertainty and helplessness
B. Prevalence
   1. 44.6 million people in the United States have an anxiety disorder (National Institute of Mental Health, 2003).
C. Anxiety is on a continuum, with lower levels helpful in motivating learning.
D. At higher levels, the person feels uncomfortable and has difficulty controlling the amount and frequency of his frightening thoughts or emotions.
E. Anxiety is very common in oncology patients and can vary.
   1. Situational anxiety is related to what they are experiencing, such as a test or treatment.
   2. Feelings of panic in some people can occur with or without a specific situation.
   3. People with pancreatic cancer can experience a great deal of anxiety that is related physiologically to their cancer (Green & Austin, 1993).
F. Differential Diagnosis
   1. Major depression (see section above on Major Depression)
   2. Delirium (see Chapter 24)
   3. Substance abuse
   4. Other possible causes
      a. Akathisia or restlessness secondary to neuroleptics or other medications (compazine, metoclopramide)
      b. Medical conditions: Congestive heart failure, pulmonary embolism and arrhythmias

G. Symptoms
   1. Excessive worry with difficulty in controlling emotions or changing patterns of thought. The patient can appear angry or irritable as well as tearful, wringing hands, or hyperalert.
   2. Difficulty concentrating, irritability, sleep disturbance, restless, muscle tension, or easily fatigued.
   3. Gastrointestinal discomfort, such as loss of appetite, nausea, diarrhea.
   4. Physical symptoms can vary and are multiple (eg, heart palpitations, rapid breathing, tremors, increased reflexes or startle response and insomnia).
   5. These symptoms cause the person to experience distress or impairment in functioning.
H. Interventions for Anxiety (see section above on Demoralization)
   1. Rate the degree of anxiety with 10 the highest and 1 the least.
   2. Have patient state what is a comfortable level, determine if this is a realistic amount of anxiety and use this number as the patient's goal.
   3. Encourage verbalization of concerns.
   4. Assist with ideas. As level of anxiety increases, patients' problem solving decreases.
   5. Encourage distraction through the use of music, TV, calling friends, and so forth.
   6. If appropriate, use social work, pastoral care, and psychiatric consult.
   7. Teach relaxation exercises or the use of relaxation tapes.
      a. Breathe in through the nose. Slowly say "I am." Hold for 1 second. Breathe out through the mouth and say "relaxed" to self.
      b. Repeat several times and practice this exercise when not anxious as well as to decrease anxiety.
I. Pharmacologic Treatment for Anxiety (Table 31–4)
   1. Goal of medication is to prevent anxiety from interfering with functioning and to allow the patient to use own coping strategies.
   2. Know the length of action of the antianxiety medication you are giving to ensure that the patient is receiving it frequently enough.
   3. Psychological dependence occurs more often when the onset of action is rapid ("buzz") and doses are further apart than the duration of action.

TABLE 31–4 Common Antianxiety Medication

Generic Name	Trade Name	Usual Therapeutic Dose (mg/d)	Extreme Dosage Range (mg/d)
Alprazolam	Xanax	0.25–0.5 tid	0.5–8
Clonazepam	Klonopin	0.5 tid	0.25–20
Diazepam	Valium	2–10 bid–qid	2–40
Lorazepam	Ativan	0.5–2 tid–qid	1–10
Oxazepam	Serax	10–30 tid–qid	30–120

Maxmen, J., Ward, N. & Dubovsky, S. (2002). *Psychotropic drugs fast facts* (3rd ed.). New York, NY: W.W. Norton.

4. If the patient receives several PRNs a day for anxiety, he or she should be on a standing dose. Consider a long-acting benzodiazepine for standing dose.
5. Physical dependence can develop.
   a. Inform the patient and family of possible withdrawal symptoms.
   b. The patient should not stop taking antianxiety medication without consulting the care provider because a taper may be needed.
   c. If the patient is taking the medication at home, make sure it is not suddenly stopped in the hospital.
6. Side effects can be fatigue or sedation. Patients should not drive if feeling sedated. This usually decreases with time. These medications can precipitate a delirious state (see Chapter 24).

III. Substance Abuse and Dependence

A. Definitions: Substance abuse and dependence are maladaptive patterns of substance use leading to clinically significant impairment or distress (American Psychiatric Association, 1994).
   1. Substance abuse involves recurrent use of substances that causes social, occupational, hazardous, and legal problems.
   2. Substance dependence includes recurrent use that is marked by tolerance, withdrawal, desire to cut down or control use, preoccupation of thinking and time to get substance, and continued use despite ongoing physical or psychological problems.
B. Prevalence
   1. May include 23% to 40% of cancer patients if dependence on nicotine is included.
C. Patients with cancer often are prescribed opiates and benzodiazepines to manage pain, anxiety, sleep disturbances, and nausea.
D. The presence of a history and/or current use of substances has both significant psychosocial and treatment implications.
   1. Current abuse/dependence can make the patient's medical status difficult to fully assess and interfere with the patient's ability to actively participate and comply with treatment.
   2. Behaviors often seen in patients with substance abuse/dependence (eg, seeking out various health providers to obtain medications, running out of medications early and frequently, missing appointments) can negatively impact the relationship between patients, families, and health care providers.
   3. Response to opiates/benzodiazepines or amounts needed to manage symptoms are different than in patients who haven't or don't abuse. More medication may be needed to manage symptoms.
   4. Patients with past abuse/dependence histories may be reluctant to take the medications, and they suffer needlessly.
   5. Fear and concerns on the part of health care providers in prescribing and administering these medications may result in undertreating the patient's symptoms.
   6. Intravenous (IV) drug use can place patients at high risk for comorbid illnesses, such as infections.
   7. Withdrawal could put patient at risk for significant medical complications.

▼ **BOX 31-2** | **CAGE (Quick Assessment Tool)**

- Have you ever felt you should **C**ut down on your drinking/drug use?
- Have people **A**nnoyed you by criticizing your drinking/drug use?
- Have you ever felt bad or **G**uilty about your drinking/drug use?
- Have you ever had to drink (**E**ye opener) or use other drugs first thing in the morning?

If answer "Yes" to:
  1 Further investigation
2–3 High index of suspicion
  4 Pathognomonic

---

8. Be aware that there are often comorbid psychiatric disorders (eg, depression, bipolar disorder, anxiety disorders) that need to be assessed for and treated. Make referrals as needed.

E. Assessment (Box 31–2)
   1. History and current use of substances
   2. Types, amount, frequency, route, last use
   3. History/current withdrawal symptoms, seizures, blackouts, delirium tremens
   4. Past treatment
   5. Legal issues
   6. Current interest in treatment

F. Interventions for Substance Abuse/Dependence
   1. Remember that substance abuse/dependence is an illness and that patients need to be treated with respect and care despite their behaviors.
   2. Adequately manage patients' pain, anxiety, and sleep difficulties.
      a. When appropriate, investigate alternatives to opiates, anxiolytics, hypnotics, such as relaxation, guided imagery, biofeedback.
      b. May benefit from use of antidepressants to manage anxiety and sleep (see Major Depression, I, I.1–2).
   3. Treat withdrawal symptoms (including for nicotine).
   4. Seek appropriate referrals (psychiatry, social work, pain specialists) for symptom management and/or substance abuse treatment.
   5. Educate patients and families.
      a. Symptom management.
      b. Medications.
      c. Dispel myths about addiction and treatment of symptom management.
   6. Assist in development of a team approach/plan of care with patients and families that includes or may include:
      a. All professional caregivers, with a designated prescriber of all opiates, anxiolytics, and hypnotics.
      b. Administration and management of medications by family member.

   c. Use of contracts.
     (1) Urine toxic screens to monitor for abuse
     (2) Prescribing of limited doses of medications with follow-up
        appointments before next prescription is given
     (3) Expected behaviors and consequences during treatment and
        hospitalizations

REFERENCES

American Psychiatric Association. (1994). *Diagnostic and statistical manual of mental disorders* (4th ed.). Washington, DC: Author.

Green, A. L., & Austin, C. P. (1993). Psychopathology of pancreatic cancer: A psychobiologic probe. *Psychosomatics,*[AQ] 34, 208–221.

Laraia, M., & Stuart, G. (1995*). Quick psychopharmacology reference* (2nd ed.). Baltimore, MD: Mosby-Year Book.

Maxmen, J., Ward, N., & Dubovsky, S. (2002). *Psychotropic drugs fast facts* (3rd ed.). New York, NY: W.W. Norton.

National Institute of Mental Health. (2003). Available at: http://www.nimh.nih. gov.home.cfm.

Newport, J., & Nemeroff, C. (1998). Assessment and treatment of depression in the cancer patient. *Journal of Psychosomatic Research, 45*(3), 215–237.

Schwartz, L., Lander, M., & Maxchochinov, H. (2002). Current management of depression in cancer patients. *Oncology,* 16(8), 1102–1110.

Slavney, P. (1998). *Psychiatric dimensions of medical practice.* Baltimore, MD: Johns Hopkins University Press.

Stuart, G., & Laraia, M. (1998). *Pocket guide to psychiatric nursing* (4th ed.). St. Louis, MO: Mosby.

32 Venous Access Devices

Norrie Rabinowitz-Hirsch
MiKaela Olsen

I. Definition: Approximately 150 million venous access devices (VAD) are inserted each year in the United States. Five million of these are central venous catheters. This number is predicted to increase as a result of more complex treatment capabilities, the continued shift to treatment in the outpatient area, and as our aging population continues to grow. The care and maintenance of VAD are among the largest developing areas for nurses today.

A. In the 1940s, intravenous (IV) therapy was limited to salt and dextrose solutions administered through steel needles placed peripherally. As IV therapies became more advanced, the need for larger, more durable veins that could withstand higher concentrations of potent solutions became apparent.

B. In 1949, short-term subclavian or jugular central venous catheters were first used. The catheter material at that time was polyethylene or polyvinylchloride, which was extremely stiff and associated with high rates of thrombosis.

C. In the 1970s, Broviac, Hickman, and Groshong catheters were developed, and the tunneling technique was discovered. These catheters were designed of a biocompatible Silastic material, which was much more flexible and compatible with the human body.

D. During the 1980s, the implanted venous access port was developed primarily for the oncology patient population, followed by the invention of the peripherally inserted central catheter (PICC). VAD redesign and the invention of novel strategies to protect against complications continue to be an important focus in this field. Complications continue to be problematic despite the definite advantages of VAD. The oncology patient is at an increased risk for many of the associated complications and must be managed carefully.

II. Types of VAD (Table 32–1)

A. Noncentral Lines

1. Peripheral vein infusion catheters—Short-term catheters, approximately ≤ 3 cm in length, that are inserted into peripheral veins at the bedside.

2. Midline catheters—Peripheral infusion catheter, approximately 10 to 13 cm in length (adults), placed in an antecubital fossa vein. Midline catheter duration of use is between 2 and 4 weeks.

B. Tunneled, Cuffed, Central Line Catheters

1. Hickman, Cook, Broviac central venous catheters are placed into a subcutaneous tract before entering the intended vein.

TABLE 32–1 VAD Advantages and Disadvantages

Catheter Type	Advantages	Disadvantages
Peripheral vein catheters	Placement by nurse at bedside Inexpensive Generally associated with a low incidence of infection	Frequent replacement Phlebitis, infiltration, and pain can occur Long-term use can damage veins
Midline catheter	Placement at bedside Blood sampling can be done easily Single and double lumens No radiographic study needed to verify placement	Short term catheter 2–4 weeks **Not a central line—do not use for infusion of continuous vesicants or hyperosmotic solutions** Phlebitis Associated with increased thrombosis if placed in subclavian vein
Peripherally inserted central line catheter (PICC)	Placement at bedside Reduction in risks such as pneumothorax and hemorrhage May be associated with fewer complications such as infection due to its location Useful when length of IV therapy exceeds 6 days	Patient must have palpable and visible antecubital fossa access unless ultrasound technology is available Catheter flow rates can be limiting to some protocols Mechanical phlebitis 20% to 60% insertion failure rates without the use of ultrasound Care and maintenance requires a caregiver due to catheter location
Nontunneled short-term central line catheters	Multilumen access—up to five lumens in some catheters Placement at bedside Can be replaced over a guidewire Easily removed at bedside	Lifespan is dependent on patient tolerance of central VAD and development of complications Associated with high risk of infections Sutures have to be left in for the life of the catheter Increased infection rates with internal jugular and femoral sites in adults
Nontunneled Hohn catheter	May be left in place for 6 weeks Provides large-bore access, single or double lumen Placement at bedside	Usually requires surgeon for placement Nontunneled Increased complications if left in > 6 weeks

(continued)

TABLE 32-1 VAD Advantages and Disadvantages *(Continued)*

Catheter Type	Advantages	Disadvantages
Tunneled catheters (eg, Broviac and Hickman)	Tunnel ensures a distance between the entry site where the catheter is placed into the vein and the catheter exit site, which has been shown to decrease infection risk Dacron cuff helps secure catheter and decreases antimicrobial migration in the subcutaneous tunnel Antimicrobial cuff releases silver ions at the catheter exit site after insertion Can be used for indefinite periods of time if complications are absent Single, double, or triple lumens are available Repair kits are available for external catheter damage	Placement requires surgeon in most institutions with a dedicated operating room space and requires sedation Catheter damage can occur with removal Body image changes
Tunneled catheters (Groshong)	Specialized valve allows for decreased flushing and the use of saline flushes instead of heparin Valve prevents reflux of blood into catheter No clamping required Repair kits available	Placement requires a surgeon
Implantable ports	Can be placed in chest or antecubital fossa area Position completely under the skin Increased patient satisfaction if needle can be removed when patient is not receiving treatment Minimal flushing requirements if deaccessed	Placement is in an operating room and requires sedation Costly placement and removal Occlusions can develop frequently with inadequate flushing of this device Discomfort from multiple needle sticks during accessing of port Skin necrosis and erosion of port through the skin can occur in the presence of infection, malnutrition, or drug infiltration
Apheresis/hemodialysis catheters (tunneled and nontunneled)	Large diameter allows for high flow rates for apheresis and dialysis	Often restricted for use in dialysis and apheresis May require higher concentrations of heparin to maintain catheter patency

2. Groshong tunneled catheter has a unique closed end, which has a valve at the distal end. The valve remains closed when no pressure is applied. The valve opens inward with aspiration and outward with infusion through the catheter. The valve prevents reflux of blood into the tip of the catheter.

3. Implantable ports. A port is a self-sealing reservoir that is placed into a subcutaneous pocket. The catheter is attached to the port and placed into a central vein. Ports can be placed in the chest or the antecubital fossa.

C. Hemodialysis/Apheresis Central Catheters—Large French-size central catheters used for dialysis and apheresis procedures where a higher flow rate is essential.

D. Nontunneled Central Line Catheters

1. Hohn short-term, central catheter has a duration of use approximately 6 weeks long. This central catheter can be placed at the bedside by a trained surgeon.

2. Peripherally inserted central catheter (PICC) is placed into a vein in the antecubital fossa such as the cephalic, basilic, or median vein. The basilic vein is ideal because it is larger and straighter. Specially trained nurses often place PICC lines.

3. Groshong PICC uses the closed end and valve.

4. Short-term central venous catheters (eg, Arrow) are typically inserted into subclavian, jugular, and femoral veins. These catheters are composed of a stiff material that makes insertion easier. Multiple-lumen catheters are associated with increased infection risks.

III. Indications/Rationale for Use

A. Patients with limited peripheral access; multiple therapies including antibiotics, blood products, nutrition, and chemotherapy, hemodialysis, or apheresis; and/or frequent blood sampling are candidates for a central VAD.

B. Other indications include the prevention of venous or tissue damage, patient comfort, and patient preference.

IV. Insertion Techniques

A. Placement of a central VAD is done by way of a large vein such as the internal and external jugular and subclavian veins for long-term and short-term central lines. The cephalic, basilic, or median veins are commonly used for PICC catheters (Fig. 32–1). The catheter tip of a central line VAD should ideally be placed in the junction of the superior vena cava and right atrium. The catheter tip should not be placed or allowed to migrate into the heart. Malpositioned catheters can cause pneumothorax, cardiac perforation, and other complications. Placement of any central line VAD should be done according to institutional guidelines using maximum sterile barrier technique (ie, cap, mask, sterile gown, sterile gloves, and large sterile drape) to decrease bloodstream infection rates.

B. Special considerations—Skin problems (eg, burns, dermatitis), previous mastectomy, history of radical neck dissection, previous VAD sites, prior history of thoracic surgery, previous radiation to the chest, presence of myelosuppression, coagulation study results.

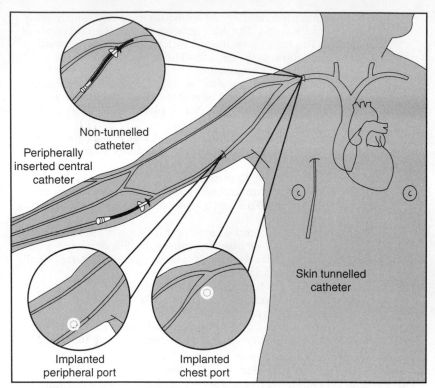

Figure 32–1. Insertion site for central venous access devices. (Dougherty, L. [2000]. Central venous access devices. *Nursing Standard, 14*, 43, 45–50.)

V. Catheter-Related Complications

A. Occlusions—Occlusions can be classified as either partial or complete. Partial occlusions exist when the catheter can be infused through but the ability to withdraw blood is absent. A less common partial occlusion can exist when the ability to infuse into the catheter is absent and the catheter does allow withdrawal of blood. A complete occlusion is the inability to aspirate or withdraw blood. Signs of occlusion include inability to aspirate, sluggish infusion, complete inability to flush or infuse, or increasing occlusion alarm incidence with electronic infusion pumps. Patency of catheters should be maintained at all times. Occlusions predispose patients to serious complications, such as infection and treatment delays.

1. Catheter-related thrombotic occlusions—59% of all obstructions

a. Intraluminal thrombus—Causes inadequate blood flow through the vein. This can be a result of inadequate flushing, after blood draws or for maintenance of the catheter, increased intrathoracic pressure from vomiting, sneezing, coughing, or forceful flushing.

b. Mural thrombus—Formation of thrombi caused by the presence of the catheter. Patients at high risk include those with venous stasis, increased blood coagulopathies, and trauma to the vessel being used for the central VAD. Venous stasis can be seen in patients who are dehydrated, hypotensive, immobile, with intrapulmonary disease, or with heart failure. Mural thrombi eventually obstruct venous flow. The thrombi typically exist at the point where the catheter enters the vein. One example is a superior vena cava thrombus, which can lead to superior vena cava syndrome (see Chapter 38). Mural thrombus can also lead to deep vein thrombosis.

c. Fibrin sheath—Fibrin adheres to the external surface of the catheter, making it difficult or impossible to withdraw and/or flush. The human body reacts almost immediately to any foreign body that is present. In the case of a VAD, the body sees the catheter as a foreign object and attempts to isolate it by producing fibrin around the catheter sheath. Virtually all catheters are totally fibrin covered within 4 to 5 days of insertion. Fibrin has the potential to grow along the catheter and extend past the catheter tip. Withdrawal occlusions or extravasation of IV fluids may occur, causing serious injury and possibly even life-threatening complications. Bacteria embedded in fibrin increase the risk of persistent catheter-related sepsis.

d. Fibrin tail—Fibrin adheres to the end of the catheter and acts like a flap on the end of the catheter. This can sometimes permit the infusion of substances but prevent aspiration.

2. Catheter-related mechanical/nonthrombotic occlusions—42% of all obstructions

a. Malposition or catheter migration—Inability to infuse or aspirate from the catheter position. Excessive vomiting or coughing can cause catheters to migrate. Malposition can occur at the time of catheter insertion if the incorrect vein is cannulated. Patient may experience ear or neck pain on the side of the VAD placement. Patients may experience a gurgling noise in the ear on the side the VAD is placed; this suggests malposition into the internal jugular vein.

b. Pinch-off syndrome—Occurs when the catheter is placed too medially to the midclavicular line, which causes pinching of the catheter between the first rib and clavicle (Fig. 32–2). Presentation includes a change in flow of the catheter as the patient changes position. Often, the catheter will flush easily when the patient raises the arm on the side where the catheter is placed, relieving pressure on the catheter. A catheter left in this position can develop a partial or complete fracture, which can lead to life-threatening catheter emboli. Extravasation of fluids can occur if catheter fracture is present.

c. Chemical precipitate—Inability to infuse or aspirate. Drug crystallization, drug-drug incompatibilities, or lipid residue can accumulate inside the lumen of the catheter (Table 32–2).

(1) Alkaline

(2) Acidic

(3) Lipid

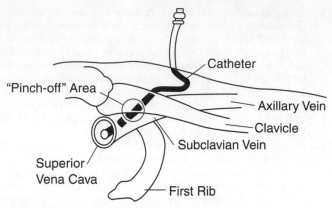

Figure 32–2. The pinch-off syndrome. (Aitken, D. R., Minton, J. P. [1984]. The "pinch-off sign": A warning of impending problems with permanent subclavian catheters. *American Journal of Surgery, 148,* 633–636.)

B. Infection—Over 400,000 catheter-related infections occur annually. Each year, 40,000 to 80,000 deaths occur as a result of these infections. Infections in central VAD are classified as local or bloodstream infections. Infections of long-term VAD are usually a result of microorganisms that enter the catheter through the hub and lumen (Crnich & Maki, 2002).
   1. Types
      a. Local
         (1) Exit site—Within 2 cm of catheter exit site in the absence of bacteremia. Signs include redness, tenderness, and/or purulence.
         (2) Tunnel—Occur in tunneled central catheters, >2 cm from the exit site of a catheter. Signs include redness, tenderness, and/or purulence.
         (3) Pocket infection—Occurs with implanted ports. Signs include redness, tenderness, and/or purulence at the subcutaneous port pocket. Infection of the port pocket can lead to erosion of the port through the skin.

TABLE 32–2 Chemical Precipitates*

Precipitate	Clearing Agent
Lipid residue	70% ethanol or sodium hydroxide
Low-pH drug (pH 1–5)	Hydrochloric acid (0.1% N)
High-pH drug (pH 9–12)	Sodium bicarbonate ($NaHCO_3$)
Calcium-phosphate	Hydrochloric acid (0.1% N)
	Cysteine hydrochloride

*For volume and concentration, refer to manufacturers' guidelines.
Infusion Nurses Society. (2002). *Policies and procedures for infusion nursing* (2nd ed.). Norwood, MA: Author.

b. Bloodstream infection (BSI)—BSI in oncology patients are the most serious and life-threatening complications of VAD. BSI is defined in the CDC guidelines as a "bacteremia/fungemia in a patient with an intravascular catheter with at least one positive blood culture and with clinical manifestations of infections (ie, fever, chills, and/or hypotension) and no apparent source for the bloodstream infection except the catheter or any of the following:

(1) A positive semiquantitative or quantitative culture whereby the same organism is isolated from the catheter segment and peripheral blood.

(2) Simultaneous quantitative blood cultures with a ≥5:1 ratio (VAD vs. peripheral).

(3) Differential time period of VAD culture vs. peripheral blood culture positivity of >2 hours (O'Grady et al., 2002).

c. The most common organisms implicated in catheter-related bloodstream infections are coagulase-negative *Staphylococcus*, *Staphylococcus aureus*, aerobic gram-negative bacilli, and *Candida albicans* (Mermel et al., 2001).

(1) Risk factors

(a) Myelosuppression

(b) Prolonged catheterization

(c) Frequent manipulation of catheter

(d) Improper aseptic technique during catheter insertion and care

(e) Multiple lumens

(f) Type of device placed and site

(g) Primary diagnosis of patient

(h) Catheter maintenance

(i) Malnutrition

(j) Immunosuppressive medications

(2) Possible causes

(a) Contaminated catheter hub

(b) Breach in aseptic technique

(c) Thrombosis

(d) Lack of education related to care of catheter

(e) Contaminated infusate

(f) Hematogenous seeding from a remote source of infection

(3) Assessment—Thorough and frequent assessments of VAD should be done. A phlebitis scale can be a useful assessment tool for monitoring VAD (Table 32–3). Cultures of site and/or blood from catheter and peripheral sites should be done if infection is suspected.

(4) Treatment—In neutropenic patients (absolute neutrophil count ≤500 mm³), local and systemic infections are usually treated with IV antibiotics in conjunction with diligent site care. Organism-specific antibiotics of choice are determined per institutional guidelines based on efficacy and resistance.

(5) Infection prevention

(a) Specially coated catheters impregnated with chlorhexidine, antibiotics, and silver sulfadiazine are under inves-

TABLE 32-3 Phlebitis Scale

Grade	Clinical Criteria
0	No symptoms
1	Erythema at access site with or without pain
2	Pain at access site with erythema and/or edema
3	Pain at access site with erythema and/or edema
	Streak formation
	Palpable venous cord
4	Pain at access site with erythema and/or edema
	Streak formation
	Palpable venous cord >1 inch in length
	Purulent drainage

Infusion Nurses Society. (2002). *Policies and procedures for infusion nursing* (2nd ed.). Norwood, MA: Author.

tigation and may prevent catheter-related bloodstream infections.

(b) Subcutaneous cuffs
- Dacron cuff—Host tissue grows in a 2- to 6-week timeframe over the cuff, creating a mechanical barrier in the tract of a tunneled catheter.
- Silver-impregnated cuffs assist in prevention of insertion tract infections.

(c) Biopatch chlorhexidine-impregnated sponge dressing, applied to exit site of catheter.

(d) Antiinfective hubs (Sefur-Lock)—Connecting chamber contains iodinated alcohol.

(e) Antibiotic locks—Practice of flushing a small amount of antibiotic into the catheter lumen and allowing it to dwell. This practice is under investigation. Potential risks, such as antimicrobial resistance, are being studied.

(f) Securing devices—StatLock (Venetec International) is used to secure PICC. This device is used in place of sutures. This device has been shown to decrease infection in PICC lines placed in adults (Schears et al., 2001).

(6) Indications for removal or treatment of a known catheter-related infection depend on the specific organism involved, patient factors, such as neutropenia, and institutional guidelines.

C. Other Catheter-Related Complications

1. Catheter-related air emboli—Caused by air entering the vascular system. The air can form bubbles and block pulmonary capillaries. Care should be taken when manipulating catheter or tubing to prevent air entry. Nursing interventions if an air embolus is suspected include lying patient on left side in Trendelenburg's position, administering oxygen, and notifying physician immediately. The left-sided position may help trap air in the right atrium and prevent it from traveling into the lung.

2. Phlebitis—Mechanical or chemical irritation or injury to the vein wall. Treatment involves rest, elevation, and application of warm compresses. Catheter may need to be removed.

3. Pneumothorax—Caused by air or blood entering the pleural space. Usually associated with catheter insertion. Signs and symptoms include pain with inspiration, dyspnea, apprehension, and decreased breath sounds on the side of insertion. Obtain physician order for a radiographic view of the chest; support patient with oxygen if needed. Patient may require a chest tube.

4. Bleeding at exit site—An exit site hematoma can be caused by traumatic insertions or in a patient with coagulopathies or thrombocytopenia. Apply local pressure with sterile gauze and notify physician.

5. Extravasation—The leakage of infusate from a vein into the subcutaneous space is a relatively infrequent complication of central venous catheters. The most common cause is needle dislodgment from ports. The greatest risk is associated with the infusion of vesicants. Antineoplastic medications are the obvious vesicants. Other solutions that can cause tissue destruction include electrolytes such as potassium chloride and calcium, antibiotics such as vancomycin and nafcillin, and vasopressors such as dopamine (see Chapter 6).

6. Catheter fracture—Tear or cut in the catheter either internally or externally. Internal tears can occur with activities such as golfing or backpacking. Catheters can develop tears when pulled or stretched beyond their limit.

7. Catheter dislodgment—Can occur if not secured properly. Most frequently occurs with new VAD. If this occurs, apply pressure to site with a dry, sterile gauze and notify physician.

8. Damaged catheter—External cuts or tears can occur while attempting to secure catheter to clothing. Patients should not secure catheters with pins because accidental puncture can easily occur. Catheters can also be damaged with infusion of fluids through syringes that are <10 mL. In general, the smaller the catheter, the more likely that it cannot withstand the pressure of small syringes or mechanical pressure injectors, such as those used in certain dye studies. Catheter repair kits are available for select catheters, and manufacturers will supply them for use.

9. Other complications—Cardiac arrhythmias, endocarditis, and osteomyelitis are additional complications of VAD.

VI. Patient Management
A. Assessment (Table 32–4)
1. Appearance
   a. Type of catheter
   b. Number of lumens
   c. Integrity of catheter
   d. Entry site (new tunneled catheters)
      (1) Sutures intact, removed per institutional guidelines ~7 days after catheter insertion
   e. Integrity of dressing
      (1) Occlusiveness
      (2) Presence of moisture
      (3) Presence of drainage

TABLE 32-4 Catheter Selection Considerations

- Does the patient need short- or long-term therapy?
- What types of therapies will be used?
- Does the patient need continuous or intermittent therapy?
- How many lumens are necessary?
- Does the patient have: lymphedema, mastectomy, scarring from other chest or neck surgeries, or any pertinent fractures?
- Does the patient have a history of thrombus, catheter-related problems, anticoagulation therapy, or a clotting disorder?
- Can the patient tolerate the VAD procedure under consideration?
- Does the patient have an increased risk of infection?
- What is the patient's allergy history?
- Does the patient have cardiovascular abnormalities, such as a pacemaker?

     f. Catheter exit site
       (1) Presence of sutures if applicable. Remove per institutional guidelines ~ 21 days after catheter insertion.
       (2) Redness.
       (3) Swelling.
       (4) Drainage.
       (5) Bleeding.
       (6) Tenderness.
     g. Function
       (1) Ability to infuse and aspirate all lumens.
       (2) Assess for sluggishness or resistance.
       (3) Assess for patient complaints such as pain, ringing in the ear.
B. General Catheter Care and Maintenance
  1. Flushing
     a. Heparin versus saline—Depends on catheter type. Heparin-induced thrombocytopenia (HIT) can occur and should be considered in patients receiving heparin.
     b. Frequency and amount—Follow institutional guidelines for specific catheter flushing and volumes. Chills or hypotension during or after flushing of a VAD may indicate bacteremia and should be reported immediately.
     c. Pulsatile technique—A push–pause technique for flushing catheters provides turbulent flow and is important in maintaining VAD patency.
     d. Positive-end pressure technique—Clamping the VAD while maintaining the syringe pressure during flushing to create a positive pressure in the catheter, thus minimizing blood reflux and subsequent intraluminal occlusion.
     e. Use of positive pressure valves that prevent reflux of blood.
     f. Infusion pressure should not exceed 25 psi.
  2. Dressing changes—The dressing primarily serves to decrease contamination of the site and to stabilize the device.
     a. Consistent aseptic technique is one of the most important considerations.

    b. Transparent dressings provide for inspection of the insertion site, and many are waterproof.

    c. Moisture-permeable transparent dressing allows moisture to escape from the VAD site and require less frequent dressing changes.

    d. Gauze dressings can retain moisture and, therefore, should only be used for sites that are oozing, diaphoretic patients, and in other situations where frequent dressing changes are necessary.

    e. Avoid topical ointments—Ointments have been shown to increase the risk of catheter colonization by *Candida* species (Mermel et al., 2001).

    f. Goals of any VAD dressing—Prevention of infection and prevention of catheter dislodgment.

3. Cleansing

    a. Hand washing is required before dressing change.

    b. Aseptic technique.

    c. Cleansing of the VAD site should include an antiseptic agent containing chlorhexidine or povodone iodine.

    d. Use a skin preparation agent such as alcohol before the primary antiseptic agent to remove excess oil.

4. Catheter removal (for nontunneled catheters only)

    a. Gather supplies: suture removal kit, sterile gloves, 4×4 sterile gauze pad, sterile hemostat, and a cleansing agent.

    b. Obtain physician order.

    c. By a trained and competent RN.

    d. Risk factors

        (1) Air embolism can occur during central line catheter removal. The patient should hold breath to create a positive pressure in the intrathoracic space. This will minimize the risk of air entry as the catheter is removed.

        (2) Bleeding—Apply pressure with dry sterile gauze after removal to prevent bleeding.

    e. Follow manufacturer's guidelines and institutional guidelines for catheter removal.

    f. Consider culturing catheter tip if line infection is suspected.

    g. Inspect tip and measure catheter length to ensure it is removed intact.

C. Diagnostic Parameters

1. As mentioned, proper placement of VAD is essential before use. Tip location should be verified by way of radiologic resources and documented in the patient record. A dye study is useful in determining if leakage, catheter damage, or clots exist and is often used when catheters are malfunctioning.

D. Nursing Diagnoses

1. Catheter-related thrombotic occlusion

    a. *Problem:* Inadequate function of catheter

    b. *Interventions*

        (1) Thrombolytic therapy is used to reestablish patency of central VAD in the presence of a fibrin sheath or an intraluminal clot. Institutional guidelines should be followed for catheter clearance (Table 32–5). A radiologic examination

TABLE 32-5 **Thrombolytic Therapy***

Clearing Agent	Dose
Retavase (Reteplase)	0.4 units
CathFlo activase (Alteplase)	2 mg

*For volume and concentration, refer to manufacturers' guidelines.

of the chest (CXR) should ideally be obtained before initiation of thrombolytic therapy to ensure catheter position is correct.

   (2) Systemic thrombolytic therapy may be required for a major vessel thrombus. The catheter may need to be removed in some cases.

  c. *Desired outcome:* Catheter function will be restored.

2. Catheter-related mechanical/nonthrombotic occlusion
  a. *Problem:* Inadequate function of catheter
  b. *Interventions*
   (1) Malpositioned catheters or ones that have migrated from their original placement can sometimes be rewired. May require removal and reinsertion.
   (2) Pinch-off syndrome—Instruct patient to raise arms over head and flush the catheter with the patient sitting upright. This can be diagnosed using a CXR or dye study. The syndrome should not be overlooked. Serious harm can occur if the catheter fractures. Catheter emboli could occur. Requires catheter removal in most cases.
   (3) Chemical precipitate (see Table 32-2).
  c. *Desired outcome:* Catheter function will be restored.

3. Potential for catheter-related infection
  a. *Problem:* The most frequent complication of VAD is infection.
  b. *Interventions*
   (1) Assess site carefully for infection.
   (2) Signs and symptoms may be absent in a neutropenic patient.
   (3) Provide care to catheter following institutional guidelines using aseptic technique. Obtain blood cultures and monitor carefully. A decision to remove the line or treat through is made on an individual basis factoring in the severity of the illness, the specific organism involved, and the catheter type and location.
   (4) Instruct patient and family in care and maintenance of catheter.

REFERENCES

Aikin, D. R., & Minton, J. P. (1984). The "pinch off sign": A warning of impending problems with permanent subclavian catheters. *American Journal of Surgery, 148,* 633–635.

Crnich, C. J., & Maki, D. G. (2002). The promise of novel technology for the prevention of intravascular device-related bloodstream infection. II. Long term devices. *Clinical Infectious Diseases, 34,* 1362–1368.

Crosby, C., & Mares, A. (2001). Skin antisepsis, past, present and future. *Journal of Vascular Access Devices, Spring,* 1–6.

Dougherty, L. (2000). Central venous access devices. *Nursing Standard, 14*(43), 45–50.

Infusion Nurses Society. (2002). *Policies and procedures for infusion nursing* (2nd ed.).

Kaufman, J. (2001). The interventional radiologist role in providing long-term central venous access. *Journal of Intravenous Nursing, 24*(3, Suppl.), 523–527.

Luptak, P. (2001). Management of catheter occlusion with Cath-Flo Activase. *Spectrum, 13*(4), 1–20.

Mayo, D. (2001). Catheter-related thrombosis. *Journal of Intravenous Nursing, 24*(3, Suppl.), 513–522.

Mermel, L. (2001). New technologies to prevent intravascular catheter-related blood stream infections. *Emerging Infectious Diseases, 7*(2), 197–199.

Mermel, L., Farr, B., Sherertz, R., et al. (2001). Guidelines for the management of intravascular catheter-related infections. *Infection Control and Hospital Epidemiology, 22*(4), 222–242.

O'Grady, N., Alexander, M., Dellinger, E., et al. (2002). Guidelines for the prevention of intravascular catheter-related infections. Centers for Disease Control and Prevention. *MMWR, 51,* RR-10.

Oncology Nursing Society. (1996). *Access device guidelines: Recommendations for nursing practice and education.*

Raad, I., & Bodey, G. (1992). Infectious complications of indwelling vascular catheters. *Clinical Infectious Diseases, 15,* 197–210.

Schears, G. J., Liebeig, C., Frey, A. M., et al. (2001). *StatLock catheter securement device significantly reduces central venous catheter complications. National Patient Safety Foundation compendium on best practice.* Chicago, IL: Joint Commission on Accreditation of Healthcare Organizations.

Schulmeister, L., & Camp-Sorrell, D. (2000). Chemotherapy extravasation from implanted ports. *Oncology Nursing Forum, 27*(3), 1–9.

Silberzweig, J., Sacks, D., Khorsandi, A., et al. (2000). Reporting standards for central venous access. *Journal of Vascular and Interventional Radiology, 11,* 391–400.

Wickham, R., Purl, S., & Welker, D. (1992). Long-term central venous catheters: Issues for care. *Seminars in Oncology Nursing, 8*(2), 133–147.

UNIT V

ONCOLOGIC EMERGENCIES

33 Disseminated Intravascular Coagulation (DIC)

Brenda K. Shelton

I. Definition: Disseminated intravascular coagulation (DIC) is defined as accelerated activation of the coagulation cascade disproportionate to normal feedback mechanisms, which results in thrombi formation throughout the microvasculature.

    A. Clotting is normally triggered by tissue injury, vessel injury, or the presence of a foreign body in the blood. In DIC, normal mechanisms of abrogating an excessive clotting response are disabled, and the process of clotting is not balanced by normal fibrinolysis.

    B. Because the primary pathophysiology is thrombotic, the major clinical consequence is systemic ischemia.

    C. Hemorrhage results from the depletion of clotting factors and ongoing stimulation of fibrinolysis.

    D. DIC may present as two distinct clinical syndromes with divergent prognostic implications—acute and chronic DIC.

        1. *Acute DIC* is rapid in onset, and severe in clinical symptomatology. This is a more common presentation in acutely ill or septic patients and carries a mortality rate in excess of 50%.

        2. *Chronic DIC* often manifests as a chronic low-level clotting stimulus that may only be recognizable by mild to moderate organ dysfunction and blood component consumption. This clinical presentation is not unusual in patients with large, solid tumors that cause chronic tissue damage and release of thromboplastin. These patients are plagued with persistent clinical symptoms but do not usually die of this syndrome.

    E. The goal of treatment must be to remove or treat the trigger. If that is not possible, the goal of therapy becomes supportive.

II. Etiology

    A. DIC is always secondary to an underlying predisposing condition.

    B. Common etiologies of DIC are linked to strong clotting stimuli or triggering of clotting by way of multiple mechanisms (tissue injury, vessel injury, foreign body in bloodstream).

        1. Severe illness with strong clotting stimulus: Cardiopulmonary arrest, shock, burns, traumatic injury.

        2. Sepsis is the most common etiology of DIC. Gram-negative bacteria release endotoxins, enhancing the clotting stimulus and risk of DIC, although infection with any organisms may cause vascular endothelial or tissue damage resulting in DIC.

C. Cancer is a common etiologic mechanism for DIC.
   1. Large tumors erode normal tissue, causing release of tissue thromboplastin and enhanced clotting.
   2. Rapidly proliferating tumors (eg, acute leukemia, Burkitt's lymphoma) cause autolysis of tumor cells, and the fragmented cells act as foreign bodies within the bloodstream that stimulate clotting.
   3. Some cancers release procoagulants that enhance clotting.
      a. Mucin-producing adenocarcinomas enhance clotting tendencies (eg, breast, colon, primary gastric cancer, pancreatic, prostate, ovarian, renal cell).
      b. Urologic tumors (prostate, renal) release urokinase, which can stimulate clotting.
      c. Brain tissue contains high levels of tissue factor, and brain tumors or procedures (eg, surgery) cause its release with increased clotting.
   4. Progranulocytic leukemia contains granules with procoagulant, and, when leukemic cells lyse, they result in abnormal coagulation.
D. Obstetric complications cause DIC by a variety of causes, but because DIC is often associated with toxemia, endothelial inflammation is thought to be the major triggering mechanism.

III. Management

A. Assessment: The clinical findings in DIC are associated with either the thrombotic pathology, or bleeding due to an inadequate reserve of coagulation factors. Thrombosis and bleeding pathology coexist simultaneously, and, consequently, clinical symptoms are mixed, even within the same organ system. A summary of the clinical findings of DIC are described in greater detail within Table 33–1.
B. Hallmarks of DIC
   1. Thrombosis that involves both veins and arteries.
   2. Demarcation cyanosis demonstrating the total occlusion of microvessels. This is evident by a line separating perfused and nonperfused tissue. It is more common in the digits (fingers and toes) but may also occur in other distal, poorly perfused areas such as earlobes.
   3. Thromboses within the body organs may only present as subclinical organ dysfunction.
   4. Bleeding is a manifestation of later disease where clotting factors have been depleted and are unavailable for simple hemostasis.
C. Potential Complications of DIC
   1. Seizures, intracranial bleed
   2. Pulmonary embolism, pulmonary hemorrhage
   3. Angina/acute myocardial infarction, hemorrhagic cardiac tamponade
   4. Bowel infarction, gastrointestinal bleed
   5. Renal failure, hemorrhagic cystitis
D. Diagnostic Tests. Serum laboratory tests are used for both presumptive and definitive diagnosis (Table 33–2). Some diagnostic tests are significant because they are early, but nonspecific, indicators of the presence of DIC.
   1. Thrombocytopenia occurs first as the platelets are consumed with production of massive intravascular platelet plugs.

TABLE 33-1 Signs and Symptoms of Disseminated Intravascular Coagulation

Body System	Thrombotic Effects	Hemorrhagic Effects
Neurologic	Focal neurologic deficits Dull, diffuse headache Visual changes—visual field cuts	Focal neurologic deficits Sudden and severe headache Visual changes—blurred vision, diplopia, floaters, sudden blindness
Respiratory	Dyspnea Hypoxemia	Dyspnea Crackles on auscultation Hemoptysis or bloody endotracheal aspirate when suctioned Hypoxemia
Cardiovascular	Chest pain Ischemia–ST depression, T wave inversion Injury/infarction—ST elevations, Q waves	Murmur followed by muffled heart sounds ECG changes of pericarditis/effusion such as low voltage, precordial lead ST elevations
Renal	Decreased urine output with pelvic or flank pain	Hematuria
Gastrointestinal	Ischemia—crampy abdominal pain, decreased bowel sounds, abdomen tender to palpation progressing to rebound tenderness Infarction—severe abdominal pain radiating to back or shoulder, rebound tenderness, absent bowel sounds, hypotension, fever, confusion	GI bleeding—heme positive, dark red-black, or frankly bloody nasogastric drainage or stool

2. Hypofibrinogenemia usually follows the decrease in platelet count and is indicative of fibrinogen being used to create massive microvascular clotting.
3. Antithrombin III and protein C levels are reduced in patients with DIC, indicating a loss of normal fibrinolytic mechanisms.
4. Some diagnostic tests are significant because they are the definitive diagnostic indicator for the presence of disease.
   a. Fibrin degradation products (FDP)/fibrin split products (FSP) become elevated with the breakdown of a large volume of clots and is the most reliable diagnostic indicator of DIC. These breakdown products have anticoagulant properties that may worsen the clinical bleeding symptoms associated with this disease.
   b. Fibrinogen D-dimer levels are elevated as plasmin breaks down fibrin.

TABLE 33-2 Diagnostic Tests Used to Assess Patients With Disseminated Intravascular Coagulation

Diagnostic Test	Normal Values	Abnormality in DIC	Rationale for Abnormal Finding
Platelet count	150,000–400,000/mm^3	↓	Early consumption to create microvascular platelet plugs
Fibrinogen level	200–400 mg/dL	↓	Moderately early consumption to create microvascular fibrin clots
Prothrombin time (PT)	11–15 s	↑	Expression of depleted extrinsic pathway factors (mostly vitamin K dependent factors)
Prothrombin time Internationalized ratio (INR)	1.0–1.2 × normal	↑	Expression of depleted extrinsic pathway factors (mostly vitamin K dependent factors)
Partial thromboplastin time (PTT)	60–70 s	↑	Expression of depleted intrinsic pathway factors (VIII, XIII)
Fibrin degradation products (FDPs)/fibrin split products (FSPs)	<10 μg/mL	↑	Indication of high levels of clot lysis relating to large clots, sudden onset of massive fibrinolysis, or excessive fibrinolytic disease
Fibrin D-dimer	<50 μg/dL	↑	Indication of excessive fibrinolysis
Antithrombin III level	80%–120%	↓	Depletion and reduced action in DIC
Protein C level	72%–142%	↓	Depletion and reduced action in DIC
Schistocytes of peripheral blood smear	Absent	↑	Fragmented cells are detected as schistocytes due to RBC destruction as they travel through clots or partially occluded vessels
Bilirubin level	0.1–1.2 mg/dL	↑	Intravascular red blood cell (RBC) hemolysis increases intravascular bilirubin that is cleared less efficiently by the liver
Blood urea nitrogen (BUN)	0.1–0.7 mg/dL	↑	Intravascular RBC hemolysis leads to elevated serum blood urea nitrogen until the kidneys can clear it

Bullock, B. A. & Henze, R. L. (2000). Unit 3, Appendix C: Normal blood coagulation values. In Bullock B. A., Henze R. L. (Eds.). *Focus on pathophysiology.* Philadelphia: Lippincott Williams & Wilkins, p. 398.

5. Diagnostic laboratory tests are divided into tests reflective of the specific pathophysiologic effects of DIC.
   a. Massive intravascular clotting (eg, thrombocytopenia)
   b. Secondary depletion of essential clotting factors: Prothrombin time (PT), partial thromboplastin time (PTT)
   c. Tests reflective of excessive or accelerated fibrinolysis (eg, increased FDPs)
   d. Clinical effects of microvascular clotting and accelerated cell destruction (eg, elevated bilirubin)
6. Urine or other tests: None

E. Treatment
   1. Treatment of the underlying clinical etiology of DIC is the most important therapeutic goal.
   2. General treatment and care principles
      a. Avoid vasoconstriction, which may worsen the perfusion deficit. Keep the patient covered and use vasopressor agents sparingly.
      b. Maintain adequate fluid volume so perfusion is not further impaired. Monitor intake/output and weight, administer maintenance fluids, use diuretics sparingly, and replace lost blood.
      c. Screen all medications the patient may be receiving, and discontinue any that enhance bleeding (eg, nonsteroidal antiinflammatory agents, histamine-2 blockers) or clotting (eg, estrogen).
      d. Management of underlying thrombotic disease
         (1) Heparin may be used for management of thrombotic disease, but use cautiously if the patient is already demonstrating bleeding tendencies. Effectiveness of low-molecular-weight heparin has not been established for treatment of DIC.
         (2) Action (interferes with thrombin production, thereby decreasing microcirculatory clot formation)
         (3) Administration guidelines have varied due to perceived risk of bleeding. Lower than standard doses are usually used.
      e. Nursing Management
         (1) Monitor for signs and symptoms of excessive bleeding.
         (2) Be alert for the rare complication of heparin-induced thrombocytopenia (HIT) characterized by paradoxical clotting with thrombocytopenia.
         (3) Monitor PTT at least every 8 hours for drug toxicity and platelet count, fibrinogen level, and FDP for evidence of therapy effectiveness. Do not draw coagulation studies from the line where the drug is infusing. Catheters that have been flushed with heparin solutions may require up to 20 mL of discard for accurate laboratory test results.
         (4) Maintain a current type and crossmatch with blood products on hold for patients receiving heparin for treatment of this disorder.
   3. Other investigational therapies—Defibrotide
      a. Action: A polydeoxyribonucleotide with antithrombotic, profibrinolytic, and antiinflammatory properties, which acts primarily on the vascular endothelium.

      b. Administration guidelines: Given as 400 to 1,200 mg/day orally or intravenously.

      c. Nursing management: This drug may be used in heparin-refractory patients or those with known heparin hypersensitivity, but should not be administered in conjunction with heparin. Its management is similar to any other antithrombotic or fibrinolytic agent (Falanga et al., 2003; Micromedex Healthcare Series, 2002; Pescador, Porta & Ferro, 1996).

4. Management of overt bleeding

    a. Reduce localized bleeding.

      (1) Topical hemostatics (eg, topical thrombin, Avitene, Gelfoam).

      (2) Pressure applied on vascular access sites for 15 to 30 minutes, or until bleeding has stopped completely.

      (3) Consider elevation of limb if gravitational pressure may be contributory to sustained bleeding.

      (4) Try to avoid use of cold or ice therapy, which enhances vasoconstriction.

    b. Replenish blood and coagulation products as needed to maintain perfusion.

    c. Administer antithrombolytic or antifibrinolytic agents cautiously (eg, epsilon-aminocaproic acid [EACA])

5. Nursing Diagnoses

    a. Altered tissue perfusion related to abnormal clotting

      (1) *Problem:* Systemic microvascular clotting obstructs perfusion to the tissues, leading to tissue ischemia and abnormal clotting.

      (2) *Interventions*

        (a) Assess signs of perfusion (eg, color and temperature of skin, peripheral pulses, level of consciousness, urine output, pO_2, and breath sounds).

        (b) Administer intravenous fluids to maintain circulatory flow per physician's order.

        (c) Monitor signs of fluid volume excess.

        (d) Warm the patient's extremities with blankets to avoid vasoconstriction, which can worsen perfusion deficit.

        (e) Administer heparin therapy as ordered (see III.E.).

      (3) *Desired outcomes*

        (a) Patient will be alert and oriented.

        (b) Patient will have pink, warm skin.

        (c) Patient will maintain urine output per physician's orders.

    b. Altered systemic protection related to bleeding

      (1) *Problem:* Systemic bleeding results from depletion of clotting factors and uncontrolled fibrinolysis.

      (2) *Interventions*

        (a) Assess site and amount of bleeding (eg, weigh dressings, count peripads, measure bodily drainage, heme test urine, stool, and emesis).

        (b) Monitor signs and symptoms of hypovolemic shock (eg, decreased blood pressure, increased heart rate).

        (c) Implement organ-specific assessments for bleeding.

          (i) Listen for crackles and observe for low oxygen saturation as indication of intrapulmonary bleeding.

(ii) Assess for visual changes (diplopia, blurred vision, visual field cuts) indicative of retinal thrombosis or hemorrhage.

(iii) Assess for back pain, flank pain, abdominal pain in conjunction with other symptoms of visceral organ bleeding.

(d) Monitor coagulation studies, hemoglobin level, and platelet count.

(e) Avoid invasive procedures and treatments.

(f) Consider insertion of a long-term indwelling catheter.

(g) Institute bleeding precautions.

(h) Apply pressure to sites of bleeding for at least 5 minutes; use pressure dressings or sandbags if needed.

(i) Elevate sites of active bleeding.

(j) Elevate head of bed to decrease intracranial pressure.

(k) Administer blood components as prescribed—platelets, red blood cells, fresh frozen plasma, and cryoprecipitate—to replace clotting factors and cryoprecipitate.

(l) Avoid medications that induce coagulopathies (ie, aspirin). Administer EACA as ordered.

(3) *Desired outcomes*

(a) Patient will have decreased or absent bleeding.

(b) Patient will have stable vital signs.

(c) Patient will maintain urine output per physician's orders.

(d) Patient will have normal platelet count and hematocrit.

c. Impaired skin integrity related to petechiae, purpura, and ecchymoses

(1) *Problem:* Hemorrhage into the skin and soft tissue leaves skin fragile.

(2) *Interventions*

(a) Monitor skin for signs of skin breakdown.

(b) Turn patient every 2 to 4 hours.

(c) Avoid shearing forces.

(d) Perform range of motion every shift.

(e) Use special mattress or low-air-loss bed as needed.

(f) Avoid interventions that put pressure on the skin or break skin integrity.

(3) *Desired outcomes:* Patient will have intact skin.

d. Risk for injury related to altered mental status

(1) *Problem:* Patients may be confused or somnolent due to decreased cerebral perfusion that has occurred with intracranial thrombosis or bleeding. Intracranial hemorrhage remains the most common cause of death in these patients.

(2) *Interventions*

(a) Assess patient's level of consciousness and orientation.

(b) When level of consciousness or orientation is impaired, increase the level of neurologic assessment to include muscle strength, pupillary responses, and more complex assessments of mentation, such as a mini-mental examination.

(c) Keep side rails up and bed in low position.

(d) Maintain bedrest during periods of active bleeding or low platelets. Place call bell within reach.

    (e) Clear pathways to bathroom and hall.
    (f) Provide assistance with activities of daily living, as needed.
    (g) Check patient frequently, especially for toileting.
    (h) Reorient patient to time, place, and person.
    (i) Avoid use of medications that may cause altered mental status and affect ability to assess the patient for intracranial bleeding or thrombosis.
    (j) Use mechanical restraints as a last resort, checking for skin integrity every 15 minutes.
   (3) *Desired outcome:* Patient will be oriented to person, place, and time, and free of neurologic impairment.
  e. Pain related to poor tissue perfusion or hemorrhage into the tissues
   (1) *Problem:* Poor tissue perfusion may lead to tissue ischemia with discomfort. Hemorrhage into tissues may cause pressure and subsequent pain.
   (2) *Interventions*
    (a) Assess level of pain using a scale of 1 to 10 or other assessment measure.
    (b) Correlate pain with signs and symptoms of internal hemorrhage.
    (c) Apply warmth to area of discomfort (per physician approval) to promote vasodilation and decrease ischemic pain.
    (d) Administer pain medications as ordered.
    (e) Elevate painful extremities.
   (3) *Desired outcome:* Patient will have reduction or total elimination of pain as documented on a pain assessment scale.
 F. Discharge Planning and Patient Education
  1. Teach patient and family to report signs and symptoms of bleeding.
  2. Teach bleeding precaution measures.
  3. Teach signs and symptoms of bleeding that should be reported to health care providers.
  4. Teach measures to prevent thrombophlebitis.
  5. Plan follow-up assessment of laboratory parameters and need for blood component transfusions (especially pertinent in chronic DIC).
  6. Make referrals for sensory and motor deficits requiring rehabilitation.
  7. Give patient written emergency phone numbers and instruction.

REFERENCES

Barbui, T., & Falanga, A. (2001). Disseminated intravascular coagulation in acute leukemia. *Seminars in Thrombosis and Hemostasis, 27*(6), 593–604.

Bick, R. L. (2002). Disseminated intravascular coagulation: A review of etiology, pathophysiology, diagnosis, and management: Guidelines for care. *Clinical Applications in Thrombosis and Hemostasis, 8*(1), 1–31.

Bullock, B. A., & Henze, R. L. (2000). Unit 3, Appendix C: Normal blood coagulation values. In B. A. Bullock & R. L. Henze (Eds.), *Focus on pathophysiology* (p. 398). Philadelphia: Lippincott Williams & Wilkins.

DeSancho, M. T., & Rand, J. H. (2001). Bleeding and thrombotic complications in critically ill patients with cancer. *Critical Care Clinics, 17,* 599–622.

Falanga, A., Vignoli, A., Marchetti, M., & Barbui, T. (2003). Defibrotide reduces procoagulant activity and increases fibrinolytic properties of endothelial cells, *Leukemia, 17*(8), 1636–1642.

Fischer, D. (2002). Disseminated intravascular coagulation. *Advance for Nurses, 4*(17), 17–20.

Gobel, B. H. (1999). Disseminated intravascular coagulation. *Seminars in Oncology Nursing, 15,* 174–182.

Hambleton, J., Leung, L. L., & Levi, M. (2002). Coagulation: Consultative hemostasis. *Hematology, 1,* 335–352.

Kwaan, H. C., Wang, J., & Boggio, L. N. (2002). Abnormalities in hemostasis in acute promyelocytic leukemia. *Hematology and Oncology, 20*(1), 33–41.

Letsky, E. A. (2001). Disseminated intravascular coagulation. *Best Practices and Research in Clinical Obstetrics and Gynecology, 4,* 623–644.

Levi, M. (2001). Cancer and DIC. *Haemostasis, 31*(Suppl. 1), 47–48.

Levi, M., & de Jonge, E. (2000). Current management of disseminated intravascular coagulation. *Hospital Practice (Off. Ed.), 35*(8), 59–66, quiz 92.

Levi, M., de Jonge, E., & Meijers, J. (2002). The diagnosis of disseminated intravascular coagulation. *Blood Reviews, 16,* 217–223.

Levi, M., de Jonge, E., & van der Poll, T. (2002). Therapeutic intervention in disseminated intravascular coagulation: Have we made any progress in the last millennium? *Blood Reviews, 16*(Suppl. 1), S29-S34.

Levi, M., & ten Cate, H. (1999). Disseminated intravascular coagulation. *New England Journal of Medicine, 341*(8), 586–592.

Levi, M. M., Vink, R., & de Jonge, E. (2002). Management of bleeding disorders by prohemostatic therapy. *International Journal of Hematology, 76*(Suppl. 2), 139–144.

Maxson, J. H. (2000). Management of disseminated intravascular coagulation. *Critical Care Clinics of North America, 12*(3), 341–352.

Messmore, H. L., & Wehrmacher, W. H. (2002, March). Disseminated intravascular coagulation. A primer for primary care physicians. *Postgraduate Medicine* [Web Exclusive]. Available: www.postgradmed.com/issues/2002/03/0302/messmore.htm.

Micromedex Healthcare Series. (2002). *Drugdex drug evaluations: Defibrotide.* Available: http://jhmcis.jhmi.edu/mdxcgi/display.

Pescador, R., Porta, R., & Ferro, L. (1996). An integrated view of the activities of defibrotide. *Seminars in Thrombosis and Hemostasis, 22*(Suppl. 1), 71–75.

Yu, M., Nardella, B. S., & Pechet, L. (2000). Screening tests of disseminated intravascular coagulation: Guidelines for rapid and specific laboratory diagnosis. *Critical Care Medicine, 28,* 1777–1780.

Wada, H., Mori, Y., Okabayashi, K., Gabazza, E. C., Kushiya, F., Watanabe, M., Nishikawa, M., Shiku, H., & Nobori, T. (2003). High plasma fibrinogen level is associated with poor clinical outcome in DIC patients. *American Journal of Hematology, 72,* 1–7.

34 Hypercalcemia

MiKaela Olsen
Joanne P. Finley

I. **Definition:** Corrected serum calcium greater than 11.0 mg/dL.
   A. Normal serum calcium is 8.6 to 10.5, and normal ionized calcium is 1.13 to 1.32 mmol/L.
   B. Calcium distribution within the body: 99% of body's calcium is stored in the bone, and 1% of the total body calcium is located in the serum.
      1. Of the 1% located in the serum, half is bound to protein and the other half is considered active and is ionized.
      2. Most of the calcium bound to protein is bound to albumin.
      3. Cancer patients often have preexisting hypoalbuminemia that will influence the amount of active calcium that is present in the serum. A formula to calculate corrected calcium is shown in Box 34–1.
      4. When interpreting laboratory values, it is important to note that a decrease in albumin results in an increase in unbound or ionized calcium.
   C. Calcium is necessary for the formation and maintenance of bones and teeth, transmission of nerve impulses, maintenance of normal clotting mechanisms, and contractility of cardiac, smooth, and skeletal muscle.
   D. Normal levels of plasma calcium are maintained in the body by three major hormones: parathyroid hormone (PTH), 1,25-dihydroxyvitamin D, and calcitonin. These individual hormones respond when necessary to maintain a steady normal level of calcium in the body.

II. **Etiology**
   A. Cancer is the most common cause of hypercalcemia in hospitalized patients and occurs in 10% to 20% of cancer patients in the United States. Eighty percent of cases are with solid tumor cancers, such as breast, lung, head and neck, bladder, thyroid, and renal. Twenty per-

---

▼ **BOX 34-1** | **Corrected Serum Calcium**

Calculation of Corrected Serum Calcium
Formula:
Corrected serum calcium = [(4.0 − serum albumin) × 0.8] + serum calcium level
Example:
Patient labs: Albumin 2.5, serum calcium 11.5
Answer: [(4.0 − 2.5) × 0.8] + 11.5 = 12.7 (corrected serum calcium)

---

cent are hematologic cancers, such as multiple myeloma, leukemia, and lymphoma.

B. Common nonmalignant causes of hypercalcemia include hyper-parathyroidism, and hyperthyroidism.

C. The two primary mechanisms associated with hypercalcemia in cancer are humoral and osteolytic.

1. Humoral mechanisms are responsible for about 80% of all hypercalcemia of malignancy (Kaplan, 1994). Humoral hypercalcemia of malignancy has been defined as an increase in calcium levels above normal with absence of skeletal metastasis (Grill & Martin, 2000). Research is continuing to determine whether humoral and osteolytic hypercalcemia can coexist in patients, and the impact of multiple mechanisms on the clinical course of the complication (Grill & Martin, 2000). Tumor production of a parathyroid hormone-like substance (PTH), increased production of 1,25-dihydroxyvitamin D, or increased secretion of certain growth factors such as tumor necrosis factor, interleukin 6, and interleukin-1 are humoral mechanisms that have been identified.

   a. The body can be tricked into believing that the calcium levels are low when tumors secrete a PTH–like substance. PTH typically functions to bring calcium levels back to normal when low. PTH does this by affecting three organs: bone, intestines, and kidneys. PTH stimulates osteoclast activity, which breaks down bone, causing the release of stored calcium into the bloodstream. PTH also stimulates the kidneys to increase excretion of phosphorus, causing serum calcium levels to rise to maintain its inverse relationship with phosphorus. The kidneys are unable to excrete the large amounts of calcium being released from bone. Intestinal reabsorption of calcium also occurs as a result of PTH secretion, thereby raising the calcium.

   b. Intestinal stimulation to increase the production of 1,25-dihydroxyvitamin D, consumption of vitamin D–enriched foods, and exposure to natural sunlight all serve to increase calcium levels in the blood. Increased production of 1,25-dihydroxyvitamin D is a common cause of hypercalcemia in lymphoma and leukemia.

   c. Growth factors and cytokines (eg, tumor necrosis factor, interleukins, interferons) stimulate osteoclast resorption of bone, resulting in elevated serum calcium levels.

2. Osteolytic causes include tumors that result in skeletal metastases or arise in the bone.

D. Other Medical Causes

1. Immobilization causes increased release of calcium into the bloodstream, which can potentiate hypercalcemia.

2. Dehydration causes the body to retain water and decrease calcium excretion through the kidneys.

3. In the presence of renal insufficiency, patients are unable to excrete excess calcium from the body.

4. Medications such as thiazide diuretics, calcium carbonate, hypervitaminosis D and A, theophylline toxicity, lithium, estrogen, and antiestrogen, and progestin therapies may cause or potentiate hypercalcemia.

III. Patient Management

A. Assessment: The following signs and symptoms are related to the actual calcium level, the general health of the patient, and the rapidity of onset of hypercalcemia. Elderly patients tend to have more symptoms with less severe increases in calcium (Table 34–1).

  1. Neuromuscular: Fatigue, weakness, lethargy, confusion, apathy, and hyporeflexia are secondary to decreased neuromuscular excitability.

  a. In severe cases, psychotic behaviors, visual changes, and seizures can occur.

  b. Stupor, coma, and death can occur in severe cases left untreated.

  c. Bone pain or achiness, skeletal fractures, and deformities can result from the increased osteoclast activity causing bone destruction.

  2. Cardiovascular: Bradycardia or heart block can occur due to depressed cardiac contractility. Waveform changes may include shortened QT interval, prolonged PR interval, and flat, widened, or inverted T waves. Increased digitalis sensitivity may also be present. Hypercalcemia can also cause hypertension, related to renal dysfunction or direct vasoconstriction.

  3. Gastrointestinal (GI): Anorexia, constipation, nausea, and vomiting are the result of decreased smooth muscle contractility and decreased motility of the GI tract. Development of a paralytic ileus is not an uncommon complication.

  4. Genitourinary: Glomerular filtration of high calcium levels causes disruption of tubular filtering mechanisms, leading to increased fluid excretion and polyuria. Excess calcium salt precipitation in the renal tubules may lead to renal calculi that present as abdominal or flank pain. Renal insufficiency or renal failure may occur in extreme cases.

TABLE 34–1 Hypercalcemia

Mild (Corrected Serum Calcium <12 mg/dL)	Moderate (Corrected Serum Calcium 12–13.5 mg/dL)	Severe (Corrected Serum Calcium >13.5 mg/dL)
Oral hydration	IV hydration with 0.9% normal saline	IV hydration with 0.9% normal saline
Sodium-restricted diet	Sodium-restricted diet	Sodium-restricted diet
Ambulation if applicable	Ambulation if applicable	Ambulation if applicable
	Administer diuretics	Administer diuretics
	Initiate pharmacologic agents	Initiate pharmacologic agents
	Consider dialysis for patients with worsening or unresponsive hypercalcemia and renal failure	Consider dialysis for patients with worsening or unresponsive hypercalcemia and renal failure
Treat malignancy	Treat malignancy	Treat malignancy

Davidson, T. G. (2001). Conventional treatment of hypercalcemia of malignancy. *American Journal of Health System Pharmacy, 58*(Suppl. 3), S8–S15.

5. Polydipsia and weight loss are related to increased urine output.

B. Diagnostic Parameters

    1. Serum blood tests

        a. Serum calcium and albumin levels using the corrected calcium formula (see Box 34–1).

        b. Ionized calcium can be used alone or in combination with the corrected serum calcium to evaluate hypercalcemia.

        c. Serum phosphorus is decreased due to increased urinary excretion enhanced by the high calcium levels.

        d. BUN and creatinine are increased due to decreased glomerular filtration rate secondary to polyuria and subsequent dehydration.

        e. Other serum electrolyte levels can be decreased (eg, magnesium and potassium).

    2. Urine test: Urinary calcium is elevated due to renal excretion of increased calcium load.

    3. Other tests: Electrocardiogram shows dysrhythmias, shortened QT interval, wide T wave, and prolonged PR interval (Figure 34–1).

C. Treatment: The most important factor after stabilization of acute symptoms is treatment of the underlying cause. Primary treatment of the cancer causing the hypercalcemia is the most successful long-term management strategy. The major tenets of treatment include:

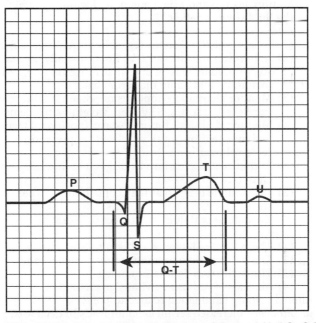

Figure 34–1. ECG changes in hypercalcemia. (Ruppert, S.D. Kernicki, J.G., & Dolan, J.T. [Eds.]. *Dolan's critical care nursing: Clinical management through the nursing process* [2nd ed., p. 210]. Philadelphia: F.A. Davis).

1. Expansion of extracellular and intravascular fluid volume
   a. Several liters of fluid are usually required to replenish fluid loss through polyuria.
   b. Fluid administration can also cause hemodilution, thereby lowering the calcium level.
   c. Normal saline 0.9% is preferred because salt enhances urinary excretion of calcium.
2. Enhancement of calcium excretion from the kidneys. Fluid repletion alone may be sufficient in mild or moderately symptomatic hypercalcemia. Administration of loop diuretics can enhance this process.
3. Reduction of calcium resorption from bones primarily through the use of bisphosphonates.
4. Pharmacologic therapies (Table 34–2).
5. Control of the malignancy
D. Nursing Diagnosis and Related Interventions and Outcomes
   1. Fluid volume deficit related to polyuria, anorexia, nausea, and vomiting
      a. *Problem:* Increased serum calcium and increased urinary calcium cause an osmotic diuresis and increased urine output, resulting in decreased circulating blood volume. After sodium and water reabsorption in response to the dehydration, there is increased calcium reabsorption, compounding the elevated serum calcium. Decreased GI smooth muscle contractility and motility lead to anorexia, nausea, and vomiting, which potentate the fluid volume deficit.
      b. *Interventions*
         (1) Assess body fluid status (eg, skin turgor, mucosal moistness).
         (2) Administer intravenous (IV) fluids, usually normal saline solution, to increase glomerular filtration rate, restore hydration, and dilute the serum calcium.
         (3) Monitor signs and symptoms of potential fluid volume excess (eg, crackles, S3 gallop, weight gain, edema).
         (4) Monitor vital signs for orthostasis (positional tachycardia and hypotension, low central venous pressure) to guide fluid replenishment plan.
         (5) Administer medications as ordered to decrease serum calcium (see Table 34–2).
         (6) Discontinue drugs that may contribute to hypercalcemia, such as diuretics and estrogens.
         (7) Encourage oral fluids to correct dehydration.
      c. *Desired outcomes*
         (1) The patient will have good skin turgor.
         (2) The patient will have moist mucous membranes.
         (3) The patient's weight will stabilize.
         (4) Absence of orthostatic vital sign changes.
   2. Altered urinary elimination related to polyuria
      a. *Problem:* Increased serum calcium leads to decreased ability of kidneys to concentrate urine and subsequent polyuria.
      b. *Interventions*
         (1) Assess urine color and specific gravity.
         (2) Monitor electrolyte values.

(3) Administer IV normal saline.

(4) Maintain strict intake and output.

(5) Weigh patient every day. Report any weight change from the patient's baseline weight.

(6) Administer diuretics per order to maintain urine output at 100 to 150 mL/h and promote calcium diuresis, which follows sodium diuresis.

(7) Monitor patient on dialysis if needed.

  c. *Desired outcomes*

(1) The patient will have normal serum calcium.

(2) The patient will maintain urine output per physician's orders.

3. Impaired physical mobility related to bone pain and weakness

  a. *Problem:* Bone pain and muscle weakness are common symptoms associated with hypercalcemia. These symptoms influence the patient's motivation to remain mobile. Decreased physical mobility increases bone resorption of calcium. It also leads to complications such as constipation.

  b. *Interventions*

(1) Assess patient's level of pain using established visual analogue scales.

(2) Administer pain medications and alternative therapies before activity (see Chapter 33).

(3) Encourage and assist patient with physical mobility. Ambulation is the most preferable activity because it is weight bearing and reduces bone resorption of calcium due to immobility. Passive and active range-of-motion exercises may reduce muscle atrophy and physical mobility problems.

(4) Use transfer devices as needed.

(5) Make referrals to physical therapy as needed.

  c. *Desired outcome:* The patient will maintain or improve mobility.

4. Risk for injury related to altered mental status

  a. *Problem:* Hypercalcemia induces mental status changes, such as confusion, lethargy, and neuromuscular weakness, which place the patient at risk for injury.

  b. *Interventions*

(1) Assess patient's level of consciousness and orientation.

(2) Place bed in a low position with side rails elevated.

(3) Maintain patient on bedrest if patient is severely confused.

(4) Place call bell within reach.

(5) Monitor patient frequently and assist with ambulation.

(6) Reorient patient to time, place, and person.

(7) Instruct patient not to smoke alone.

(8) Clear hall and bedside of obstacles.

(9) Assist with activities of daily living, as needed.

(10) Use restraints as a last resort, checking skin integrity frequently.

(11) Place patient on seizure or aspiration precautions as appropriate.

  c. *Desired outcome:* The patient will be free of injury.

TABLE 34-2 Pharmacologic Agents for Hypercalcemia Treatment Administration

Drug	Action	Dosage Guidelines	Nursing Considerations
Furosemide	Blocks calcium reabsorption in the ascending loop	20–40 mg q12h slow IV push If over 100 mg, give at 10 mg/min to reduce tinnitus.	Monitor potassium, phosphorus, magnesium, and calcium levels and supplement if necessary. Assess for signs of dehydration.
Glucocorticoids (eg, hydrocortisone)	Increase urinary calcium excretion Inhibit vitamin D–related calcium absorption	Orally 100–300 mg qd Slow onset	Monitor serum glucose. Advise patient to take with milk or food.
Calcitonin	Inhibits bone resorption Promotes renal excretion Rapid onset ~2 h Erratic and unpredictable patient response	4–12 IU/kg IM or SQ q6–12h *Note:* Administer test dose before therapy if ordered.	Monitor nausea, vomiting, and signs of allergic reaction.
Plicamycin	Inhibits bone resorption Peak response = 48–72 h after administration	25 µg/kg IV over 4–6 h May repeat in 1 week or longer.	Monitor for thrombocytopenia and leukopenia, GI upset, and blood pressure. Monitor renal and liver function. Use vesicant extravasation precautions. Rarely used.

Etidronate disodium	Reduces bone formation Slow onset Effect not sustained	7.5 mg/kg/day IV for 3–7 days 20 mg/kg/day PO dilute in at least 250 mL. Administer over 2–4 h.	Assess renal function and GI upset. Rapid administration can result in renal insufficiency.
Pamidronate disodium	Inhibits bone resorption Response is seen in ~2 days.	60–90 mg IV over 2–24 h May repeat after 7 days Oral 1,200 mg/day in divided doses	Monitor temperature and renal function. Monitor IV site.
Zoledronate	Inhibits bone resorption Response is seen in ~2 days.	4 mg IV over 15 min May repeat Q month or in 7 days if no response Do not administer faster than 15 min in patients with renal insufficiency.	Monitor patient for flulike symptoms and GI symptoms.
Gallium nitrate	Inhibits bone resorption Response seen in 48 h, but duration is short.	200 mg/m²/day for 5 days by way of continuous infusion	Assess renal function. Hydrate first and use caution with con- current aminoglycosides.

5. Constipation related to the effects of hypercalcemia on smooth muscles controlling peristalsis

    a. *Problem:* Hypercalcemia induces constipation by depressing neuromuscular transmission to the GI tract, thereby decreasing GI motility.

    b. *Interventions*

        (1) Monitor frequency and character of stools.

        (2) Encourage oral fluids (at least 3 to 4 L/day).

        (3) Increase physical activity to highest tolerable level.

        (4) Encourage patient to include high-fiber foods in diet.

        (5) Administer stool softeners and laxatives, as prescribed.

        (6) Provide privacy for elimination needs.

    c. *Desired outcome:* The patient will maintain a normal pattern of bowel elimination.

E. Discharge Planning and Patient Education: Both are especially important due to the high incidence of recurrence. The recurrence of the malignancy is often associated with a recurrence of the hypercalcemia as well.

  1. Teach patient and family the risk factors for hypercalcemia.

  2. Teach patient and family the signs and symptoms of hypercalcemia to report.

  3. Instruct patient and family about the importance of hydration and mobility.

  4. Calcium and vitamin D supplements should be avoided. However, low-calcium diets are difficult for cancer patients to tolerate and are not believed to be helpful in treating hypercalcemia of malignancy. If the hypercalcemia exists in a lymphoma patient with excessive 1,25-dihydroxyvitamin D secretion, then enhanced intestinal calcium absorption may occur, and calcium intake should be limited (Myers, 2001).

  5. Teach safety measures for home.

  6. Give patient and family written emergency phone numbers and instructions.

REFERENCES

Davidson, T. G. (2001). Conventional treatment of hypercalcemia of malignancy. *American Journal of Health System Pharmacy, 58*(Suppl. 3), S8–S15.

Deftos, L. J. (2002). Hypercalcemia in malignant and inflammatory diseases. *Endocrinology and Metabolism Clinics, 31*(1), 1–14.

Grill, V., & Martin, T. J. (2000). Hypercalcemia of malignancy. *Reviews in Endocrine & Metabolic Disorders, 1,* 253–263.

Hotte, S. J., Hirte, H. W., Rabbani, S. A., Carling, T., Hendy, G. N., & Major, P. P. (2002). Hypercalcemia of malignancy. Pathophysiology, diagnosis and treatment. *American Journal of Cancer, 1*(3), 179–187.

Kaplan, M. (1994). Hypercalcemia of malignancy: A review of advances in pathophysiology. *Oncology Nursing Forum, 21*(6), 1039–1048.

Major, P. (2002). The use of zoledronic acid, a novel, highly potent bisphosphonate, for the treatment of hypercalcemia of malignancy. *The Oncologist, 7*(6), 481–491.

Major, P., Lortholary, A., Hon, J., Abdi, E., Mills, G., Menssen, H. D., et al. (2001). Zoledronic acid is superior to pamidronate in the treatment of hypercalcemia of malignancy: A pooled analysis of two randomized, controlled clinical trials. *Journal of Clinical Oncology, 19*(2), 558–567.

Myers, J. (2001). Oncologic complications. In S.E. Otto (Ed), *Oncology nursing* (4th ed.). St. Louis: Mosby.

Naco, G. J., & von Gunten, C. (2002). Refractory neuropathic pain from chronic cord compression. *Journal of Palliative Care Medicine, 5*(3).

Singer, F. R., & Minoofar, P. N. (1995). Biophosphonates in the treatment of disorders of mineral metabolism. *Advances in Endocrinology & Metabolism, 6,* 259–288.

Warrell, R. P. (2001). Metabolic emergencies. In V. DeVita, S. Hellman, & S. A. Rosenberg (Eds.), *Cancer: Principles and practice of oncology* (6th ed.). Philadelphia: Lippincott-Raven.

35 Neoplastic Cardiac Tamponade

Brenda K. Shelton

I. Definition: Cardiac tamponade is a syndrome of pericardial constriction that does not permit the normal expansion of the heart, impeding venous blood return and ventricular filling.

    A. Intrapericardial pressure is normally subatmospheric, allowing the inflow of low-pressure venous blood into the right heart. When the pericardium is constricted by fibrous bands or filled with fluid, the pressure in the pericardial sac is raised to a level that exceeds the normal filling pressure of the ventricle.

        1. The initial pathophysiology is venous congestion caused by obstruction to inflow of blood into the heart.

        2. When ventricular filling is more severely impaired, there is no blood inflow and, therefore, no subsequent cardiac output. This is called cardiac tamponade.

    B. Three terms are used to describe the clinical conditions of increased intrapericardial pressure typical of this syndrome.

        1. Pericarditis is an inflammation of the lining surrounding the heart that may be fibrous or exudative.

        2. Pericardial effusion refers to excessive fluid accumulation within the pericardial sac and involves serous, purulent, bloody, or malignant exudates.

        3. Pericardial tamponade (cardiac tamponade) is fluid accumulation in the pericardial sac that is so great that normal contraction and ejection capabilities fail.

II. Etiology: The etiologies of pericardial tamponade depend on the mechanism of action or type of exudate. For a listing of common etiologies of tamponade according to their pathophysiologic mechanism, see Table 35–1.

    A. Transudative effusions are due to alterations in capillary permeability.

    B. Exudative effusions occur due to malignant cell invasion of the pericardium.

    C. Traumatic injury causes hemorrhagic tamponade (which rarely occurs in cancer patients).

    D. Infectious diseases (not the usual etiologic factor): Fluid collection related to infection may be purulent and harboring infective organisms, or serous and related to the inflammatory response of the pericardium.

III. Patient Management

    A. Assessment

        1. Signs and symptoms may depend on the type of pericardial disorder or may be a reflection of the chronicity of the problem.

TABLE 35–1   Etiologies of Cardiac Tamponade

Pathophysiologic Mechanism	Examples of Etiologies
Capillary permeability induced fluid extravasation into the pericardium	Leukemia Cytokine arabinoside Inflammatory cytokines given as anticancer therapy: interleukin-2, tumor necrosis factor
Severe chest venous congestion and obstruction of normal lymphatic fluid removal	Cardiomyopathy Myocardial infarction Thoracic lymph duct obstruction due to pulmonary infection or tumor
Hemorrhage into the pericardium	Traumatic injury (eg, motor vehicle accident) Central venous catheter insertion After cardiac surgery Renal failure Misplaced superior vena cava stent Severe thrombocytopenia
Infectious disorder	Candida Nocardia Toxoplasmosis Tuberculosis
Malignant involvement	Breast cancer Endometrial cancer Gastric cancer Head and neck cancer Hepatocellular cancer Hodgkin's and non-Hodgkin's lymphomas Kaposi's sarcoma Leukemia Lung cancer Melanoma Mesothelioma Ovarian cancer Prostate cancer Sarcoma Teratoma

    a. For differentiation of signs and symptoms according to their relation to pericarditis, effusion, or tamponade, see Table 35–2.

    b. Rapidly developing effusions may present symptomatically with minimal fluid accumulation (ie, 50 to 80 mL).

    c. Patients with slow-developing effusions compensate for a lower cardiac output and may not demonstrate signs or symptoms until there is more than 1,000 mL of fluid accumulation.

  2. Inflammation of the pericardium often causes pain in the chest that is exacerbated by movement, deep breathing, or lying flat. When pericarditis without fluid is present, pain is most severe, sharp, and localized. This severe discomfort may be partially relieved by sitting up and leaning forward, which displaces the heart within the chest and allows freer movement for ventricular filling. As an effusion

TABLE 35–2 Clinical Presentation of Pericardial Disorders

Clinical Finding	Pericarditis: Inflammation of the Pericardial Lining	Pericardial Effusion: Excess Fluid Collection Within the Pericardial Sac	Pericardial Tamponade: Pericardial Fluid Resulting in Reduced Cardiac Contraction and Ejection
Chest pain	Severe, with deep breath; relieved by sitting up and leaning forward	Less intense; more dull and aching; less positional	Absent or faint
Cough	Not present	New onset of cough often related to heart failure	Variable
Heart sounds	Rub present and related to inflammation; best heard with heart close to chest wall; location may change with position change	Distant, faint, or muffled heart sounds; heard best with the patient positioned on left side, or sitting and leaning forward	Muffled or absent heart sounds in all positions
Point of maximal impulse (PMI)	Normal placement and intensity of PMI	PMI displaced laterally, and may be weaker than normal	Faint, barely discernible PMI in displaced position
Peripheral pulses	Normal	Weak, thready; upper extremities stronger than femoral or lower extremity pulses	Faint or absent lower extremity pulses, with slight but weak carotid or upper extremity pulses
Jugular venous pulsations/distention	Normal	Increased	Severe jugular venous distention, cannon A waves
Blood pressure (BP)	Narrow pulse pressure with rising diastolic BP and/or mild hypotension	Progressive hypotension with worsening narrowed pulse pressure, and falling systolic BP; pulsus paradoxus >10 mmHg	Frank hypotension with minimal difference between systolic and diastolic blood pressures

develops, the pain becomes more dull and diffuse, but less positional. When tamponade is present, pain is more often described as chest heaviness, or pain is not present at all.

3. Pericardial rub or muffled heart sounds are revealed on cardiac auscultation.

   a. A pericardial rub is an abrasive scratching sound heard throughout systole and diastole. It may be auscultated at any anatomic site because it reflects inflammation or irritation between the myocardium and pericardial sac. Most pericardial rubs are heard best at the apex when the patient is lying down, and at the base of the heart when the patient is sitting up and leaning forward. Having the patient lie on the left side to facilitate the heart's shift toward the chest wall may also make this abnormal sound more discernible.

   b. Muffled or distant heart sounds are noted when excess pericardial fluid diffuses the normal valve closure sounds. Muffled heart sounds do not always indicate cardiac effusion or tamponade; they also occur with large people, barrel-chested people, severe pleural effusions, or with poor cardiac function.

4. Displacement of the point of maximal impulse (PMI) of the heart reflects an enlarged heart with the strongest contraction at the apex being shifted.

   a. The PMI is usually located in the fifth intercostal space, along the midclavicular line.

   b. In pericardial effusion and tamponade, the PMI reflects the larger cardiac diameter and is shifted to the left (toward the axilla) or downward (toward the sixth intercostal space).

5. The strength of the central and peripheral pulses will be diminished according to the degree of compromised cardiac output.

   a. In pericarditis and effusion, the cardiac output is decreased, but it first feeds the proximal branches of the aortic arch that perfuse the brain and upper extremities.

   b. As a consequence, head (carotid) and upper extremity (brachial, radial) pulses will be stronger than lower extremity pulses (femoral, pedal).

   c. This differs from other decreased cardiac output states where the femoral pulse is usually stronger than the radial pulse.

6. Jugular venous pressure (JVP) increases due to resistance to flow of blood into the heart. The waves of JVP can be seen by examining the neck above the midclavicular line and by measuring the number of centimeters the wave extends above the clavicle when the patient is in a semi-Fowler's position. These pulsations can be so prominent as to produce a large continuous wave up the neck to the chin (called cannon a wave) when cardiac tamponade is present. Jugular venous distention (JVD), often referred to as bulging neck veins, is present bilaterally in severe effusion or impending tamponade.

   a. The amount of venous pressure may also be measured by right atrial (RA) or central venous pressure (CVP) readings.

   b. In pericardial effusion and tamponade, the RA pressure will exceed 6 mmHg (transduced pressure) or 10 cm of water (water manometer).

7. Peripheral edema, hepatomegaly, and splenomegaly are other symptoms of venous congestion that may be present, particularly if the onset of effusion or tamponade is insidious.

8. Cough is only present with pericardial effusion if the backflow of venous blood and congestive heart failure are prominent features.

9. Hypotension occurs in effusion and tamponade because of decreased cardiac output and increased vascular resistance due to a sympathetic vasoconstriction.

   a. First, the diastolic pressure rises; then the systolic pressure decreases.

   b. Patients usually have a narrow pulse pressure (systolic and diastolic pressures are nearly equal) due to equalization of the pressure within and around the heart.

   c. The presence of a pulsus paradoxus >10 mmHg signifies resistance to the inflow of blood into the heart. Pulsus paradoxus may be present in less severe conditions of increased thoracic pressure, such as with chronic lung disease; however, it is rarely absent in impending cardiac tamponade. Of clinical significance is that the lower systolic blood pressure is the actual perfusing blood pressure (see Interventions in Section III.D.1.b).

   d. Cardiac dysrhythmias are almost always present, although the prevalent pathophysiologic manifestations predict whether tachycardia or bradycardia is present.

   e. Tachycardia is the first heart rate response to decreased cardiac output and is considered an early symptom.

   f. Patients with impending tamponade will have such high thoracic resistance that blood does not fill the ventricles or the coronary arteries during inspiration, and bradycardia, heart block, or short periods of asystole may occur during the inspiratory phase of breathing.

10. Dyspnea occurs due to poor lung blood flow and compromised oxygen exchange or occurs with the congestion present with obstructed venous return. It is the most common, although the least specific, symptom.

11. Alterations in mental status may be present if blood flow to the brain is impaired.

12. Oliguria is often an early indicator of compromised cardiac output.

B. Diagnostic Parameters: There are no laboratory or urine tests used to diagnose neoplastic cardiac tamponade; however, there are other tests that can indicate the presence of the condition.

   1. Echocardiogram analysis will show fluid in the pericardial sac and distorted or inadequate ventricular expansion. In impending tamponade, one or both ventricles are collapsed/closed due to high intrapericardial pressure (van Steijn, et al, 2002).

   2. Chest x-rays show symmetric cardiac enlargement, with the cardiac diameter exceeding half the chest, with a water bottle silhouette of the heart, and with clear lung fields.

   3. Electrocardiograms (ECG) most often reveal low-voltage QRS complexes and tachycardia (early) or bradycardia/heart block (late). Electrical alternans (alternating positive- and negative-deflected QRS complexes) occurs in a small number of patients, but almost always

signifies impending cardiac tamponade (Lau, Civitello, Hernandez & Coulter, 2002).

C. Treatment (see Table 35–3 for detailed information)

  1. Emergency care is supportive, although the definitive treatment of fluid removal from the pericardium should be implemented as rapidly as possible after diagnosis.

  2. Initial treatment is aimed at raising the pressure of returning venous blood by administration of large volumes of fluid. This provides temporary venous return to allow for ejection of fluid.

  3. Hypoxemia is the consequence of low cardiac output. Oxygen therapy is commonly implemented, but endotracheal intubation with mechanical support (by way of ambu bagging or mechanical ventilation) should be avoided if possible.

   a. Assisted ventilation induces higher thoracic pressures that impede venous return, further compromising cardiac output.

   b. High thoracic pressures with sudden compromise in venous return are likely to cause pulseless electrical activity or bradyarrhythmias.

  4. Pericardial drainage can be categorized as temporary or permanent. Temporary fluid removal by way of pericardial catheter drainage is highly effective at alleviating immediate symptoms, although recurrence occurs in about 40% of the patients (Martinoni et al., 2000). More permanent resolution is seen with surgical procedures such as pericardial window; however, the safety and recovery time period for these procedures may prohibit its immediate use as initial treatment.

  5. Palliative care: Symptoms can rarely be managed conservatively without pericardial drainage, although there are a few therapeutic strategies that may be employed if pericardial drainage is not feasible or desired. Radiosensitive tumors may demonstrate a clinical response in 3 to 4 days and may be employed if the situation is urgent, but not an emergency. Colchicine has also been employed as an antiinflammatory with some success noted in 5 to 14 days for patients with end-stage multiple myeloma (Ng, Gatt, Pagliuca, & Mufti, 2000).

D. Nursing Diagnosis and Related Interventions and Outcomes

  1. Decreased cardiac output related to fibrous pericardial lining or increased pericardial fluid

   a. *Problem*: Intrapericardial fluid causes a more positive pressure around the heart and impedes the inflow of low-pressure venous blood. Obstruction to the inflow of blood results in venous congestion. Less blood inflow also leads to decreased cardiac output.

   b. *Interventions*

    (1) Assess heart sounds and PMI for evidence of altered contraction or heart size.

    (2) Implement continuous cardiac monitoring. Tachycardia occurs early with lowered cardiac output. Bradycardia or heart block occurs with inspiration when pericardial pressure impedes inflow of blood and feeding of the conduction system. Asystole or pulseless electrical activity occurs with cardiac tamponade.

(Text continues on page 530)

TABLE 35–3 Treatment of Neoplastic Cardiac Tamponade

Treatment	Indications	Methodology	Nursing Implications
Massive fluid administration	Emergency management of hypotension, cardiac arrest, pulseless electrical activity	Use a large vessel, preferably central vessel, to administer large volumes of intravenous fluids as quickly as possible until venous exceeds pericardial pressure.	Have multiple lines available when possible. Some physicians prefer colloids (eg, plasma, blood) to expand blood volume. Use infusion pumps or pressure bags as needed to increase the rate of infusion.
Radiation therapy	Progressive malignant effusion with a known radiosensitive tumor	Low-dose daily fractionated radiation therapy to cardiac region	Assess for previous anthracycline therapy, because risk of cardiomyopathy may be worsened with radiation therapy to the heart. Lung fields may also receive radiation exposure, so assess for findings indicative of radiation pneumonitis.
Chemotherapy	Progressive malignant effusion with a known chemosensitive tumor	Single- or multiple-dose intravenous chemotherapy administration that has been established as effective against tumor. Chemotherapy administration into the pericardial sac—still investigational.	Usual nursing implications of chemotherapy. Nurses do not administer chemotherapy into the pericardium; physicians do.
Pericardial catheter	Short-term emergent removal of slow- or rapid-developing effusion; can be performed emergently with echocardiogram or fluoroscopic guidance	Fluoroscopy-directed pericardial catheter with drainage and sclerosing	Preprocedural preparation: minor sedating at bedside or procedure room, light meal permitted if clinical condition warrants.

Maintenance of catheter patency:

Maintain a closed system.

Account for drainage quantity, color, and consistency each shift.

Keep drainage bag below the level of the heart.

Sudden cessation of drainage may indicate misplacement or clotting of the catheter.

Observe the patient for recurrent tamponade; a sudden increase in catheter drainage may indicate a clotting abnormality.

Report a change in drainage to the physician. Flushing the catheter with approximately 3 mL of preservative-free normal saline may be performed by physician or nursing staff every 4 to 8 h as needed. If the drainage is extremely bloody, low-dose heparin may be used.

Exit site care:

Catheter is not sutured in place; it has a curled tip that should help to keep it in the pericardial sac.

Maintain sterile dressing over the exit site.

(*continued*)

TABLE 35–3   Treatment of Neoplastic Cardiac Tamponade *(Continued)*

Treatment	Indications	Methodology	Nursing Implications
			Nursing during administration of sclerosing agent: Administer pain medication if doxycycline is used. Administer antipyretics if bleomycin is used. Clamp catheter for 2 to 4 h after administration of sclerosing agent. Refer to the preprocedure preparation for pericardial catheter above. Monitor for recurrent tamponade symptoms.
Balloon pericardotomy	Short-term emergent removal of slow- or rapid-developing effusion	Catheter inserted into pericardial sac and balloon inflated to open a hole in the pericardial sac; catheter is immediately removed and pericardial fluid drains into the mediastinum	
Pericardial window	Chronic, severe effusions in a patient with otherwise good performance status; must be able to tolerate a thoracoscopic procedure	Thoracostomy or thoracotomy surgical wound with resection of lower section of pericardial sac; screenlike grid placed to allow pericardial fluid drainage into mediastinum. A variation of this procedure is used to create a peritoneal-pericardial window.	*Preoperative preparation:* Follow regular operative procedure with anesthetic. *Postoperative thoracotomy:* Prevent pulmonary complications by encouraging coughing and deep breathing.

		Mediastinal chest tube care: Monitor drainage (no bubbling from mediastinal chest tube); tube is positioned in the epigastric region, usual chest tube exit site care. Teach patient and significant other about symptoms of occlusion and reaccumulation.
Pericardectomy	Chronic, severe effusions in a patient with good performance status; must be able to tolerate a thoracotomy procedure; used only after other interventions have failed	Patients have permanent elimination of problem. Constrictive pericarditis may occur due to fibrous scar tissue on the outside of the heart.
Pericardial stripping		
Pericardiocentesis	Life-threatening cardiac tamponade in presence of moderate/large pericardial effusion; occurs when open procedure cannot be performed promptly	Have emergency equipment (crash cart, defibrillator) nearby during procedure. Use ECG machine whenever possible to avoid removal of intracardial blood. Save fluid aspirated. Pericardial fluid should not clot, but if blood is withdrawn from the ventricle, it will clot in the syringe. Monitor return or strengthening of pulses during procedure.
	Emergency bedside insertion of needle into pericardial sac for removal of fluid: Long, cardiac needle is attached to alligator clamp that is connected to the V chest lead of the ECG machine; needle is inserted subxiphoid and pointed toward the left shoulder; when injury curve occurs on ECG machine, needle is backed off and fluid is aspirated.	

(3) Assess pulse strength and equality, blood pressure, skin temperature, and skin color to ascertain adequacy of perfusion.

(4) Assess characteristics of chest pain and response to interventions. Evaluate ECG for evidence of ischemia or impending tamponade.

(5) Assess for pulsus paradoxus and report paradoxus >10 mmHg.
   (a) Lower cuff pressure while patient breathes normally.
   (b) Note pressure when first systolic sound is heard.
   (c) Continue to lower the cuff pressure until sounds can be heard throughout the respiratory cycle.
   (d) Note blood pressure reading (second systolic sound).
   (e) Subtract the second pressure from the first measurement.
   (f) Evaluate the pulsus measurement for an elevation >10 mmHg, indicating a significant paradoxical pulse indicative of increased thoracic pressure that is characteristic, but not conclusive, for clinically symptomatic pericardial effusion.

(6) Monitor for jugular venous distention/pulsations or elevated CVP readings. Other signs/symptoms of venous congestion include edema, pulmonary crackles, hepatomegaly, and splenomegaly.

(7) Maintain patient nothing by mouth (NPO) until diagnostic tests rule out the need for emergent surgical interventions.

(8) Assist in obtaining chest x-rays used to monitor progression of effusions. Be sure to use consistent technique when obtaining chest x-rays. Upright position is preferred; posterior-anterior (not available by portable x-ray), as well as lateral pictures are also most sensitive to cardiac enlargement.

(9) Assist with patient preparation and positioning for echocardiograms, used to diagnose or monitor effusions.

(10) Provide personal care and perform activities of daily living so oxygen demands are minimized.

(11) Provide for rest periods between care to minimize oxygen demands.

(12) Administer low doses of sedatives as needed to reduce oxygen demands.

(13) In symptomatic tamponade, administer fluid challenges as ordered. Increasing vascular volume increases venous pressure so that it exceeds pericardial pressure, permitting inflow of venous blood.

(14) Administer vasopressor agents as ordered for severe hypotension.

(15) Assist with catheter or surgical aspiration of fluid (see Table 35–3).

(16) Assist with emergency bedside pericardiocentesis as ordered (Figure 35–1).

c. *Desired outcomes*
   (1) The patient will have normal blood pressure.
   (2) The patient will not have pulsus paradoxus.
   (3) The patient will not have cardiac dysrhythmias.
   (4) The patient will not have excess pericardial fluid seen on chest x-ray.

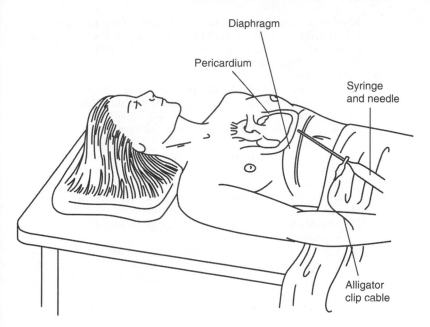

Figure 35–1. Proper needle placement for pericardiocentesis.

      (5) The patient will have a normal ventricular filling, seen on echocardiogram.
2. Altered thought processes related to inadequate brain perfusion
    a. *Problem*: Decreased cardiac output will compromise brain circulation, leading to altered cerebral function. Level of consciousness is the most sensitive indicator of cerebral perfusion.
    b. *Interventions*
      (1) Assess wakefulness and orientation for evidence of poor perfusion from decreased cardiac output.
      (2) Reorient with clock, calendar, and verbal reinforcement as needed.
      (3) Provide a safe environment.
      (4) Restrain protectively as needed, but avoid chemical restraints (eg, sedatives) that make it difficult to assess mental status and further compromise the airway.
    c. *Desired outcomes*
      (1) The patient will remain oriented to person, place, and time.
      (2) The patient will have normal wakefulness, cognition, and appropriateness of affect and conversation.
3. Altered tissue integrity related to decreased cardiac output and poor perfusion
    a. *Problem*: Decreased cardiac output causes compensatory blood shunting to the major organs (heart, lungs, brain) and dimin-

ished flow to less essential organs (kidneys, GI tract, periphery). Decreased peripheral blood flow results in soft tissue ischemia or necrosis. Decreased blood flow to the GI tract leads to decreased digestion and peristalsis.

  b. *Interventions*
   (1) Assess noninvasive parameters reflecting tissue oxygenation (eg, pulse oximetry, oxygen saturation monitoring, urine output).
   (2) Assess inner eyelid or lip mucosa for early symptoms of cyanosis.
   (3) Assess for weak or thready peripheral pulse, sluggish capillary refill, cool skin temperature, and altered skin color for signs and symptoms of blood shunting (eg, cool extremities, cyanosis) away from the periphery and less essential organs.
   (4) Avoid using distal extremities for intravenous (IV) access.
   (5) Provide warm coverings or warm packs to extremities to reduce risk of tissue necrosis.
   (6) Use strict aseptic technique for invasive procedures because poor peripheral circulation increases the risk of infection.
   (7) Assess for decreased bowel sounds indicative of blood shunting.
   (8) Evaluate tolerance of diet or tube feedings. Supplement nutrition intravenously as needed.
   (9) Monitor for low urinary output; report according to physician-ordered parameters.

  c. *Desired outcomes*
   (1) The patient's extremities will be warm, dry, and pink.
   (2) The patient will not experience cyanosis of the skin and mucous membranes.
   (3) The patient will have normal bowel and kidney function.

4. Ineffective breathing pattern related to hypoxemia and increased thoracic pressure

  a. *Problem*: Decreased pulmonary blood flow causes reduced oxygenation. The body's first response to hypoxia is to produce tachypnea, although dyspnea and more labored breathing often follow.

  b. *Interventions*
   (1) Provide supplemental oxygen as ordered and indicated.
   (2) Position in reverse Trendelenburg's or high Fowler's position as the blood pressure permits to enhance lung expansion and oxygenation.
   (3) Administer sedatives or bronchodilators as ordered to enhance oxygenation.
   (4) Provide ventilatory assistance as ordered for hypoxemia or hypercarbia. Positive pressure ventilation is used as a last resort because it increases thoracic pressure and may exacerbate cardiac compromise.

  c. *Desired outcomes*
   (1) The patient will have unlabored respirations of 12 to 22 breaths per minute.
   (2) The patient will maintain partial pressure oxygen >80 mmHg, measured on arterial blood gas.

(3) The patient will maintain partial pressure carbon dioxide between 35 and 45 mmHg, measured on arterial blood gas.

5. Alteration in elimination: urine output less than normal related to poor kidney perfusion

   a. *Problem*: Decreased cardiac output leads to blood shunted away from the kidneys. Decreased renal blood flow slows glomerular filtration, decreases urine production, and results in reduced elimination of wastes.

   b. *Interventions*

     (1) Assess intake and output every 1 to 2 hours.

     (2) Insert Foley catheter as ordered to accurately monitor urine output.

     (3) When a dramatic urine output decrease occurs, assess for catheter patency by checking for bladder distention and flushing the catheter.

     (4) Monitor serum creatinine, blood urea nitrogen, potassium, phosphate, and uric acid as ordered to assess renal excretion of metabolic wastes.

     (5) Administer potentially nephrotoxic medications with caution.

   c. *Desired outcomes*

     (1) The patient's urine output will be at least 30 mL/h.

     (2) The patient will have normal serum blood urea nitrogen and creatinine.

6. Altered comfort related to chest pain or dyspnea

   a. *Problem*: Inadequate venous blood return and low cardiac output states produce chest discomfort, dyspnea, and a sense of air hunger. These sensations make the patient more anxious/restless and may increase oxygen consumption, worsening the problem.

   b. *Interventions*

     (1) Administer sedatives or analgesics to reduce oxygen demand or consumption. Give in small increments until therapeutic effects are achieved, but respiratory depression or hypotension is not apparent. Morphine may be most helpful because of histamine-stimulating effects and vasodilation with lowering of diastolic blood pressure.

     (2) Provide emotional support to patient. Allow family members who are positive and supportive to have liberal visitation.

     (3) Explain all procedures (reason for procedure, expected sensations, expected outcome) to allay the patient's anxiety.

   c. *Desired outcomes*

     (1) The patient verbalizes relief of chest discomfort and dyspnea.

     (2) The patient displays both the ability to rest and minimal anxious behaviors.

E. Discharge Planning and Patient Education

   1. Teach patients who are at risk for or experiencing early signs and symptoms of pericardial effusion important reportable symptoms that may signify worsening of the condition. For many patients with cancer, the malignant effusion develops slowly and is more likely to present as gradual right heart failure with edema, jugular venous pulsations, and hepatomegaly. The subtle worsening of these symp-

toms or addition of cardiopulmonary symptoms, such as chest pain or dyspnea, often heralds impending tamponade.

2. Teach patients who have been treated for pericardial effusion with catheter or needle aspiration and pericardial window about the risks for recurrence if the fluid reaccumulates and is not drained into the mediastinum. These patients may have continuous symptoms and must be aware of subtle changes in their dyspnea, such as needing three pillows instead of one to sleep at night.

3. Explain to the patient that, although neoplastic cardiac tamponade was once viewed as an irreversible complication related to extensive or metastatic cancer, it can now be effectively abrogated.

REFERENCES

Atar, S., Chiu, J., Forrester, J. S., & Siegel, R. J. (1999). Bloody pericardial effusion in patients with cardiac tamponade: Is the cause cancerous, tuberculous, or iatrogenic in the 1990's? *Chest, 116*(6), 1564–1569.

Bastian, A., Meibner, A., Lins, M., Siegel, E. G., Moller, F., & Simon, R. (2000). Pericardiocentesis: Differential aspects of a common procedure. *Intensive Care Medicine, 26,* 572–576.

Beauchamp, K. A. (1998). Pericardial tamponade: An oncologic emergency. *Clinical Journal of Oncology Nursing, 2,* 85–95.

Camione, A., Cacchiarelli, M., Ghiribelli, C., Caloni, V., D'Agata, A., & Gotti, G. (2002). Which treatment in pericardial effusion? *Journal of Cardiovascular Surgery, 43*(5), 735–739.

Flounders, J. A., (2003). Cardiovascular emergencies: Pericardial effusion and cardiac tamponade. *Oncology Nursing Forum* On-line exclusive, *30*(2): www.ons.org/xp6/ ONS/Library.xml/ONS Publications.xml/ONF.xml/ONF2003?M, accessed 12/20/03.

Gibbs, C. R., Watson, R. D. S., Singh, S. P., & Lip, G. Y. H. (2000). *Postgraduate Medical Journal, 76,* 809–813.

Goyle, K. K., & Walling, A. D. (2002). Diagnosing pericarditis. *American Family Physician, 66*(9), 1695–1702.

Hawley, J., Dreher, H. M., & Vasso, M. (2003). Under pressure: Treating cardiac tamponade. *Nursing Management, 34*(2), 44D–44H.

Karam, N., Patel, P., & deFilippi, C. (2001). Diagnosis and management of chronic pericardial effusions. *American Journal of the Medical Sciences, 322*(2), 79–87.

Keefe, D. L. (2000). Cardiovascular emergencies in the cancer patient. *Seminars in Oncology, 27*(3), 244–255.

Kirsner, K. (2003). Cancer: New therapies and new approaches to recurring problems. *AANA Journal, 71*(1), 55–62.

Knoop, T., & Willenberg, K. (1999). Cardiac tamponade. *Seminars in Oncology Nursing, 15,* 168–173.

Lau, T. K., Civitello, A. B., Hernandez, A., & Coulter, S. A. (2002). Cardiac tamponade and electrical alternans. *Texas Heart Institute Journal, 29*(1), 66–67.

Martinoni, A., Cipolla, C. M., Civelli, M., Cardinale, D., Lamantia, A., Colleoni, M., DeBraud, F., Susini, G., Martinelli, G., Goldhirsh, A., & Fiorenti, C. (2000). Intrapericardial treatment of neoplastic pericardial effusions. *Herz, 25*(8), 787–793.

Mueller, X. M., Tevaearai, H. T., Hurni, M., Ruchat, P., Fische, A. P., Stumpe, F., & von Segesser, L. K. (1997). Long-term results of surgical subxiphoid pericardial drainage. *Thoracic and Cardiovascular Surgery, 45*(2), 65–69.

Ng, T., Gatt, A., Pagliuca, A., & Mufti, G. J. (2000). Colchicine: An effective treatment for refractory malignant pericardial effusion. *Acta Hematologica, 104,* 217–219.

Palacios, I. F. (1999). Pericardial effusion and tamponade. *Current Treatment Options in Cardiovascular Medicine, 1*(1), 79–89.

Rabinovici, R., Szewczyk, D., Ovadia, P., Greenspan, J. R., & Sivalingham, J. J. (1997).

Candida pericarditis: Clinical profile and treatment. *Annals of Thoracic Surgery, 63,* 1200–1204.

Retter, A. S. (2002). Pericardial disease in the oncology patient. *Heart Disease,*[AQ] 4(6), 387–391.

Sagrista-Sauleda, J., Merce, J., Permanyer-Miralda, G., & Soler-Soler, J. (2000). Clinical clues to the causes of large pericardial effusions. *American Journal of Medicine, 109,* 95–101.

Shepherd, F. A. (1997). Malignant pericardial effusions. *Current Opinion in Oncology, 9*(2), 147–148.

Spodick, D. H., (2003). Acute cardiac tamponade. *New England Journal of Medicine, 329*(7), 684–690.

Spodick, D. H. (2003). Acute pericarditis. Current concepts and practice. *Journal of the American Medical Association, 289*(9), 1159–1159.

Totaro, P., Lorusso, R., Ceconi, C., & Zogno, M. (2002). Transperitoneal approach for pericardial drainage. *Journal of Cardiovascular Surgery, 43*(5), 671–673.

Tsang, T. S. M., Enriquez-Sarano, M., Freeman, W. K., Barnes, M. E., Sinak, L. J., Gersh, B. J., Bailey, K. R., & Seward, J. B. (2002). Consecutive 1127 therapeutic echocardiographically guided pericardiocenteses: Clinical profile, practice patterns, and outcomes spanning 21 years. *Mayo Clinic Proceedings, 77*(5), 429–436.

van Steijn, J. H., Sleijfer, D. T., van der Graaf, W. T., van der Sluis, A., & Nieboer, P. (2002). How to diagnose cardiac tamponade. *Netherlands Journal of Medicine, 60*(8), 334–338.

36 Pleural Effusions

Brenda K. Shelton
Beth Kozak Onners

I. Definition

A. Excess fluid accumulation in the pleural space (Antunes et al., 2003)

  1. *Large effusion* is defined as more than two thirds of the hemithorax involved.

  2. *Massive effusion* is defined as complete or almost complete opacification of the hemothorax.

B. The pathophysiologic effects are:

  1. Collapse of alveoli and impaired oxygenation.

  2. Increased work of breathing due to changes in the intrapleural pressures.

C. Incidence

  1. Affects about 15% of patients with cancer sometime during the course of their disease (American Thoracic Society, 2000).

  2. Significant association with metastatic disease

    a. Over 50% with metastatic disease develop pleural effusion (Pollack et al, 2001).

    b. Average life expectancy of a patient with cancer after diagnosis of pleural effusion is 3 to 12 months (Antunes & Neville, 2000; Shoji, Tanaka, Yanagihara, Inui & Wada, 2002).

  3. Dyspnea, often from pleural effusions, is described as one of top three distressing symptoms in patients with advanced cancer (Campbell, Draper, Reid & Robinson, 2001; Sahn, 2001)

II. Etiology

A. Normal pleural mechanics (Antony, 2003)

  1. Pleura cover the lungs and adhere to the inner chest wall, serving as a protective barrier for the lungs.

  2. The potential "space" between the visceral and parietal pleura contains 5 to 30 mL of fluid at any given time, but circulates 1 to 2 L of fluid a day through a pumping action produced when the lungs expand and relax.

  3. The pressure in the pleural space is normally negative, allowing for easy inflow of air when the diaphragm and intercostal muscles are contracted and pull the pleura against the chest wall.

  4. Passive exhalation occurs with relaxation of the chest muscles.

  5. Increased pleural fluid increases the pressure within the pleural space, increasing the work of breathing.

  6. Symptoms of pleural effusion usually begin with increased work of breathing to maintain the same "oxygenation standard," but, as pleural fluid becomes excessive, alveoli are unable to fully expand, and oxygenation is impaired.

B. Both malignant and nonmalignant etiologies of pleural effusions exist, but more than 50% of all symptomatic pleural effusions presenting for treatment are related to malignancy (Antunes & Neville, 2000).

1. Etiologies can be listed by pathophysiologic triggers.

   a. Excess pleural fluid production—Most pleural fluid production occurs in the apex, and abnormalities in this area may increase the risk of effusion (Antunes et al., 2003).

      (1) Inflammation—Infection, malignant infiltration of the pleura

      (2) Fluid overload

   b. Inadequate pleural fluid drainage—Pleural fluid is drained by way of parietal cells located in the mediastinum and diaphragm, so diseases causing injury or pressure in these areas may obstruct pleural fluid drainage (Antunes et al., 2003).

      (1) Lymphatic obstruction

      (2) Altered pleural dynamics due to masses

      (3) Diaphragmatic irritation (eg, hepatomegaly, pancreatitis)

2. Most common malignant associations.

   a. Most common cancers—Lung, mesothelioma, breast, lymphoma.

   b. Any cancer with enlarged mediastinal lymph nodes may obstruct lymph drainage from thoracic duct.

   c. Other commonly noted malignant etiologies:

      (1) Ovarian cancer

      (2) Sarcoma

   d. Certain chemo/biotherapy agents (Micromedex, 2003).

      (1) Aldesleukin (interleukin-2)

      (2) Cytosine arabinoside

      (3) Docetaxel—Decreased incidence if treated before or after therapy with dexamethasone (Markman, 2003)

      (4) Gemtuzumab (Mylotarg)

      (5) Interferon

      (6) Oprelvekin (Neumega)

      (7) Trastuzumab (Herceptin)

      (8) Vinca agents: Vinblastine, Vincristine, Vindesine

3. Nonmalignant conditions that may cause pleural effusion

   a. Amyloidosis

   b. Cirrhosis—Called hepatic hydrothorax; more common if ascites is also present (Hayes, 2001)

   c. Congestive heart failure—Presents as unilateral right-sided, or bilateral with equal fluid distribution, usually associated with left ventricular failure, not right ventricular failure (Mitrouska, 2002)

   d. Hypothyroidism

   e. Human immunodeficiency virus (HIV) disease (Miller, Howling, Reid & Shaw, 2000)

   f. Infections (Ferrer et al., 1999; Miller et al., 2000)

      (1) Anthrax

      (2) *Cryptococcus*

      (3) *Legionella*

      (4) *Nocardia*

        (5) *Pneumococcus*

        (6) *Pneumocystis carinii*

        (7) Tuberculosis

     g. Nephrotic syndrome

     h. Pancreatitis (usually left-sided)

III. Patient Management

  A. Assessment

     1. Patient history for risk factors

       a. Concomitant diseases associated with pleural effusion

       b. Malignant disease of the chest or one of high-risk malignancies

       c. Exposure to medications that enhance capillary permeability (eg, biologic therapies, cytosine arabinoside)

       d. Hypoalbuminemia

     2. Physical complaints

       a. Severity of symptoms relate to how fast fluid has accumulated and the severity of compromise to lung expansion.

       b. Related to fluid collection in the pleural space.

         (1) Increased effort to breathe, use of accessory muscles.

         (2) Dyspnea.

           (a) Most common and distressing symptom

           (b) Not present in 15% to 25% of patients (Antunes et al., 2003)

           (c) Positioning for best breathing is sitting up and leaning forward

         (3) Pleuritic chest pain.

         (4) Cough is stimulated as the brain detects atelectasis and attempts to stimulate alveolar expansion.

       c. Related to increased work of breathing

         (1) Fatigue and weight loss are common due to the energy expenditure used for breathing.

         (2) Difficulty focusing or concentrating.

       d. Related to hypoxemia

         (1) Anxiety, restlessness, emotional lability

         (2) Headache, feeling of fullness in the head

     3. Physical findings

       a. Signs of alveoli collapse

         (1) Diminished breath sounds in lower lung fields

         (2) Unequal chest excursion or, if severe, total absence of chest wall movement on the affected side

       b. Signs of resultant hypoxemia

         (1) Cyanosis, cool extremities

         (2) Oliguria

         (3) Decreased bowel sounds, constipation

       c. Signs of pleural space expansion within the chest

         (1) Trachea deviated away from the side with the pleural effusion.

         (2) Displaced point of maximal impulse (apical pulse) shifted, especially if pleural effusion is on the left.

  B. Diagnostic Tests

     1. Initial screening

       a. Chest x-ray

(1) Anterior-posterior view usually adequate unless effusion is loculated in a single area, then lateral decubitus x-ray may be helpful (Antunes et al., 2003).

(2) Best results if taken with patient in the upright position; supine x-rays will cause the fluid to track the length of the lung field and appear as haziness rather than a fluid filling the base of the lung.

(3) Reveals blunted diaphragmatic dome, reduced opacity in the lung field due to alveolar collapse, fluid meniscus with possible tracking up the side of the pleural space.

b. Clinical examination

(1) Confirms severity as determined by chest excursion

(2) Assists the clinician to determine the work of breathing the patient is exerting to achieve compensation and a marginally normal oxygenation

(3) Assists in assigned severity of symptomatology to the diagnostic test finding

2. Definitive diagnosis

a. Chest tomography (CT) scan.

(1) Helpful to differentiate interstitial and pleuritic processes that may be occurring simultaneously

(2) Identifies loculated effusions; may allow external skin marking for needle thoracentesis localization

b. Ultrasound is especially helpful at localization of small effusions.

3. Histopathologic diagnosis

a. Thoracentesis fluid collection

(1) Transudative versus exudative—It is unclear whether existing criteria for defining effusions in these two categories can be used as a definitive diagnostic tool, or to even guide therapeutic decisions; however, it is considered standard management to send pleural fluid for chemistry to classify the effusion characteristics. An overview of the defining features of transudative and exudative effusions is included in Table 36–1.

TABLE 36–1 Transudative Versus Exudative Effusions

Characteristic	Transudative Effusion	Exudative Effusion
Etiology	Cirrhosis Left ventricular heart failure Pulmonary embolism Chest mass	Infectious pneumonia (bacteria, tuberculosis, certain other microbes) Malignant cell infiltration
Color	Clear, straw color	Cloudy, milky, or bloody
Fluid pH	Alkaline (>7.45)	Acidic or normal (<7.45)
Pleural fluid LDH	< 200 IU/L	> 200 IU/L
Plasma protein level	< 3 g/dL	> 3 g/dL
White blood cells	< 8/mm^3	> 8/mm^3
Red blood cells	< 8/mm^3	> 8/mm^3
Alkaline phosphatase level	< 75 mg/dL	> 75 mg/dL

(a) Light's criteria are considered the gold standard, although other factors have been assessed to determine if these variables or constituents could be more predictive. None have shown equal sensitivity or specificity.

(b) Light's criteria—Presence of one of the following: Pleural fluid-to-serum protein ratio >0.5, LDH >200 IU, pleural fluid-to-serum LDH ratio >0.6 (Light, 1972).

(c) Reagent strip for serum protein has a 93% sensitivity, but low specificity (50%) for detection of exudates. It may be helpful as a quick screen for an infectious etiology, permitting start of antimicrobials while awaiting culture and chemistry results (Azoulay et al., 2000).

(2) Cytology for presence of malignant cells may be considered the definitive diagnostic tool for actual malignant infiltration, although many effusions that are related to malignancy do not actually involve the pleura with malignant cells.

(3) Pleural fluid for tumor markers—Carcinoembryonic antigen (CEA), CA-9–19 for pancreatic cancer. These are inconsistently present, with many false-negative findings (Garcia-Pachon, 2002).

(4) Amylase may be found in the pleural fluid if related to pancreatitis or esophageal rupture, but rarely present otherwise (Branca et al., 2001)

b. CT- or ultrasound-guided thoracentesis is especially useful in small or loculated effusions that may be difficult to tap, or obtain an adequate specimen for evaluation. Studies suggests the complication rate may also be lower than in traditional blind needle thoracenteses (Jones et al., 2003; Perkins & Thickett, 2003).

C. Treatment

1. Observation and supportive care is indicated when the etiology may be easily resolved, or the patient is not yet symptomatic (Hayes, 2001).

2. Therapeutic thoracentesis may be performed for both diagnostic purposes and symptom relief.

a. In patients with a very limited life expectancy, repeated thoracenteses may be the treatment of choice.

b. Patients requiring thoracenteses more than two to three times a week with fluid removal in excess of 1,000 mL each time may be a candidate for chest catheter drainage or a thoracoscopic procedure (Antunes et al., 2003).

c. Repeated thoracenteses may cause pleural inflammation and cause a transudative effusion to become exudative, causing some confusion if using the transudative and exudative criteria to help identify malignant effusion (Antunes et al., 2003).

3. Intrapleural chemotherapy or radiation to the tumor bed may be effective, especially if the effusion is related to a large tumor obstructing the outflow of pleural fluid. Chemotherapeutic agents that are reported to have been instilled into the pleural space include cisplatin, interferon, 5-FU (Antunes et al., 2003; Shoji et al., 2002).

4. Chest catheter drainage involves the placement of a chest tube/catheter for drainage of the pleural space.

   a. Traditional chest drainage dictates using a large tube so obstruction is less likely, but because pleural fluid does not normally clot, this has been debated.

   b. Small-bore, soft chest catheters have been developed that are more comfortable and may permit patients to remain at home for the time period of chest drainage (Carroll, 2002; Parulekar, Di Primio, Matzinger, Dennie & Bociek, 2001; Sahn et al., 2000).

5. Chemical pleurodesis. (See Table 36–2 for specific details about assisting with this therapeutic intervention.)

   a. A procedure used to cause inflammatory adherence of the visceral and parietal pleura to each other so fluid can not reaccumulate within the pleural space.

   b. Indications

   (1) Recurrent pleural effusions despite multiple thoracenteses.

   (2) Suspected or known malignant cells in pleural fluid.

   (3) When there is less than 150 mL pleural fluid drainage from the chest tube in the previous 24 hours (chemical pleurodesis).

   (4) This is effective about 67% of the time, but an additional 10% to 15% can be gained if the procedure is repeated (Sahn, 2001).

   c. Mechanical (surgical) pleurodesis (also called poudrage)

   (1) Thoracoscopic surgical maneuver that historically was a manual/mechanical scraping, but now usually involves blowing talc into the pleural space.

   (2) May be preferred if the patient's chest drainage never decreases to below 150 mL within a 24-hour period, or if chemical pleurodesis has been unsuccessful.

6. Loculated pleural effusions have been treated successfully with instillation of a thrombolytic such as streptokinase, but no routine management guidelines exist to instruct on this practice.

7. Pleurectomy (also called decortication) is removal of the pleura and is reserved for patients with recurrent symptomatic pleural effusions and a long life expectancy.

8. Long-term indwelling implanted catheters or pleuroperitoneal shunts have been used for recurrent effusions with some success (Pien, Gant, Washam & Sternman, 2001; Pollack, 2002).

D. Nursing Diagnoses

   1. Impaired gas exchange related to accumulation of pleural fluid

   a. *Problem:* Pleural fluid accumulation from a variety of etiologies impairs gas exchange and increases the work of breathing.

   b. *Interventions*

   (1) Assist patients to determine position of comfort.

   (2) Assess respiratory rate, respiratory effort, chest excursion, and breath sounds every shift or with every clinic visit.

   (3) Plan with physician for routine monitoring of pleural effusions—when clinical evaluation is adequate, routine chest x-ray or CT scans.

   (4) Assist with thoracenteses as needed

TABLE 36-2 Assisting With Pleural Sclerosis

Type of Pleurodesis	Method	Nursing Implications and Care
Chemical pleurodesis— Instillation of a pleural irritant into the pleural space, causing inflammation and sclerosing the pleural membrane together. About 60% effective on the first attempt, but the cumulative success rate with multiple attempts is 75% to 80%.	1. Agent chosen by physician: Bleomycin 60–120 Units Doxycycline 500 mg diluted in 30 mL of saline. Talc slurry 50–75 mL followed by 30–50 mL saline 2. Decision whether to use lidocaine made by physician (two 50-mL bottles of 1%). 3. If lidocaine is not used, 100 of normal saline should be drawn into a syringe. 4. Take down chest tube dressing to make certain there is no leaking of fluid at the tube exit site. This could result in loss of sclerosing agent, or severe tissue extravasation if bleomycin is used. 5. Patient pretreatment with antipyretic or analgesic determined by agent used. 6. Sclerosing agent instilled by physician. 7. Normal saline/lidocaine is instilled by physician.	1. If an antineoplastic is used, hazardous precautions are observed. 2. Lidocaine is thought to decrease discomfort but may interfere with efficacy. 4. Bleomycin is a vesicant that can cause necrosis of soft tissue if it leaks out of the tube. 5. Bleomycin causes fever; doxycycline causes pleural pain.

8. The tube is clamped for 2–4 hours, and suction remains off for 4–5 hours.

9. Observe drainage after unclamping; drainage should slow or be near absent.

10. Obtain chest x-ray 24 hours after pleurodesis, then after chest tube is changed to water seal.

Mechanical pleurodesis—

Thoracostomy or thoracoscopic approach into pleura, with manual abrasion of the visceral pleura or insufflation with talc

The success rate of this procedure is 87% to 93%.

8. Patient rotation while the tube is clamped with the sclerosing agent instilled is not supported by research, but the patient may turn side to side as tolerated (Antunes et al., 2003).

Patients may experience considerable post-operative pain, particularly with manual abrasion.

1. Usual preoperative preparation.

2. Patient will have a pleural chest tube postoperatively.

3. Care of the chest tube is unchanged from usual standards, but pleural drainage should be minimal.

(a) Position patient upright, leaning forward and with shoulders elevated on a table, if possible, for best lung expansion and intercostal separation.

(b) Obtain supplies. Thoracentesis kits may have safety needles, but some physicians prefer large-bore and long (eg, 1.5- to 2-inch) intravenous needles, syringes for specimen collection, laboratory specimen bottles/vials, culture media, xylocaine for intradermal injection, vacuum bottles, noncollapsible tubing.

(c) Plan for follow-up chest x-ray after procedure, having it read, and not having patients leave clinic until the results are evaluated.

(d) If the patient is leaving the clinic in less than 2 to 4 hours after the procedure, teach symptoms of pneumothorax that require immediate medical evaluation—sudden dyspnea, air hunger, increased work to breathe, chest pain/tightness, unequal chest movement.

(5) Assist with chest catheter insertion and management as needed.

(a) This procedure usually requires sedation if a large-bore catheter is placed.

(b) Chest catheters are connected to a drainage system. Some institutions use traditional chest tube set-ups, and others use ambulatory sets after the majority of fluid is drained dry.

(c) Chest drainage for pleural effusion usually does not have an air leak unless the lung is nicked during insertion. The presence of an air leak necessitates suction.

(d) Have clamps, petrolatum gauze, regular gauze, and occlusive tape at the bedside.

(6) After large amounts of pleural fluid drainage, reexpansion pulmonary edema may occur. Nurses should be alert for this complication and provide supportive interventions (Adegboye, Falade, Osinusi & Obajimi, 2002).

(a) In patients at high risk, clamp drainage at 1000 mL and assess respiratory status for tolerance of fluid removal.

(b) Administer oxygen as needed.

(c) Encourage coughing, deep breathing, and mobility, if possible.

(d) Discuss benefits and risks of treatment with diuretics, and, if used, monitor blood pressure carefully.

(e) Avoid administering large amounts of fluid or blood products in the first 12 hours after drainage when this is the greatest risk.

c. *Desired outcomes*

(1) Pleural effusions are managed so patient experiences minimal clinical symptoms.

(2) Patient is able to maintain the normal activities of daily living.

2. Potential fluid volume deficit due to fluid shifts

a. *Problem:* Drainage of large amounts of fluid from the pleural space causes a compensatory shift of fluids from the vascular space into the pleura, causing hypovolemia and hypotension.

b. *Interventions*
    (1) After 1,000 mL of fluid drainage, clamp and observe heart rate and vital signs for 15 to 30 minutes before resuming fluid removal.
    (2) If not possible to clamp after 1,000 mL (eg, thoracentesis), observe vital signs carefully and have a bed or recliner readily available for the patient if he or she becomes hypotensive.
    (3) Assess laboratory tests for hypoalbuminemia, which increases the patient's risk for this complication. When possible, boost albumin level before performing thoracentesis.
c. *Desired outcome:* Absence of hypovolemia and hypotension

3. Potential altered nutrition due to work of breathing from pleural fluid collection
    a. *Problem:* Weight loss is a common clinical finding in patients with pleural effusion, and relates mostly to anorexia, and difficulty having the energy to eat when the work of breathing is so great. The malnutrition worsens the hypoalbuminemia, which, in turn, worsens the pleural effusion.
    b. *Interventions* (see Chapter 28)
    c. *Desired outcomes*
        (1) Normal serum albumin
        (2) Absence of altered nutrition

IV. Discharge Planning and Patient Education

A. Teach high-risk patients important symptoms of pleural effusion and the available treatment methods.
B. Ascertain the patient's understanding of the etiology and prognosis associated with pleural effusion and, refer to mental health professionals as appropriate.
C. Reinforce importance of maintaining physical activity to minimize pleural effusions.
D. Provide information about home chest drainage symptoms, and refer to home care services as needed. Patient will need to be taught management of the catheter, and given supplies (clamps, petrolatum gauze) to emergently manage complications such as disconnection or accidental removal.

REFERENCES

Adegboye, V. O., Falade, A., Osinusi, K., & Obajimi, M. O. (2002). Reexpansion pulmonary oedema as a complication of pleural drainage. *Nigerian Postgraduate Medical Journal, 9*(4), 214–220.

American Thoracic Society. (2000). Management of malignant pleural effusions. *American Journal of Respiratory Care and Medicine, 162,* 1987–2001.

Ang, P., Tan, E., Leong, S., Koh, L., Eng, P., Agasthian, T., & Cheah, F. K. (2001). Primary intrathoracic malignant effusion. A descriptive study. *Chest, 120,* 50–54.

Antony, V.B. (2003). Immunological mechanisms in pleural disease. *European Resiratory Journal, 21*(3), 539–544.

Antunes, G., & Neville, E. (2000). Management of malignant pleural effusions. *Thorax, 55,* 981–983.

Antunes, G., Neville, E., Duffy, J., Ali, N., on behalf of the BTS Pleural Disease Group, a subgroup of the BTS Standards of Care Committee. (2003). BTS guidelines for the management of malignant pleural effusions. *Thorax, 58*(Suppl. II), II29-II38.

Azoulay, E., Fartoukh, M., Galliot, R., Baud, F., Simmonneau, G., Le Gall, J. R.,

Schlemmer, B, & Chevret, S. (2000). Rapid diagnosis of infectious pleural effusions by use of reagent strips. *Clinical Infectious Disease, 31*(4), 914–919.

Bernard, A., de Dompsure, R. B., Hagry, O., & Favre, J. P. (2002). Early and late mortality after pleurodesis for malignant pleural effusion. *Annals of Thoracic Surgery, 74*(1), 213–217.

Branca, P., Rodriguez, R. M., Rogers, J. T., Ayo, D. S., Moyers, J. P., & Light, R. W. (2001). Routine measurement of pleural fluid amylase is not indicated. *Archives of Internal Medicine, 161*(2), 228–232.

Cardillo, G., Facciolo, F., Carbone, L., Regal, M., Corzani, F., Ricci, A., Di Martino, M., & Martelli, M. (2002). Long-term follow-up of video-assisted talc pleurodesis in malignant recurrent pleural effusions. *European Journal of Cardio-thoracic Surgery, 21,* 302–306.

Carroll, P. (2002). A guide to mobile chest drains. *RN, 65*(5), 56–60.

Craggun, W. H. (2002). Pleural effusion prediction failures. *Chest., 122*(5), 1503–1504.

De Campos, J. R. M., Vargas, F. S., Werebe, E. dC., Cardoso, P., Teixeira, L. R., Jatene, F. B., & Light, R. W. (2001). Thoracoscopy talc poudrage. A 15 year experience. *Chest, 119,* 801–806.

Erikson, K. V., Yost, M., Bynoe, R., Almond, C., & Nottingham, J. (2002). Primary treatment of malignant pleural effusions: Video-assisted thoracoscopic surgery poudrage versus tube thoracostomy. *American Surgery, 68*(11), 955–959.

Ferrer, A., Osset, J., Alegre, J., Surinach, J. M., Crespo, E., Fernandez de Sevil, T., & Fernandez, F. (1999). Prospective clinical and microbiological study of pleural effusions. *European Journal of Clinical Microbiology and Infectious Disease, 18*(4), 237–241.

Garcia-Pachon, E. (2002). Tumor markers for diagnosing malignant pleural effusion? *Chest, 121*(1), 302–303.

Hayes, D. D. (2001). Stemming the tide of pleural effusions. *Nursing, 31*(5), 49–52.

Jones, P. W., Moyers, J. P., Rogers, J. T., Rodriguez, R. M., Lee, Y. C., & Light, R. W. (2003). Ultrasound-guided thoracentesis: Is it a safer method? *Chest, 123*(2), 418–423.

Joseph, J., Badrinath, P., Basran, G. S., & Sahn, S. A. (2001). Is the pleural fluid transudate or exudates? A revisit of the diagnostic criteria. *Thorax, 56*(11), 867–870.

Light, R. W. (2002). Clinical practice. Pleural effusion. *New England Journal of Medicine, 346*(25), 1971–1977.

Light, R.W., Macgregor, M.I., Luchsinger, P.C., & Ball, W.C., Jr. (1972). Pleural effusions: The diagnostic separation of transudates and exudates. *Annals of Internal Medicine, 77*(4), 507-513.

Lone, M. A., Wahid, A., Saleem, S. M., Dhobi, G. N., & Shahnawaz, A. (2003). Alkaline phosphatase in pleural effusions. *Indian Journal of Chest Disease and Allied Science, 45*(3), 161–163.

Mager, H., Maesen, B., Verzijlbergen, F., & Schramel, F. (2002). Distribution of talc suspension during treatment of malignant pleural effusion with talc pleurodesis. *Lung Cancer, 36,* 77–81.

Markman, M. (2003). Taxane toxicities. *Supportive Care in Cancer, 11*(3), 144–147.

Maskell, N. A., Gleeson, F. V., & Davies, R. J. (2003). Standard pleural biopsy versus CT-guided cutting-needle biopsy for diagnosis of malignant disease in pleural effusions: A randomised controlled trial. *Lancet, 361*(9366), 1326–1330.

Micromedex Healthcare Series. (2003). *Drugdex drug evaluations.* Available: http://jhmcis.jhmi.edu/mdxcgi/display.

Miller, R. F., Howling, S. J., Reid, A. J., & Shaw, P. J. (2000). Pleural effusions in patients with AIDS. *Sexually Transmitted Infections, 76*(2), 122–125.

Mitrouska, I. (2002). The trans-exudative pleural effusion. *Chest, 122*(5), 1503–1504.

Mohamed, K. H., Mobasher, A. A., Yousek, A. I., Salah, A., Ramadan, M. A., Emam, A. K., Alhayawan, H. M., & Light, R. W. (2000). Pleural lavage: A novel diagnostic approach for diagnosing exudative pleural effusion. *Lung, 178*(6), 371–379.

Parulekar, W., Di Primio, G., Matzinger, F., Dennie, C., & Bociek, G. (2001). Use of small-bore vs large-bore tubes for treatment of malignant pleural effusions. *Chest, 120,* 19–25.

Perkins, G. D., & Thickett, D. (2003). CT-guided biopsy for diagnosis of malignant disease in pleural effusions. *Lancet, 362*(9378), 173, author reply 174.

Pien, G. W., Gant, M. J., Washam, C. L., & Sternman, D. H. (2001). Use of an implantable pleural catheter for trapped lung syndrome in patients with malignant pleural effusion. *Chest, 119,* 1641–1646.

Pollack, J. S. (2002). Malignant pleural effusions: Treatment with tunneled long-term drainage catheters. *Current Opinion in Pulmonary Medicine, 8,* 302–307.

Pollack, J. S., Burdge, C. M., Rosenblatt, M., Houston, J. P., Hwu, W., & Murren, J. (2001). Treatment of malignant pleural effusions with tunneled long-term drainage catheters. *Journal of Vascular Interventional Radiology, 12,* 201–208.

Porcel, J. M., & Vives, M. (2003). Etiology and pleural fluid characteristics of large and massive effusions. *Chest, 124*(3), 978–983.

Prevost, A., Costa, B., Elamarti, R., Nazeyrollas, P., Mallet, F., Yazbek, G., & Cauchois, A. (2001). Long-term effect and tolerance of talc slurry for control of malignant pleural effusions. *Oncology Report, 8*(6), 1327–1331.

Reeder, L. B. (2001). Malignant pleural effusions. *Current Treatment Options in Oncology, 2*(1), 93–96.

Sahin, U., Unlu, M., & Ornek, Z. (2001). The value of small-bore catheter thoracostomy in the treatment of malignant pleural effusions. *Respiration, 68,* 501–505.

Sahn, S. (2001). Management of malignant pleural effusions. *Monaldi Archives for Chest Disease, 56*(5), 394–399.

Schulze, M., Boehle, A. S., Kurdow, R., Dohrmann, P., & Henne-Burns, D. (2001). Effective treatment of malignant pleural effusion by minimal invasive thoracic surgery: Thoracoscopic talc pleurodesis and pleuroperitoneal shunts in 101 patients. *Annals of Thoracic Surgery, 71,* 1809–1812.

Schwartz, R. E., Posner, M. C., Ferson, P. F., Keenan, R. J., & Landreneau, R. J. (1998). Thoracoscopic techniques for the management of intrathoracic metastases. Results. *Surgical Endoscopy, 12*(6), 842–845.

Shoji, T., Tanaka, F., Yanagihara, K., Inui, K., & Wada, H. (2002). Phase II study of repeated intrapleural chemotherapy using implantable access system for management of malignant pleural effusion. *Chest, 121,* 821–824.

Spiegler, P.A, Hurewitz, A. N., & Groth, M. L. (2003, June). Rapid pleurodesis for malignant pleural effusions. *Chest, 123*(6), 1895–1898.

Tang, A. (1999). A regional survey of chest drains: Evidence-based practice? *Postgraduate Medicine, 75,* 471–474.

Taubert, J. (2001). Management of malignant pleural effusion. *Nursing Clinics of North America, 36*(4), 665–683, vi.

37 Spinal Cord Compression

Brenda K. Shelton

I. Definition: Spinal cord compression (SCC) is a disorder caused by direct pressure or compromised vascular supply to the spinal cord or cauda equina.
   A. Approximately 5% to 10% of patients with metastatic cancer develop SCC.
   B. Although more commonly associated with metastatic disease, 8% to 35% of cases of SCC present as the initial manifestation of cancer.
   C. Patients rarely die from SCC; however, it is considered a medical emergency because delay in treatment can result in irreversible paralysis and loss of voluntary and involuntary sphincter control.
   D. Once a severe neurologic deficit has occurred, treatment is unlikely to reverse the deficit. In one large study, 90% of patients who were nonambulatory at the time of diagnosis remained paraplegic after treatment.

II. Etiology
   A. Cord ischemia or necrosis with neurologic impairment occurs by three processes.
      1. Direct compression of the spinal cord or cauda equina
         a. The most common means of compression is progressive tumor expansion within the vertebral column with later invasion of the epidural space either by direct extension, lymph node growth through the epidural space, or by hematogenous spread.
         b. This pathophysiology is most typical of cancers of the lung, prostate, breast, and kidney.
      2. Interference in vascular supply to the spine
      3. Compression due to pathologic fracture and vertebral collapse: Direct tumor extension into the vertebral body occurs with lymphomas, multiple myeloma, and neuroblastoma.
   B. SCC can occur anywhere along the spinal cord and is related to the location of the primary or metastatic tumor causing cord injury.
      1. The frequency of distribution in cord compression cases is: cervical (10%), thoracic (70%), and lumbosacral (20%).
      2. Common malignant associations (occurring in >10% of patients)
         a. Multiple myeloma
         b. Lung cancer
         c. Prostate cancer
         d. Breast cancer
         e. Renal cell cancer
      3. Infrequent but possible malignant associations
         a. Lymphoma
         b. Malignant melanoma
         c. Head and neck cancer

III. Patient Management

  A. Assessment: Signs and symptoms of SCC vary based on the site and extent of infiltration. The symptomatology of SCC is consistent, regardless of the originating tumor. The time interval from the diagnosis of the primary cancer to that of SCC depends on the type of tumor and its metastatic potential.

  1. The location of pain, sensory, and motor symptoms depends on the site of compression and on the nerves involved. Table 37–1 depicts a summary of clinical symptoms according to site of involvement.

  2. Localized or radicular back pain is the earliest and most common symptom, preceding other symptoms by several months.

      a. The onset of pain is usually gradual and progressive and can be focal, radicular (resulting from compression of a nerve root), or referred.

      b. The distribution of radicular pain is contingent on the level of spinal involvement.

      c. Pain associated with SCC is usually unremitting and is exacerbated over an affected area or in the dermatome of the affected nerve root.

      d. Pain can be elicited by having the patient, while in a supine position, flex the neck or raise legs straight.

      e. Back pain associated with SCC is also unique because it can be exacerbated by manual palpation of the area.

  3. Sensory deficits include numbness and paresthesias.

      a. Patients complain of numbness and tingling or feelings of coldness in the affected area. Often, a sensation of "heaviness" in the affected extremities accompanies these symptoms.

      b. Numbness typically begins in the toes and gradually ascends to the level of spinal cord involvement.

  4. Most patients experience weakness by the time SCC is diagnosed; it chronologically occurs after sensory changes.

      a. Because most cord compression is at or below the thoracic area, lower extremity weakness is most common.

      b. Motor weakness may present in the form of an unsteady gait, ataxia, or favoring the affected extremity.

  5. Approximately half of patients exhibit autonomic dysfunction, such as bowel or bladder difficulties, at diagnosis; this is associated with a poorer prognosis.

      a. Constipation is an early indication of neurologic impairment, resulting from decreased neurologic stimulus for peristalsis; however, loss of sphincter control with intractable constipation occurs as cord compression worsens. Diminished urge to defecate and inability to bear down are initial signs of autonomic dysfunction involving the bowel, which contributes to constipation, obstipation, and, finally, incontinence.

      b. Urinary dysfunction begins with hesitancy and incomplete voiding and progresses to urinary retention and, finally, incontinence, when the bladder is filled to capacity and unable to empty. Increased postvoid volume after catheterization may be an indication of early autonomic dysfunction.

TABLE 37–1 Signs and Symptoms of Spinal Cord Compression

Location of Lesion	Physical Symptoms	Autonomic Symptoms
Cervical spine	Radicular pain in the neck, occipital region, and shoulders (pain is many times provoked by neck movement) Quadriplegia Upper extremity weakness (may be spastic or atrophy) Sensory loss in area of weakness Weakness or paralysis of the diaphragm may occur with lesion at or above C4 (may be unilateral or bilateral)	Hypotension Bradycardia Loss of temperature autoregulation Autonomic hyperreflexia Gastric hypersecretion and paralytic ileus Reflex bowel, bladder, and penile erection Hoffman's sign (flicking of the middle finger induces flexion of the ipsilateral thumb or index finger)
Thoracic spine	Pain (may be local, radicular, or both) Paraplegia Sensory loss below the level of the lesion Reflex abnormalities distal to the lesion	Venous stasis and associated complications Reflex bowel, bladder, and penile erection
Lumbar spine	Bowel and bladder dysfunction Extensor plantar response	Venous stasis and associated complications Reflex bowel, bladder, and penile erection
Cauda equina	Pain (may be local, referred, or radicular) Sphincter disturbances Loss of buttock and leg sensation Lower extremity weakness/paralysis	Areflexic bowel, bladder, and erection

From Byrne, T. N., & Waxman, S. G. (1990). Clinical pathophysiology of spinal signs and symptoms. In *Spinal cord compression* (pp. 49-54). Philadelphia: F. A. Davis; Garner, C. (1999). Cancer-related spinal cord compression. *American Journal of Nursing, 99*(7), 34-35; Glaser, J. A., Cure, J. K., Bailey, K. L., Morrow, D. L. (2001). Cervical spinal cord compression and the Hoffmann sign. *Iowa Orthopedic Journal, 21,* 49-52; Rude, M. (2000). Selected neurologic complications in the patient with cancer. Brain metastases and spinal cord compression. *Critical Care Nursing Clinics of North America, 12*(3), 269-279; Wilson, S. (1993). Acute spinal cord injury. In J. E. Wright & B. K. Shelton (Eds.), *Desk reference for critical care nursing* (p. 328). Boston: Jones & Bartlett.

6. SCC can also affect the nerves controlling penile erection or ejaculation, causing altered sexual function in many patients.

B. Diagnostic Parameters: There are no serum or urine tests used to diagnose spinal cord compression; however, other tests can indicate the condition.

　1. Spinal x-rays are performed to show bone deformities (eg, necrotic bone lesions from metastatic tumor). Although these are not specifically diagnostic for SCC, they are used to validate a potential etiologic factor in the presence of suspicious symptoms.

　2. Magnetic resonance imaging (MRI) is used to identify precisely the location of all lesions. MRI is sensitive to neurologic tissue and has the ability to distinguish between extradural, intradural, and extramedullary lesions. The disadvantage of this diagnostic test is that it requires the patient to remain motionless for approximately 1 hour in a small, confined space. If the patient moves during the examination, it results in poor imaging.

　3. Myelogram of the spine is the injection of dye into the epidural space. It can be used to diagnose SCC. The flow of dye and any obstructions encountered will show up on a nuclear scan of the area. This diagnostic test has been replaced by MRI for diagnosis of SCC because MRI (1) is noninvasive, (2) is more sensitive diagnostically, (3) images the entire spine, and (4) can indicate the presence of SCC as well as presence of paraspinal masses. The benefits of a myelogram are that cerebrospinal fluid sampling can occur, enabling meningeal carcinomatosis to be ruled out. The myelogram can be used when MRI assessment cannot explain neurologic deficits.

C. Treatment

　1. Corticosteroids are immediately administered intravenously to reduce inflammation and edema. An initial bolus of 16 to 100 mg dexamethasone (Decadron) is given, followed by 4 mg four times a day for about 14 days. A comparable steroid potency dose of hydrocortisone may be used as an alternative to dexamethasone.

　2. Radiation therapy is the best treatment for SCC because response rates are equivalent to those with surgery, but with less morbidity. Treatment must be implemented immediately for optimal reversal of neurologic deficits.

　　a. Maximal tolerated lifetime radiation exposure of the spine is 6,000 Cy.

　　b. Each treatment for SCC uses about 2,000 to 3,000 Cy.

　　c. Single daily dosing has been proven equally effective as hyperfractionation several times a day.

　　d. Patients often develop recurrent SCC that can no longer be treated with radiation.

　3. Surgical decompression (such as partial resection of the tumor or laminectomy), with or without Harrington rod stabilization, is performed in the patient with minimal or slow-growing tumor or when the patient is in good health. It is used for patients with rapidly progressing dysfunction or radioresistant tumors and for those who have had previous maximal radiation to the involved area.

    a. Because most vertebral lesions are positioned on the anterior surface, the anterior surgical approach may be necessary to achieve vertebroplasty or laminectomy. This thoracic approach carries significant risk of morbidity and a prolonged recovery period.

    b. The posterior (back) approach is less invasive and preferred whenever feasible.

    c. Newer posterolateral thoracoscopic approaches have been used with reduced morbidity and enhanced recovery.

  4. Multimodal therapy often combines, such as laminectomy with implantation of ^{125}I seeds

D. Nursing Diagnosis and Related Interventions and Outcomes

  1. Altered comfort due to back pain

    a. *Problem:* Compression on the spine and spinal nerves increases the local ischemia, causing localized pain or pain in the nerve root. When pain occurs in the nerve root, it is referred down the length of the spinal nerve and its dermatome.

    b. *Interventions*

      (1) Assess quantity and quality of pain with each clinic visit or at each shift during inpatient stay.

        (a) Obtain numeric pain rating.

        (b) Document exacerbating and alleviating factors.

        (c) Document quality of pain (eg, burning, sharp).

        (d) Document pain radiation.

        (e) Assess whether there is vertebral tenderness.

        (f) Note if pain is worsened by flexing neck or straight leg raising.

      (2) Administer analgesics as ordered, and assess response of pain to interventions. Antidepressants and anticonvulsants may be helpful adjuncts for neuropathic pain.

      (3) Provide nonpharmacologic suggestions for pain relief (eg, relaxation exercises, diversionary activity).

      (4) Administer short-acting corticosteroids for possible spinal cord compression immediately after ordered. Edema from the tumor or inflammation can worsen ischemia and cord injury. Pain is the indicator of ischemia. A rapid-acting corticosteroid will decrease inflammation, and pain may be partially relieved as well.

      (5) Assist patient in finding a position of comfort. Patients often find lying on their sides and/or leaving their feet uncovered to be more comfortable.

    c. *Desired outcome:* The patient will be free of pain.

  2. Altered sensory perception due to injury to the spinal cord and spinal nerves

    a. *Problem:* As the spinal cord and nerves become ischemic, pain and sensory changes are the first to occur. The numbness and tingling that are present alter other perceptions, such as touch, acute pain, and temperature. These altered sensations increase risk of injury.

    b. *Interventions*

      (1) Ensure spine stabilization (eg, neck brace, back brace) and bedrest until diagnostic tests validate the location and severity of cord compression. Activity limitations may be lifted if the spine is viewed as structurally stable.

(2) Caution patient to wear shoes or firm slippers when walking to avoid possible inadvertent injury to the toes and feet. Wearing supportive foot coverings also provides support for walking because altered sensation will blunt normal sensations that produce a smooth walking pattern.

(3) If the patient is out of bed, provide devices to assist in walking as ordered by physician.

(4) Provide pain medications that are particularly helpful for neuropathic pain (eg, antidepressants) as ordered.

(5) Assess sensory response to pain (eg, blunt-tipped, sharp object) and temperature (warm or cold) during every clinic visit or shift to assess progressive sensory changes. Perform assessment progressing from feet upward to highest level of sensory changes, or along the affected dermatome.

(6) Assess whether other specific measures alleviate discomforting sensations.

(7) Teach patient or family to inspect the patient's feet daily for injury and potential sites of infection.

c. *Desired outcomes*
(1) The patient has a complete return of peripheral sensation to touch and temperature.
(2) The patient is free of injury related to altered sensation.

3. Altered mobility due to injury to the spinal cord and spinal nerves
a. *Problem:* When SCC is severe, weakness or paralysis (particularly in the lower extremities) is common. This major physiologic change alters the patient's mobility and ability to perform usual activities of daily living.

b. *Interventions*
(1) Assess degree of weakness at every clinic visit or shift. Weakness of the feet can be assessed by flexor and extensor strength. Upper leg muscle strength can be assessed by asking patients to raise their knees or lift their legs off the bed.

(2) Provide passive range of motion at least twice daily to paretic extremities. Sometimes, patients can perform some of these exercises themselves.

(3) Treat limb spasticity with application of warmth.

(4) Refer patient to physical therapy to develop a plan to maintain joint mobility and any remaining muscle strength.

(5) Refer patient to occupational therapy to plan for home, vehicle, or work alterations that will allow the patient maximum independence.

(6) Refer patient to social worker for assessment of home and financial resources to cope with changes in lifestyle.

c. *Desired outcomes*
(1) The patient achieves complete recovery of mobility or adapts to alternate means of activity.
(2) The patient is able to return to pre-illness activities of daily living.

4. Potential altered urinary elimination due to injury to the spinal cord and spinal nerves

  a. *Problem:* When the spinal cord is compressed above the second lumbar vertebra, bladder dysfunction usually occurs. Reduced innervation of the bladder leads to sphincter relaxation and urinary retention. Later, spasticity, or an overfilled bladder, can lead to urinary incontinence.

  b. *Interventions*

  (1) Assess for urinary symptoms indicative of autonomic bladder dysfunction such as hesitancy, urgency, frequency, difficulty initiating urine stream, and stopping mid-stream

  (2) If autonomic bladder is suspected, perform postvoid catheterization. If the residual volume is >100 mL, there is bladder dysfunction.

  (3) Use an indwelling Foley catheter in the acute stage of SCC, until permanence of dysfunction is established.

  (4) If permanent bladder dysfunction occurs, teach the patient or significant other about straight catheterization for home. In the hospital, postvoid catheterization is performed at least twice daily.

  (5) Monitor for fever or cloudy urine indicative of urinary tract infection, which is common with urinary retention and which may occur with frequent or unclean catheterizations.

  (6) Treat with parasympathomimetics (cholinergic agents) to possibly increase bladder emptying. Some commonly used agents are bethanechol and Diprivan.

  c. *Desired outcomes*

  (1) The patient will have normal urine output by way of normal structures or catheterization.

  (2) The patient will be free of urinary tract infection.

5. Potential altered gastrointestinal elimination due to injury to the spinal cord and spinal nerves

  a. *Problem:* When the spinal cord is compressed above the first lumbar vertebra, some bowel dysfunction usually occurs. Reduced innervation of any of the intestines leads to decreased peristalsis and constipation. In the later stages of SCC, sphincter relaxation leads to an inability to evacuate stool. Patients often do not even have the urge to defecate.

  b. *Interventions*

  (1) Monitor for decreased bowel sounds indicating decreased peristalsis due to reduced innervation of the gastrointestinal (GI) tract.

  (2) Assess for abdominal distention and other symptoms of autonomic bowel dysfunction.

  (3) Monitor frequency and characteristics of stool. In early SCC, hard and dry stools are a common problem. Failure to defecate despite stool formation occurs later in the disorder. Stools should occur at least every 3 days.

  (4) Encourage fluid and fiber intake, which will increase the stimulus for normal peristalsis.

  (5) Administer stool softeners for patients with hard, dry stools.

(6) Try manual rectal stimulation to enhance rectal evacuation of stool.

(7) If manual stimulation is unsuccessful in producing stool output, schedule enema administration to induce stool evacuation.

  c. *Desired outcome:* The patient will have normal quantity and consistency of stool output by way of normal physical means or bowel stimulation.

6. Potential for altered sexual function due to injury to the spinal cord and spinal nerves

  a. *Problem:* Ischemia and injury to spinal nerves above the lumbar region lead to decreased innervation of the blood supply to the penis and inability to achieve erection. If spasticity has occurred, inability to ejaculate may be a problem as well.

  b. *Interventions*

  (1) Educate patient and significant other about possible sexual dysfunction related to SCC, but reassure them that it should be reevaluated after completing therapy because reversal of spinal ischemia may lead to return of previous function.

  (2) Assess the patient's normal sexual activity and ability to function at the conclusion of therapy.

  (3) Explore alternative methods of intimacy with patient and significant other.

  (4) Refer patient to mental health professional for counseling as needed.

  c. *Desired outcomes*

  (1) The patient will engage in alternate methods of expressing intimacy or sexual activity as established by patient and significant other.

  (2) The patient demonstrates effective coping mechanisms with lifestyle change.

7. Activity intolerance due to weakness or paraplegia/quadriplegia from spinal cord compression

  a. *Problem:* Weakness and paralysis that occur with SCC alter normal activity patterns and require increased dependence on the health care provider or family caregiver.

  b. *Interventions*

  (1) Forewarn the patient that he or she will be physically challenged with complications of SCC.

  (2) Schedule activities to allow for rest periods when there are no interruptions.

  (3) Refer patient to occupational therapy for items to assist with normal activities, such as eating and bathing, and special implements (eg, a wheelchair) to enhance independence.

  c. *Desired outcomes*

  (1) The patient will return to independent activities of daily living.

  (2) The patient will accept and implement assistive devices that enhance independent activities.

8. Potential for altered skin integrity and wound healing with spinal radiation or surgery

    a. *Problem:* Patients with SCC receive high doses of corticosteroids throughout their treatment. These reduce cord edema, but also increase the risk of altered skin integrity and infection.

    b. *Interventions*

        (1) Assess the skin daily or at each clinic visit to detect skin lesions and any abnormal wound healing.

        (2) Provide frequent turning using log-roll technique and massage the skin to preserve resilience to minimize potential spinal injury.

        (3) Ensure adequate nutritional intake with vitamins and minerals (eg, zinc, selenium) to aid in maintenance of intact skin integrity.

        (4) Report to the physician any unhealed, draining, red, or tender skin lesions.

    c. *Desired outcome:* The patient's skin that is affected by the radiation field or postsurgical wound will remain intact.

9. Potential for impaired swallowing related to cervical or thoracic radiation

    a. *Problem:* Esophagitis, dysphagia, and hypersalivation occur approximately 5 to 8 days after the start of treatment in patients receiving cervical or thoracic radiation therapy for SCC.

    b. *Interventions*

        (1) Change to a mechanical soft diet when dysphagia is present.

        (2) Monitor caloric intake and encourage high-calorie liquid supplements (eg, milkshakes), as tolerated.

        (3) Assess for stridor or evidence of severe esophageal edema causing airway incompetence.

        (4) Assess for bleeding in oral secretions.

        (5) Provide oral suction as needed to clean oropharynx and reduce aspiration risk.

        (6) Implement aspiration precautions (eg, head of bed elevations, liquid diet) as outlined by specific institutional guidelines.

        (7) Administer topical anesthetics to alleviate the situation and to assist the patient back to independence.

    c. *Desired outcomes*

        (1) The patient will maintain normal nutritional status.

        (2) The patient will have no evidence of aspiration.

10. Potential for impaired gas exchange due to spinal cord or nerve damage and hypoventilation

    a. *Problem:* When SCC occurs at or above the fifth cervical vertebra, inadequate innervation of the diaphragm or intercostal muscles can result in hypoventilation with respiratory acidosis.

    b. *Interventions*

        (1) When spinal cord lesions are equal to or above C5, assess and monitor the respiratory status of the patient (respiratory rate and rhythm, pulse oximetry, bedside spirometry to assess inspiratory effort).

        (2) Employ aggressive pulmonary toileting (cough, deep breathing, incentive spirometry) to avoid pulmonary complications.

    c. *Desired outcomes*

      (1) The patient will have a normal breathing pattern and oxygen saturation level >90%.

      (2) The patient will have normal chest excursion with breathing.

E. Discharge Planning and Patient Education

  1. Continue frequent assessment of the cancer patient for SCC and implement preventive strategies to minimize neurologic compromise.

  2. Recognize the increased risk of spinal cord compression in patients with bone metastases and recommend bisphosphonate therapy to prevent or control bone metastases.

  3. Initiate periodic home visits for patients who are not admitted and who do not attend the clinic. The home nurse determines the need for further treatment of SCC.

  4. Teach the patient and significant other to immediately report back pain occurring in the pattern typical of SCC. Early intervention preserves neurologic function and enhances quality of life for these people.

  5. Provide information about analgesic therapy as needed for chronic SCC.

  6. Teach infection control precautions for patients with SCC who receive long-term corticosteroids.

  7. Encourage preventive measures to compensate for constipation or urinary infection due to retention associated with autonomic dysfunction. This may include a diet high in fluids and fiber.

REFERENCES

Arce, D., Sass, P., & Abul-Khoudoud, H. (2001). Recognizing spinal cord emergencies. *American Family Physician, 64*(4), 631–638.

Baines, M. J. (2002). Spinal cord compression—A personal and palliative care perspective. *Clinical Oncology, 14*(2), 135–138.

Bayley, A., Milosevic, M., Blend, R., Logue, J., Gospodarowicz, M., Boxen, I., Warde, P., McLean, M., Catton, C., & Patton, P. (2001). A prospective study of factors predicting clinically occult spinal cord compression in patients with metastatic prostate carcinoma. *Cancer, 92,* 303–310.

Benjamin, R. (2002). Neurologic complications of prostate cancer. *American Family Physician, 65*(9), 1834–1840.

Bucholtz, J. D. (1999). Metastatic epidural spinal cord compression. *Seminars in Oncology Nursing, 15,* 150–159.

Byrne, T. N., & Waxman, S. G. (1990). Clinical pathophysiology of spinal signs and symptoms. In *Spinal cord compression* (pp. 49–54). Philadelphia: F. A. Davis.

Camp-Sorrell, D. (1998). Clinical focus. Spinal cord compression. *Clinical Journal of Oncology, 2*(1), 112–113.

Chen, T. C. (2001). Prostate cancer and spinal cord compression. *Oncology, 15*(7), 841–855.

Cher, L. M. (2001). Cancer and the nervous system. *Medical Journal of Australia, 175*(5), 277–282.

Chong, C. C., Kneebone, A., & Sheridan, M. (2001). Managing malignant spinal cord compression. *Australian Family Physician, 30*(9), 859–861.

Donato, V., Bonfili, P., Bulzonetti, N., Santarelli, M., Osti, M. F., Tombolini, V., Banelli, E., & Enrici, R. M. (2001). Radiation therapy for oncological emergencies. *Anticancer Research, 21*(3C), 2219–2224.

Eke, N. (2001). Symptomatic spinal cord involvement in prostate cancer. *Central African Journal of Medicine, 47*(2), 49–53.

Flounders, J. A., & Ott, B. B. (2003). Oncology emergency modules: Spinal cord compression. *Oncology Nursing Forum, 30*(1), E17-E23.

Garner, C. (1999). Cancer-related spinal cord compression. *American Journal of Nursing, 99*(7), 34–35.

Glaser, J. A., Cure, J. K., Bailey, K. L., & Morrow, D. L. (2001). Cervical spinal cord compression and the Hoffmann sign. *Iowa Orthopedic Journal, 21*, 49–52.

Hardy, J. R., & Huddart, R. (2002). Spinal cord compression—What are the treatment standards? *Clinical Oncology, 14*(2), 132–134.

Hashimoto, S., Shirato, H., Kaneko, K., Ooshio, W., Nishioka, T., & Miyasaka, K. (2001). Clinical efficacy of telemedicine in emergency radiotherapy for malignant spinal cord compression. *Journal of Digital Imaging, 14*(3), 124–130.

Husband, D. J. (1998). Malignant spinal cord compression: Prospective study of delays in referral and treatment. *British Medical Journal, 317*, 18–21.

Husband, D. J., Grant, K. A., & Romaniuk, C. S. (2001). MRI in the diagnosis and treatment of suspected malignant spinal cord compression. *British Journal of Radiology, 74*, 15–23.

Janjan, N. (2001). Bone metastases: Approaches to management. *Seminars in Oncology, 28*(4, Suppl. 11), 28–34.

Kienstra, G. E., Terwee, C. B., Dekker, F. W., Canta, L. R., Bostlap, A. C., Tijssen, C. C., Bosch, D. A., & Tijssen, J. G. (2000). Prediction of spinal epidural metastases. *Archives of Neurology, 57*(5), 690–695.

Maher DeLeon, M. E., Schnell, S., & Rozental, J. M. (1998). Tumors of the spine and spinal cord. *Seminars in Oncology Nursing, 14*, 43–52.

Malcolm, G. P. (2002). Surgical disorders of the cervical spine: Presentation and management of common disorders. *Journal of Neurosurgical Psychiatry, 73*(Suppl. 1), i34-i41.

McLain, R. F. (2001). Spinal cord decompression: An endoscopically assisted approach for metastatic tumors. *Spinal Cord, 39*, 482–487.

Myers, J. S. (2001). Oncologic complications. In S. E. Otto (Ed.), *Oncology nursing* (4th ed., pp. 498–581). St. Louis: C. V. Mosby.

Naco, G. J., & von Gunten, C. (2002). Refractory neuropathic pain from chronic cord compression. *Journal of Palliative Care Medicine, 5*(3), 433–436.

Nielsen, O. S. (2001). Present status of palliative radiotherapy. *European Journal of Cancer, 37*(Suppl. 7), S279-S288.

Preciado, D. A., Sebring, L. A., & Adams, G. L. (2002). Treatment of patients with spinal metastases from head and neck neoplasms. *Archives of Otolaryngology, Head and Neck Surgery, 128*(5), 539–543.

Rades, D., Heidenreich, F., & Karstens, J. H. (2002). Final results of a prospective study of the prognostic value of the time to develop motor deficits before irradiation in metastatic spinal cord compression. *International Journal of Radiation, Oncology, Biology, Physics, 53*(4), 975–979.

Rades, D., Karstens, J. H., & Alberti, W. (2002). Role of radiotherapy in the treatment of motor dysfunction due to metastatic spinal cord compression: Comparison of three different fractionation schedules. *International Journal of Radiation, Oncology, Biology, Physics, 54*(4), 1160–1164.

Rogers, C. L., Theodore, N., Dickman, C. A., Sonntag, V. K. H., Thomas, T., Lam, S., & Speiser, B. L. (2002). Surgery and permanent ^{125}I seed paraspinal brachytherapy for malignant tumors with spinal cord compression. *International Journal of Radiation, Oncology, Biology, Physics, 54*(2), 505–513.

Rude, M. (2000). Selected neurologic complications in the patient with cancer. Brain metastases and spinal cord compression. *Critical Care Nursing Clinics of North America, 12*(3), 269–279.

Schoeggl, A., Reddy, M., & Matula, C. (2002). Neurological outcome following laminectomy in spinal metastases. *Spinal Cord, 40*, 363–366.

Seol, H. J., Chung, C. K., & Kim, H. J. (2002). Surgical approach to anterior compression in the upper thoracic spine. *Journal of Neurosurgery, 97*(3 Suppl.), 337–342.

Soerdjbalie-Maikoe, V., Pelger, R. C., Lycklama a Nijeholt, G. A., Arndt, J. W., Zwinderman, A. H., Papapoulos, S. E., & Hamdy, N. A.(2002). Strontium-89 (metastron) and the bisphosphonate olpadronate reduce the incidence of spinal cord compression in patients with hormone refractory prostate cancer metastatic to the skeleton. *European Journal of Medicine and Molecular Imaging, 29*(4), 494–498.

Solti, M., Kumar, D., & Abraksia, S. (2001). Unusual sites of involvement by hematologic malignancies. Case 2. Meningeal myeloma with cord compression. *Journal of Clinical Oncology, 19*(19), 3991–3993.

Walker, J. (2002). Caring for patients with a diagnosis of cancer and spinal metastatic disease. *Nursing Standard, 16*(42), 41–44.

Wilson, S. (1993). Acute spinal cord injury. In J. E. Wright & B. K. Shelton (Eds.), *Desk reference for critical care nursing* (p. 328). Boston: Jones & Bartlett.

38 Superior Vena Cava Syndrome

Brenda K. Shelton

I. Definition: Superior vena cava syndrome (SVCS) is a disorder defined by internal or external obstruction of the superior vena cava (SVC), leading to reduced venous blood return into the right heart. The presence of this complication is an ominous prognostic sign, carrying a life expectancy of 4 to 6 months in recurrent malignant disease (Anderson & Coia, 2000; Tanigawa et al., 1998; Wilson, Lyn, Lynn & Khan, 2002).

    A. When less blood returns to the heart, cardiac output is compromised.

    B. The primary clinical outcomes are venous congestion and low cardiac output.

II. Etiology: When more than one potential mechanism of vena caval obstruction is involved, the risk of this complication is proportionately increased. The degree of obstruction and the speed of onset will be reflected in the severity of signs and symptoms.

    A. Direct Tumor Involvement: Malignancies associated with tumor involvement of the SVC are more likely to involve the mediastinum, and particularly the vasculature.

        1. The most prevalent malignant cause of SVCS is bronchogenic lung carcinoma (may be small-cell or adenocarcinoma, occasionally large-cell lung cancer). This accounts for about 80% of all cases.

        2. Breast cancer and lymphoma are the two other tumors that comprise the majority of the remaining 20% of cases.

        3. Other tumors identified as metastasizing to the chest vessels and causing SVCS include head and neck cancers, renal cell carcinoma, and malignant melanoma.

        4. Five-year survival rate after diagnosis of SVCS due to mediastinal tumor is 0% to 5% (Roberts, Bueno & Sugarbaker, 1999).

    B. Extrinsic Compression: The SVC is a low-pressure vessel anatomically positioned between two immovable bone structures, the clavicle and scapula. When mediastinal structures become edematous or when mass-occupying lesions are introduced, there is insufficient room for all structures, and the soft-walled vena cava becomes occluded.

        1. Many lymph nodes in the region (~20) can become enlarged with infection or malignancy.

        2. A tumor in this region can compress the vena cava, causing obstruction of venous return. In addition to the most common malignancies associated with SVCS, lung metastases from tumors such as thymoma, thyroid cancer, myxoma, prostate, and Wilms' have caused extrinsic compression of the vena cava.

        3. Adhesions from previous radiation therapy, centrally placed venous access devices (eg, implanted ports), mediastinal devices (eg, pacing or internal defibrillator wires), or cavitating infections (eg, aspergillosis, tuberculosis) may increase the risk of SVCS.

4. There are a number of reported cases of cardiovascular or thoracic surgical interventions that have caused vena caval obstruction. This is a particularly common etiology among children. Occlusion of vena caval filters (eg, Greenfield filter) placed for recurrent thromboemboli has also caused SVCS syndrome when multiple clots are trapped in the device.

5. Nonmalignant conditions causing benign masses (eg, lipoma), or mass-occupying lesions (eg, cystic fibrosis, sarcoidosis, amyloidosis) can cause compression of the vena cava.

C. Intraluminal Thrombosis: This is the most common benign etiology of SVCS (Morales, Comas, Trujillo & Dorta, 2000). When an indwelling venous catheter is positioned in the vena cava, it occupies space normally used by the flow of blood, slowing the blood flow and enhancing the risk of blood stagnation and thrombosis around the catheter. This thrombosis reduces venous inflow and cardiac filling, causing SVCS.

1. Catheter variables increasing the risk of thrombosis include large lumen size and multiple lumens.

2. Host variables increasing the risk of SVCS in patients include hypercoagulability, multiple previous central venous catheter placements, and tumor involvement of the vena cava.

3. About one third of cases of SVCS involve thrombosis in addition to other etiologic factors.

4. A hypercoagulable tendency will also increase the risk of venous thrombosis. Hypercoagulability is enhanced by mucin-producing tumors (ie, any adenocarcinomas), procoagulants produced by myelocytic leukemias, hyperviscosity as seen in abnormal immunoglobulins with multiple myeloma, and other tumors associated with hypercoagulable states (eg, lymphoma or glioblastoma). Hypercoagulability leading to possible superior vena cava thrombosis is enhanced with infection, disseminated intravascular coagulation (DIC), and Trousseau's syndrome.

III. Patient Management

A. Assessment: Most assessment findings in SVCS occur in the head, neck, and upper extremities and are related to the backflow of venous blood, normally drained by the SVC, into other body organs. Many of these physiologic symptoms persist even after the SVCS has resolved, particularly if symptoms have been prolonged and permanent vascular changes have occurred.

1. Dyspnea is the most common symptom of SVCS. It occurs because of venous congestion and cardiac failure due to inadequate blood volume.

2. If blood flow through the coronary arteries is compromised, reduced cardiac output will produce weak peripheral pulses, cool extremities, central cyanosis, and bradydysrhythmias.

3. A feeling of fullness in the head, headaches, neck swelling, distended neck veins, facial edema with flushing, conjunctivitis, and conjunctival hemorrhage occur due to venous congestion in the head and neck region.

4. Difficulty swallowing and hoarseness reflect congestion with edema of the neck and indicate a greater risk of airway obstruction.
5. Sensory disturbances, such as blurred vision and tinnitus, occur due to the excess venous blood in the head region.
6. Lethargy or somnolence, confusion, and enlarged or sluggish papillary response occur when venous congestion is severe enough to cause increased intracranial pressure. Papilledema on fundoscopic eye examination is also detectable in patients with increased intracranial pressure.
7. Headache or visual disturbances may be present due to head and neck congestion.
8. Veins in the chest will be distended, tortuous, and prominent due to venous congestion. Although more common on the right side, they may be present diffusely across the thorax.
9. Veins in the upper extremities, especially on the right side, will be distended and prominent, and edema of that extremity will range from mild to severe. This will be most noticeable in the brachial area.
10. Blood pressure will be elevated in the arm most affected, usually the right side.

B. Diagnostic Parameters: There are no serum or urine tests used to diagnose SVCS; however, other tests assist in diagnosis of the condition.
1. Chest x-ray is not diagnostic but is used to complement key clinical presentation cues.
   a. Show mediastinal masses in the hilar region that may contribute to SVCS.
   b. Show the right middle lobe congestion that is typical in SVCS.
   c. Lateral x-rays can show masses and enlarged nodes between the clavicle and scapula.
2. Computed tomography (CT) scans
   a. More precisely show the location and size of tumors or enlarged lymph nodes.
   b. Better demonstrate whether the vessel is externally compressed or has tumor growth into the vessel.
   c. A spiral CT scan is thought to best show the multiple dimensions needed to precisely define the perimeters and involvement of tumor near and within the vena cava.
3. When the spiral CT scan is inconclusive, venogram is performed to clarify whether there is a venous thrombosis causing or contributing to the SVCS.
   a. Most patients with SVCS demonstrate some degree of thrombosis, even if the main etiologic factor is external compression of the vena cava.
   b. The confirmation of thrombosis through venogram validates the decision to add thrombolytic therapy to the treatment plan.
   c. Doppler flow studies may replace the use of venogram in patients with significant blood flow disturbances (Panzironi, Rainaldi, Ricci, Casale & Macciucca, 2003).
   d. Transesophageal echocardiography has been used to diagnose vena caval thrombi, with reported success exceeding other noninvasive diagnostic methods (Shapiro, Johnson & Feinstein, 2002).

C. Treatment: SVCS is best treated by definitive antineoplastic therapy. The nature of this therapy will depend on the tumor type and its responsiveness to radiation therapy and chemotherapy.

1. Radiation therapy is used on radiosensitive tumors such as Hodgkin's disease and thyroid cancer.

a. Patients receive 3,000 to 5,000 Cy of radiotherapy, given as 300 to 400 Cy for the first 2 to 4 days, then 150 to 200 Cy daily until the total dose is given.

b. Hyperfractionation schedules have not been proven superior to traditional 3- to 4-week therapy plans (Anderson & Coia, 2000).

2. Chemotherapy is administered when radiation therapy is not likely to succeed, when patients have received the maximum tolerated dose of radiation, or when patients have chemosensitive tumors (eg, small-cell lung cancer).

3. Endovascular stenting of the vena cava (Lanciego et al., 2001)

a. Stents may be made of flexible wire (self-expandable) or Silastic.

b. Placement percutaneously by interventional cardiovascular specialists.

c. Potential adverse effects include pulmonary emboli, hemorrhage, pericardial tamponade, stent malposition, and recurrence of SVCS.

d. Rapid return of venous blood into the heart after stenting procedure may cause transient congestive heart failure due to sudden increased workload on the heart. This is more likely if SVCS has been long-standing and severe (Yamagami, Nakamura, Kato, Iida & Nishimura, 2002).

e. Long-term patency rates are not well established, but range from 20 days to 6 months. One study shows an 83% 6-month patency rate for single stenting procedures (Thony et al., 1999).

4. Superior vena caval bypass graft may be used, but is used more often for treatment of SVCS due to nonmalignant conditions (Panneton, Andrews & Hofer, 2001).

5. High-dose, rapid-acting corticosteroids have been used to reduce inflammation related to the syndrome and patient responses to treatment, but have not been proven beneficial (Rowell & Gleeson, 2001).

6. Anticoagulant or thrombolytic therapy may be indicated if thrombosis of the SVC is present. Most clinicians advocate simultaneous treatment of other risk factors for SVCS, and most suggest thrombolytic therapy is more effective than anticoagulant therapy (Morales et al., 2000).

D. Nursing Diagnoses

1. Decreased cardiac output related to reduced venous blood return to the heart

a. *Problem:* Reduced venous return decreases ventricular filling and reduces cardiac output to the body.

b. *Interventions*

(1) Assess heart rate and blood pressure for tachycardia, dysrhythmias, and hypotension, which indicate cardiac compromise.

(2) Assess pulse quality for threadiness, pulsus alternans, or pulse deficit between apical and peripheral pulses; all reflect decreased cardiac output.

      (3) Assess urine output frequently. Oliguria is a sensitive indicator of decreased renal blood flow.

      (4) Assess skin and mucous membranes for cyanosis or pallor indicative of poor peripheral perfusion.

      (5) Note skin temperature for coolness or clamminess, indicative of poor perfusion.

      (6) Monitor for alterations in mental status indicative of poor perfusion.

      (7) Assist in care of the patient receiving antineoplastic therapy to correct SVCS.

      (8) Administer inotropes (eg, dopamine, digoxin) as ordered to improve cardiac output.

      (9) Monitor fluid status. Report intake greater than output because it worsens venous congestion.

     (10) Administer preload reduction agents (nitroglycerin, diuretics) cautiously as ordered. Too much venodilation or volume reduction will decrease ventricular filling pressures and may decrease blood pressure.

     (11) Provide care in small increments, allowing frequent rest periods to improve tolerance of low cardiac output.

     (12) Administer sedation, as ordered, to reduce oxygen demands related to anxiety or restlessness in face of reduced cardiac output.

     (13) Check electrocardiogram (ECG) for ischemic changes.

  c. *Desired outcomes*

      (1) The patient will show evidence of normal tissue perfusion—pink and warm skin, normal capillary refill, normal urine output, normal mentation.

      (2) The patient will not experience upper extremity edema.

2. Altered gas exchange

  a. *Problem:* Reduced venous return decreases ventricular filling and reduces blood flow through the lungs, which decreases oxygen and carbon dioxide exchange.

  b. *Interventions*

      (1) Assess pulse oximetry continuously when patient is seriously ill to detect hypoxemia; otherwise, spot-check frequently.

      (2) Monitor arterial blood gases as ordered for hypoxemia, hypercarbia (elevated $Paco_2$), or metabolic acidosis.

      (3) Monitor breath sounds for increased crackles, indicative of worsening pulmonary edema, or stridor, indicative of upper airway obstruction.

      (4) Monitor and report hoarseness or dysphagia, which are indicative of upper airway obstruction.

      (5) Monitor skin and mucous membranes for cyanosis, pallor, coolness, or clamminess, which are indicative of oxygen deficit.

      (6) Place patient in position to best facilitate breathing and oxygenation (reverse Trendelenburg's or high-Fowler's position is recommended).

      (7) Provide care in small increments to reduce oxygen demand. Administer sedation as ordered to reduce oxygen demand related to anxiety or restlessness.

(8) Administer oxygen therapy as ordered.

(9) Administer corticosteroids as ordered to reduce laryngeal edema that may result in airway obstruction.

(10) Provide a patent airway with an oral or nasopharyngeal airway if the patient is severely neurologically impaired.

(11) Assist with endotracheal intubation as needed to provide adequate oxygenation.

c. *Desired outcomes*

(1) The patient will maintain normal PaO_2 and $PaCO_2$ as seen on arterial blood gas.

(2) The patient will not experience cyanosis or organ dysfunction, which indicate inadequate gas exchange.

3. Ineffective breathing pattern due to venous congestion and altered secretions from chest radiation therapy

a. *Problem:* Congestive heart failure causes pulmonary crackles and pulmonary edema, causing tachypnea, dyspnea, and excess secretions. Radiation therapy to the chest causes initial hypersecretion of the airways, but later produces a cough with dry airways.

b. *Interventions*

(1) Assess respiratory rate, effort, and breath sounds. Crackles are indicative of pulmonary edema. When hypersecretion occurs, gurgles and excess sputum are common within the first 3 to 7 days of chest irradiation.

(2) Encourage coughing and deep breathing to maintain a patent airway and to enhance secretion expectoration.

(3) Position patient in reverse Trendelenburg's or high-Fowler's position to facilitate ventilation and to reduce the risk of secretion aspiration.

(4) Suction oral, nasotracheal, and endotracheal airways as needed to maintain patient airway. Use 80 to 120 mmHg suction to minimize trauma to the airways.

(5) Provide additional humidification with oxygen therapy for patients receiving radiation. After 5 to 10 days of radiation therapy, airways become dry and are at high risk to bleed. Increased secretions may occur 2 to 3 weeks after radiation begins.

(6) Administer cough suppressants cautiously and only when breath sounds are clear.

(7) Monitor chest x-ray results for evidence of pulmonary edema, radiation pneumonitis, or infectious pneumonitis.

(8) Culture sputum as ordered to assess for pneumonia.

c. *Desired outcomes*

(1) The patient's respirations will be 12 to 24 breaths per minute and unlabored.

(2) The patient's breath sounds will remain clear to auscultation.

4. Altered mental status

a. *Problem:* Venous congestion causes increased blood backup in the head and neck region. Excess blood in this area can cause increased intracranial pressure with alterations in mental status.

    b. *Interventions*

        (1) Assess cognition, wakefulness, and ability to follow commands; look for early signs and symptoms of neurologic impairment.

        (2) Assess for signs and symptoms of increased intracranial pressure: hypertension, bradycardia, mental status changes, headache, vomiting, and irregular respiration patterns.

        (3) Elevate head of bed and avoid Trendelenburg's position, which increases intracranial pressure.

        (4) Administer corticosteroids as ordered to reduce potential increased intracranial pressure.

        (5) Implement seizure and aspiration precautions.

        (6) Monitor fluid intake and output, and report excessive intake, which may worsen venous congestion and increase intracranial pressure.

        (7) Provide a safe environment.

    c. *Desired outcomes*

        (1) The patient remains oriented to person, place, and time and answers questions appropriately.

        (2) The patient will not experience symptoms of increased intracranial pressure.

5. Altered sensory perception

    a. *Problem*: Venous congestion causes increased blood backup in the head and neck region. Excess blood in this area can cause altered sensory perceptions of the eyes (diplopia), ears (tinnitus), and peripheral skin sensory receptors (paresthesias).

    b. *Interventions*

        (1) Assess patient's visual acuity and hearing ability for sensory changes.

        (2) Assess patient's sensitivity to touch in upper extremities, chest, neck, and face.

        (3) Provide a safe environment to reduce risk of injury resulting from altered sensory perceptions.

        (4) Assist patient with activities of daily living to reduce risk of injury due to sensory alteration.

        (5) Avoid use of hot or cold packs that may cause inadvertent skin injury due to the patient's altered perception.

        (6) Assist with or provide a mirror for grooming, to avoid inadvertent injury.

        (7) Use electric razors only.

    c. *Desired outcomes*

        (1) The patient will maintain normal vision.

        (2) The patient will maintain normal hearing without auditory hallucinations.

        (3) The patient will maintain normal sensory perception to touch, pressure, and temperature on the head, neck, chest, and arms.

6. Activity intolerance

    a. *Problem*: Venous congestion and decreased cardiac filling lead to reduced cardiac output and limitations in activities of daily living.

b. *Interventions*
  (1) Provide care in small increments to avoid exhaustion or exacerbation of oxygen compromise.
  (2) Involve the patient in prioritization of activities.
  (3) Assist patient with bathing, dressing, or eating as needed to meet basic needs.
  (4) Encourage isometric exercise or progressive muscle relaxation to enhance muscle tone.
  (5) Ensure frequent position changes to protect from skin breakdown during period of reduced activity.
c. *Desired outcomes*
  (1) The patient will be able to perform self-care activities.
  (2) Congestive heart failure symptoms are not exacerbated by physical activity.

7. Altered body image
   a. *Problem*: Venous congestion of the upper body causes severe edema with distortion of the normal facial features.
   b. *Interventions*
     (1) Reassure patient that edema will resolve as SVCS lessens.
     (2) Encourage patient to try aesthetic improvements to lessen body image noticeability (eg, long-sleeves, turtlenecks)
     (3) Provide skin care to prevent skin breakdown or infection that occurs with edema.
     (4) Encourage verbal social encounters, such as by telephone, which can be less threatening than physical encounters and can keep patient in contact with social circle.
   c. *Desired outcome:* The patient verbalizes recognition of the time-limited nature of altered body image and adjusts to temporary image changes.

8. Potential for bleeding related to thrombolytic therapy
   a. *Problem:* Because many patients with SVCS have accompanying thrombosis, thrombolytics are administered. Thrombolytic administration increases the patient's risk of bleeding.
   b. *Interventions*
     (1) Confirm/check if institution requires physician to administer the bolus doses of the agent.
     (2) Administer thrombolytics through the central venous catheter, unless ordered to do otherwise.
     (3) Verify dosage with another nurse before hanging or adjusting doses.
     (4) Institute bleeding precautions. A second intravenous line may be placed to permit blood drawing from a line where thrombolytics are not simultaneously infusing.
     (5) Institute fall precautions. To reduce the risk of bleeding due to injury, assist patient whenever he or she is out of bed.
     (6) Perform neurologic examination every 8 hours. Increase to every 4 hours if platelets are less than $20,000/mm^3$ or if infusion is extended beyond 72 hours. Intracranial bleeding may be life-threatening and is best monitored through assessment of cognition, wakefulness, orientation, and motor and sensory evaluation.

(7) Test excretions for occult or overt blood.

(8) Assess the integument frequently. Document evidence of new or extending bruising and bleeding tendency.

(9) Note visual or sensory disturbances (headache, dizziness, perceptual difficulties, paresthesias) that may indicate increased intracranial pressure or intracranial bleeding.

(10) Measure the arm circumference if enlarged, making note if size is increased.

(11) Document coagulation test results (usually fibrinogen levels and thrombin time), which are normally performed every 6 hours during infusion and 12 hours after completion of infusion.

c. *Desired outcomes*

(1) The patient will show no evidence of overt bleeding.

(2) The patient will have reduced thrombus as evidenced by clinical manifestations and follow-up venogram.

9. Altered comfort due to edema, dyspnea, and headache

a. *Problem:* The symptoms of SVCS alter normal body structure and function, limiting the ease with which patients can perform normal activities. Edema expands the skin, causing aching, itching, and a feeling of heaviness. Venous congestion causes difficulty breathing and a sense of air hunger, which is often distressing to the patient.

b. *Interventions*

(1) Provide analgesics as ordered for headaches or other minor discomforts.

(2) Provide frequent skin care with massage and emollients to reduce discomfort.

(3) Position patient in a comfortable position, using pillows or bed adjustments.

(4) Encourage use of behavioral interventions, such as imagery or progressive muscle relaxation, to enhance rest and alleviate discomfort.

(5) Encourage diversionary activity to allay attention to discomforts.

c. *Desired outcome:* The patient verbalizes comfort with breathing and movement.

E. Discharge Planning and Patient Education

1. Patients exhibit residual signs and symptoms despite resolution of the clinical syndrome. Neck, thoracic, and arm vein distention may persist, but edema and heart failure should be resolved.

2. Teach at-risk patients and their families the reportable signs and symptoms of SVCS. For many patients, subtle symptoms such as tight shirt collars, weakness or tingling of the right arm, and dyspnea on exertion may signal recurrent SVCS.

3. Be sensitive to potential poor prognostic significance of SVCS in recurrent malignant disease.

4. Patients may require social work referral or support in finding transportation for daily radiation therapy even after discharge from the hospital. Visual disturbances and respiratory complications may preclude them traveling alone.

5. Advise patients of potential adverse effects of short-term high-dose corticosteroids, such as insomnia, high glucose, and acne.

REFERENCES

Anderson, P. R., & Coia, L. R. (2000). Fractionation and outcomes with palliative radiation therapy. *Seminars in Radiation Oncology, 10*(3), 191-199.

Arya, L. S., Narain, S., Tomar, S., Thavaraj, V., Dawar, R., & Bhargawa, M. (2002). Superior vena cava syndrome. *Indian Journal of Pediatrics, 69*(4), 293-297.

Bilyeu, J. A. (2001). Superior vena cava syndrome. *Journal of Insurance and Medicine, 33*(4), 349-352.

Courtheoux, P., Alkofer, B., Al Refai, M., Gervais, R., Le Rochais, J. P., & Icard, P. (2003). Stent placement in superior vena cava syndrome. *Annals of Thoracic Surgery, 75*(1), 158-161.

Donato, V., Bonfili, P., Bulzonetti, N., Santarelli, M., Osti, M. F., Tambolini, V., Banelli, E., & Enrici, R. M. (2001). Radiation therapy for oncological emergencies. *Anticancer Research, 21*(3C), 2219-2224.

Gupta, R., & Gupta, S. (2002). Oncologic emergencies: Superior vena cava syndrome. *Cleveland Clinic Journal of Medicine, 69*(10), 744.

Haapoja, I. S., & Blendowski, C. (1999). Superior vena cava syndrome. *Seminars in Oncology Nursing, 15*(3), 183-189.

Hemann, R. (2001). Superior vena cava syndrome. *Clinical Excellence in Nurse Practice, 5*(2), 85-87.

Lanciego, C., Chacon, J. L., Julian, A., Andrade, J., Lopez, L., Martinez, B., Cruz, M., & Garcia-Garcia, L. (2001). Stenting as first option for endovascular treatment of malignant superior vena cava syndrome. *American Journal of Roentgenology, 177*, 585-593.

Marcy, P. Y., Magne, N., Bentolila, F., Drouillard, J., Bruneton, J. N., & Descamps, B. (2001). Superior vena cava obstruction: Is stenting necessary? *Supportive Care in Cancer, 9*(2), 103-107.

Markman, M. (1999). Diagnosis and management of superior vena cava syndrome. *Cleveland Clinic Journal of Medicine, 66*(1), 59-61.

Morales, M., Comas, V., Trujillo, M., & Dorta, J. (2000). Treatment of catheter-induced thrombotic superior vena cava syndrome: A single institution's experience. *Supportive Care in Cancer, 8*(4), 334-338.

Panneton, J. M., Andrews, J. C., & Hofer, J. M. (2001). Superior vena cava syndrome: Relief with a modified saphenojugular bypass graft. *Journal of Vascular Surgery, 34*(2), 360-363.

Panzironi, G., Rainaldi, R., Ricci, F., Casale, A., & Macciucca, M de V. (2003). Gray-scale and color doppler findings in bilateral internal jugular vein thrombosis caused by anaplastic carcinoma of the thyroid. *Journal of Clinical Ultrasound, 31*(2), 111-115.

Porte, H., Metois, D., Finzi, L., Lebuffe, G., Guidat, A., Conti, M., & Wurtz, A. (2000). Superior vena cava syndrome of malignant origin. Which surgical procedure for which diagnosis? *European Journal of Cardiothoracic Surgery, 17*(4), 384-388.

Queen, J. R., & Berlin, J. (2001). Superior vena cava syndrome. *Journal of Emergency Medicine, 21*(2), 189-191.

Roberts, J. R., Bueno, R., & Sugarbaker, D. J. (1999). Multimodality treatment of malignant superior vena cava syndrome. *Chest, 116*, 835-837.

Rowell, N. P., & Gleeson, F. V. (2001). Steroids, radiotherapy, chemotherapy, and stents for superior vena cava obstruction in carcinoma of the bronchus. *Cochrane Database Systematic Review, 4*, CD001316.

Shapiro, M. A., Johnson, M., & Feinstein, S. B. (2002). A retrospective experience of right atrial and superior vena caval thrombi diagnosed by transesophageal echocardiography. *Journal of the American Society of Echocardiography, 15*(1), 76-79.

Sharafuddin, M. J., Sun, S., & Hoballah, J. J. (2002). Endovascular management of venous thrombotic diseases of the upper torso and extremities. *Journal of Vascular Interventional Radiology, 13*(10), 975-990.

Smayra, T., Otal, P., Chabbert, V., Chemla, P., Romero, M., Joffre, F., & Rousseau, H. (2001). Long-term results of endovascular stent placement in the superior vena caval venous system. *Cardiovascular Interventional Radiology, 24*(6), 388-394.

Stockton, P. A., Ledson, M. J., & Walshaw, M. J. (2001). Persistent superior vena caval syndrome due to totally implantable venous access systems. *Journal of the Royal Society of Medicine, 94*(11), 584–585.

Tanigawa, N., Sawada, S., Mishima, K., Okuda, Y., Mizukawa, K., Ohmura, N., Toita, T., Ogawa, K., Kobayashi, M., & Kobayashi, M. (1998). Clinical outcome of stenting in superior vena cava syndrome associated with malignant tumors. Comparison with conventional treatment. *Acta Radiologica, 39*(6), 669–674.

Thony, F., Moro, D., Witmeyer, P., Angiolini, S., Brambilla, C., Coulomb, M., & Ferretti, G. (1999). Endovascular treatment of superior vena cava obstruction in patients with malignancies. *European Radiology, 9*(5), 965–971.

Wilson, E., Lyn, E., Lynn, A., & Khan, S. (2002). Radiological stenting provides effective palliation in malignant central venous obstruction. *Clinical Oncology, 14*(3), 228–232.

Wudel, L. J. Jr., & Nesbitt, J. C. (2001). Superior vena cava syndrome. *Current Treatment Options in Oncology, 2*(1), 77–91.

Yamagami, T., Nakamura, T., Kato, T., Iida, S., & Nishimura, T. (2002). Hemodynamic changes after self-expandable metallic stent therapy for vena cava syndrome. *American Journal of Roentgenology, 178*, 635–639.

Yin, C. D., Sane, S. S., & Bjarnason, H. (2000). Superior vena cava stenting. *Radiology Clinics of North America, 38*(2), 409–424.

CHAPTER

39 Syndrome of Inappropriate Antidiuretic Hormone (SIADH)

MiKaela Olsen
Joanne P. Finley

I. Definition: SIADH is a syndrome resulting from the abnormal production of antidiuretic hormone (ADH), causing excessive water retention, dilutional hyponatremia, and increased excretion of sodium.
  A. Normally, the primary function of ADH is to retain water when the body needs it. Its release is regulated by a negative feedback mechanism.
  B. Without the presence of ADH, one would need to ingest 10 to 20 L of water per day to match urinary losses.
  C. ADH is released by the posterior pituitary in response to increased plasma osmolality or decreased plasma volume.
  D. ADH causes increased water reabsorption at the distal renal tubules and collecting ducts, thereby diluting the blood and returning plasma osmolality to normal levels.
  E. Ectopic (outside of the pituitary gland) ADH does not follow this normal feedback mechanism and is released uncontrollably, leading to excess ADH and chronically diluted blood.
  F. The predominant etiology of clinical symptoms with this disorder is related to its hyponatremia.
    1. Normal sodium levels are 135 to 145 mEq/L.
    2. Sodium is the primary electrolyte in the extracellular fluid.
    3. Severe hyponatremia of acute onset leads to cellular swelling, which can have dangerous consequences if left untreated.

II. Etiology
  A. Cancer is the most frequent cause of ectopic ADH production. This abnormal production of ADH confuses the body into believing that it needs to hold onto more water. Small-cell lung cancer is responsible for the majority of SIADH cases (80%). Other cancers that are associated with SIADH include the tumors of the pancreas, prostate, brain, lymphatic system, and duodenum. Any tumor that can metastasize to the lungs can also cause SIADH (see C. below).
  B. Central nervous system disease, such as meningeal infection or brain tumors, may also trigger SIADH due to its direct or indirect effects on the pituitary gland.
  C. Pulmonary conditions, such as tuberculosis (TB), chronic obstructive pulmonary disease (COPD), lung abscesses, or pneumonia and positive pressure ventilation can stimulate ADH receptors in the lungs, causing the release of ADH.

571

D. Drugs that most notably induce or potentiate SIADH include the thiazide diuretics, antidepressants, antipsychotics, morphine, and oral hypoglycemic agents. Antineoplastics agents such as vincristine, cisplatin, bleomycin, and cyclophosphamide have also been associated with this syndrome.

III. Patient Management

A. Assessment

1. The severity of symptoms greatly depends on the onset of sodium depletion and severity of the water retention (Table 39–1).
   a. Acute onset SIADH with sodium levels
   b. Patients with chronic SIADH may be asymptomatic despite sodium levels

2. Hyponatremia occurs because of increased water reabsorption at the distal renal tubules, thereby diluting the contents of the blood and increasing the concentration of sodium in the urine. This results in decreased serum osmolality, increased urinary osmolality, and the development of cellular swelling (cellular water intoxication). Clinical manifestations of SIADH are usually related to one of three mechanisms.
   a. Cellular swelling and cerebral edema. Signs and symptoms include:
   (1) Confusion
   (2) Irritability
   (3) Headache
   (4) Muscle weakness cramps
   (5) Lethargy
   (6) Seizures
   (7) Coma
   (8) Death
   b. Increased water reabsorption occurs because of abnormal ADH production, which stimulates increased water reabsorption at the distal renal tubules. Signs and symptoms include:
   (1) Decreased urine output
   (2) Weight gain
   (3) Increased specific gravity
   (4) Edema

TABLE 39–1 Signs and Symptoms Relative to Sodium Serum Levels

Mild (125–134 mEq/L)	Moderate (115–124 mEq/L)	Severe (<114 mEq/L)
Mental status changes	Lethargy	Lethargy
Headache	Mental status changes	Seizures
Fatigue	Nausea/vomiting	Coma
Anorexia	Weakness	Death
Weight gain	Weight gain	
Muscle cramps	Oliguria	

    c. Decreased gastrointestinal motility occurs because of hyponatremia and fluid imbalance. Signs and symptoms include:

      (1) Nausea and vomiting

      (2) Anorexia

B. Diagnostic Criteria (Table 39–2)

  1. Serum tests

    a. Serum sodium is decreased due to renal sodium loss and serum dilution by inappropriate water reabsorption.

    b. Serum osmolality is decreased due to inappropriate water reabsorption.

    c. BUN and creatinine are normal.

    d. Potassium, calcium, and magnesium are decreased due to dilution from inappropriate water reabsorption.

  2. Urine tests

    a. Urine sodium is increased due to normal renal perfusion and excretion of sodium despite decreased serum sodium.

    b. Urine osmolality is increased due to water reabsorption at the tubules despite decreased serum osmolality.

    c. Urine specific gravity is increased above the normal range of 1.002 to 1.028 due to less water and higher levels of solutes. Specific gravity measures the kidney's ability to concentrate or dilute urine in relation to plasma. Because urine is a solution containing minerals, salts, and compounds dissolved in water, the normal specific gravity is greater than 1.000. The more concentrated the urine, the higher the urine specific gravity.

  3. Other tests

    a. The water-loading test may be used to assess the body's ability to adjust urine output to fluid intake. For this test, the patient drinks 20 mL of water per kg (~1,500 mL) over 15 to 20 minutes. Urine is collected hourly for 5 hours and tested for specific gravity and osmolality. Normally, greater than 80% of the water should be excreted in the first 5 hours; the urine specific gravity and osmolality will be low to normal. If SIADH is present, less than 80% of the water will be excreted, the urinary sodium will rise, and the urine specific gravity and osmolality are increased, showing a lack of dilution. *Note:* This test must not be done until the sodium is greater than 125 mEq/L. Patients who fail to excrete the water given in this test should receive additional fluid restriction the remainder of the day.

TABLE 39–2 Criteria for Diagnosis of SIADH

Serum sodium	<130 mEq/L
Serum osmolality	<280 mOsm/kg
Urine osmolality	>330 mOsm/kg
BUN and creatinine	WNL
Urine sodium	>20 mEq/L
Adrenal function	WNL
Thyroid function	WNL

WNL = within normal limits.

      b. Adrenal and thyroid function tests should be normal but are performed to rule out other causes of hyponatremia.

C. Treatment

   1. The underlying cause of SIADH, such as cancer, must be treated after the patient is stabilized.

   2. The most important initial treatment for SIADH is free water fluid restriction.

   3. Other pharmacologic agents are used to treat SIADH (Table 39–3)

D. Nursing Diagnoses

   1. Fluid volume excess related to increased water reabsorption

      a. *Problem:* Inappropriate ADH release causes increased water reabsorption.

      b. *Interventions*

         (1) Assess for signs and symptoms of water retention (eg, edema, weight gain, decreased urine output, confusion, irritability, headache, pulmonary crackles).

         (2) Restrict free water to 500 to 1,000 mL/day based on severity of hyponatremia.

            (a) Teach patient the need for restriction and assist patient to divide amounts over a 24-hour period.

            (b) Consider palatable methods for fluid restrictions (eg, ice or Popsicles that may quench thirst and be less fluid volume).

            (c) Concentrate all intravenous (IV) fluids.

            (d) Maintain strict intake and output records.

         (3) Consider pharmacologic agents for patients unable to comply with fluid restriction (see Table 39–3).

         (4) For severe hyponatremia, administer 3% hypertonic saline solution as ordered (Box 39–1). Administration of a hypertonic solution should be done with extreme caution to prevent too rapid or overcorrection of hyponatremia, which may lead to seizures.

         (5) Irrigate nasogastric tubes with normal saline solution.

         (6) Switch IV flush bottles to normal saline solution.

      c. *Desired outcomes*

         (1) The patient will maintain or return to normal weight.

         (2) The patient will have no edema or crackles.

   2. Risk for injury related to change in mental status

      a. *Problem:* Confusion and lethargy may occur due to water intoxication and low sodium. Severe hyponatremia may also cause generalized seizures.

      b. *Interventions*

         (1) Assess level of consciousness, orientation, strength, pupillary responses, visual defects at least once every shift.

         (2) Neurologic checks every 4 hours for severe hyponatremia.

         (3) Place bed in a low position with side rails up.

         (4) Check patient frequently.

         (5) Provide assistance with activities of daily living, answer call lights promptly, and implement mechanical restraints as a last resort.

         (6) Orient patient at least every shift.

TABLE 39-3 Pharmacologic Agents for SIADH Treatment Administration

Drug	Action	Administration Guidelines	Nursing Care
Demeclocycline	Interferes with ADH action on the renal tubules Takes 5–7 days to become effective	600–1,200 mg/day PO, divided; 1 h before and 2 h after meals	Teach patient to avoid the sun and use sunscreen. Monitor signs and symptoms of infection, GI upset, and impaired renal function.
Lithium	Decreases renal sensitivity to ADH	600–900 mg/day PO	Monitor thyroid function tests. Assess for tremors, weakness, GI upset, and cardiac changes.
Urea	Promotes diuresis	30–60 g PO q day	No need for fluid restriction. Monitor GI upset.

▼ BOX 39-1 | **Guidelines for Administration of 3% Hypertonic Saline Solution**

Action
Increases water movement from tissues to plasma.

Administration Guidelines
Give slowly over 2–3 h to increase fluid excretion.*
Gentle diuresis—Furosemide is usually given at the same time to prevent fluid overload.
The serum sodium should not increase faster than 1–2 mEq/L/h.

Nursing Care
Monitor fluid and electrolyte balance, especially sodium, and vital signs.

*Administering hypertonic saline too quickly can result in increased edema and heart failure.

      (7) Institute seizure precautions for sodium less than 125 mEq/L.
      (8) Elevate head of bed to reduce risk of increased intracranial pressure and aspiration.
   c. *Desired outcome:* The patient will be free of injury.
  3. Altered urinary elimination
   a. *Problem:* Urine output is decreased due to abnormally increased water reabsorption.
   b. *Interventions*
      (1) Assess urine amount, color, and specific gravity.
      (2) Monitor serum and urine sodium and osmolality.
      (3) Weigh patient every day, or more frequently as warranted. Report weight gains above goal weight.
      (4) Administer pharmacologic agents as prescribed (see Table 39–3).
   c. *Desired outcomes*
      (1) The patient will maintain urine output per physician's orders.
      (2) The patient will maintain normal urine specific gravity.
      (3) The patient will have normal serum sodium and osmolality.
  4. Altered oral mucous membranes related to fluid restriction and nausea/vomiting
   a. *Problem:* Fluid restriction and vomiting decrease moisture in the mouth.
   b. *Interventions*
      (1) Assess oral cavity every shift.
      (2) Assist patient with frequent mouth care. Teach patient to rinse without swallowing.
      (3) Administer antiemetics as needed.

      (4) Provide sugar-free gum or candy as tolerated.

      (5) Teach patient not to use commercial alcohol-based mouthwashes or lemon glycerine swabs that dry the mouth.

   c. *Desired outcome:* The patient will have pink, moist, intact oral mucosa.

 5. Potential for altered skin integrity related to edema and excess extracellular fluid

   a. *Problem:* Excess extracellular fluid causes interstitial swelling and higher risk for skin excoriation.

   b. *Interventions*

      (1) Maintain clean and dry skin.

      (2) Encourage mobilization and frequent position changes to reduce the risk of skin breakdown.

      (3) Optimize nutrition to reduce the risk of skin breakdown.

      (4) Elevate edematous dependent extremities as needed.

      (5) Apply sequential compression devices to lower legs to reduce risk of deep vein thrombosis.

      (6) Discuss with physician potential need for prophylactic anticoagulant therapy.

      (7) Provide skin lotion to maintain supple and intact skin.

      (8) Use skin barrier protection as indicated.

   c. *Desired outcomes*

      (1) Absence of edema

      (2) Absence of skin excoriation and breakdown

E. Discharge Planning and Patient Education

 1. Teach patient signs and symptoms of SIADH and the need to report weight gain and decreased urine output.

 2. Reinforce need for fluid restrictions and the importance of fluid records.

 3. Instruct patient about medications and side effects.

 4. Consider dietary consult as needed.

 5. Teach patient and family appropriate safety precautions.

 6. Teach patient and family skin care guidelines to prevent breakdown.

 7. Give patient written emergency numbers and instructions.

REFERENCES

Adrogue, H. J., & Madias, N. E. (2000). Hyponatremia. *New England Journal of Medicine, 342,* 1581–1589.

Batcheller, J. (1994). Syndrome of inappropriate antidiuretic hormone secretion. *Critical Care Nursing Clinics of North America, 6*(4), 687–692.

Bryce, J. (1994). SIADH: Recognizing and treating syndrome of inappropriate antidiuretic hormone secretion. *Nursing, 24*(4), 33.

Ezzone, S. A. (1999). SIADH. *Clinical Journal of Oncology Nursing, 3*(4), 187–188.

Gerber, R. B. (2002). Paraneoplastic syndromes associated with bronchogenic carcinoma. *Clinics in Chest Medicine, 23*(1), 257–264.

Tan, S. J. (2002). Recognition and treatment of oncologic emergencies. *Journal of Infusion Nursing, 25*(3), 182–188.

40 Tumor Lysis Syndrome

Kristen L. Ambrosio

I. Definition: Tumor lysis syndrome (TLS) is an oncologic emergency in which metabolic imbalance occurs as a consequence of tumor cell kill, causing rapid release of normal intracellular products.

    A. Death of malignant cells results in large amounts of intracellular contents such as potassium, phosphorus, and nucleic acids being released into circulation.

    B. The syndrome includes hyperkalemia, hyperphosphatemia, and hyperuricemia (from the conversion of nucleic acid to uric acid).

        1. This may lead to hyperuricemia-induced acute renal failure.

        2. Hypocalcemia results from the binding of increased phosphorus with calcium to form calcium phosphate salts (Table 40–1).

    C. Timing

        1. The syndrome may occur spontaneously (autolysis) or begin 1 to 5 days after the initiation of therapy (chemotherapy, radiation therapy, or biologic therapy).

        2. It ends in about 5 to 7 days, when cell lysis resolves.

    D. TLS can be anticipated, treated, and even prevented before life-threatening complications develop.

II. Etiology

    A. Cancers with a high growth fraction (rapidly dividing and more sensitive to antineoplastic therapy), large size (especially bulky abdominal tumors), and elevated lactate dehydrogenase (indirectly indicates tumor burden) commonly cause TLS.

        1. Lymphomas (especially Burkitt's, bulky disease, or treatment with rituximab)

        2. Multiple myeloma—has been reported even with a single dose of corticosteroids and is thought to be more prevalent when concomitant renal dysfunction is also present.

TABLE 40–1 Laboratory Values in Tumor Lysis Syndrome

Tumor Lysis Labs	Expected Finding
Potassium	Increased
Phosphorus	Increased
Uric acid	Increased
BUN/creatinine	Increased
Magnesium	Decreased
Calcium	Decreased

3. Leukemias—patients who present with lymphoblasts (eg, acute lymphocytic leukemia) have four times more intracellular organic and inorganic phosphates, putting them at even greater risk to develop tumor lysis syndrome (Ezzone, 1999).
4. Small-cell lung cancer, due to rapid proliferation rate.
5. Other malignancies in which TLS has been a reported complication—breast cancer (particularly treated with biologic therapy), hepatocellular cancer after chemoembolization, choriocarcinoma, testicular cancer, gastric cancer, pancreatic cancer, malignant melanoma

   B. Volume depletion enhances electrolyte concentration, especially hyperkalemia and hyperphosphatemia.
   C. Renal insufficiency places the patient at higher risk for tumor lysis syndrome because the kidneys are the route of elimination for potassium, uric acid, and phosphorus.

III. Patient Management

A. Assessment: Table 40–2 lists the common signs and symptoms of TLS affecting cardiovascular, renal, neuromuscular, and gastrointestinal systems. These systems are affected due to the electrolyte abnormalities, hyperuricemia, and acidosis produced when intracellular components are released into the serum.
B. Diagnostic Parameters
   1. Serum tests
      a. The serum chemistry panel indicates increased potassium, phosphorus, uric acid, blood urea nitrogen, and creatinine, and decreased calcium. Magnesium may also be decreased in response to elevated serum phosphorus levels. Some institutions differentiate between serum electrolyte profiles and comprehensive metabolic panels that include phosphorus and uric acid.
      b. Arterial blood gas analysis may be performed to assess the severity of acidosis that has occurred due to excess uric acid or renal insufficiency.
   2. Other tests: Electrocardiogram (ECG) is performed routinely to assess the severity of ECG waveform changes that have occurred due to hyperkalemia or hypocalcemia (Figs. 40–1 and 40–2).
C. Treatment (Table 40–3)
   1. TLS may be prevented in high-risk people with aggressive hydration and conservative diuresis. Dilution of electrolytes reduces the severity of imbalance and, in normally functioning kidneys, enhances excretion. Diuretics must be administered cautiously to avoid volume depletion and dangerously low calcium and magnesium levels.
   2. Medications are administered to prevent or reduce the severity of specific metabolic defects (eg, phosphate-binding antacids to reduce phosphorus, allopurinol to decrease uric acid levels).
   3. Hydration with a balanced intravenous (IV) fluid such as dextrose 5% and 0.9% normal saline at a rate of 250 to 500 mL/h is recommended once TLS has been confirmed. The solution may be changed to dextrose with bicarbonate in the presence of severe acidosis.
   4. Renal replacement therapy (dialysis therapies) may be indicated for electrolyte abnormalities despite preventive therapies, or when renal failure is induced.

TABLE 40–2 Common Signs and Symptoms of Tumor Lysis Syndrome

Body System	Common Signs/ Symptoms	Rationale for Physical Alteration
Cardiovascular	Dysrhythmias	Increased irritability (ectopic beats, atrial dysrhythmias) occurs due to hyperkalemia >6.5 mEq/L. Bradycardia and heart blocks may occur with severe acidosis or hypoxemia. Cardiac arrest is not uncommon if electrolyte levels are poorly controlled.
	Altered ECG waveform	Hyperkalemia causes peaked T waves and flattened P waves, followed by prolonged PR interval, then widening of the QRS complex. Hypocalcemia is characterized by shortened PR and QRS intervals or tachycardia.
Neuromuscular	Muscle twitching Tetany Cramping	Increased muscle tone is the consequence of hypocalcemia. Increased contractility and deep tendon reflexes are usually the predominant neuromuscular finding.
	Weakness	Occurs due to hyperkalemia and hyperphosphatemia. May manifest as diaphragmatic weakness and hypoventilation.
	Lethargy Confusion Seizures	Acidosis and hypocalcemia can cause abnormal neuronal discharges, and seizure activity.
	Paresthesias	Hyperphosphatemia alters peripheral nerve conducion, affecting sensory perception.
Renal	Oliguria Flank pain Hematuria	Hyperuricemia can cause uric acid crystallization within the kidney tubules, resulting in obstruction of urine, pain in the kidney region, and enlargement of the kidney. Severe crystallization may also erode into the endothelial walls and cause hematuria.
	Weight gain Edema	Decreased renal clearance and production of urine results in retention of fluid. Increased intravascular fluid causes high hydrostatic pressure, increased vascular permeability, and increased perivascular fluid.
Gastrointestinal	Nausea/vomiting Anorexia Diarrhea	Associated with both hyperkalemia and hyperphosphatemia, although renal insufficiency may also cause gastrointestinal distress.

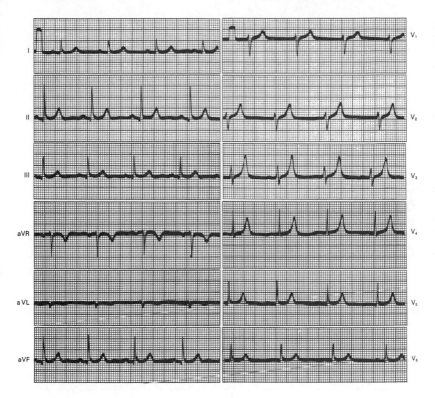

Figure 40-1 Electrocardiographic effects of hyperkalemia. (Note that all V leads are shown at half standard voltage.) (Bernreiter, M. [1963]. *Electrocardiography* [p. 155]. Philadelphia: J. B. Lippincott.)

    a. Hemodialysis is the initial treatment of choice because it rapidly removes potassium, uric acid, and phosphate from the serum and corrects hypocalcemia.

    b. Peritoneal dialysis is no longer considered a desirable treatment because of its slow correction of electrolytes. It is also a perforation risk for patients with abdominal tumors and an infection risk for those with low white blood cell counts.

    c. Continuous renal replacement therapies (eg, continuous arteriovenous hemofiltration and dialysis [CAVHD], continuous venovenous hemofiltration and dialysis [CVVHD]) are being used more frequently. CAVHD uses a patient's arterial blood pressure to continuously filter blood by convective transport (Nicolin, 2002). CVVHD uses a blood pump to provide filtration pressure without using arterial access (Nicolin, 2002). These forms of treatment slowly and continuously correct electrolyte abnormalities, an added advantage while the patient is continually lysing

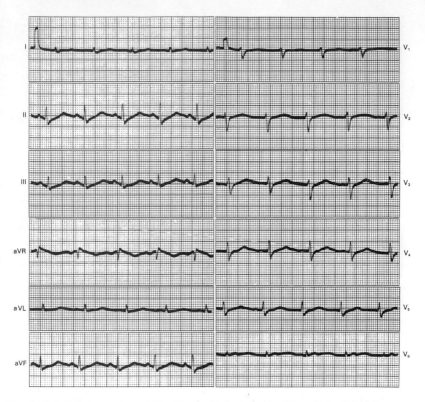

Figure 40-2 Electrocardiographic effects of hypokalemia. (Note that all V leads are shown at half standard voltage.) ((Bernreiter, M. [1963]. *Electrocardiography* [p. 162]. Philadelphia: J. B. Lippincott.)

tumor cells. Predominantly, hemodialysis is instituted first to immediately correct electrolyte abnormalities, then continuous therapies may be used to maintain stable electrolyte levels during the time of tumor lysis.

5. Blood transfusions during the period of TLS can be a risk for enhanced hypocalcemia, hyperkalemia, and acidosis for the patient.

   a. Blood banks add an acidic anticoagulant called sodium citrate to the preservative fluid of red blood cells to preserve 2,3-diphosphoglycerate, a molecule that releases oxygen to the tissues (Corazza & Hranchook, 2000). This can worsen existing acidosis.

   b. During a large-volume blood transfusion, citrate binds to calcium, resulting in hypocalcemia.

   c. The refrigeration of banked blood inactivates the sodium-potassium pump, causing potassium levels to increase (Corazza & Hranchook, 2000).

D. Nursing Diagnoses
  1. Altered urinary elimination related to increased need for excretion of tumor byproducts
   a. *Problem:* Increased elimination of tumor byproducts (eg, potassium, phosphorus, uric acid) results in renal tubular damage and decreased urinary elimination. Uric acid can crystallize within the tubules, obstructing outflow of urine.
   b. *Interventions*
     (1) Monitor and maintain urinary output (>100 mL/h), absence of hematuria, color, specific gravity (<1.010), and urinary pH (>7.0) at least every 4 hours, but more frequently if oliguria is present.
     (2) Monitor serum electrolyte values every 6 to 12 hours during the high-risk period.
     (3) Administer IV fluids before and after cancer treatment. IV fluids containing sodium bicarbonate (5% dextrose + 100 mEq $NaHCO_3$/L) are used to increase the solubility of uric acid and prevent crystal formation. IV fluids also increase the glomerular filtration rate, thereby increasing the excretion rate of toxic byproducts.
     (4) Administer allopurinol as prescribed (see Table 40–3).
     (5) Administer aluminum hydroxide as prescribed (see Table 40–3).
     (6) Administer cation-exchange resins as prescribed (see Table 40–3).
     (7) Assist with renal replacement therapies as needed.
     (8) Teach the patient to restrict foods high in potassium (green vegetables, citrus fruits) and phosphorus (organ meats, beans) and to increase fluid intake.
   c. *Desired outcomes*
     (1) The patient will maintain urine output per physician's order.
     (2) The patient's serum potassium, phosphorus, calcium, uric acid, BUN, and creatinine levels will be within normal limits.
  2. Potential fluid volume excess related to decreased renal function
   a. *Problem:* The patient is at risk for fluid volume excess due to compromised renal function. IV fluid administration to dilute toxic byproducts may also place the patient at risk for fluid volume excess.
   b. *Interventions*
     (1) Assess for dependent edema. An increase in hydrostatic pressure will force fluid into the tissue areas. The influence of gravity causes fluid to settle in dependent areas such as the ankles or sacrum.
     (2) Auscultate breath sounds. Crackles may be a sign of pulmonary edema due to increased hydrostatic pressure in the pulmonary capillaries forcing fluid into the pulmonary alveoli.
     (3) Monitor cardiovascular vital signs and hemodynamics. Tachycardia, hypertension, increased central venous pressure, and an S3 gallop may be signs of fluid overload.

TABLE 40–3 Pharmacologic Agents for Tumor Lysis Syndrome Management

Drug	Action	Guidelines	Nursing Care
Allopurinol	Blocks xanthine oxidase, an enzyme necessary to convert methyl-xanthine to uric acid	Usually 300–800 mg/day orally, or 200–400 mg/m² /day IV from before start of treatment until 3–5 days after the end of treatment. IV use preferred for patients with endotracheal intubation, continuous emesis, or impaired GI absorption.	Assess for rash, fever, GI upset.
Rasburicase	Promotes excretion of uric acid byproducts in the urine	Based on the patient's weight: 0.20 mg/kg IV, over 30 min from the start of treatment until about the 7th day. FDA labeled for use with only pediatric patients.	Monitor closely for hypersensitivity reactions, anaphylaxis, fever, nausea/vomiting, rash, diarrhea, and headache. Assess for glucose-6-phosphate dehydrogenase deficiency, which is a contraindication for use due to risk of hemolytic anemia with concomitant administration. Antibodies may develop from exposure to this agent. Second course must be monitored carefully. Administer by a dedicated line.

Agent	Action	Dose/Route	Nursing Considerations
Aluminum hydroxide	Binds phosphate in small intestine to promote fecal excretion of excess phosphate	30–60 mL PO every 4–6 h from the first to 5th to 7th day of treatment.	Monitor for constipation.
Cation exchange resins	Binds to potassium in GI tract and is excreted through the stool to reduce serum potassium levels	PO is preferred route, but may be given rectally as an enema	May chill oral suspension or give as a cookie for greater palatability. Monitor for hypomagnesemia, hypocalcemia, and constipation.
Diuretics (commonly loop diuretic such as furosemide)	Inhibits sodium reabsorption at the renal tubules, thereby increasing sodium excretion with water. Also promotes potassium excretion.	Usually PO or IV by slow IV push. Usual dose begins at 20–60 mg, but doses up to 160 mg may be administered.	If dose is over 100 mg, give at 10 mg/min to reduce tinnitus and hearing loss. Continuous infusion up to 10–14 mg/h may be more effective without adverse effects of higher IV push doses. Monitor potassium, magnesium, and calcium levels for enhanced excretion. Monitor for orthostatic heart rate and blood pressure and signs of dehydration (eg., poor skin turgor, thirst, dry mucous membranes).

(4) Maintain strict intake and output every 4 hours because oliguria and fluid overload may have a rapid onset, and rapid volume hydration is usually being administered.

(5) Establish an ideal or goal weight. Weigh patient one to three times a day (dependent on diuretic and fluid administration regimen) and report any weight above the goal weight.

(6) Administer diuretics (usually loop diuretics such as furosemide) as ordered, but cautiously to avoid excessive dehydration. Continuous infusion diuretics have been shown effective in chronic renal insufficiency and have been used by some clinicians for management of renal compromise in TLS.

c. *Desired outcomes*

(1) The patient will not exceed goal weight.

(2) The patient will have no clinical signs of excess interstitial fluid (eg, crackles, edema).

(3) The patient will not display clinical signs of cardiovascular decompensation.

3. Risk for injury related to mental status changes

a. *Problem:* Lethargy, confusion, altered cognition, and seizures may occur with electrolyte and acid-base disturbances. These altered mental states place the patient at risk for falls or self-inflicted injury.

b. *Interventions*

(1) Assess mental status (including orientation, judgment, motor strength, and sensation) at least once a shift.

(2) Implement safety measures for changes in level of consciousness—call light within patient reach, room lighting, frequent reorientation, bed in low position and bed side rails in up position, bed alarm systems turned on, tubes or lines covered to prevent the patient from removing them.

(3) Maintain patient on bedrest or constant supervision if TLS symptomatology is severe.

(4) Implement mechanical restraints according to institutional policy and as indicated.

(5) Implement seizure precautions.

(6) Avoid administration of mind-altering medications if possible (eg, opiates, benzodiazepines, some antiemetics).

c. *Desired outcomes*

(1) The patient will be free of injury.

(2) The patient will not exhibit seizures.

4. Potential decreased cardiac output related to dysrhythmias

a. *Problem:* Hyperkalemia and hypocalcemia are common causes of dysrhythmias and altered depolarization/repolarization of the heart that can decrease cardiac output and reduce essential tissue perfusion.

b. *Interventions*

(1) Monitor the ECG rhythm for altered waveform. Observe for shortened or widened intervals (PR, QRS, QT) or amplitude changes (peaked T waves, flattened P waves). If electrolytes

produce waveform variations, continuous cardiac monitoring is recommended.

(2) Obtain serum chemistry panel every 6 to 12 hours to assess
for abnormal electrolytes.

(3) Obtain 12-lead ECG daily to monitor for cardiac ischemia.

(4) Obtain heart rate, blood pressure, respirations, and pulse
oximetry every 2 to 4 hours to assess for changes in tissue
perfusion.

(5) Thoroughly evaluate all patient complaints of palpitations,
chest pain, dyspnea.

(6) Have emergency antidote/counteracting medications immediately available for hyperkalemia, hypocalcemia, and acidosis (sodium bicarbonate, dextrose 50% + insulin, Kayexalate,
calcium gluconate).

(7) Have emergency cardiovascular support available for management of dysrhythmia-related arrest (eg, ambu bag, defib-
rillator).

   c. *Desired outcomes*

     (1) The patient will have normal heart rate and rhythm.

     (2) The patient will have a normal blood pressure.

E. Discharge Planning and Patient Education

  1. Teach patient and family to report signs and symptoms of TLS,
especially if the patient is being managed in the ambulatory setting.
Provide emergency contact information.

  2. Instruct the patient to increase intake of oral fluids, but to avoid
high-electrolyte drinks such as sport drinks. Calcium-containing fluids (eg, milk products) are only recommended if the phosphate level
is stabilized.

  3. Teach the patient importance of maintaining allopurinol and phosphate-binding agent schedule and provide patient with written
instructions and adverse effects of all prescribed medications.

REFERENCES

Agha-Razii, M., Amyot, S. L., Pichette, V., Cardinal, J., Ouimet, D., & LeBlanc, M.
(2000). Continuous veno-venous hemodiafiltration for treatment of spontaneous
tumor lysis syndrome complicated by acute renal failure and severe hyperuricemia.
Clinical Nephrology, 54(1), 59–63.

Altman, A. (2001). Acute tumor lysis syndrome. *Seminars in Oncology, 28*(2, Suppl. 5), 3–8.

Beriwal, S., Singh, S., & Garcia-Young, J. A. (2002). Tumor lysis syndrome extensive-
stage small-cell lung cancer. *American Journal of Clinical Oncology, 25*(5), 474–475.

Brant, J. M. (2002). Rasburicase: An innovative new treatment for hyperuricemia associated with tumor lysis syndrome. *Clinical Journal of Oncology Nursing, 6*(1), 12–16.

Corazza, M. L., & Hranchook, A. M. (2000). Massive blood transfusion therapy. *AANA
Journal, 68*(4), 311–314.

Doane, L. (2002). Overview of tumor lysis syndrome. *Seminars in Oncology Nursing,
18*(3), 2–5.

Ezzone, S. A. (1999). Tumor lysis syndrome. *Seminars in Oncology Nursing, 15*(3),
202–208.

Holmes-Gobel, B. (2002). Management of tumor lysis syndrome: prevention and treatment. *Seminars in Oncology Nursing, 18*(3), 12–16.

Jeha, S. (2001). Tumor lysis syndrome. *Seminars in Hematology, 38*(4, Suppl. 10), 4–8.

Jones, D. P., Mahmoud, H., & Chesney, R. W. (1995). Tumor lysis syndrome: Pathogenesis and management. *Pediatric Nephrology, 9*(2), 206–212.

Kaplow, R. (2002). Pathophysiology signs and symptoms of acute tumor lysis syndrome. *Seminars in Oncology Nursing, 18*(3), 6–11.

Kunkel, L., Wong, A., Maneatis, T., et al. (2000). Optimizing the use of rituximab for treatment of B-cell non-Hodgkin's lymphoma: A benefit-risk update. *Seminars in Oncology, 27*(6, Suppl. 12), 53–61.

Nicolin, G. (2002). Emergencies and their management. *European Journal of Cancer, 38,* 1365–1377.

Pui, C. H. (2001). Urate oxidase in the prophylaxis or treatment of hyperuricemia: The United States experience. *Seminars in Hematology, 38*(4, Suppl. 10), 13–21.

Schetz, M. (1999). Non-renal indications for continuous renal replacement therapy. *Kidney International, 72*(Suppl.), S88-S94.

Smalley, R. V., Guaspari, A., Hasse-Statz, S., et al. (2000). Allopurinol: Intravenous use for prevention and treatment of hyperuricemia. *Journal of Clinical Oncology, 18*(8), 1758–1763.

Index

Note: Page numbers followed by f, t, and b indicate figures, tables, and boxed material, respectively.